Experimental Brain Research Supplementum 6

The Cerebellum–
New Vistas

Edited by
S. L. Palay and V. Chan-Palay

With 264 Figures and 16 Tables

Springer-Verlag
Berlin Heidelberg New York 1982

Papers from a Conference
Held May 15–17, 1980 at the National
Institutes of Health, Bethesda, MD, USA

Sanford L. Palay, Ph. D., M. D.
Victoria Chan-Palay, Ph. D., M. D.

Harvard Medical School
25 Shattuck Street, Boston, MA 02115, USA

ISBN-13: 978-3-642-68562-0 e-ISBN-13: 978-3-642-68560-6
DOI: 10.1007/978-3-642-68560-6

Library of Congress Cataloging in Publication Data. Main entry under title: The Cerebellum: new vistas. (Experimental brain research. Supplement; 6) "Papers from a conference held May 15–17, 1980 at the National Institutes of Health, Bethesda, MD" – T. p. verso. Bibliography: p. Includes index. 1. Cerebellum-Congresses. I. Palay, Sanford L. II. Chan-Palay, Victoria. III. Series. [DNLM: 1. Cerebellum-Congresses. W1 EX485B v.6 1981/WL 320 C4145 1981] QP379.C45 599.01'88 82-5641 AACR2

Softcover reprint of the hardcover 1st edition 1982

Typesetting, printing and binding: K. Triltsch, Würzburg.
2125/3140-543210

For Alf Brodal
and Janos Szentágothai

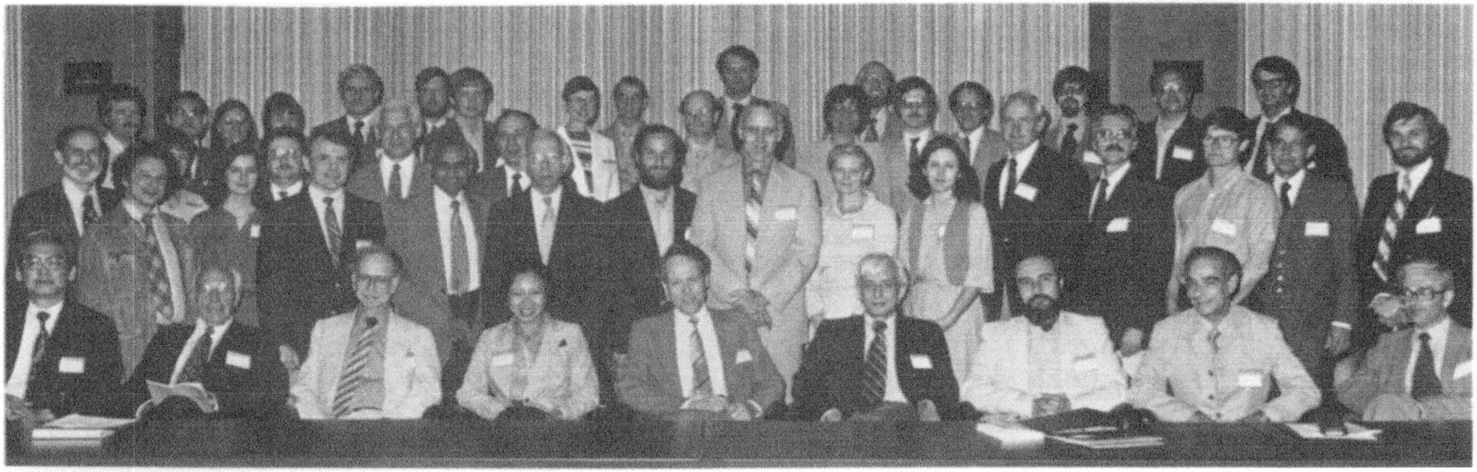

Participants

Seated, Left to Right
M. Ito, J.C. Eccles, S.L. Palay, V. Chan-Palay, G. Grant, R. Llinás, C. Sotelo, R. Balazs, J. Voogd

Standing, First Row
H. Korn, J.S. King, A.G. Gona, R.S. Snider, S.G. Lisberger, G.F. Martin, M.-L. Oster-Granite, B.B. Gould, K.C. Marshall, D.E. Haines, P. Brodal, W. Lange, J. Mallet

Second Row
E. Mugnaini, J. Altman, M.B. Carpenter, V. Friedrich, P. Satrulee, L.T. Robertson, G.W. Patrick, J. Simpson, T. Thach

Third Row
N.-I. Mano, G. Bishop, K. Krnjevic, W. Oertel, D.L. Tolbert, A.J. Beitz

Preface

The present volume consists of papers prepared for a conference on the cerebellum which was held at the National Institutes of Health in Bethesda on 15–17 May 1980. This was the first general conference on the cerebellum since the 1972 symposium in Portland, Oregon, which was convened to celebrate the publication of the last volume of the *Comparative Anatomy and Histology of the Cerebellum* by Larsell and Jansen.

In organizing the 1980 Conference, we elected to emphasize advances in neuroanatomy over other aspects because, in our view, morphological investigation continues to play a large and essential role in the developing understanding of cerebellar function, and, despite the general impression that cerebellar anatomy is better known than any other part of the nervous system, our information on this topic is far from complete. Nevertheless, the cerebellum offers the best model we have for analyzing the vertebrate central nervous system. The correlation of anatomical, cytological, developmental, physiological, chemical, and pharmacological data on this relatively simple and uniform structure, which has persisted with remarkable conservatism through vertebrate evolution, still holds a rich store of answers to the most penetrating questions concerning the functional organization of the brain. Naturally, within the limits of time, space, and our resources we could not pretend to include everything that has been learned about the cerebellum in the past decade. We tried to select representative areas that promise to develop further in the next decades. We recognize that certain topics have been omitted or have received scant attention in this book – for example, the interposed and lateral deep cerebellar nuclei – but these have been dealt with extensively in other publications.

The objective reader will find much of interest in this book, from the cellular mechanisms of development to the chemical signatures of the pathways in the cerebellum, from the ascending and descending connections to the intracerebellar circuits. The large number of unanswered questions raised surely suggests that much remains to be learned and that the cerebellum will remain a fertile field of neuroscientific endeavor for a long time.

The editors acknowledge with gratitude the support of the Fogarty International Center for Advanced Study in the Health Sciences and the National Institute of Neurological and Communicative Disorders and Stroke which made this conference possible. The senior editor is especially grateful to the Fogarty International Center for an appointment as Fogarty Scholar-in-Residence at the National Institutes of Health during which the conference was organized and this volume was edited.

Boston, March 15, 1982

Sanford L. Palay
Victoria Chan-Palay

Contents

List of Senior Authors

Altman, J.
Department of Biological Sciences, Purdue University, Life Science Building, West Lafayette, IN 47907, USA

Armstrong, D. M.
Department of Physiology, The Medical School, University of Bristol, University Walk, Bristol BS8 1TD, United Kingdom

Axelrad, H.
Inserm, U3, Laboratoire de Physiologie, C.H.U. Pitié-Salpétrière, 91, Boulevard de l'Hôpital, 75634 Paris Cedex 13, France

Balazs, R.
MRC Developmental Neurobiology Unit, Institute of Neurology, 33 John's Mews, London WC1N 2NS, United Kingdom

Beitz, A. J.
Department of Veterinary Biology, University of Minnesota, 1988 Fitch Avenue, St. Paul, MN 55108, USA

Brodal, P.
Anatomical Institute, University of Oslo, Karl Johansgt. 47, Oslo 1, Norway

Carpenter, M. B.
Department of Anatomy, Uniformed Services University, 4301 Jones Bridge Road, Bethesda, MD 20014, USA

Chan-Palay, V.
Department of Neurobiology, Harvard Medical School, 25 Shattuck Street, Boston, MA 02115, USA

Eccles, J. C.
6611 Contra (Ticino), Switzerland

Grant, G.
Department of Anatomy, Karolinska Institutet, 104 01 Stockholm, Sweden

Haines, D. E.
Department of Anatomy, West Virginia University School of Medicine, Medical Center Drive, Morgantown, WV 26506, USA

Ito, M.
Department of Physiology, Faculty of Medicine, University of Tokyo, 7-3-1 Hongo, Bunkyo-ku, Tokyo 113, Japan

Krnjević, K.
Departments of Anaesthesia Research and Physiology, McGill University, McIntyre Medical Building, 3655 Drummond Street, Montreal PQ H3G 1Y6, Canada

Lange, W.
Department of Anatomy, Rheinisch-Westfälisch Technische Hochschule Aachen, Melatener Straße 211, 5100 Aachen, Germany

Lisberger, S. G.
Division of Neurobiology, Department of Physiology, School of Medicine, University of San Francisco, San Francisco, CA 94141, USA

Llinás, R.
Department of Physiology and Biophysics, New York University Medical Center, New York, NY 10016, USA

Mallet, J.
Institut de Microbiologie, Université Paris-Sud, 91405 Orsay, France

Mano, N.
Department of Neurophysiology, Tokyo Metropolitan Institute for Neurosciences, Musashidai 2–6, Fuchu-shi, Tokyo 183, Japan

Marshall, K. C.
Department of Physiology, University of Ottawa, Ottawa, Ontario K1N 9A9, Canada

Martin, G. F.
Department of Anatomy, The Ohio State University, College of Medicine, 1645 Neil Avenue, Columbus, OH 43210, USA

Oster-Granite, M. L.
Department of Anatomy, University of Maryland School of Medicine, 655 W. Baltimore Street, Baltimore, MD 21201, USA

Palay, S. L.
Department of Anatomy, Harvard Medical School, 25 Shattuck Street, Boston, MA 02115, USA

Snider, R. S.
Department of Neurology, Health Sciences Center, University of Arizona, Tucson, AZ 85723, USA

Sotelo, C.
Laboratoire d'Histologie Normale et Pathologique du Système Nerveux, Unité U-106 de l'I.N.S.E.R.M., Centre Médico-Chirurgical Foch, 42 rue Desbassayns de Richemont, 92150 Suresnes, France

Thach, W. T.
Department of Anatomy and Neurobiology, School of Medicine, Washington University, 660 South Euclid Avenue, St. Louis, MO 63110, USA

Tolbert, D. L.
Murphy Neuroanatomy Research Laboratory, Department of Anatomy and Division of Neurosurgery, Department of Surgery, St. Louis University School of Medicine, 1402 South Grand Boulevard, St. Louis, MO 63104, USA

Voogd, J.
Department of Anatomy, University of Leiden, Wassenaarseweg 62, 2333 Al Leiden, The Netherlands

Walberg, F.
Anatomical Institute, University of Oslo, Karl Johansgt. 47, Oslo 1, Norway

Current Status of Neuroanatomical Research in the Cerebellum

S. L. Palay

The cerebellum is often cited as that part of the brain about which we know the most. Certainly the cerebellum has figured in every technical and conceptual advance in neurology during the past 160 years. In the 1830s it provided one of the first nerve cell types to be recognized and described [27]. In the 1850s it provided a model for the reticularist theory [17], and in the 1890s it was a prime model for the neuronists [29,30]. It was in the cerebellum that Cajal [28] discovered nerve endings and dendritic spines and conceived of axosomatic and axodendritic synapses, although he did not use this word. For the cerebellum he constructed the first neuronal circuits in the central nervous system and reconstructed for the first time the developmental history of nerve cells. The cerebellum was also a favored subject of Golgi and his followers, and we may mention the classic division of nerve cells into two types according to their axonal trajectories and patterns of arborization which Golgi [18] instituted on the basis of his cerebellar studies.

Cajal's analysis of the circuitry in the cerebellar cortex, with his discovery of the mossy fibers and the climbing fibers, parallel fibers, and baskets, has remained for almost a century the most satisfactory model for the morphological analysis of the central nervous system [29]. Only in the hippocampus has it been emulated and this achievement, too, was largely due to Cajal and his students. The rest of the nervous system, even those parts that are usually considered to be relatively simple, such as the spinal cord and the retina, are only now beginning to yield the secrets of their organization under the pressure of new methods and interdisciplinary investigation.

Cajal's analysis of the cerebellum was hardly challenged during all this time, and except for the perceptive study of climbing fibers by the Scheibels in 1954 [31], very little of any significance was added until the past two decades. An attempt of the Scheibels [22] in 1958 to reinterpret the circuitry of the cortex on the basis of their new Golgi preparations was shown to be misconceived by subsequent electron microscopic studies, which confirmed in almost frightening detail the skillful descriptions and deductions of Cajal [26].

At the same time and without more than the most superficial obeisance to the structure of the cerebellum, a large literature grew up around the physiology of this organ, to a great extent motivated by a desire to understand the symptomatology of experimental ablations and such human diseases as intracranial tumors, congenital hypoplasia, and chronic alcoholism. A relationship between the cerebellum and equilibration, the maintenance of muscle tone, and certain types of tremor was early established. The organ was divided into lobes on the

Experimental Brain Research, Suppl. 6

basis of intersecting transverse and parasagittal planes and the different motor syndromes following selective ablations were ascribed to the loss of participation by the excised or disconnected lobes. Early studies by Jansen and Brodal [21, 22] linking these lobes with different central or vestibular nuclei gave this gross physiological analysis a modicum of morphological credibility. But the precise role of the cerebellum in the regulation of movement, and especially the relationship between the exquisite architectonics of the cerebellar cortex and function, remained elusive. The well-known lectures and books by John Fulton [16] during this period testify to this discrepancy between knowledge and understanding, and a large compendium of cerebellar physiology and anatomy published in 1958 by Dow and Moruzzi [14] shed little light on these important problems. As late as 1964 at an international meeting on the cerebellum in Amsterdam, a well-known physiologist, who had devoted his life to the cerebellum, confessed that although he could understand how the cortex might be some kind of timing device – one of the plausible suggestions of the period – the function of the deep cerebellar nuclei completely eluded him.

But help was already on the way. In the same year (1964) Eccles [3, 15] and a succession of colleagues began to publish their brilliant physiological dissection of the cells and fibers in the cerebellar cortex, and Ito [19, 20] and his colleagues discovered the inhibitory action of the Purkinje cell projection upon the deep cerebellar nuclei. In just a few years the circuitry of the cerebellar cortex, which had seemed so blandly repetitious and uninteresting since its discovery 70 years earlier, suddenly came alive [15]. Now it became important once again to confirm that the neuronal elements in the cerebellum really were arranged as described. Fortunately, neurocytologists had been early attracted to the cerebellum exactly because of its regular architecture and the limited number of its cell types. Many of the cells and synaptic junctions had already been identified at the electron microscope level [25] and during the next decade the entire population of the cerebellar cortex became familiar to neuroanatomists and neurophysiologists as the best model of correlated structure and function in the central nervous system. Success in understanding the cerebellar cortex at the ultrastructural level contributed to the revival of interest in the Golgi method and the widespread application of all morphological methods to other parts of the nervous system and to a variety of species.

At the same time, some new problems were uncovered. Electron microscopy showed that the elaborate and beautifully sculptured dendritic tree of the Purkinje cell, so dramatically displayed in Golgi preparations, is indeed a field for precisely localized excitatory and inhibitory synapses from a variety of sources, each with its delimited zone of distribution. Cajal had demonstrated that the dendritic tree developed according to a regular sequence, which proceeded along with the parallel development of the afferent fibers and their parent cells. How does this pattern develop? What controls the shape, branching, and extent of the dendritic arborization? Why is it flat? Why is it in the parasagittal plane? What would happen if the afferent fibers failed to arrive at the usual time? How would the Purkinje cell dendritic tree develop in the absence of parallel fibers? Are the famous dendritic spines dependent on the synaptic terminals that are seated on them? All these and many more questions became subjects for experimental study as methods for differential X-irradiation were developed [1, 2]. But there are also natural experiments produced by defective genetic complements that allow the Purkinje cell to express its innate morphogenetic capability, and these suggest that each cell type has a great potential to develop or maintain its classic morphology even in the absence of the usual cellular environment [33]. Studies of cerebellar explants in organ culture have also borne this out.

Another problem illuminated by modern studies is the nature and function of the articulation between the basket cell axon and the Purkinje cell. This intricate synapse was shown to be inhibitory by the neurophysiologists and with some difficulty was proved to use γ-aminobutyric acid as its transmitter. But there are some complications. Branches of the basket cell axons not only twine around the branches of the lower dendritic tree and form a basket around the Purkinje cell body, but also dangle loosely beneath the cell body in a terminal formation that is known as the pinceau [26]. Although the branches engage in many synapses en passant along the surfaces of dendrites and the cell body, they form hardly any synapses on the initial segment of the Purkinje cell axon, around which they are disposed beneath the cell body. According to a serial section study by Somogyi and Hámori [32] no more than one to three synapses occur between these axons and the initial segment, and since 7–15 different basket cells contribute to any single basket (the number varies in different species) it must be clear that many axons do not succeed in making a terminal synapse with any particular Purkinje cell axon. The peculiar formation of the pinceau has long puzzled neurocytologists, but it has only recently attracted the serious attention of neurophysiologists [23]. The free terminal segments of the basket axons are bound together by means of strange intercellular junctions [34] and their membranes are studded with GABA receptors [11]. What properties do these terminal axon segments contribute to the inhibition that the basket cells exert over Purkinje cells?

Cajal made clear that in the mature cerebellum each Purkinje cell receives a single climbing fiber, but he could not define its source. The answer to this question became a matter for much dispute. Beginning with an experimental study by Szentágothai and Rajkovitz [35], a large body of morphological evidence has been marshalled to prove that the contralateral inferior olive is the exclusive source of climbing fibers. No one would deny that the inferior olive gives rise to climbing fibers, and a detailed topographic map has been constructed of the projection of inferior olivary fibers onto the cerebellar cortex and the deep nuclei. But it is still not established that the olive is the exclusive source of climbing fibers. The distribution of the regular parasagittal bands in the cortex revealed by labeling of both olives with radioactive amino acids [12] strongly suggests that there must be another source of climbing fibers, but none has been found yet.

A related but less controversial issue is the revision that has become necessary in the old assumption that each climbing fiber impinges upon only one Purkinje cell. If it is true that all climbing fibers originate from the inferior olive, then the number of olivary cells should equal the number of Purkinje cells, but they differ by about an order of magnitude. Therefore each climbing fiber should give rise to about ten terminal arborizations. Physiological studies indicate that the branching seems to occur in the central white matter and that the terminal arbors lie in different folia within the same parasagittal band [6].

This brings me to the question of the parasagittal organization of the cerebellum. Of course, the classic subdivision of the cerebellum into the midline vermis, lateral hemispheres, and intermediate lobes suggested a parasagittal organization. But the long-standing preoccupation with the comparative anatomy and homologies of the ten transverse lobules into which the folia could be grouped tended to overshadow the longitudinal divisions. Jansen and Brodal [21, 22] connected the parasagittal lobes with the three pairs of central nuclei and added the lateral vestibular nucleus as a fourth central nucleus for the ancient flocculonodular lobe. But really it was not until Voogd's studies on the cerebellum of the cat [36] and the ferret that the parasagittal organization achieved the attention it deserves. Voogd noted that the myelinated fibers in the medullary rays of the folia were clustered in alternating groups according to transverse diameter. By careful reconstruction of serial sections he discovered that the groups in one folium lay in register with the corresponding groups in other folia, so that each group could be considered as lying within a compartment, which included a parasagittal band of the cerebellar cortex, the underlying white matter, and a zone of the pertinent central nucleus. What Voogd had discovered is an orderly parasagittal arrangement of the cerebellum, based upon the arborization pattern of both afferent and efferent fibers and thus corresponding in principle to the columnar arrangement of the cerebral cortex, discovered by physiologists and now confirmed by anatomical studies. In the case of the cerebellum, the discovery was anatomical and was confirmed by detailed and careful physiological work. We see then that the cerebellum has multiple representations of the afferent pathways, each one probably signifying something different and making the appearance of uniform simplicity, traditionally ascribed to the cerebellum, both specious and bewildering.

In view of the fact that the cerebellar cortex can exercise its influence on the rest of the brain only through its projection upon the central nuclei, including the lateral vestibular nucleus, it is extraordinary how little attention was paid to the deep cerebellar nuclei until very recently. The pathways from the nuclei had been studied with degeneration techniques [4, 5, 8, 13]. These studies had revealed that the projections of the nuclei were vastly more extensive than was imagined before. Even these results did not prepare us for the pervasiveness of the cerebellar projections revealed in recent years by the techniques of axoplasmic transport with horseradish peroxidase or tritiated amino acids [10]. If we can say now that the cerebellum receives inputs from all sensory systems and from nearly all parts of the central nervous system, it seems also to project its output into all parts again. The input-output connections, although often indirect, seem to be generally reciprocated. Many of these relations will be discussed in the chapters of this book.

But beyond these projections almost no attention was paid to the architecture of the central nuclei themselves between the time of the classic but rather superficial description by Cajal and half a dozen years ago. The nuclei were considered to be a uniform population of relay cells. But the discovery that the output of the cortical computer was inhibitory directed attention to the central nuclei. A major exploration of the lateral nucleus in the rat and the monkey was carried out by Chan-Palay and published in a magnificent book in 1977 [10]. Electron microscopy, Golgi procedures, autoradiography, horseradish peroxidase, and cytochemistry were all applied to the problem of deciphering the architecture of the nucleus. A similar analysis of the other deep nuclei needs to be done and some progress in that direction has already begun.

I have left to the last, reference to the one entirely new area that has issued from neuroanatomical work of the past decade. An entirely new and unexpected category of afferent nerve fibers was discovered in the cerebellar cortex in the late 1960s and early 1970s. These fibers were not recognized by Cajal or anyone else using the classical methods. They could only have been identified by a method that specifically detected their chemical idiosyncrasy. These are the fiber systems first recognized by Bloom and his colleagues [7] which contain the monoamines, either catecholamines or indoleamines. Although Bloom's discovery at first met with considerable skepticism, improved methods have securely established these afferent systems. The catecholamine fibers originate from the locus coeruleus while the indoleamine pathway arises from certain serotonin neurons in five of the raphe nuclei, principally the raphe dorsalis. The forms of these fibers have been described in considerable detail in a variety of species at the light microscopic and electron microscopic levels by Chan-Palay [9], Mugnaini and Dahl [24], and others. Both locus coeruleus and raphe projections contribute to each of three fiber systems. Some of the fibers terminate as mossy fibers in the granular layer; others pass up into the molecular layer where they divide T-fashion and mingle with the classical parallel fibers. These two groups tend to make classical synapses with granule cells and with Purkinje cells as well as others. But a third category ramifies sparsely through the granular layer and more richly in the molecular layer and rarely terminates in synaptic relation with any recognizable postsynaptic formation. This latter class displays numerous varicosities and pursues a trajectory that is inconsistent with any of the classically recognized fibers. It represents a new class – a type of nonsynaptic nerve fiber that apparently releases its transmitter en passant into the interstitial space without respect for precise and localized postsynaptic structures. Similar nonsynaptic monoamine afferents have been described in the cerebral cortex. Their role and their importance all wait to be discovered.

In this admittedly impressionistic summary I have tried to review some of the most challenging aspects of cerebellar neuroanatomy, and I have tried to show that far from being a closed chapter in modern neuroscience, it is still productive of new discoveries and insights into the organization of the nervous system. Still the greatest challenge remains to be met, and that is to unravel the mysterious relationship between the architecture of the cerebellum and its role in movement. We understand neither the mission of the cerebellum nor how it works, and until the mystery is elucidated it will hold its fascination for all of us.

References

1. Altman J (1973) Experimental reorganization of the cerebellar cortex. III. Regeneration of the external germinal layer and granule cell ectopia. J Comp Neurol 149:153–180
2. Altman J, Anderson WJ (1973) Experimental reorganization of the cerebellar cortex. II. Effects of elimination of most microneurons with prolonged X-irradiation started at four days. J Comp Neurol 149:123–152
3. Andersen P, Eccles JC, Voorhoeve PE (1964) Postsynaptic inhibition of cerebellar Purkinje cells. J Neurophysiol 27:1138–1153
4. Angaut P (1969) Étude anatomique expérimentale des afférences cérébelleuses ascendentes. Analyse électroanatomique des projections cérébelleuses sur le noyau ventral latéral du thalamus. PhD thesis, Paris
5. Angaut P, Browsher D (1970) Ascending projections of the medial cerebellar (fastigial) nucleus: An experimental study in the cat. Brain Res 24:49–68
6. Armstrong DM, Harvey RJ, Schild RF (1966) Branching of individual olivo-cerebellar axons to terminate in more than one subdivision of the feline cerebellar cortex. J Physiol (Lond) 187:553–574
7. Bloom FE, Hoffer BJ, Siggins GR (1971) Studies on norepinephrine containing afferents to Purkinje cells of rat cerebellum. I. Localization of the fibers and their synapses. Brain Res 25:501–521
8. Carpenter MB, Stevens GH (1957) Structural and functional relationships between the deep cerebellar nuclei and the brachium conjunctivum in the rhesus monkey. J Comp Neurol 107:109–163
9. Chan-Palay V (1975) Fine structure of labelled axons in the cerebellar cortex and nuclei of rodents and primates after intraventricular infusions with tritiated serotonin. Anat Embryol 148:235–265
10. Chan-Palay V (1977) Cerebellar dentate nucleus, organization, cytology and transmitters. Springer, Berlin Heidelberg New York
11. Chan-Palay V, Palay SL (1978) Ultrastructural localization of γ-aminobutyric acid receptors in the mammalian central nervous system by means of [^{3}H]muscimol binding. Proc Natl Acad Sci USA 75:2977–2980
12. Chan-Palay V, Palay SL, Brown JT, Van Itallie C (1977) Sagittal organization of olivocerebellar and reticulocerebellar projections: Autoradiographic studies with ^{35}S-methionine. Exp Brain Res 30:561–576
13. Cohen D, Chambers WW, Sprague JM (1958) Experimental study of the efferent projections from the cerebellar nuclei to the brainstem of the cat. J Comp Neurol 109:233–259
14. Dow RS, Moruzzi G (1958) The physiology and pathology of the cerebellum. University of Minnesota Press, Minneapolis
15. Eccles JC, Ito M, Szentágothai J (1967) The cerebellum as a neuronal machine. Springer, Berlin Heidelberg New York
16. Fulton JF (1949) Functional localization in the frontal lobes and cerebellum. Oxford University Press, London
17. Gerlach J (1858) Mikroskopische Studien aus dem Gebiete der menschlichen Morphologie. Enke, Erlangen
18. Golgi C (1882) Sulla fina anatomia degli organi centrali del sistema nervoso. I. Note preliminari sulla struttura, morfologia e vicendevoli rapporti delle cellule gangliari. Riv Sper Freniat 8:165–195
19. Ito M, Yoshida M (1964) The cerebellar-evoked monosynaptic inhibition of Deiters' neurones. Experientia 20:515–516
20. Ito M, Yoshida M, Obata K (1964) Monosynaptic inhibition of the intracerebellar nuclei induced from the cerebellar cortex. Experientia 20:575–576
21. Jansen J, Brodal A (1940) Experimental studies on the intrinsic fibers of the cerebellum II. The corticonuclear projection. J Comp Neurol 73:267–321
22. Jansen J, Brodal A (1958) Das Kleinhirn. In: Bargmann W (ed) Handbuch der mikroskopischen Anatomie des Menschen, vol 4, part 8. Springer, Berlin Göttingen Heidelberg
23. Korn H, Axelrad H (1980) Electrical inhibition of Purkinje cells in the cerebellum of the rat. Proc Natl Acad Sci USA 77:6244–6247

24. Mugnaini E, Dahl AL (1975) Mode of distribution of aminergic fibers in the cerebellar cortex of the chicken. J Comp Neurol 162:417–432
25. Palay SL (1964) The structural basis for neural action. In: Brazier MAB (ed) Brain function vol 2. RNA and brain function; memory and learning. University of California Press, Los Angeles, pp 69–108
26. Palay SL, Chan-Palay V (1974) Cerebellar cortex: cytology and organization. Springer, Berlin Heidelberg New York
27. Purkinje JE (1837) Neueste Untersuchungen aus der Nerven- und Hirn-Anatomie. In: Sternberg K, von Krombholtz JV (eds) Bericht über die Versammlung deutscher Naturforscher und Ärzte in Prag im Sept, 1837, pp 177–180
28. Ramón y Cajal S (1888) Sobre las fibras nerviosas de la capa molecular del cerebelo. Rev Trimestr Histol No. 2:33–44
29. Ramón y Cajal S (1909–1911) Histologie du système nerveux de l'homme et des vertébrés. Maloine, Paris. Translated by L Azoulay
30. Ramón y Cajal S (1934) Les preuves objectives de l'unité anatomique des cellules nerveuses. Trab Lab Invest Biol (Madrid) 29:1–137
31. Scheibel ME, Scheibel AB (1954) Observations on the intracortical relations of the climbing fibers of the cerebellum. J Comp Neurol 101:733–763
32. Somogyi P, Hámori J (1976) A quantitative electron-microscopic study of the Purkinje cell axon initial segment. Neuroscience 1:361–365
33. Sotelo C (1975) Anatomical, physiological, and biochemical studies of the cerebellum from mutant mice. II. Morphological study of cerebellar cortical neurons and circuits in the weaver mouse. Brain Res 94:19–44
34. Sotelo C, Llinás R (1972) Specialized membrane junctions between neurons in the vertebrate cerebellar cortex. J Cell Biol 53:271–289
35. Szentágothai J, Rajkovits U (1959) Über den Ursprung der Kletterfasern des Kleinhirns. Z Anat Entwicklungsgesch 121:130–141
36. Voogd J (1964) The cerebellum of the cat. Structure and fibre connexions. Van Gorcum & Co, Assen

Morphological Development of the Rat Cerebellum and Some of Its Mechanisms

J. Altman

Introduction

The ontogeny of the cerebellum has been studied with cytological techniques for about 100 years. Contributions were made to the subject in the 1880s by Bellonci, Larousse, Obersteiner, and Vignal, and in the following decade by Athias, Azoulay, Lugaro, Lui, Popoff, Ramón y Cajal, Retzius, and Schaper [25]. It was generally accepted by the turn of the century that the cerebellum originates from the bilateral eminence in the metencephalon, the cerebellar plate. It was also assumed that a secondary germinal matrix located superficially over the cerebellar cortex, the external granular layer, originates at some stage of development from the primary matrix of the cerebellar plate. The picture that emerged was that the neurons of the cerebellum migrate to their final locations from two directions: from the region of the fourth ventricle outward and from the surface of the cerebellum inward. It seemed reasonable to assume that the neurons of the deep nuclei, and possibly the Purkinje cells, followed the outward course and there was evidence available from Golgi studies that the granule cells descended from the surface. But it was not possible to test this hypothesis or similar schemes until the technique of thymidine radiography became available to label multiplying cells. This technique made it possible to obtain answers to the questions: When and where do identifiable cell types originate and what course do they follow to reach their final settling sites? The pioneering autoradiographic studies of cerebellar neurogenesis were carried out in the mouse by Uzman [34] and Miale and Sidman [30]. The technique was used profitably in the ensuing years by many anatomists who studied the ontogeny of the cerebellum in a variety of species, ranging from frogs to primates. This review will be restricted to the development of the cerebellum in the rat and will be based largely on studies from our own laboratory. It is reasonable to assume that the major steps in cerebellar neurogenesis are similar in most mammalian species.

Prenatal Cytogenesis and Histogenesis

Time of Origin of the Macroneurons of the Cerebellar System

The quantitative determination of the birth dates of neurons of the cerebellum and of several structures intimately related to it was based on thymidine radiog-

Experimental Brain Research, Suppl. 6

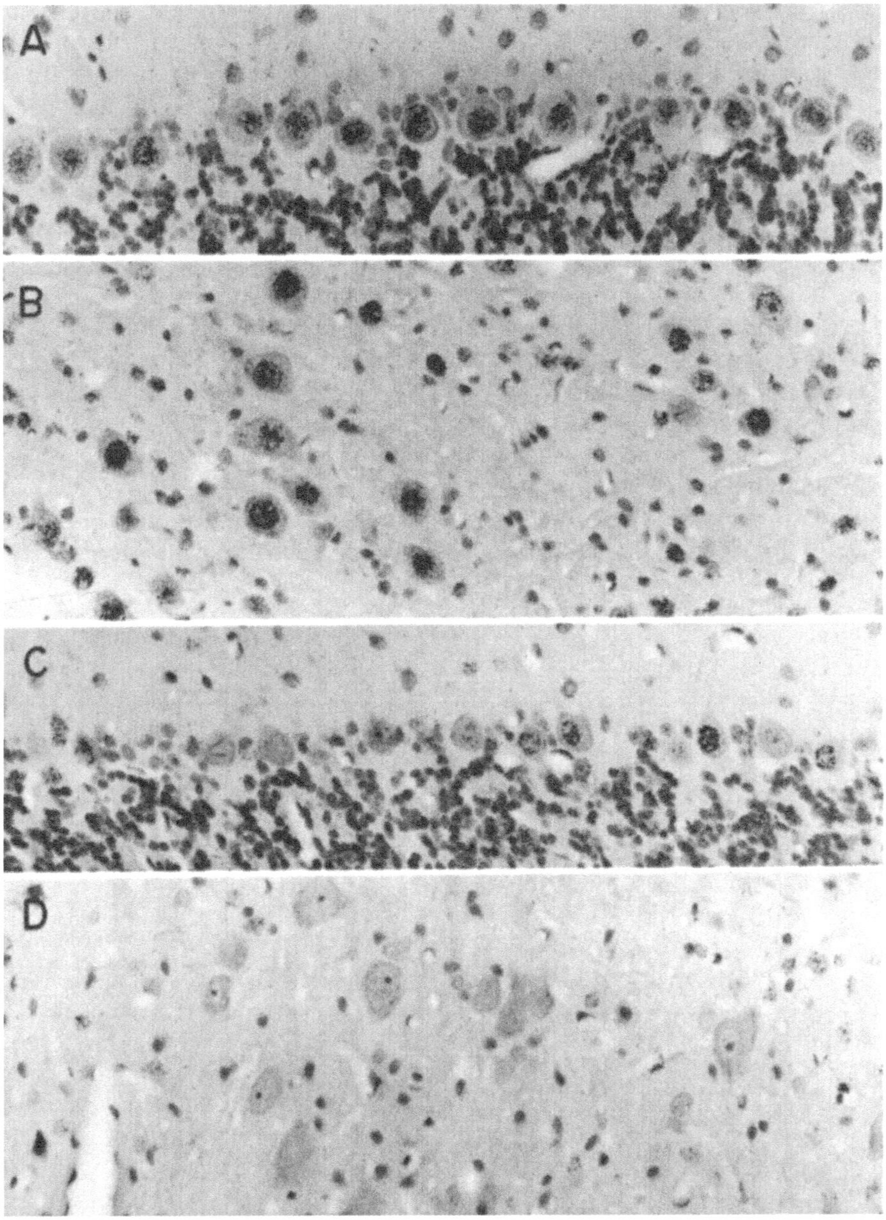

Fig. 1 A–D. All Purkinje cells (**A**) and deep nucleus neurons (**B**) are labeled in the animal which received ^{3}H-thymidine on days E 13 + 14. Many of the Purkinje cells (**C**) but none of the large deep nucleus neurons (**D**) are labeled in the animal which received the radiochemical on days E 15 + 16

raphy with the progressively delayed cumulative labeling procedure. Groups of pregnant rats were injected with two successive daily doses of ^{3}H-thymidine from gestational day 12 and 13 (E 12+13) until the day before parturition (E 21+22), and their offspring were killed at 60 days of age. This double-labeling procedure leads to the labeling of all (or virtually all) cells in most brain structures as long as their precursors are proliferating (Fig. 1). The percentage of cells that can no longer be labeled as a result of daily delays in starting the cumulative injections is used to determine the proportion of neurons generated on specific days (Fig. 2).

It was established that in the rat cerebellum the neurons of the deep nuclei are generated between days E 13 and E 15 with a peak production of about 60% of the cells on day E 14. The Purkinje cells are generated between days E 13 and E 16 with a peak on day E 15 (Fig. 2). The production of Golgi cells begins on day E 19 and extends into the perinatal period [13]. These results showed that the three large types of cerebellar neurons are produced sequentially, the output neurons being first and the interneurons (Golgi cells) last.

Figure 3 summarizes the chronology of neuron production in the cerebellum (macroneurons), in six structures that supply the cerebellum with afferents, and

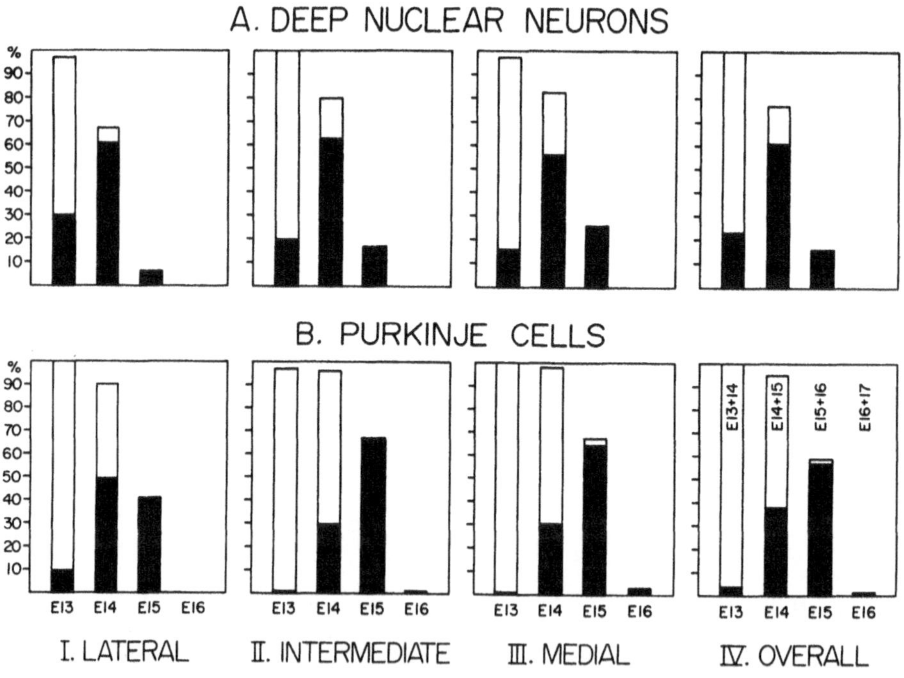

Fig. 2. **A** Proportion of labeled neurons in the dentate (I), interpositus (II), and fastigial (III) nuclei, and their average (IV). **B** Proportion of labeled Purkinje cells at the same sagittal levels and their average. *Empty bars* show the actual proportion of labeled cells in the E 13+14, E 14+15 and E 15+16 groups (six animals in each group), respectively. *Solid bars* indicate the inferred proportion of cells produced on specific days, as specified on the abcissa. Altman and Bayer [13]

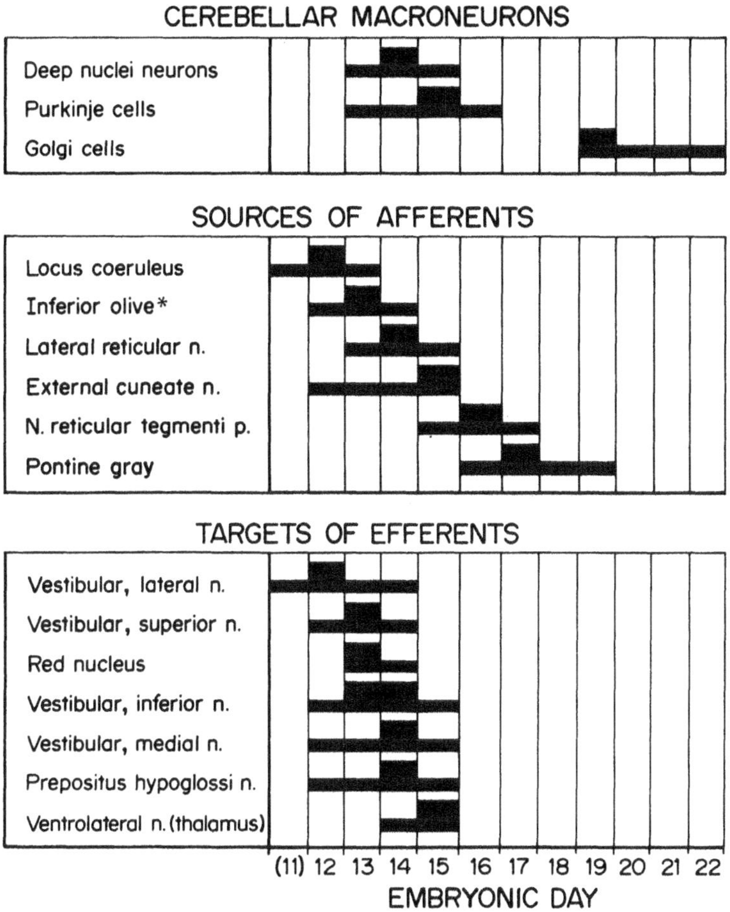

Fig. 3. Time of origin of neurons in the cerebellum (macroneurons only) in relation to the production of neurons in six structures that are sources of cerebellar afferents and in seven structures that receive cerebellar efferents. The time span of neuron production is exact. The proportion of cells produced on specific days is schematic; *tall bars* indicate day of peak production time. (Data based in the following refs.: 13–19.) *Asterisk:* the production of neurons in the inferior olive on day E 12 is inferential. Day E 11 in brackets implies day E 11 or earlier

in seven structures that receive cerebellar afferents. The neurons of the structures that send afferents to the cerebellum are produced sequentially. The neurons of the locus coeruleus and of the inferior olive are produced before cerebellar neurogenesis is in full swing. The production of neurons in four major sources of mossy fibers to the cerebellum overlaps with or follows the generation of deep neurons and Purkinje cells, but they antedate the Golgi cells. The neurons of the pontine gray, which relay cortical input to the cerebellum, are the last elements of this system to be produced. We have also determined the time of neuron origin in seven structures that receive cerebellar efferents. With the exception of the neurons of the medial vestibular nucleus and the prepositus nucleus, which are produced simultaneously [18], we again see a sequential order. The neurons of the red nucleus and the lateral vestibular (Deiters) nucleus, which may be considered major cerebellar relays to the spinal cord, are produced before the deep neurons and the Purkinje cells and before the neurons of the inferior olive and the other precerebellar nuclei. The neurons of the ventrolateral thalamic nucleus, which is the cerebellar relay to the cortex, are the elements produced last in this group.

Prenatal Histogenesis of the Cerebellum

The cerebellar plate is clearly recognizable on day E 13. Its medial portion is composed exclusively of neuroepithelial cells with mitotic nuclei near the lumen of the metencephalon (Fig. 4). Some differentiating cells are recognizable dorsally in the vertical curvature of the neuroepithelium in the anterior part of the cerebellar plate both medially and laterally. The medial neurons (Fig. 4B) must be the early differentiating cells of the locus coeruleus, which are generated predominantly on day E 12. These cells are associated with a small fiber

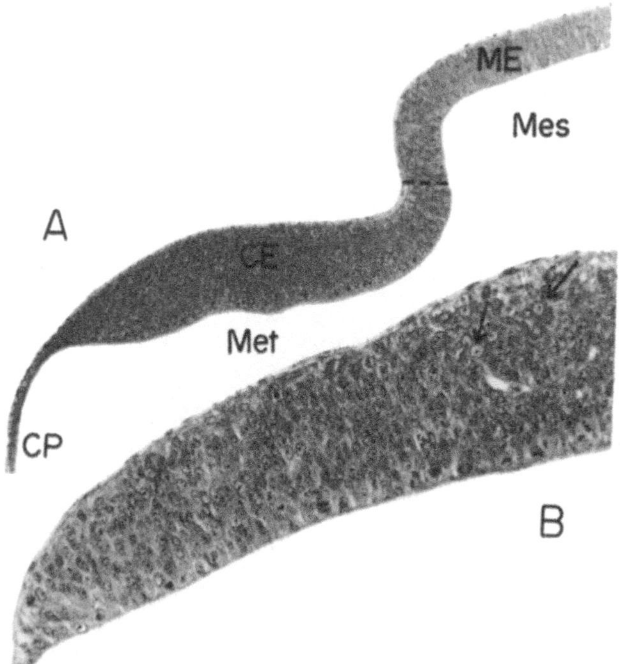

Fig. 4. **A** The cerebellar plate (*CE*) in sagittal section in a day E 13 embryo. *Broken lines* indicate the approximate rostral boundary with the neuroepithelium of the mesencephalon (*ME*). **B** *Arrows* point to differentiating large neurons dorsally in the rostral aspect of the cerebellar plate. These cells are considered to be the early differentiating neurons on the locus coeruleus. *CP*, primordium of the choroid plexus; *Mes*, mesencoele; *Met*, metencoele

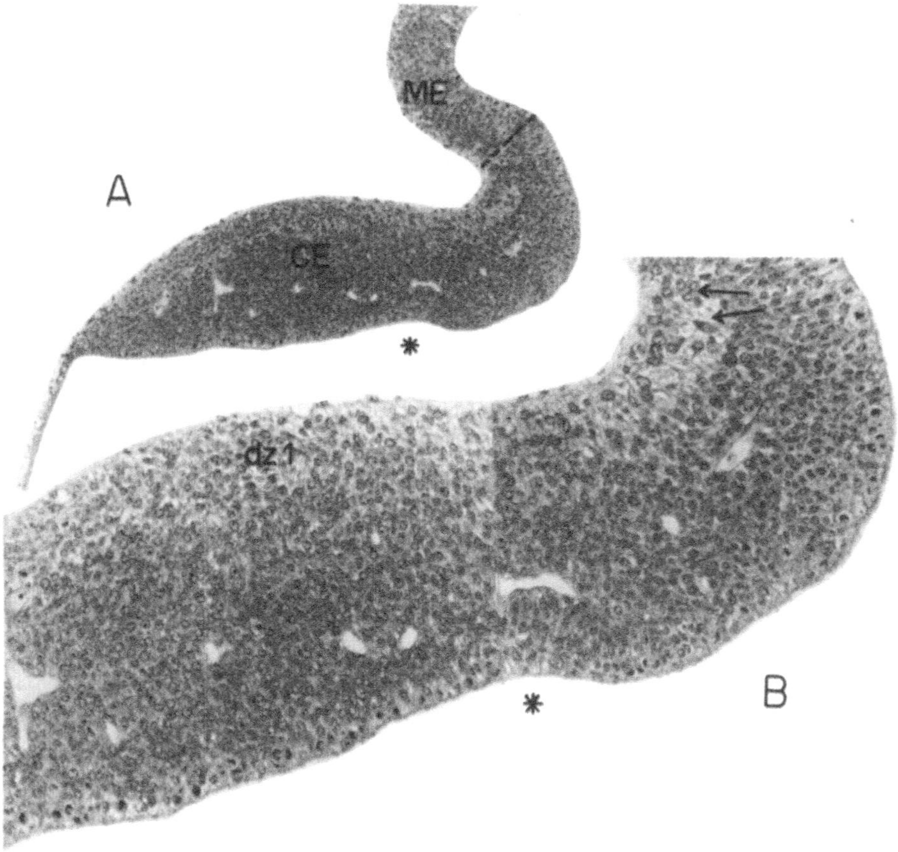

Fig. 5. **A** The cerebellar plate (*CE*) in a day E 14 embryo. *Broken lines* indicate approximate boundary with the neuroepithelium of the mesencephalic (*ME*) neuroepithelium. *Asterisk* indicates the approximate rostral boundary of the cerebellar plate that is believed to be the source of cerebellar neurons. **B** The small cells of the first differentiating zone (*dz 1*) are presumed to be the early differentiating deep nuclei neurons. *Arrows* point to the larger young neurons, and the fiber plexus surrounding them, in the dorsal region of the rostral cerebellar plate. On the basis of radiographic datings and the embryonic tracing of the fate of these cells (Fig. 6), they are considered to be the neurons of the locus coeruleus

bundle by the same day; this bundle becomes more visible by day E 14 (Fig. 5B). A larger group of differentiating cells is seen laterally in the rostral part of the cerebellar plate on day E 13 and E 14. Our tracings of these cells on the subsequent days (Fig. 6) suggested that these large neurons are those of the vestibular nuclei, presumably mostly neurons of the Deiters nucleus and of the superior vestibular nucleus.

Apparently the cells generated in the rostral part of the cerebellar plate do not differentiate as neurons of the cerebellum. However, in the posterior aspect of the cerebellar plate a horizontal zone of differentiating cells is seen in day E 14 embryos (Fig. 5). This zone becomes larger and more clearly separated from

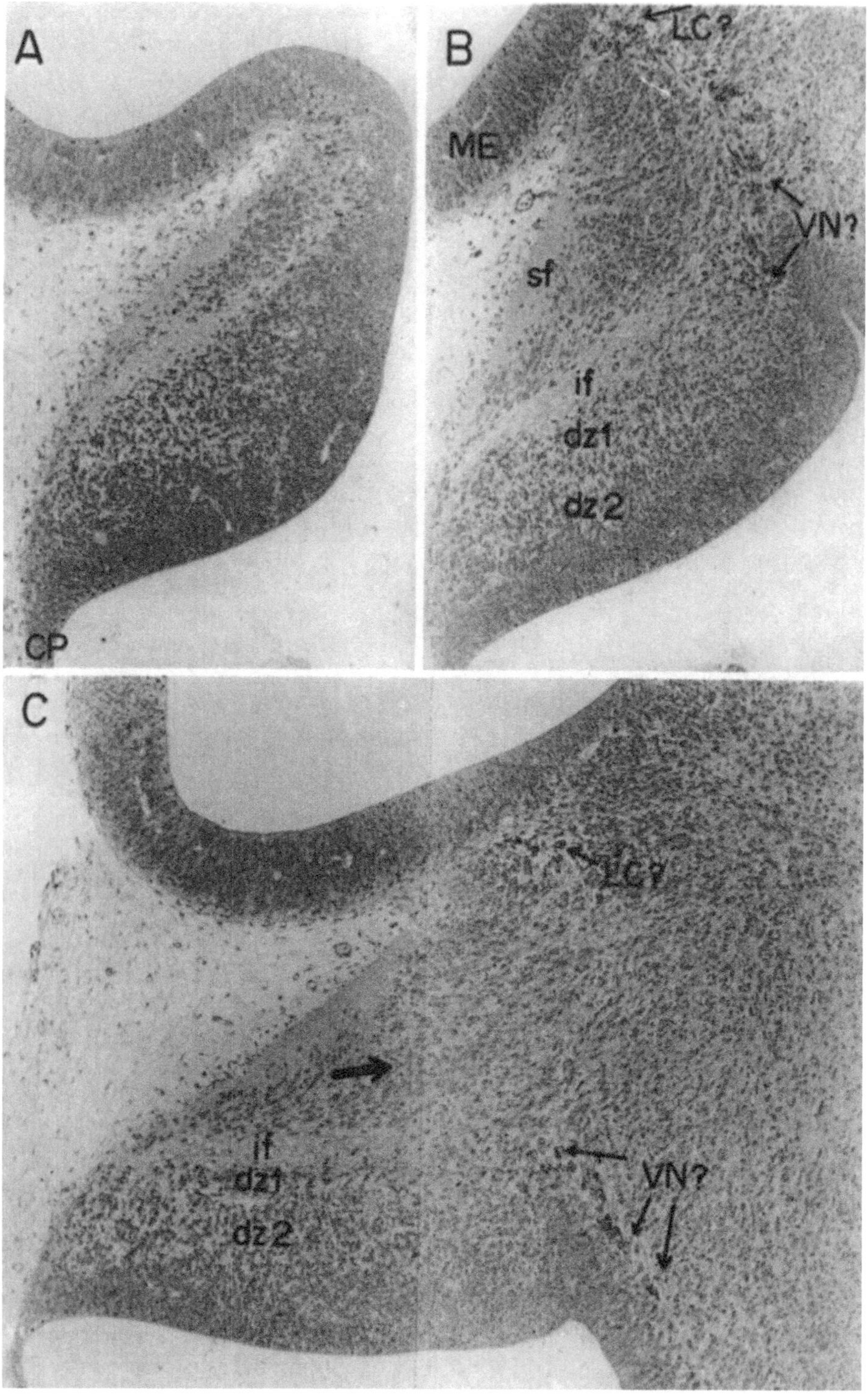
A
CP
B
LC?
ME
VN?
sf
if
dz1
dz 2
C
LC?
if
dz1
dz 2
VN?

the underlying neuroepithelium by day E 15. On the basis of our radiographic datings we identify these as the young neurons of the deep cerebellar nuclei. Beginning on day E 15, and more clearly on day E 16, this superficial zone of differentiating cells becomes segregated by a fibrous band from a new zone of differentiating cells adjacent to the neuroepithelium. This second wave of differentiating cells, situated beneath the presumed zone of deep nuclei neurons, are identified as the young Purkinje cells. (The several differentiating structures seen by this time in the rostral and dorsal aspects of the cerebellar plate will not be considered further.) With the cessation of the production of Purkinje cells the first phase in cerebellar development comes to an end on day E 16.

The second phase of cerebellar development begins on day E 17 and ends before birth. It is marked by two major events: (a) the formation of the external germinal layer (EGL), which heralds a new stage in cerebellar cytogenesis, and (b) the migration of Purkinje cells toward the surface, which is the beginning of cerebellar corticogenesis. The EGL arises on day E 17 as one of the prongs of the "germinal trigone" in the posteroventral aspect of the cerebellum. On the succeeding days it spreads rostrally over the surface of the cerebellum and reaches its anterior pole by days E 20–21 (Fig. 7). This process is associated with the progressive lining up of Purkinje cells beneath the spreading EGL and a layer of fibers that separates the two. The implication of this reconstruction is that the Purkinje cells migrate from their original site near the neuroepithelium through the ranks of the deep neurons in order to reach the surface. Spindle-shaped cells have been seen in abundance beneath the primitive cortex (Fig. 8). The partial differentiation of Purkinje cells is suggested by their resistance to X-irradiation (Fig. 8 B), since migrating primitive cells are radiosensitive [22]. The three elements of the primitive cerebellar cortex (the EGL, the Purkinje cells, and the fibrous layer between them) form a fused canopy over the underlying cerebellum and this may be the major process in the fusion of the initially separate cerebellar primordia. The major steps in the prenatal development of the rat cerebellum are summarized in Fig. 9.

Some Unresolved Questions on the Prenatal Development of the Rat Cerebellum

It is conceivable that the Purkinje cells spin their axons as they move through the field of deep nuclei neurons and establish some form of contact. However, the evident growth of Purkinje cell somata does not begin until after birth. The

Fig. 6 A–C. The cerebellar plate in a day E 16 embryo from **A** medial to **C** lateral. The differentiating zone (*dz 1, dz 2*) in the caudal aspect of the cerebellar plate has grown considerably and may be divisible into two parts. The second differentiating zone is postulated to be composed of Purkinje cells that are leaving the neuroepithelium. The intermediate fibrous layer (*if*) marks the future dorsal surface of the cerebellum over which the cells of the EGL will disperse from the next day onward (Fig. 7). *LC?*, presumed large neurons of the locus coeruleus; *ME*, mesencephalic neuroepithelium; *sf*, superficial fibrous layer; *VN?*, presumed large neurons of the vestibular nuclei. *Thick arrow:* presumed migrating cells

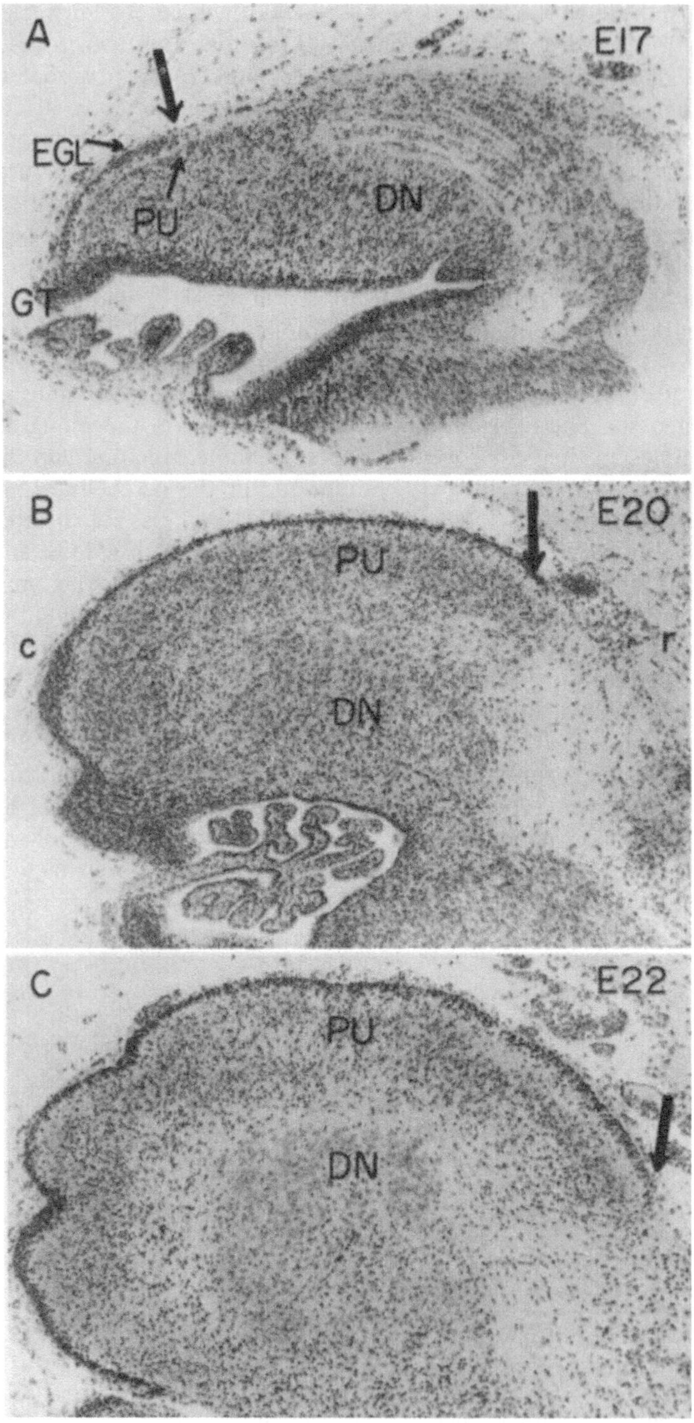
A
E17
EGL
PU
DN
GT
B
E20
PU
c
r
DN
C
E22
PU
DN

Fig. 7 A–C. The spread of the EGL from the germinal trigone (*GT*) caudally (*c*) towards the rostral (*r*) pole of the primitive cerebellum. The morphological differentiation of the deep neurons (*DN*) is evident by day E 20. *Thick arrows* point to the rostral boundary of the EGL. *PU*, Purkinje cell layer

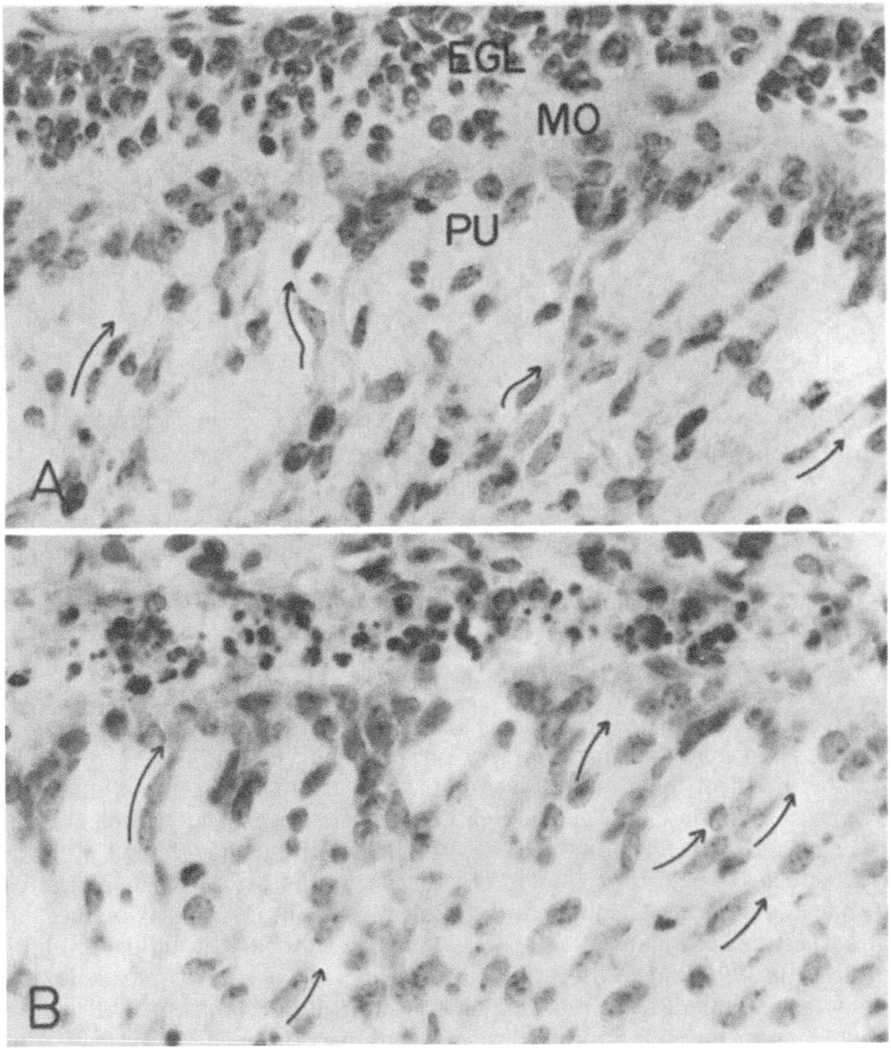

Fig. 8. A Spindle-shaped (*arrows*), apparently migrating, young Purkinje cells beneath the formative Purkinje cell layer (*PU*) in a day E 20 normal rat. The EGL is separated from the Purkinje cell layer by the primitive molecular layer (*MO*), possibly composed of climbing fibers. **B** This E 20 rat was irradiated with 200 R X-rays before it was killed to destroy the undifferentiated cells of the cerebellum. Pyknotic cells are abundant in the EGL, but few of the migrating Purkinje cells are affected, presumably because their cytological differentiation is in progress

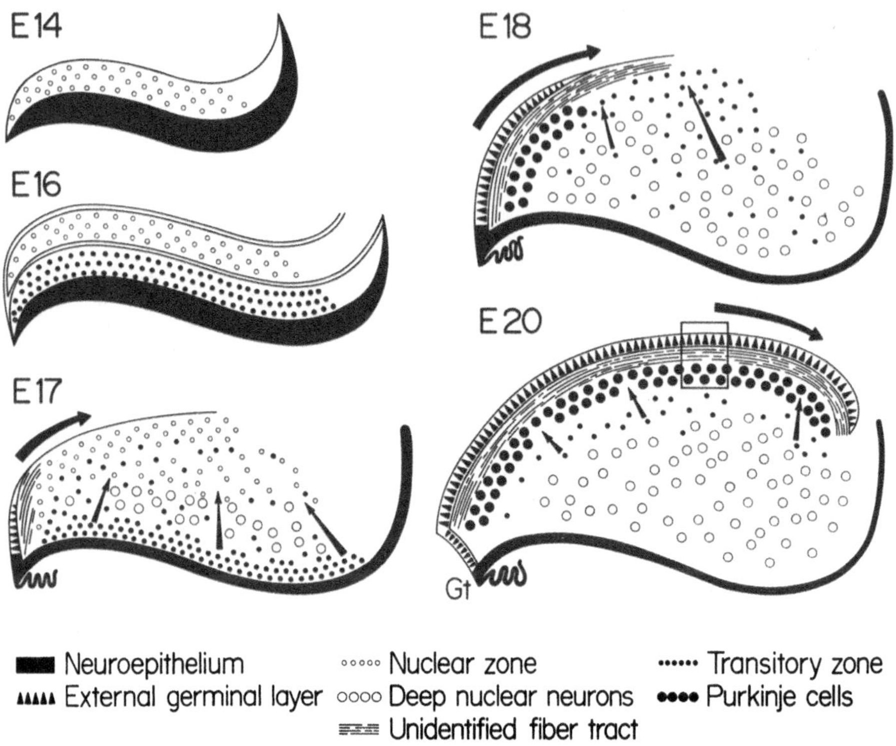

Fig. 9. Summary diagram of the major steps in the prenatal development of the cerebellum. The deep nucleus neurons are postulated to derive from the earlier generated and differentiating nuclear zone. The Purkinje cells are initially gathered in a transitory zone and then migrate to the surface to occupy positions beneath the spreading EGL to form the primitive cortex. Altman and Bayer [13]

Golgi cells are generated during this phase of development, but they cannot be recognized in embryonic material with our present techniques.

Another problem that is unresolved is the early ontogeny of the afferent and efferent connections of the cerebellum. Afferents from the locus coeruleus could reach the nearby cerebellum by day E 14. The noradrenergic afferents of the locus coeruleus, which have a wide distribution in the brain, are demonstrable with the fluorescence technique in 11-mm embryos, approximately on day E 14 [31]. The locus coeruleus afferents could conceivably have an influence on the cytogenesis of Purkinje cells. But if climbing fibers have a developmental role it would have to be restricted to the phase of cortical development. The neurons of the inferior olive are produced in large numbers quite early (day E 13), but according to our embryological evidence they do not begin to reach their settling site in the medulla until day E 16 and the process is not completed until day E 19 [14]. If the axons begin to grow toward the cerebellum on day E 16 or thereafter, at best they could influence the maturation of the deep neurons and the development of the primitive cortex. The fact that a fibrous plexus is present by day E 17 between the external germinal layer and the gathering Purkinje cells suggested the possibility that the climbing fibers start to grow toward the cerebellum before the cell bodies have reached their settling site in the inferior olive.

Indeed, the trajectory of olivary cell migration seems to correspond to the future course of the inferior cerebellar peduncle. However, this possibility is ruled out for the neurons of the pontine gray. These late-generated cells do not begin to reach their settling site until day E 19, and the process continues until day E 22 [14]. The migrating pontine cells (though not the settling cells) are radiosensitive [14]. This suggests that they are not differentiating until they reach the region of the pons. Since the trajectory of the migratory path of pontine neurons is different from the course of the middle cerebellar peduncle, axonogenesis would have to begin after the arrival of the first contingents of pontine neurons. Our observations confirm the late formation of the brachium pontis [14]; it is very likely that these fibers of the mossy system do not reach the cerebellum until some time during the perinatal period. If so, these mossy fibers cannot have an influence on the initial phase of the development of the cerebellar cortex.

Postnatal Cytogenesis, Histogenesis, and Synaptogenesis

Time of Origin of Cerebellar Microneurons

In our initial studies of postnatal cerebellar cytogenesis we utilized mainly the single injection procedure, though occasionally we have injected animals with successive daily doses of ^{3}H-thymidine. In one experiment [2], groups of rats were injected from the day of birth (P 0) to day P 13 and were killed at intervals ranging from 1 h to 180 days following the injection. In the short-survival part of the study using single injections (Fig. 10) it was established that the external germinal layer is composed of two zones.

In animals killed 1 h after the injection the labeled cells were restricted to the upper zone; the spindle-shaped cells of the lower zone were not labeled. The latter were labeled in animals killed 6 h after injection, indicating that some of the cells synthesizing DNA divided and became translocated into the differentiating zone within 6 h. Labeled cells appeared in the molecular layer 24 h after the injection and differentiating neurons were seen both in the molecular layer and the granular layer 3 days after the injection. In another experiment utilizing multiple injections we confirmed our earlier result (a) of the sequential production of cells of the lower molecular layer (including basket cells) and of the upper molecular layer (including stellate cells). Our results (b) suggested that the majority of basket cells were produced between days P 6–7 and the majority of stellate cells on days P 8–11 (Fig. 11). Granule cells were produced in the external granular layer throughout the entire period but with considerable regional differences [1]. In the vermis, lobules I and X were among the early developing ones and lobules VI b, VII, and VIII were the last (Fig. 12). In general, granule cell production ceased earlier in the depth of the fissures than the outer regions of the folia. Granule cell production comes to an end in the rat cerebellar cortex on day P 21.

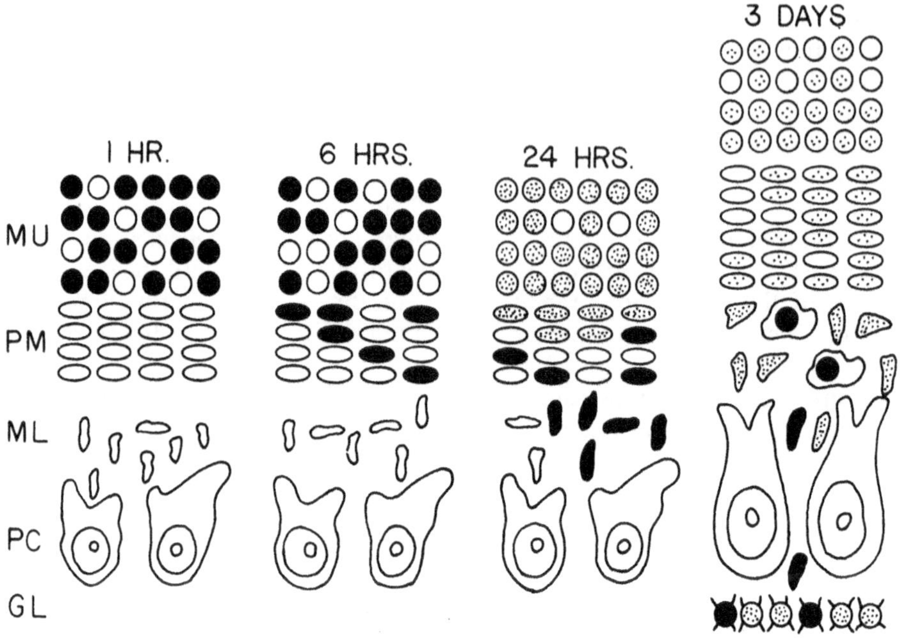

Fig. 10. Rats were injected on day P 6 with ^{3}H-thymidine and killed at different intervals (1 h to 3 days) afterwards. The fate of cells that were labeled with a single injection in the multiplying zone (*MU*) of the EGL is traced from there. After 6-h survival the labeled cells appeared among the bipolar cells in the premigratory zone (*PM*). From there the cells moved into the molecular layer (*ML*) and either settled there or continued past the Purkinje cell layer (*PC*) into the granular layer (*GL*). The originally labeled cells are opaque; their daughter cells are dotted. Altman [2]

Postnatal Histogenesis of the Cerebellum

The primitive cerebellar cortex is composed at birth of the EGL, a thin band of fibers, and a multicellular layer composed of immature Purkinje cells. Between days P 0 and P 21 [1] the midsagittal area of the vermis increases 22-fold (Fig. 13). The major histogenetic events during this period are the dispersal of Purkinje cells in a monolayer (beginning on day P 4, with regional differences), the rapid increase in the area occupied by the molecular layer and the granular layer, and the initial increase and decline in the area occupied by the EGL and its disappearance by day P 21.

Electron microscopic observations [2] confirmed earlier descriptions with the Golgi technique that the perikarya of granule cells descend from the differentiating zone of the EGL after a considerable length of the parallel fiber has been extruded by the bipolar cell (in the coronal plane in the vermis). The position of the parallel fiber thus becomes fixed after its initial formation, and parallel fibers that form later are continuously stacked on earlier fibers. As the molecular layer thickens the EGL is displaced progressively farther away from the layer of Purkinje cell somata (Fig. 14). We have suggested [20] that as the descending granule cells begin to pile up underneath the growing Purkinje cells,

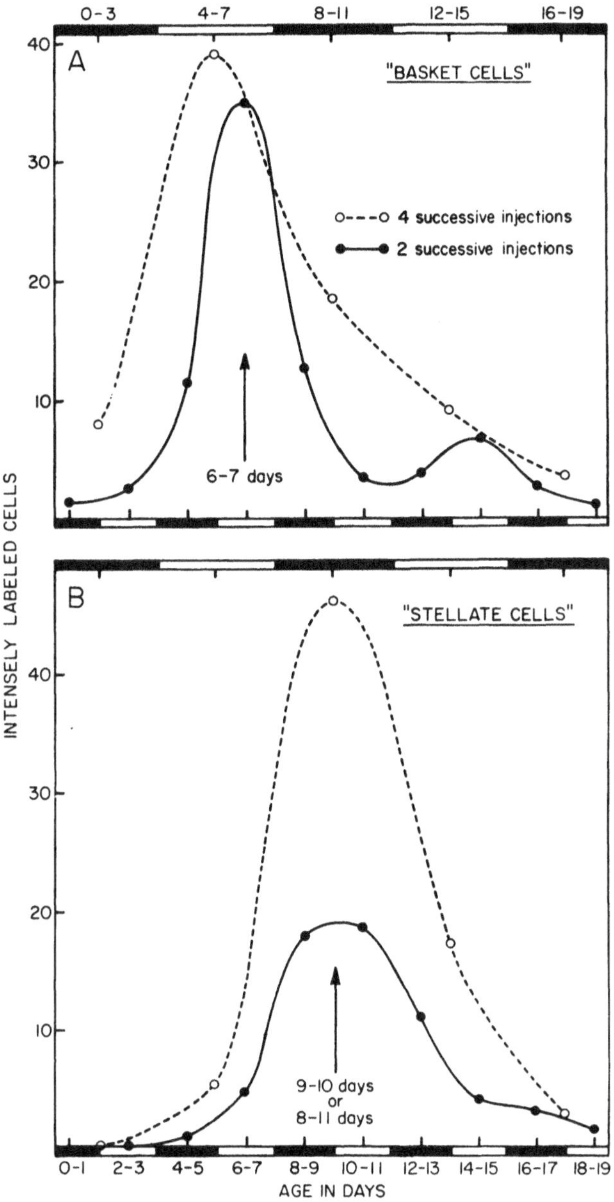

Fig. 11. Concentration of intensely labeled cells in the lower half of the molecular layer ("basket cells") and its upper half ("stellate cells") in adult rats that were injected with two or four successive daily doses of ^{3}H-thymidine between days P 0 and P 19. This study was not based on the progressively delayed cumulative labeling procedure that can be used to calculate the percentage of cells formed on a particular day. Altman [2]

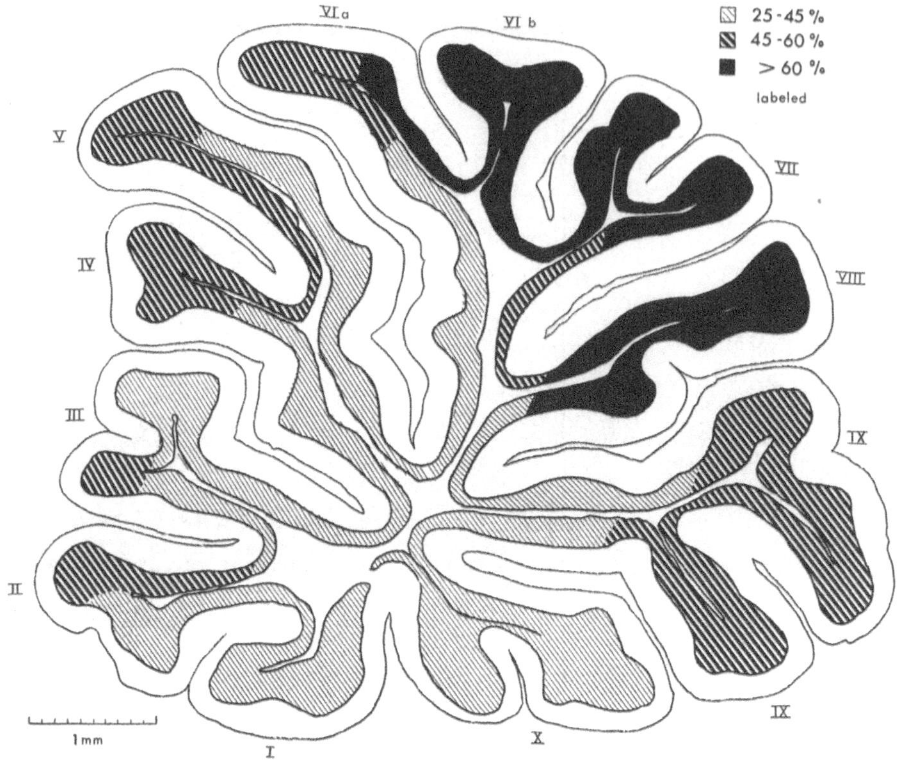

Fig. 12. Schematic presentation of the percentage of granule cells labeled in the different lobules of the vermis (I–X) in rats that were injected with multiple doses of ^{3}H-thymidine between days P 11 and P 16. Regions where less than 45% of the cells could be tagged are considered early forming while those where more than 60% of the cells were labeled are considered late forming. Altman [1]

which at this stage have blunt apical cytoplasmic "cones," and the parallel fibers form a taut barrier above them, the Purkinje cells become mechanically sandwiched between these two growing layers and are forced to form a monocellular sheet (Fig. 15) with a hexagonal arrangement of the cell bodies [20]. The stacking of parallel fibers from the bottom of the molecular layer upward is matched by a similar arrangement in the chronological order of the cells that remain in the molecular layer, as was shown earlier with autoradiography. Since the processes of basket cells are oriented at a right angle to the bed of parallel fibers we suggested [1] that their cell bodies may become arrested in their position as parallel fibers grow above them (Fig. 16).

Fig. 13. **A** Tracings of matched sagittal sections of the vermis from rats of different postnatal ages. *Outer band,* EGL; *black zone,* granular layer; *white zone* between the two, molecular layer. **B** Planimetric measurement of the areal and laminar growth of the cerebellar cortex after birth. Altman [1]

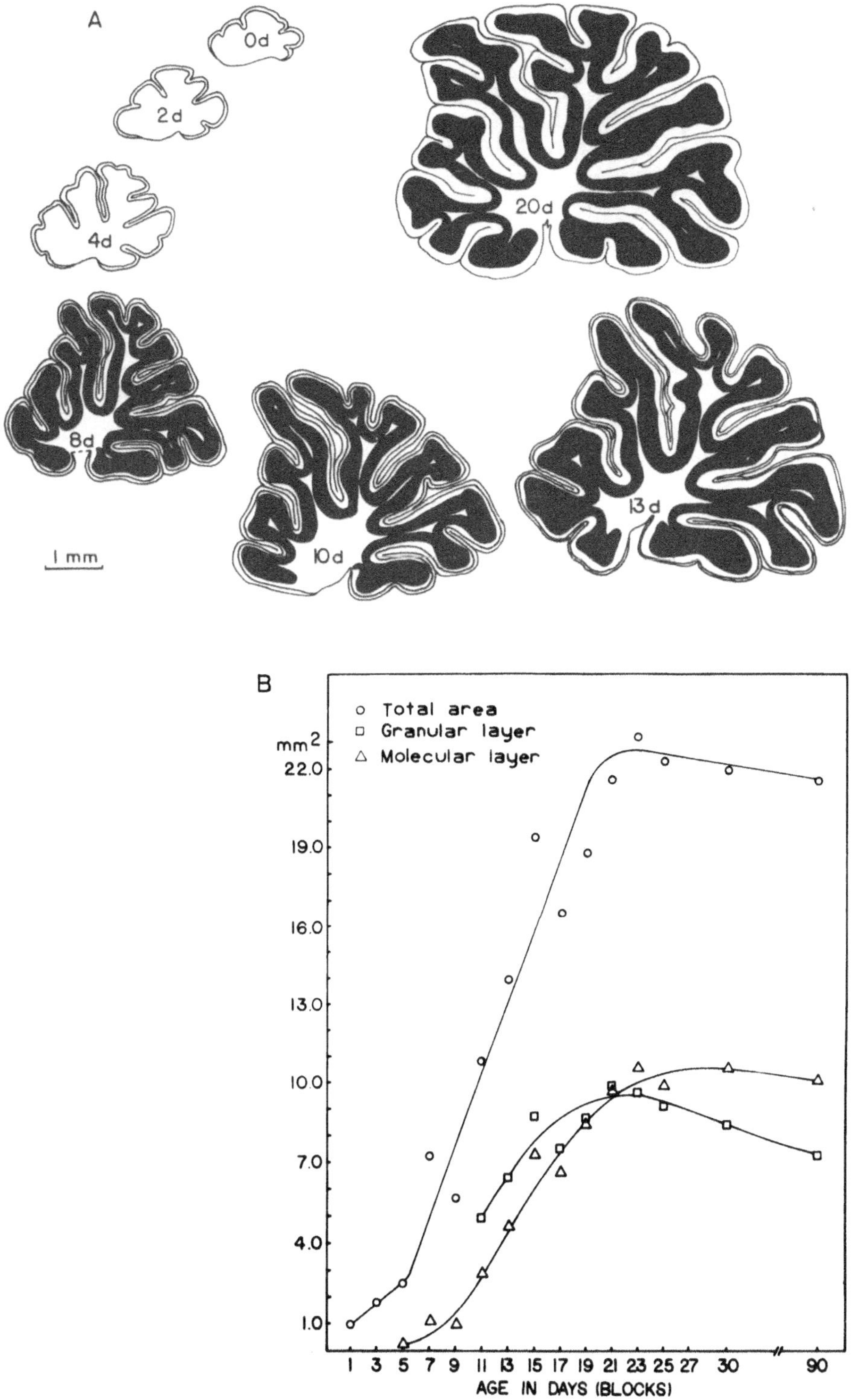
A
0d
2d
4d
20d
8d
10d
13d
1 mm
B
Total area
Granular layer
Molecular layer
mm2
22.0
19.0
16.0
13.0
10.0
7.0
4.0
1.0
1 3 5 7 9 11 13 15 17 19 21 23 25 27 30 90
AGE IN DAYS (BLOCKS)

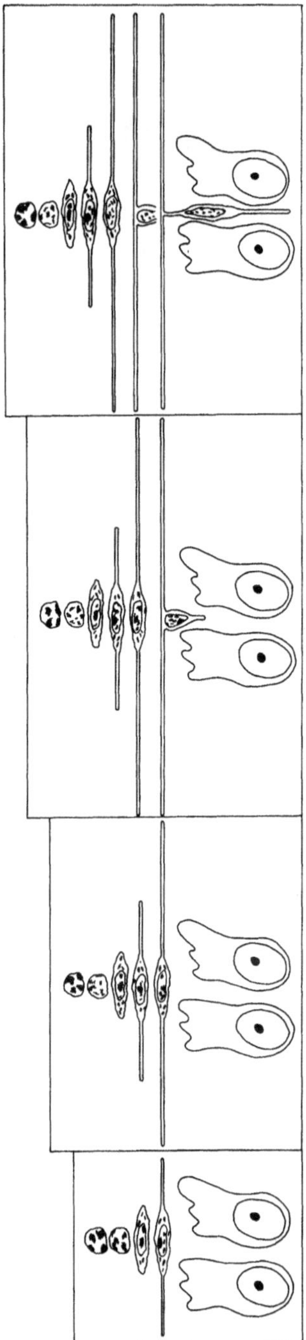

Fig. 14. Transformation of multiplying round cells in the outer EGL into differentiating bipolar cells, and the "extrusion" of the horizontal portion of the parallel fiber before the young granule cells begin their translocation into the granular layer. The effect of this process is that the parallel fibers are stacked from the bottom of the molecular layer upward as a function of their age. Altman [2]

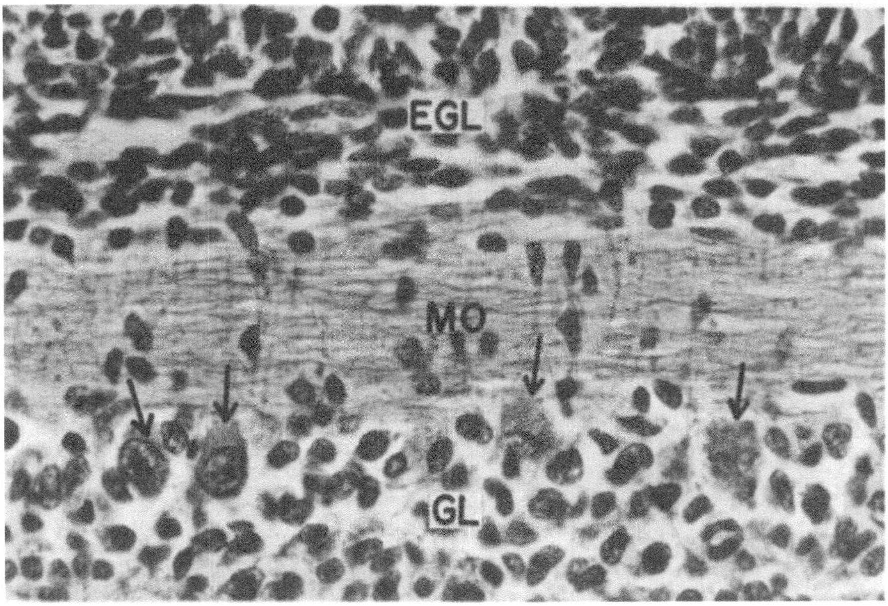

Fig. 15. The aligned pile of parallel fibers in the molecular layer (*MO*) between the EGL and the granular layer (*GL*). The large "apical cones" (*arrows*) of the maturing Purkinje cells are situated beneath the parallel fibers. From a day P 8 rat; coronal section; Bodian stain

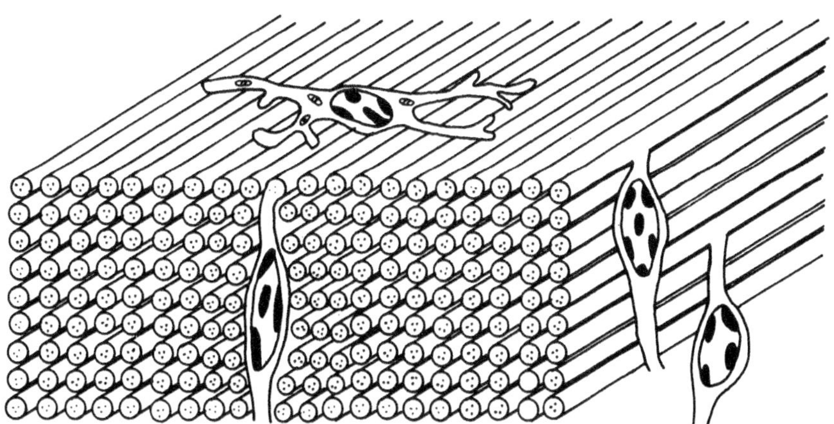

Fig. 16. A hypothesis explaining how the basket cells with processes oriented at a right angle to the parallel fibers become immobilized in the molecular layer as soon as they start to differentiate. The vertically elongated differentiating granule cells are not seriously hindered in their descent. Altman [2]

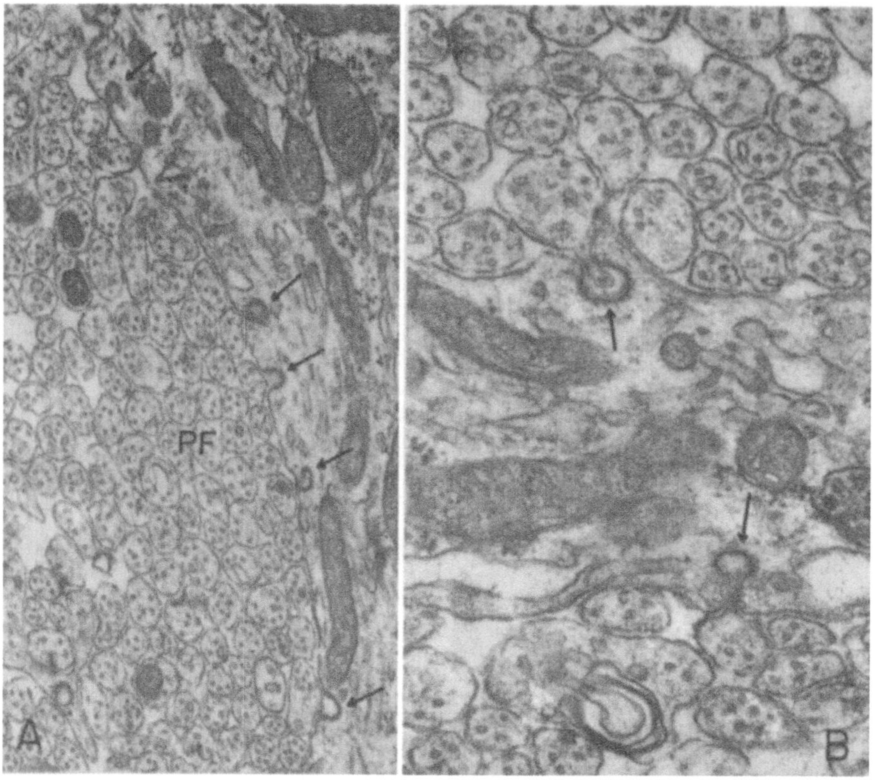

Fig. 17. A High concentration of open coated vesicles (*arrows*) in the primary dendrite of a Purkinje cell opposite parallel fibers (*PF*). **B** Portion of the parallel fiber may be "sucked" into the open coated vesicle (*arrows*). Electron micrographs from the pyramis (lobule VIII) of a day P 12 rat. Altman [3]

Synaptogenesis and Dendritic Development

Our electron microscopic observations [3] showed that the earliest synapses in the cerebellar cortex are with the transient perisomatic processes of Purkinje cells. The synapses are of the asymmetrical type, and probably the terminals are those of climbing fibers. These perisomatic processes disappear at about 1 week of age. A few days later (there are regional differences) the growth of the stem dendrite begins and symmetrical synapses appear on the rounded contours of the Purkinje cell somata; these are basket cell synapses. Asymmetrical synapses are seen a few days later on the stem dendrite and the growing secondary den-

Fig. 18. Changing proportion of parallel fiber profiles (*PP*), parallel fiber varicosities (*PV*), and dendritic spines of Purkinje cells (*DS*) in the **A** upper, **B** middle, and **C** lower portion of the molecular layer in the pyramis of a day P 21 rat. The lower portion of the molecular layer with a smaller proportion of parallel fiber profiles appears mature, the upper molecular layer with few synaptic profiles is immature. Altman [3]

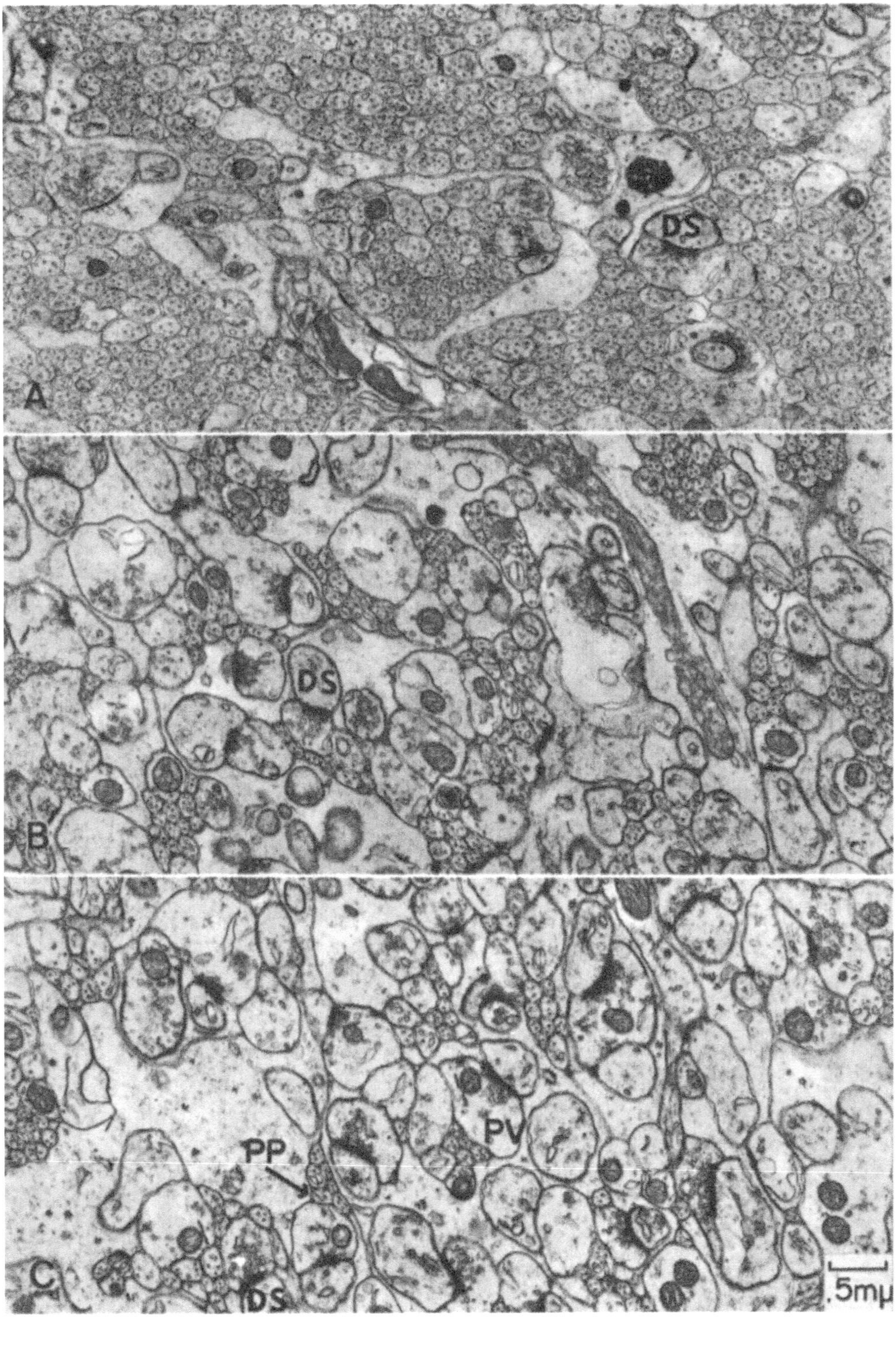
A
DS
B
DS
C
PP
PV
DS
.5mμ

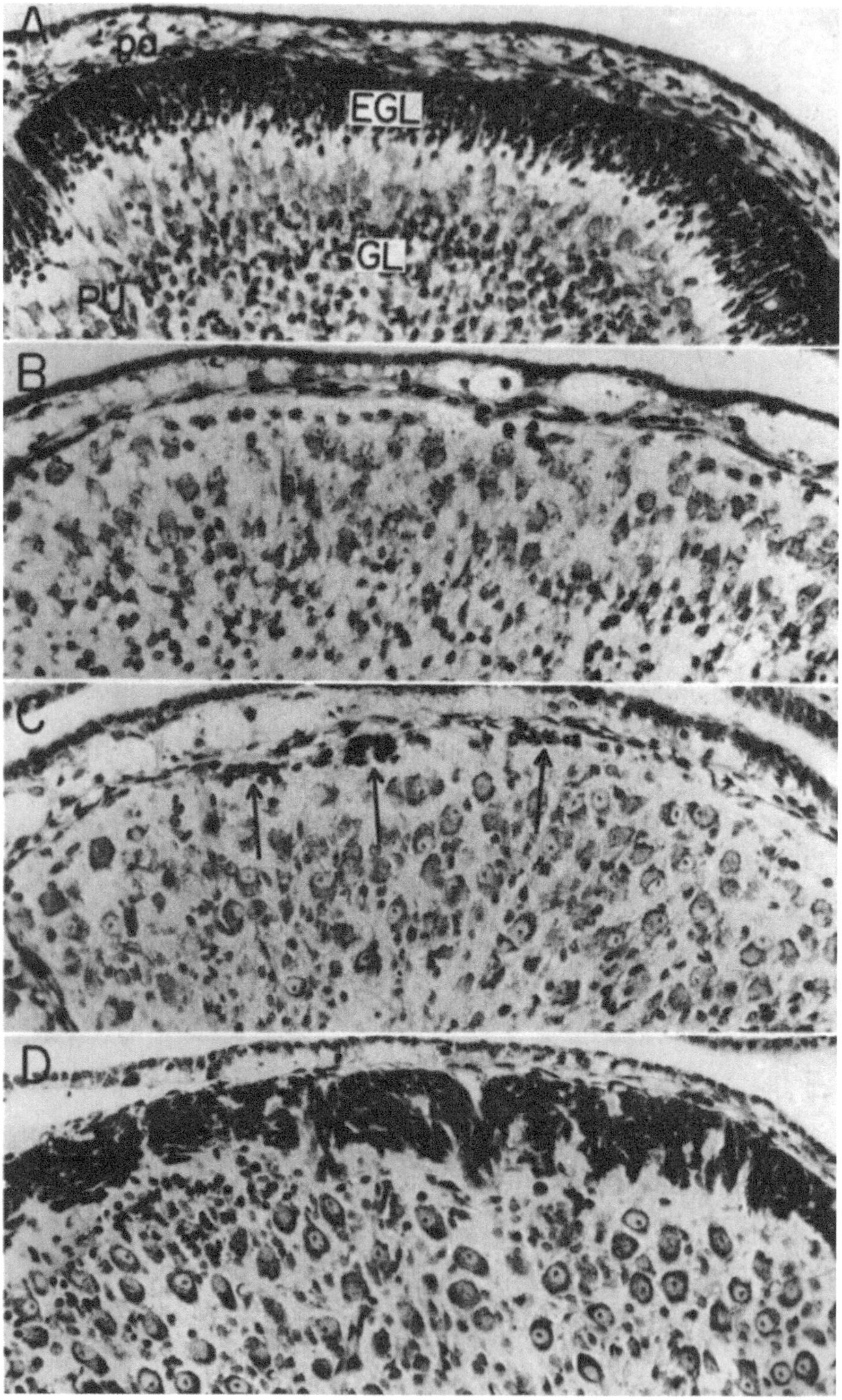
A
pa
EGL
GL
PU
B
C
D

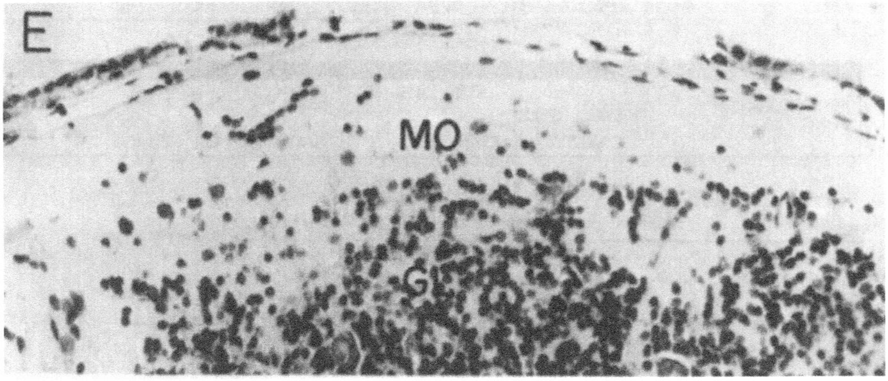

Fig. 19 A–E. Illustration of the regeneration of the EGL in vermal lobule II after X-irradiation. **A** Control, day P 4 rat. **B** Day P 4 rat in which the cerebellum was irradiated daily between days P 0 and P 4 and killed 2 h after the last exposure. EGL has disappeared except for a few cells. Subsequent photographs are from animals that received the same irradiation treatment, but survived for different periods. **C** Rat survived for 4 days after last irradiation. Note reapearance of clumps of EGL cells (*arrows*). **D** Rat survived for 6 days after last irradiation. The EGL has recovered but the arrangement of cells is irregular. **E** An irradiated day P 30 rat; the cells of the EGL have migrated into the granular layer. Many ectopic cells are seen above the Purkinje cells. *GL*, granular layer; *MO*, molecular layer; *pa*, pia-arachnoid membranes; *PU*, Purkinje cell layer. Altman et al. [24]

drites; these are interpreted as the mature, translocated climbing fiber terminals. Synapse formation with parallel fibers begins at about day P 12, and this process again follows a gradient from the bottom of the molecular layer upward.

The formation of true synapses with parallel fibers is preceded by the appearance of membrane thickenings in association with coated vesicles [3]. These coated vesicles are seen in closed or open form. The open coated vesicles had parts of the parallel fibers drawn toward them or entirely engulfed; it was postulated that the parallel fibers and future spiny dendrites exchange material before synaptogenesis (Fig. 17). Synapse formation with parallel fibers is a protracted process and such synapses were still sparse in the upper molecular layer on day P 21 (Fig. 18). Electron microscopic observations also suggested that the final step in the maturation of the molecular layer, the proliferation of glial processes, likewise followed the gradient from the bottom of the molecular layer upward. Synapse formation was also protracted in the glomeruli of the granular layer. But a topographic gradient was not evident here [4].

Experimental Studies of Cerebellar Development

Interference with Postnatal Cerebellar Cytogenesis by Focal X-irradiation

Multiplying cells are extremely radiosensitive [29], and if the brain is exposed to a source of ionizing radiation the cells of the EGL are destroyed [26, 28, 33]. We have irradiated the cerebellum with a single dose of 150 or 200 R of X-rays

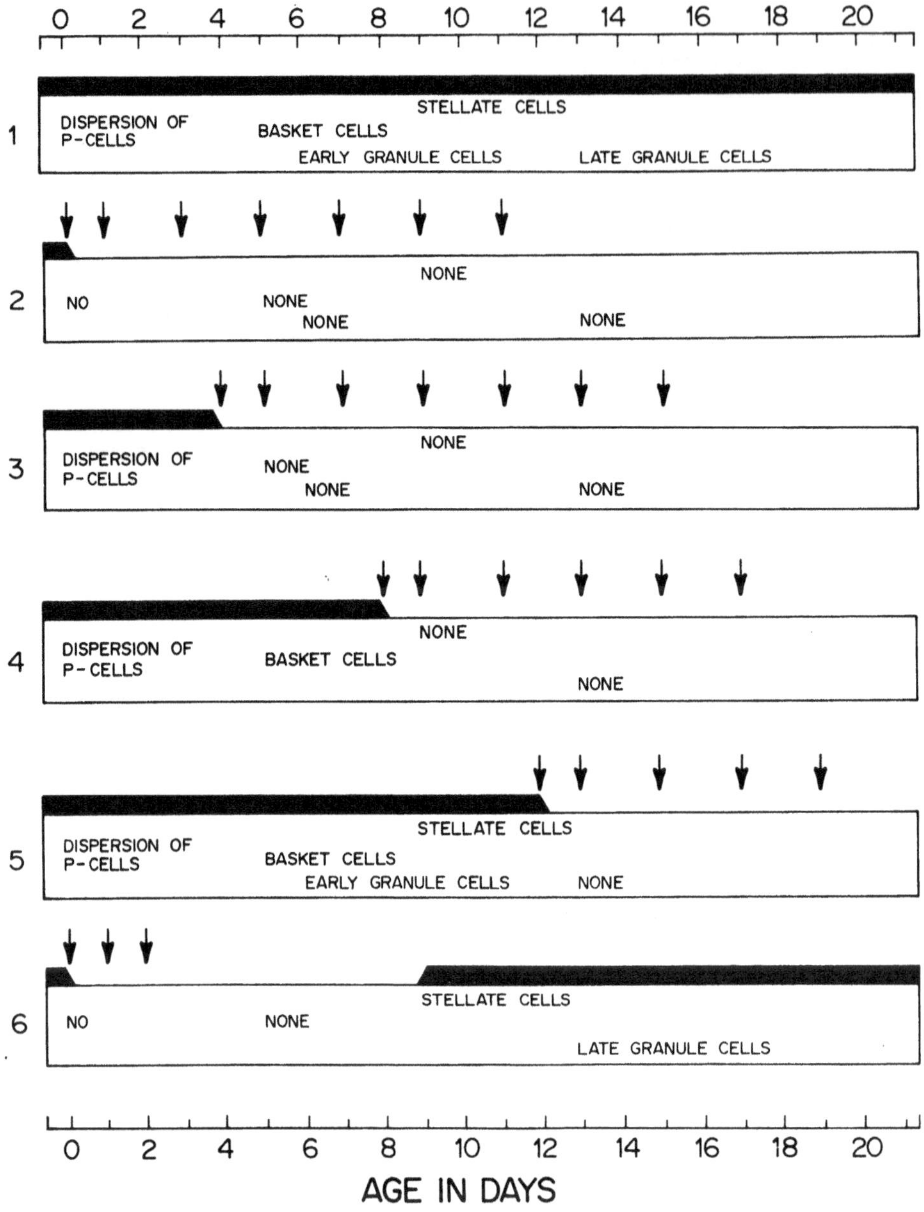

Fig. 20. Diagram illustrating the expected consequences of irradiation of the cerebellum after birth with different exposure schedules on cell acquisition in the cerebellar cortex. *Row 1* shows schematically the sequential production of different cell types in normal animals and approximate postnatal ages. *Row 2* shows that with repeated doses of X-rays (*arrows*), which destroy the cells of the EGL and prevent their regeneration, the acquisition of the postnatally forming microneurons can be prevented. *Row 3* shows that similar effects can be obtained by delaying irradiation until day P 4. However, if the exposure to X-rays is begun on day P 8 (*row 4*), the basket cells are spared, and if it is delayed until P 12 (*row 5*) the stellate cells are also spared and only the acquisition of the late granule cells is prevented. *Row 6* is an example of a schedule which permits the recovery of the EGL and the production of late-produced microneurons. Altman and Anderson [11]

and found that a high proportion of the cells of the EGL are killed without visible harm to the Purkinje cells and other mature or differentiating neurons [10, 21, 22]. Some cells of the EGL do survive such an irradiation and within 4–5 days they regenerate the EGL (Fig. 19) [23, 24]. This regeneration can be delayed by added exposures or prevented altogether if the supplementary irradiations are continued until recovery is prevented by the natural dissolution of the EGL on day P 21 [10]. With this procedure the population of the postnatally acquired granule cells can be varied from close to none (when irradiation is started on day P 0 and continued until day P 13) to a very small fraction (if only a single dose is delivered on day P 0). An alternative method [11] is to vary the starting date of irradiations (Fig. 20). For instance, if the exposure of the cerebellum is begun on day P 8, the basket cells are spared [7]. If it is delayed until day P 12 the stellate cells are also spared, but a high proportion of the late generated granule cells, those with parallel fibers in the upper molecular layer, are prevented from forming [8]. We have used these experimental procedures in a series of behavioral studies [27, 32], but our present discussion will be restricted to the morphogenetic consequences of interference with the acquisition of cerebellar microneurons on the dendritic development of Purkinje cells with which they maintain an intimate synaptic relationship.

Developmental Effects of X-irradiation with Different Schedules

If focal X-irradiation of the cerebellum is started on day P 0 and continued at intervals up to day P 13 to prevent the regeneration of the EGL, a cerebellum develops that is essentially devoid of all basket, stellate, and granule cells [11]. The somata of Purkinje cells reach normal size (Fig. 21), and their ultrastructural organization seems unaffected. However, the cell bodies are not spread out in a monolayer and the stem dendrites are oriented haphazardly. The cell bodies also retain the transient perisomatic processes with asymmetrical synapses typical of climbing fibers. In addition, synapses of mossy fibers, and others that were postulated to be of other Purkinje cells, were seen. A substantial part of the neuropil of the molecular layer was made up of dendritic "thorns" which, in addition to having true synapses, had extensive postsynaptic membrane specializations often in apposition to Purkinje cell or glia cell processes.

Essentially a similar developmental pattern was obtained if irradiation was started on day P 4 and continued until day 15 [12]. The alignment of the Purkinje cells in a monolayer and the outward orientation of the hypertrophied cytoplasm ("apical cone") that generates the dendritic arbor are established in certain folia by day P 4. But the cells became scattered again when irradiation was started on this day and the dendrites were haphazardly oriented. This suggested that developmental events occurring after day P 4 are responsible for the preservation of the monocellular distribution of Purkinje cell somata and the perpendicular, upward growth of their stem dendrites.

In a related study irradiation was started on days P 3, P 4, and P 6 and was continued for varying periods (ranging from day P 4 to day P 11) with a schedule

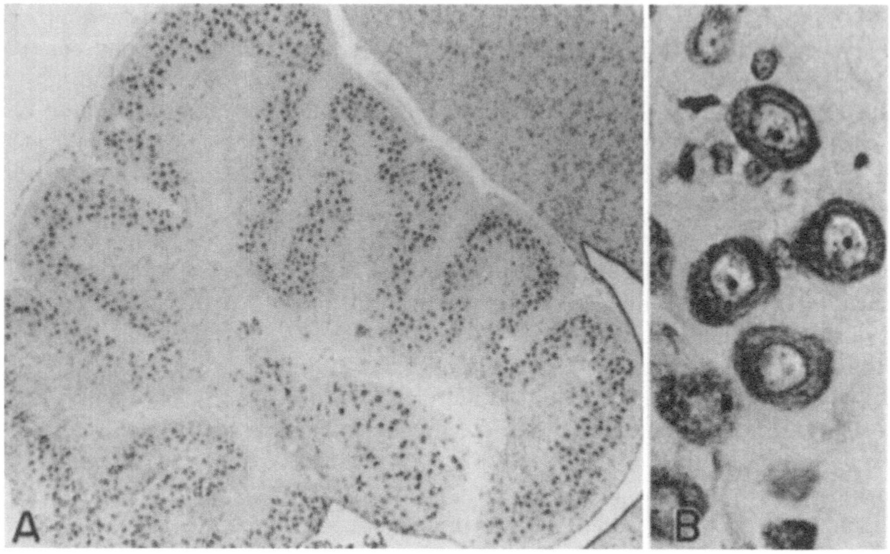

Fig. 21. A The vermis in an adult rat that received 150–200 R between days P 0 and P 13. The cerebellum is made up mostly of the prenatally produced deep nuclei neurons and Purkinje cells; few of the postnatally generated cells are present. **B** The cell bodies of Purkinje cells are essentially normal in size and shape. Altman and Anderson [11]

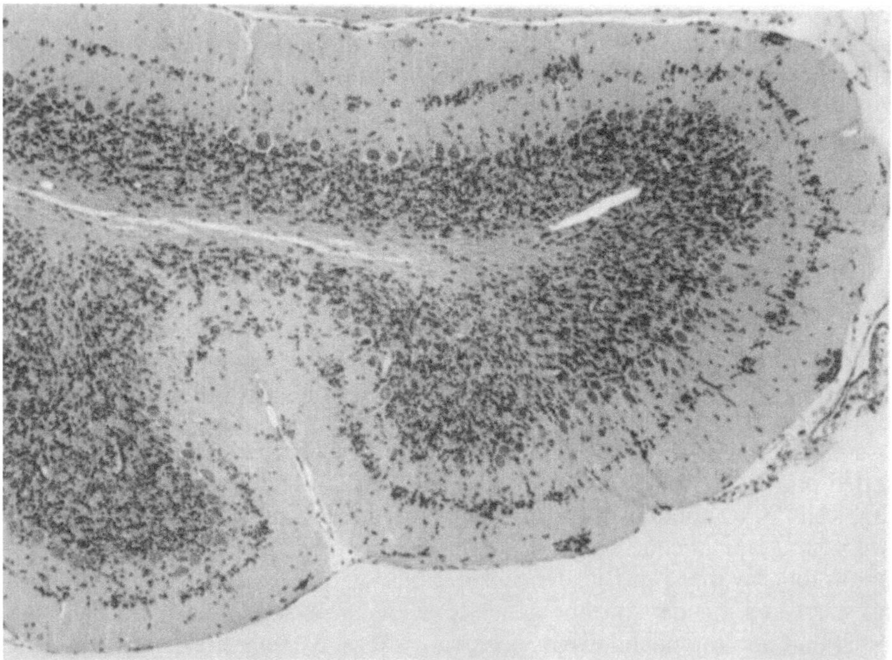

Fig. 22. Ectopic zone of granule cells in the middle of the molecular layer in vermal lobule IX of a rat that was irradiated with 150 R on days P 4, 5, 6, and 7 and was killed at day P 30. Altman [5]

that was compatible with the recovery of the EGL [5]. Under these conditions many of the granule cells that were delayed in descending from the EGL (the EGL had first to be regenerated) became arrested in the molecular layer and formed an ectopic zone there (Fig. 22). The longer regeneration was delayed, the higher in the molecular layer the granule cells became arrested in a given lobule (Fig. 23). It was postulated that the growth of the mossy fibers into the

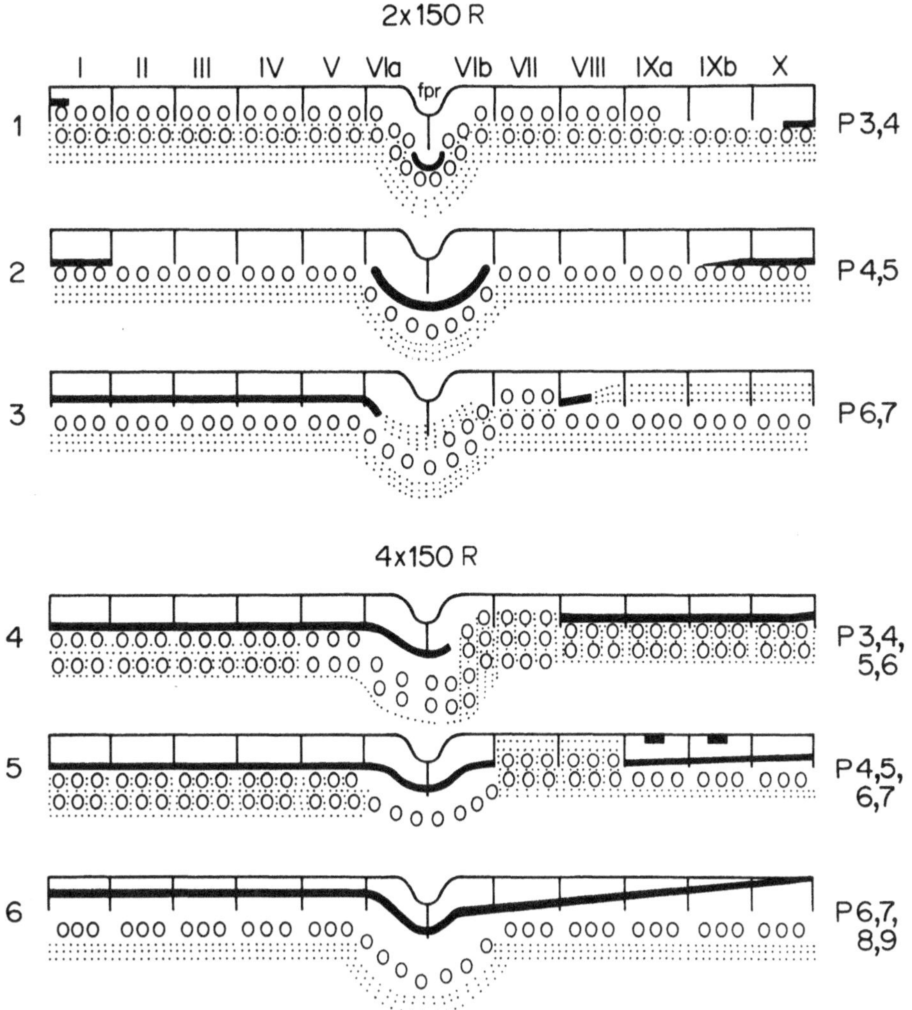

Fig. 23. Schematic survey of the pattern of granule cell ectopia (heavy black line in the molecular layer) in the lobules of vermis (rectangles designated I–X) and in the fissura prima (*fpr*) in rats that were irradiated on the days indicated (*right*) either with two or four doses of 150 R. *Circles* represent Purkinje cells. *Small dots* are granule cells located in the granular layer, either among the Purkinje cells or forming a diffuse ectopic zone in the molecular layer. The time of recovery of the EGL is a function of the last day of irradiation and the number of exposures. The longer the irradiation was continued the higher the ectopic zone was situated in the molecular layer in a given lobule. Changes in the width of the molecular layer of different irradiation groups are not indicated. Altman [5]

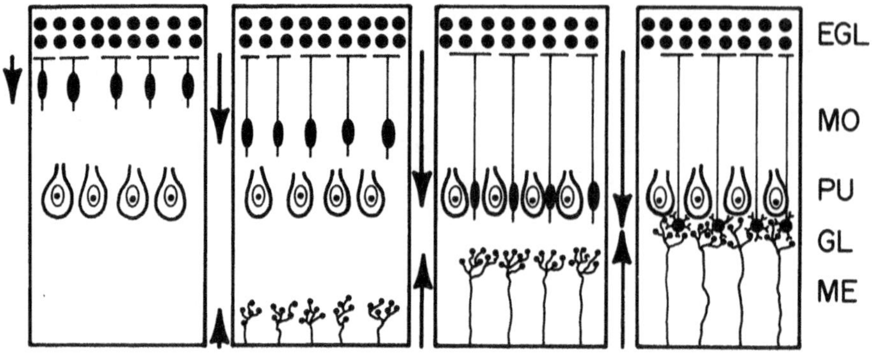

Fig. 24. Diagrammatic representation of the hypothesis of the synchronized descent of young granule cells through the molecular layer (*MO*) and past the Purkinje cell layer (*PU*) and the ascent of mossy fibers through the medullary layer (*ME*), leading to their meeting in the prospective granular layer (*GL*) where they form synapses and their movements become arrested. Altman [5]

cerebellar cortex is normally synchronized with the descent of granule cells and that the two meet beneath the layer of Purkinje cells to form the granular layer (Fig. 24). However, if the descent of granule cells is artificially delayed by irradiation, the mossy fibers grow past the layer of Purkinje cells and grow into the molecular layer. The longer the regeneration of the EGL is delayed and, therefore, the descent of granule cells, the farther the mossy fibers penetrate up into the molecular layer, and it is there that they arrest the descent of granule cells and form an ectopic zone of granule cells. Contrariwise, if irradiation is stopped sufficiently early (day P 4), and the granule cells descend in time, there is minimal or no granule cell ectopia, except in the earliest forming lobules (Fig. 23). As mentioned before, the Purkinje cells fail to develop stem dendrites directed perpendicularly into the molecular layer if irradiation is begun on day P 0 or P 4 and is continued long enough to prevent regeneration of the EGL. However, if irradiation is started on day P 8 the basket cells that are produced on the previous days are spared, and only the generation of stellate cells and the bulk of granule cells is prevented [8]. Under such conditions the somata of Purkinje cells remained aligned in a monolayer and developed singularly straight, upright stem dendrites (Fig. 25). These stout dendrites were surrounded by the descending axons of basket cells (Fig. 26). It was postulated that the perpendicular outgrowth of the primary dendrite is promoted by the basket cell axons through some inductive influence; they may also provide a channel through the bed of parallel fibers for this initial event in dendritic development. The scarcity or absence of secondary smooth branches, which normally appear a short distance above the somata of Purkinje cells, may be due to the absence of stellate cells. This was suggested by the observation that if an irradiation schedule was used that allowed the regeneration of the EGL and the production of some late stellate cells, the upper portion of the stem dendrite, which presumably grew into the regenerated part of the molecular layer, often had secondary smooth branches at its top. In other cases, or if regeneration was not allowed by using irradiations until day P 15, the stem dendrite tended to turn downward near the top (often bifurcating there) and gave off numerous downward directed tertiary spiny branchlets. These tertiary dendrites established synaptic contacts with the spared, early developing parallel fibers of the lower molecular layer; in these cerebella Purkinje cells had the appearance of "weeping willows" in Golgi-impregnated material (Fig. 27).

When irradiation was begun on day P 12 after the generation of the basket cells and many of the stellate cells, the Purkinje cells appeared stunted but otherwise of normal shape [9]. This treatment reduced the granule cell population by 40% [32] and, therefore, there was interference with the formation of the upper level of the molecular layer. This observation of stunted but normally shaped dendritic development is compatible with the hypothesis that the stellate cells are involved in the formation of secondary smooth branches. A summary of these observations is presented in Fig. 28.

Finally, evidence was obtained that the sagittal orientation of spiny branchlets in the vermis is dependent on the initial orientation of parallel fibers in the coronal plane [6]. In animals in which irradiation was begun on days 4, 5, 6, or 7 with schedules that allowed regeneration of the EGL, the bipolar cells were often oriented in planes other than the normal coronal direction. Correspondingly in adults there were often two parallel fiber zones in the molecular layer. There was a lower zone in which the parallel fibers were oriented coronally, and an upper zone (the regenerated part) where they were oriented in other directions, occasionally sagittally (Fig. 29). Where the latter kind of reorganization occurred the dendritic configuration of many Purkinje cells was profoundly affected: the orientation of the planar dendritic arbor was sagittal in the lower part of the cell and coronal in its upper part (Fig. 30). This suggested that, beyond having

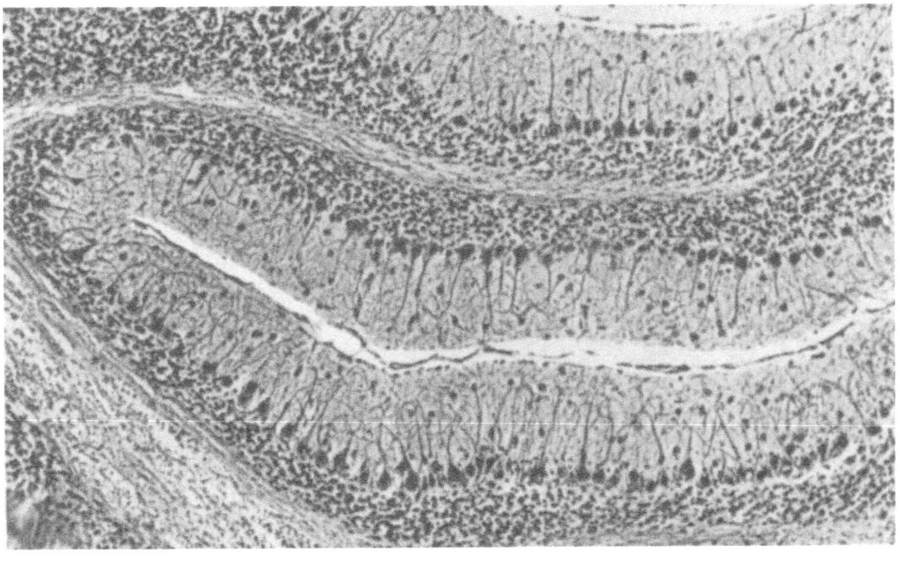

Fig. 25. Vermal lobules VIII and VII from a day P 30 rat that was irradiated between days P 8 and P 15. Purkinje cells tend to have an unarborizing, upright dendrite

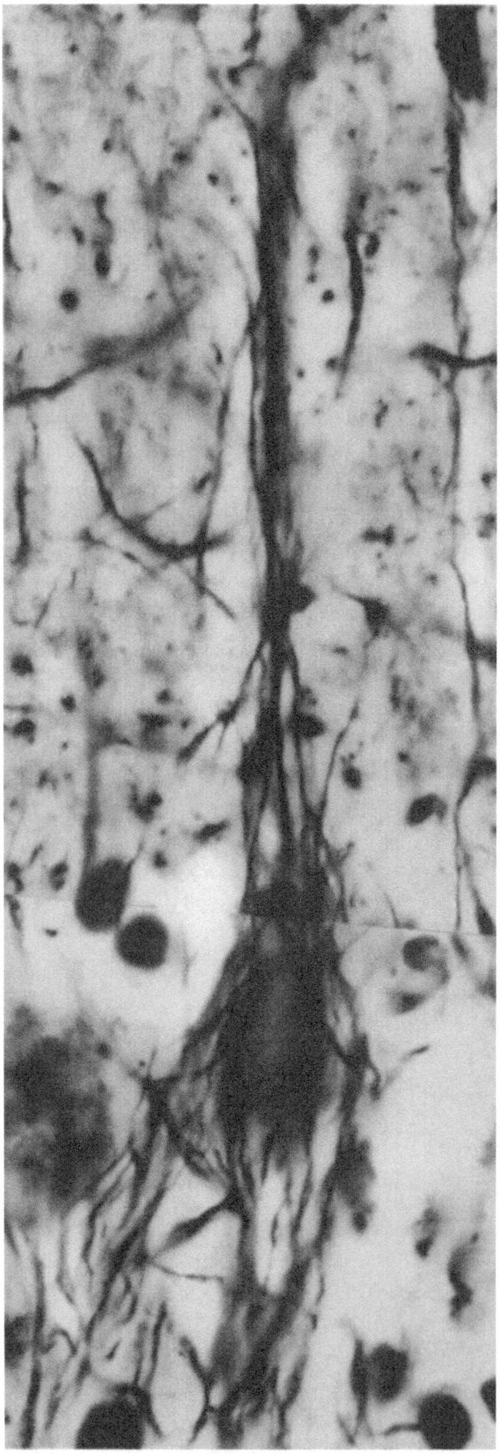

Fig. 26. Unarborizing, straight Purkinje cell stem dendrite (out of focus) with intimately apposed descending basket cell axons (Bodian impregnation), from a rat irradiated between days P 8 and P 15. Altman [8]

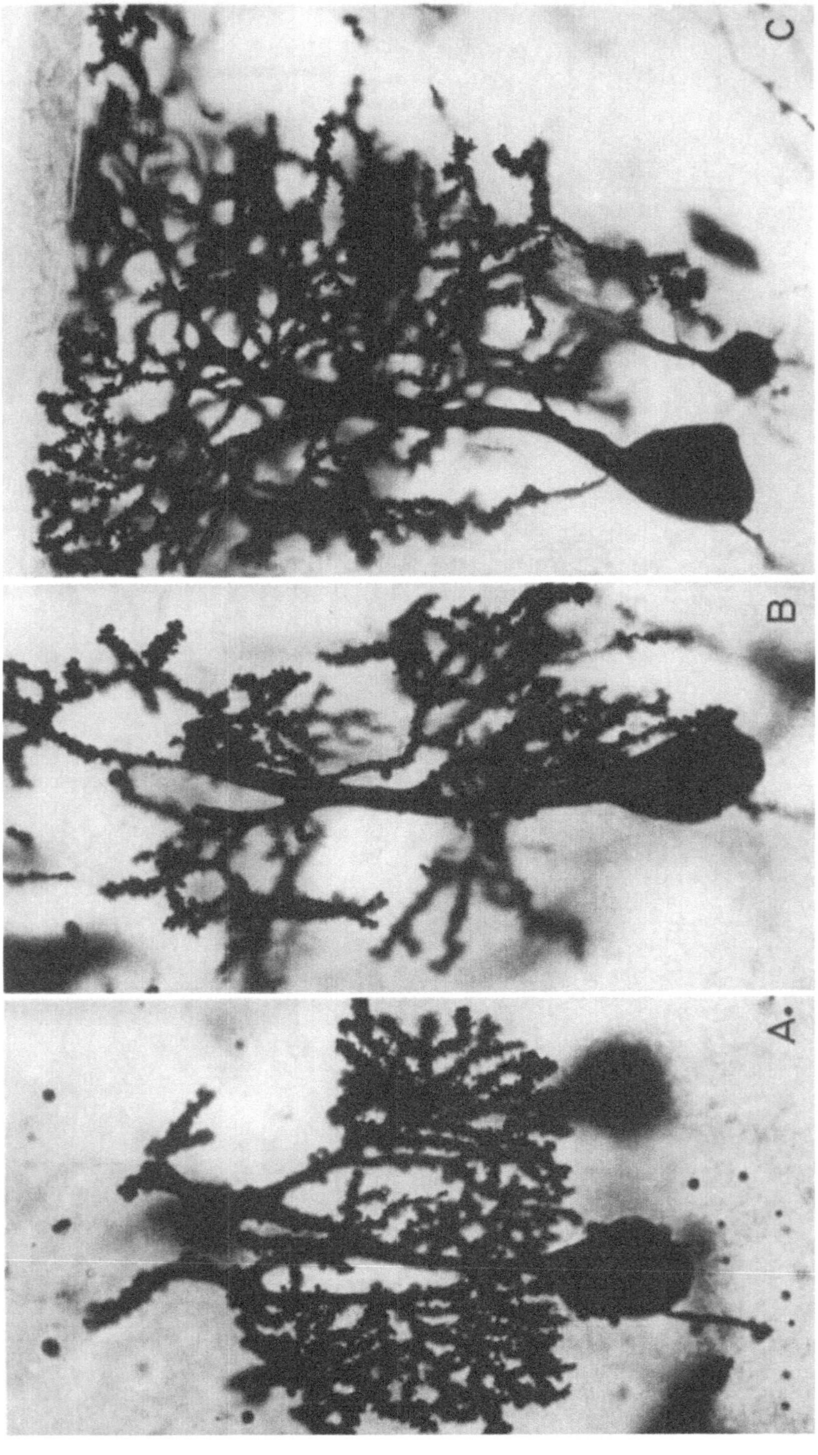

Fig. 27 A–C. Purkinje cells with upright dendrites and different patterns of dendritic arborization from rat irradiated between day P 8 and P 11. **A** A "weeping willow" type with the tertiary branchlets arborizing in the spared, lower molecular layer; **B** intermediate type; **C** this type suggests arborization in the regenerated, upper molecular layer

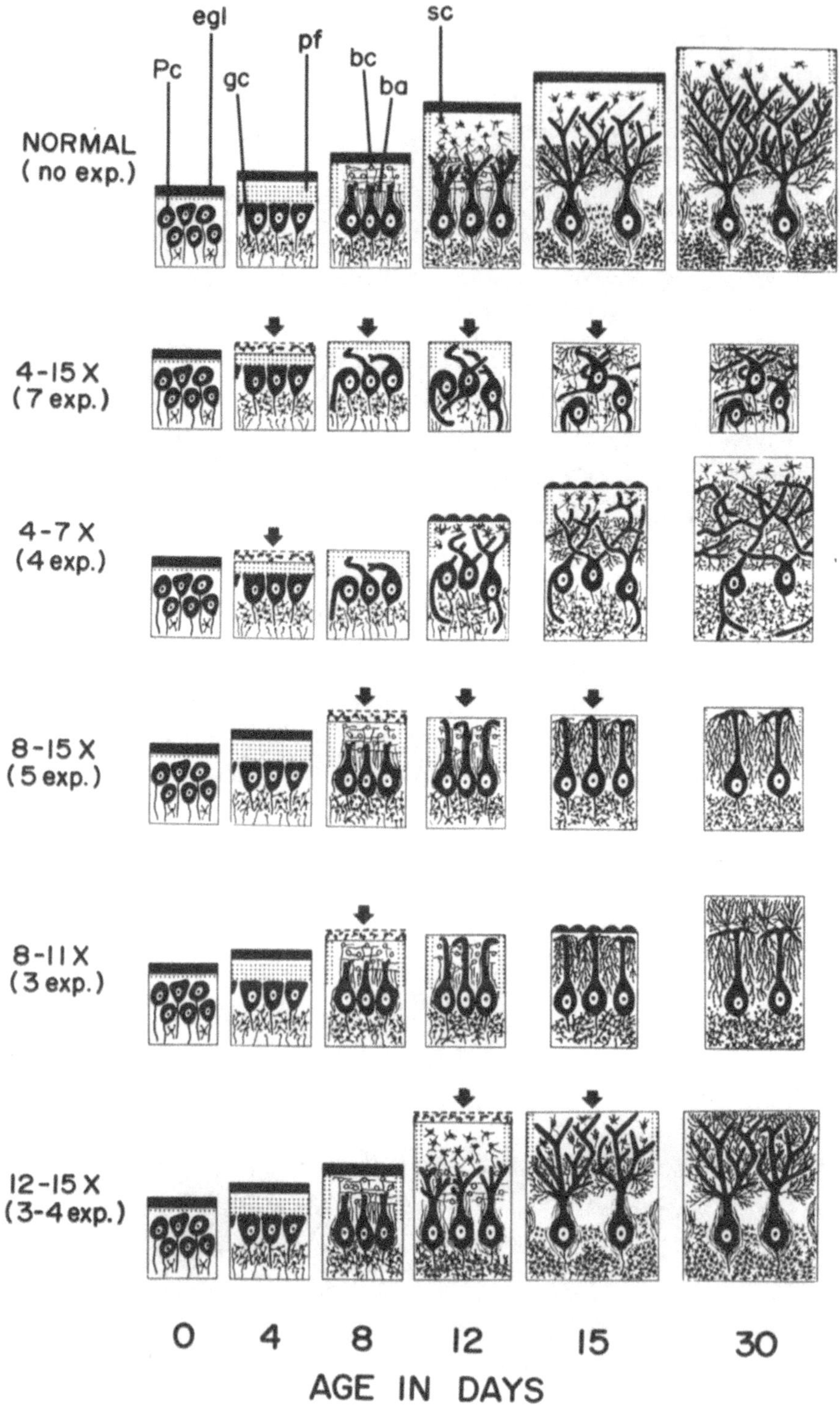
egl
sc
pf
Pc
bc
gc
ba
NORMAL
(no exp.)
4-15 X
(7 exp.)
4-7 X
(4 exp.)
8-15 X
(5 exp.)
8-11 X
(3 exp.)
12-15 X
(3-4 exp.)
0
4
8
12
15
30
AGE IN DAYS

a general role in inducing spiny branchlet formation, the parallel fibers are also involved in inducing the planar outgrowth of these tertiary elements at a right angle to the direction of the parallel fibers.

The following hypothesis was offered for the planar orientation of the spiny branchlets of the Purkinje cells at a right angle to the orientation of parallel fibers [9]. We mentioned earlier that before synapse formation occurs between the growing Purkinje cell dendrites and parallel fibers at a given level of the molecular layer, parts of the parallel fibers are drawn toward open coated vesicles in the Purkinje cell dendrite and are often engulfed (Fig. 17). This suggests material exchange between those two elements prior to synaptogenesis. We postulate that this event is the basis of an operating "exclusion principle," or contact inhibition, which precludes additional contacts between the same parallel fiber and Purkinje cell. This would discourage the parallel fiber-induced growth and proliferation of spiny branchlets in the coronal plane, but would not interfere with their growth in the sagittal plane where they can establish contact with other parallel fibers (Fig. 31). What this hypothesis does not explain is why the secondary, smooth branches, which are postulated to be controlled by stellate cells, are also growing in a planar fashion in the sagittal plane.

Genetic, Epigenetic, and Functional Factors in Cerebellar Development

Our thymidine radiographic studies revealed a great precision in the time of origin of neurons of the cerebellum and of the structures directly connected with it. Moreover, the different types of cerebellar macroneurons and microneurons are produced in a sequential order. Of the macroneurons derived from the ventricular neuroepithelium, the deep nuclei neurons, which are the major output elements of the cerebellum, are generated first. The Purkinje cells, which represent the outflow link between the deep nuclei and the cerebellar cortex, are produced next. The Golgi cells, which are interneurons of the cerebellar cortex, are produced last. A similar precisely set order operates also in the production of cerebellar microneurons derived from the EGL. The basket cells are produced before the stellate cells, and the granule cells are divisible into early elements that overlap with the basket and stellate cells and late elements that outlast them.

Fig. 28. Schematic summary of the stages and time course of Purkinje cell dendritic development in normal rats (*top row*) and in rats irradiated between the postnatal days, and the number of X-ray exposures specified in the legend column on the left. *Arrows* indicate X-irradiation; fragmented EGL symbolizes its destruction by irradiation; absence of EGL indicates its failure to recover after irradiation or its natural dissolution; corrugated EGL symbolizes its recovery after irradiation. *ba*, basket cell axons; *bc*, basket cell bodies; *egl*, external germinal layer; *exp*, exposure; *gc*, granule cells; *Pc*, Purkinje cells; *pf*, parallel fibers; *sc*, stellate cells. Altman [9]

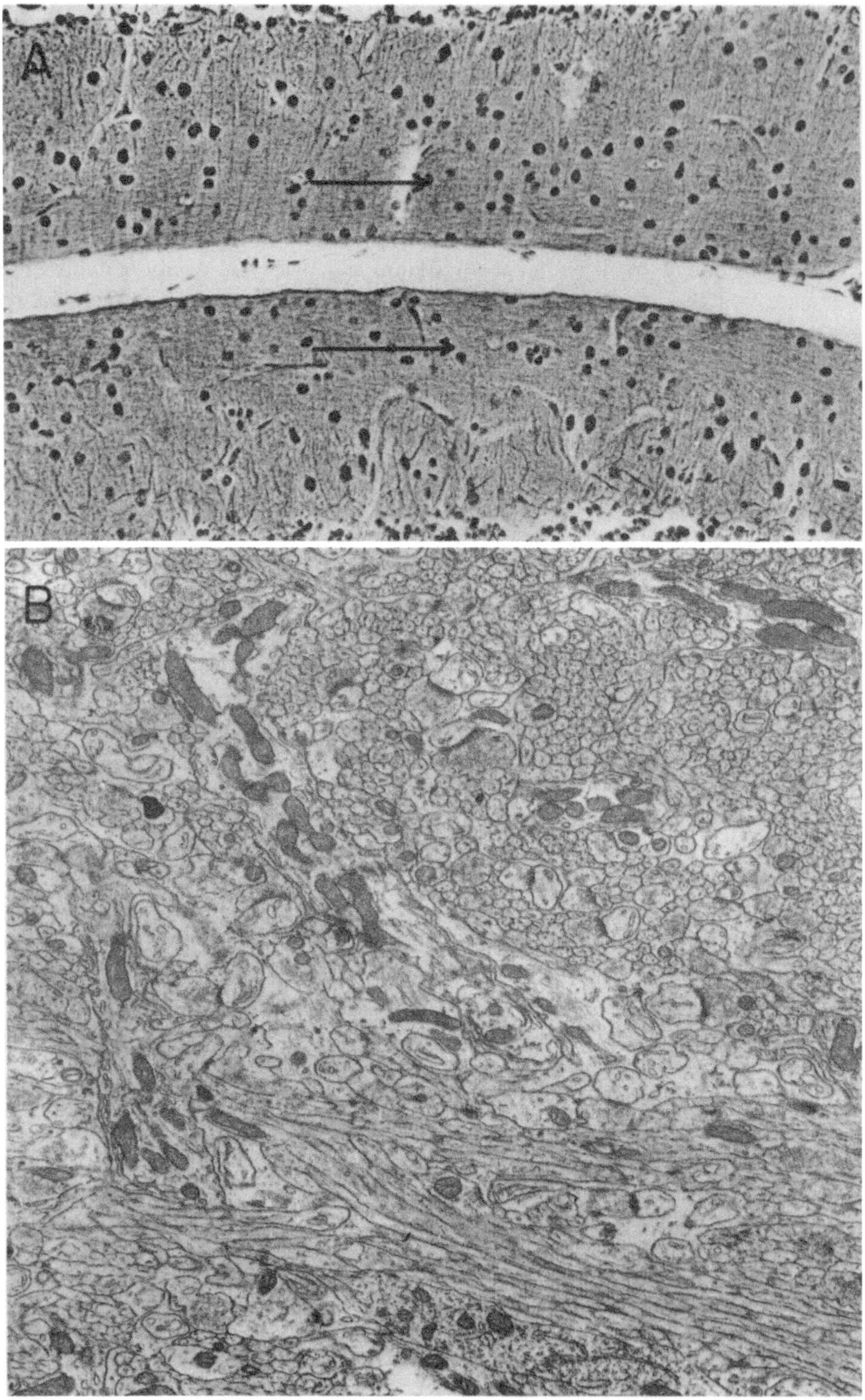
A
B

Fig. 29. **A** In the two lobules shown, the parallel fibers are cut in cross section in the lower molecular layer (normal orientation in sagittal sections), but they are cut parallel to the fiber orientation in the regenerated upper molecular layer (*arrows*). Bodian stain. **B** Transverse and parallel orientation of the parallel fibers in vermal lobule VIII. Electron micrograph. Altman [6]

Intrinsic Specification of Cytogenesis

Since cytogenesis is the first step in the development of a brain structure, it is reasonable to suspect that the precision in the order of its neuron production is an important requirement for the orderly unfolding of the subsequent steps of its morphogenesis. We have at present little information about the mechanisms regulating cell production in different cell lines of the brain, but it does not appear likely, at least in the cerebellum, that neurotrophic factors play a role in the initial phases of cytogenesis. Our datings indicate that the production of deep neurons and Purkinje cells is preceded by the production of neurons in only two structures that send fibers to the cerebellum, namely, the locus coeruleus and the inferior olive. The fibers of the locus coeruleus could reach the cerebellar plate by day E 14, possibly even earlier, at a time when the production of deep neurons is in full swing and Purkinje cell production has just begun. But the fibers of the locus coeruleus are not specific for the cerebellum and if they do exert a neurotrophic effect it is likely to be a nonspecific one. The neurons of the inferior olive are produced in time to exert such an influence by way of the climbing fibers, but we know that the olivary cells have to migrate first a considerable distance from their site of production in the dorsal medulla [14] and by the time they form the inferior olive the production of deep nuclei neurons and Purkinje cells has come to an end.

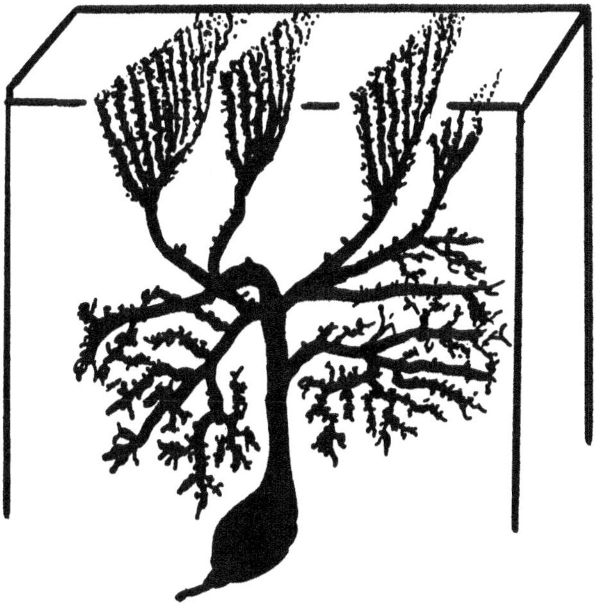

Fig. 30. Drawing of a Golgi-impregnated Purkinje cell with the dendrites oriented in two planes. The lower branches are aligned normally in the sagittal plane. But the upper branches are oriented coronally at a right angle to the rotated parallel fibers of the cells of the regenerated EGL

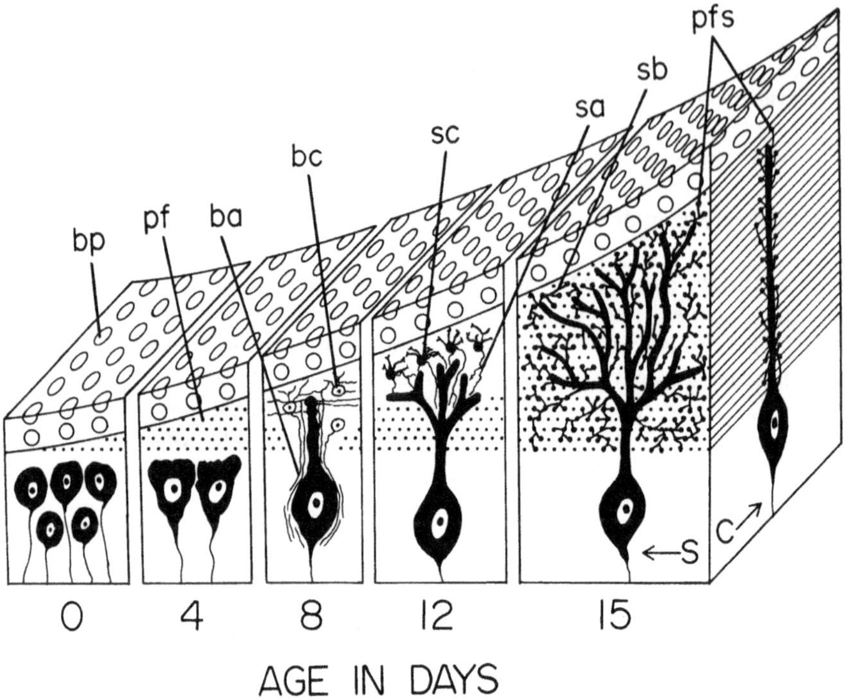

Fig. 31. Scheme of the major steps in the postnatal morphogenesis of rat Purkinje cells and of the proposal for the growth of spiny branchlets in a single plane and at a right angle to the pile of parallel fibers. An "exclusion principle", which allows a single contact between a given Purkinje cell and a parallel fiber, confines outgrowth in the coronal plane (*C*) to the vicinity of the stem dendrite. This principle does not affect growth in the sagittal plane (*S*) as contacts can be established with other parallel fibers. *ba*, basket cell axons; *bc*, basket cells; *pf*, parallel fibers; *pfs*, parallel fiber synapses; *sa*, stellate cell axons; *sb*, spiny branchlets; *sc*, stellate cells. Altman [9]

We may assume tentatively that instead of neurotrophic mechanisms, intrinsic genetic factors control the onset and cessation of cell production in the neuroepithelium that generates the deep neurons and Purkinje cells. What about the production of cerebellar microneurons? The climbing fibers are probably present when the primitive cerebellar cortex forms. There is a fibrous layer between the EGL and the layer of Purkinje cells as this primordium of the cerebellar cortex gradually spreads over the cerebellar plate from caudal to rostral. We do not know about the possible role of mossy fibers in the differentiation of the deep nuclei, but the fibers of the late-generated neurons of this system, particularly the pontine gray, must arrive too late to have an effect on early events of cerebellar differentiation.

Intrinsic Specification of Axonogenesis

In the case of the granule cells we have good evidence that the chronology in the production of neurons has an effect on the organization of their axons. We

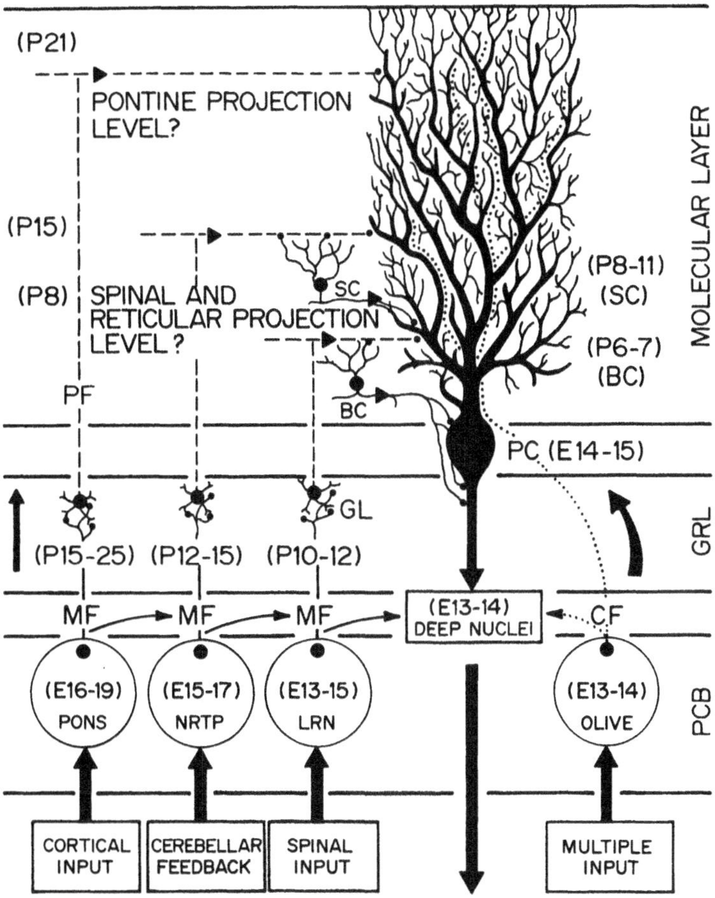

Fig. 32. Summary diagram of the temporal relationships between the cytogenesis of some precerebellar nuclei (the external cuneate nucleus not included) and the cerebellum. The dates are based on the studies described in the text; the selective connections of parallel fibers of the upper and lower molecular layer with mossy fibers of different origins are hypothetical. *BC*, basket cells; *CF*, climbing fibers; *GL*, granule cells; *GRL*, granular layer; *LRN*, lateral reticular nucleus; *MF*, mossy fibers; *NRTP*, nucleus reticularis tegmenti pontis; *PC*, Purkinje cell; *PCB*, precerebellar nuclei; *PF*, parallel fibers; *SC*, stellate cells. Altman [9]

saw that the parallel fibers are laid down in chronological order from the bottom of the molecular layer as the EGL is displaced upward. We obtained suggestive evidence that after the "extrusion" of the horizontal branches of the parallel fiber the granule cell descends until arrested by ascending mossy fibers at the level of the formative granular layer. We have hypothesized that the mossy fibers arriving earliest would be likely to establish synaptic contacts with the earliest descending granule cells and that the preferential contacts of late arriving mossy fibers would be with the later descending granule cells. We do not have information about the time of arrival of mossy fibers in the cerebellar cortex, but we do know that the neurons of the lateral reticular nucleus and external cuneate nucleus are produced substantially earlier than the neurons of the nucleus reticularis tegmenti pontis and the pontine gray. This suggests the possibility (Fig. 31) that the early descending granule cells, those that have their axons in the lower molecular layer, establish synaptic relations with the mossy fibers of the lateral reticular nucleus and external cuneate nucleus. If so, the impulses relayed to the lower domain of the molecular layer would be predominantly from the spinal cord. In contrast, the latest descending granule cells, whose parallel fibers are located in the upper molecular layer, would establish contacts preferentially with mossy fibers of the nucleus reticularis tegmenti pontis and pontine gray nuclei and, in the latter instance, would be influenced primarily from the cerebral cortex. Such a scheme suggests that the sequential production of neurons of the cerebellar cortex and of the precerebellar nuclei constituting the mossy fiber system results in the structural stratification of afferrents to the basket and stellate cells and to the dendritic expanse of Purkinje cells. Some of our behavioral studies carried out in animals that were treated with different schedules of cerebellar X-irradiation indicated that there may be a corresponding functional stratification in the molecular layer [32]. Briefly, we have observed that animals in which the development of the entire molecular layer was interfered with suffered lasting motor deficits. But this was not obtained in animals in which only the formation of the upper molecular layer was prevented; instead, these animals displayed excessive spontaneous locomotor activity.

Epigenetic Factors in Dendrogenesis and Synaptogenesis

Our considerations so far allow for the possibility that the temporal order in the generation of neurons, which is likely to be controlled by intrinsic genetic factors, also determines the temporal order in the outgrowth of their axons. But if the initial phase of axonogenesis is intrinsically specified, our evidence speaks against a similar intrinsic determination for dendrogenesis and synaptogenesis. In the case of the dendritic development of the Purkinje cell we have found, rather, that the orderly growth of the primary, secondary, and tertiary dendrites is dependent on the presence of basket, stellate, and granule cells respectively. This dependence of Purkinje cell dendritic development on neurotrophic, or extrinsic, factors might be described as an epigenetic mechanism as the successive generation of the microneurons exerting their influence upon the Purkinje cell is presumably intrinsically specified. In addition, functional, or environmentally mediated, effects may also operate. After all the basket, stellate, and granule cells exert their apparent neurotrophic effects on components of the Purkinje cell with which they have specific physiological relations. Functional effects are particularly likely on synaptogenesis which appears to be a protracted process both in the molecular layer and in the granular layer.

There is need for much more experimental work, and with techniques other than those we have used in these studies, to prove or refute the hypothesis of a sequence of genetic, epigenetic, and, possibly, functional determination in the ontogeny of the circuitry of the cerebellum. If such a scheme were to obtain further experimental support, it is conceivable that the sequential determination would be related to the uniquely stratified organization of the deep nuclei in relation to the cortex of the cerebellum and of the various cellular components of the cerebellar cortex itself. Therefore, it would not be justified to infer that a similar sequence of morphogenetic mechanisms determines the development of other brain structures that are not hierarchically organized.

Acknowledgment. Much of this research was done in collaboration with Dr. William J. Anderson and Dr. Shirley A. Bayer. The project has been supported by grants from the Atomic Energy Commission, the National Institutes of Health, and the National Science Foundation. In the preparation of this paper, I received technical assistance from William Boyle, Carol Landon, Kathy Shuster, and Mary Ward.

References

1. Altman J (1969) Autoradiographic and histological studies of postnatal neurogenesis. III. Dating the time of production and onset of differentiation of cerebellar microneurons in rats. J Comp Neurol 136:269–294
2. Altman J (1972) Postnatal development of the cerebellar cortex in the rat. I. The external germinal layer and the transitional molecular layer. J Comp Neurol 145:353–398
3. Altman J (1972) Postnatal development of the cerebellar cortex in the rat. II. Phases in the maturation of Purkinje cells and of the molecular layer. J Comp Neurol 145:399–464
4. Altman J (1972) Postnatal development of the cerebellar cortex in the rat. III. Maturation of the components of the granular layer. J Comp Neurol 145:465–514
5. Altman J (1973) Experimental reorganization of the cerebellar cortex. III. Regeneration of the external germinal layer and granule cell extopia. J Comp Neurol 149:153–180
6. Altman J (1973) Experimental reorganization of the cerebellar cortex. IV. Parallel fiber reorientation following regeneration of the external germinal layer. J Comp Neurol 149:181–192
7. Altman J (1976) Experimental reorganization of the cerebellar cortex. V. Effects of early X-irradiation schedules that allow or prevent the acquisition of basket cells. J Comp Neurol 165:31–48
8. Altman J (1976) Experimental reorganization of the cerebellar cortex. VI. Effects of X-irradiation schedules that allow or prevent cell acquisition after basket cells are formed. J Comp Neurol 165:49–64
9. Altman J (1976) Experimental reorganization of the cerebellar cortex. VII. Effects of late X-irradiation schedules that interfere with cell acquisition after stellate cells are formed. J Comp Neurol 165:65–76
10. Altman J, Anderson WJ (1971) Irradiation of the cerebellum in infant rats with low-level X-ray: Histological and cytological effects during infancy and adulthood. Exp Neurol 30:492–509
11. Altman J, Anderson WJ (1972) Experimental reorganization of the cerebellar cortex. I. Morphological effects of elimination of all microneurons with prolonged X-irradiation started at birth. J Comp Neurol 146:355–406
12. Altman J, Anderson WJ (1973) Experimental reorganization of the cerebellar cortex. II. Effects of elimination of most microneurons with prolonged X-irradiation started at four days. J Comp Neurol 149:123–152
13. Altman J, Bayer SA (1978) Prenatal development of the cerebellar system in the rat. I. Cytogenesis and histogenesis of the deep nuclei and the cortex of the cerebellum. J Comp Neurol 179:23–48
14. Altman J, Bayer SA (1978) Prenatal development of the cerebellar system in the rat. II. Cytogenesis and histogenesis of the inferior olive, pontine gray, and the precerebellar reticular nuclei. J Comp Neurol 179:49–76

15. Altman J, Bayer SA (1979) Development of the diencephalon in the rat. IV. Quantitative study of the time of origin of neurons and the internuclear chronological gradients in the thalamus. J Comp Neurol 188:455–472
16. Altman J, Bayer SA (1980) Development of the brain stem in the rat. I. Thymidine-radiographic study of the time of origin of neurons of the lower medulla. J Comp Neurol 194:1–35
17. Altman J, Bayer SA (1980) Development of the brain stem in the rat. III. Thymidine-radiographic study of the time of origin of neurons of the vestibular and auditory nuclei of the upper medulla. J Comp Neurol 194:877–904
18. Altman J, Bayer SA (1980) Development of the brain stem in the rat. IV. Thymidine-radiographic study of the time of origin of neurons in the pontine region. J Comp Neurol 194:905–929
19. Altman J, Bayer SA (1981) Development of the brain stem in the rat. V. Thymidine-radiographic study of the time of origin of neurons in the midbrain tegmentum. J Comp Neurol 198:677–716
20. Altman J, Winfree AT (1977) Postnatal development of the cerebellar cortex in the rat. V. Spatial organization of Purkinje cell perikarya. J Comp Neurol 171:1–16
21. Altman J, Anderson WJ, Wright KA (1967) Selective destruction of precursors of microneurons of the cerebellar cortex with fractionated low-dose X-rays. Exp Neurol 17:481–497
22. Altman J, Anderson WJ, Wright KA (1968) Differential radiosensitivity of stationary and migratory primitive cells in the brains of infant rats. Exp Neurol 22:52–74
23. Altman J, Anderson WJ, Wright KA (1969) Early effects of X-irradiation of the cerebellum in infant rats: Decimation and reconstitution of the external granular layer. Exp Neurol 24:196–216
24. Altman J, Anderson WJ, Wright KA (1969) Reconstitution of the external granular layer of the cerebellar cortex in infant rats after low-level X-irradiation. Anat Rec 163:453–472
25. Athias M (1897) Recherches sur l'histogénèse de l'ecorce du cervelet. J Anat Physiol Norm 33:372–404
26. Brunner H (1920) Über den Einfluß der Röntgenstrahlen auf das Gehirn. Arch Klin Chir 144:332–372
27. Brunner RL, Altman J (1973) Locomotor deficits in adult rats with moderate to massive retardation of cerebellar development during infancy. Behav Biol 9:169–188
28. Hicks SP (1958) Radiation as an experimental tool in mammalian developmental neurology. Physiol Rev 38:337–356
29. Hicks SP, D'Amato CJ (1966) Effects of ionizing radiations on mammalian development. In: Woollam DHM (ed) Advances in Teratology. Logos Press, London, pp 195–250
30. Miale I, Sidman RL (1961) An autoradiographic analysis of histogenesis in the mouse cerebellum. Exp Neurol 4:277–296
31. Olson L, Seiger Å (1972) Early prenatal ontogeny of central monoamine neurons in the rat: Fluorescence histochemical observations. Z Anat Entwicklungsgesch 137:301–316
32. Pellegrino LJ, Altman J (1979) Effects of differential interference with postnatal cerebellar neurogenesis on motor performance, activity level, and maze learning of rats. A developmental study. J Comp Physiol Psychol 93:1–33
33. Shofer RJ, Pappas GD, Purpura DP (1964) Radiation-induced changes in morphological and physiological properties of immature cerebellar cortex. In: Haley TJ, Snider RS (eds) Response of the nervous system to ionizing radiation. Little, Brown, Boston, pp 476–508
34. Uzman LL (1960) The histogenesis of the mouse cerebellum as studied by its tritiated thymidine uptake. J Comp Neurol 114:137–159

Discussion

A major point of discussion was on the comparison of Dr. Altman's results with those of experiments on genetic mutants. Dr. Sotelo indicated that the results of his Golgi studies on Purkinje cells of mutant mice did not agree with Dr. Altman's hypothesis, and he went on to elaborate this apparent discrepancy. In the *weaver* mutant, although the postmitotic granule cells die before migration, stellate cells and basket cells are present in normal numbers. In fact, because of the reduced volume of the cerebellar cortex, the density of these cell types is greater than normal. Yet, most of the Purkinje cells have dendritic trees resembling those of the rat agranular cerebellum. Dr. Sotelo also felt that the *reeler* mutant provides an ideal system for testing Dr. Altman's hypothesis. Purkinje cells, dispersed throughout the granular layer and elaborating their dendritic arborization on a variety of cellular milieux, exhibit three types of dendritic patterns. Only one of them, however, fits Dr. Altman's hypothesis, although all three of them have basket cell investment.

Dr. Altman responded as follows: "We believe that the doses of radiation used in our experiments do not directly harm the maturing Purkinje cells and the damage is restricted to the multiplying cells of the external granular layer. It is conceivable that only normal Purkinje cells can respond to the inductive influences exerted by basket, stellate, and granule cells. In those cerebellar mutants in which the Purkinje cells are also obviously affected, the trophic interactions between the microneurons and the maturing Purkinje cells could be drastically altered."

Dr. Sotelo pointed out that those who work with mutants do not agree with that view; in fact, they are inclined to believe that X-ray treatment affects more than just one population of cells, meaning that the Purkinje cells are probably affected too. Obviously realizing that this line of argument cannot lead to an objective resolution of the differing views, Dr. Altman concluded the lengthy discussion on this point by stating that, despite the advantages and disadvantages inherent in the various experimental procedures, it is good to have different approaches to study these intriguing interactions.

Another point of apparent discrepancy, raised by Dr. Chan-Palay, was on the temporal separation of the arrival of the afferent systems very early (between embryonic days 11 and 19) and the descent of granule cells much later (postnatally). Dr. Altman explained that the mossy fibers make their contacts at two levels. They make their first contacts in the deep cerebellar nuclei by about the time of birth and they are occupied there for some time. Much later, they migrate upward into the cerebellar cortex. There is indeed almost a week between these two steps. It should be pointed out that, as far as fibers are concerned, everything that was said, except concerning parallel fibers, was hypothetical. Dr. Chan-Palay then reviewed a series of experiments done in their laboratory, especially those done in collaboration with Dr. Yamamoto (Anat. Embryol. 159:1–15, 1980). These experiments involved transplantation of various monoamine-containing neuron groups, such as the raphe and locus coeruleus, into the fourth ventricle. They were able to produce ectopic granule cells and even caused the growth of new areas of what looked like the granular layer and also cause the migration of mossy fiber systems or other fiber systems. Most significantly, they found hyperinnervation by the serotonin transmitter system they were working with. The point Dr. Chan-Palay made was that the migration of the afferents appears to be very much cued in with the migration of the granule cells. Dr. Altman, however, felt that the picture is much more complicated than it may appear to be.

Dr. Voogd showed a few slides on the developing chick cerebellum to bring up an interesting point concerning Dr. Altman's description of the layering in the granular layer. When the migration of external granule cells into the internal granular layer starts, around incubation day 10, strands of cells appear in between the Purkinje cell clusters. These strands can be seen clearly until day 14, after which the migration pattern becomes increasingly diffuse. Although similar observations have been made by other investigators, Dr. Voogd reported a new observation that the spinocerebellar fibers terminate on the first arriving internal granule cells in a pattern of parallel, parasagittal strips, as one would expect if, based on Dr. Altman's suggestion, the earliest migrating granule cells are contacted by the early arriving mossy fibers.

Dr. Voogd's comments were of particular relevance to the hypothesis proposed by Dr. Llinás later at the conference on the possibility that the vertical parts of the granule cell axons may constitute the anatomical basis of the physiological organization of the cerebellar cortex in vertical columns, at right angles to the pial surface. The migration of the external granule cells as strands and the concomitant synaptic termination of the mossy fibers on these cells in a band-like manner would seem to support such a hypothesis.

Dr. Llinás brought into the discussion some physiological observations made in his laboratory. They found very clear synaptic transmission (i.e., synaptic potentials) in the 1-day-old rat which, Dr. Llinás thought, is not supposed to have any clear synapses. He raised the question as to whether clear, conventional synapses of electron microscopy are needed for neuronal communication and interaction. Dr. Altman's response was in two parts: (a) There *are* clear synapses in the 1-day-old rat cerebellum. These are the climbing fiber synapses on the perisomatic processes of Purkinje cells, seen by Mugnaini, Larramendi and many others. (b) In the immature cerebellum, there are contacts which are not synaptic in nature. These are the open coated vesicles where a Purkinje cell dendrite "sucks in" a parallel fiber. These have been seen in the rat, and Gona (1978) has seen them in the frog cerebellum. These "protosynaptic", or synaptoid, contacts could serve the function of neuronal interaction.

Dr. Mugnaini commented on the phylogenetic aspect of cerebellar development as follows: Any comprehensive theory of cellular morphogenesis should explain not only the experimental differences with time in anyone species, but also the phylogenetic differences in the dendritic patterns of Purkinje cells. For example, Purkinje cells in the amphibians, reptiles, and birds have a long apical main stem dendrite and very long spiny branchlets. Birds have typical basket cells, but frogs and turtles lack the periaxonal painter's brush. It should also be mentioned that in birds parallel fibers synapse early on the apical dendrite, although these synapses are later lost. They could have a morphogenetic role so far overlooked. The parallel fibers which were not destroyed in Dr. Altman's X-irradiation experiments might have made synaptic contacts with the main stem dendrites of Purkinje cells, exerting some influence on dendritic development.

In response to Dr. Marshall's query on the role of perisomatic processes and somatic dendrites of Purkinje cells, Dr. Altman indicated that, while the role and fate of the perisomatic processes is not clear, the apical column of organelle-rich cytoplasm of the maturing Purkinje cell migrates up through the "ceiling" of parallel fibers and, in doing so, probably exerts an inductive influence.

Dr. Grant asked if it is feasible to destroy that part of the anlage of the cerebellum which gives rise to the locus coeruleus and then study the effects on the development of the cerebellar cortex, in order to investigate the possibility that locus coeruleus has a trophic function. Dr. Altman answered that a selective destruction of the locus coeruleus by X-irradiation may be difficult to accomplish because it develops very early during embryonic growth. Dr. Llinás suggested that lesions of locus coeruleus could be attempted by a chemical approach using 6-hydroxydopamine. Dr. Balázs, who has experience in this particular area, provided information on this subject. First, 6-hydroxydopamine has secondary effects on other cell types, and so all of this work needs to be repeated using inhibitors to block the uptake by the nonselective areas. Secondly, this kind of work has not been done very early in development. To determine what kind of trophic effects, if any, the locus coeruleus may exert on the developing cerebellum, we need to go back further in ontogeny to about day 13 or 14 of development of the rat.

Dr. Snider asked (i) if the early organization of the small blood vessels has any effect on the orientation of neuronal processes, as may be suspected on the basis of Tennyson's studies on substantia nigra; (ii) if recurrent collaterals from the deep cerebellar nuclei might have any effect on the Purkinje cell dendritic development, especially on the basal dendrites. Dr. Altman's views were that it is unlikely that blood vessels have any morphogenetic effect, since some of these events occur before the capillaries invade the differentiating zones, and that the possible role of collaterals of the deep cerebellar nuclei is not readily amenable to experimental analysis.

Dr. Chan-Palay expressed concern about the dosage of X-irradiation used in Dr. Altman's experiments, which she considered were excessive. Dr. Altman indicated that the animals were irradiated as many as ten times and yet electron microscopic examination failed to show any pathology, other than a few vacuoles in Purkinje cells. Body weights were normal as long as they were fed on powdered food, which had to be done because the motor deficits precluded the animals from feeding on pellets.

Dr. Palay asked about the source of the Golgi cells of the cerebellum. Dr. Altman stated that they must arise from the neuroepithelium, rather than from the external granular layer, since they are generated by day E 19, when the external granular layer is not established yet.

Reference

1. Gona AG (1978) Ultrastructural studies on cerebellar histogenesis in the frog: The external granular layer and the molecular layer. Brain Res 153:435–447

Synaptic Remodeling in Agranular Cerebella

C. Sotelo

Introduction

The numerous morphological studies carried out on the developing cerebellum have been useful in elucidating some of the problems concerned with neuronal proliferation, migration, and differentiation [1, 9, 16, 28, 33, 34, 37, 42]. Regarding synapse formation, the analysis of normal development has provided complete information on the chronology of events taking place during the establishment of the different kinds of synapses which compose the cerebellar cortical circuitry [2, 3, 4, 23, 29, 30]. However, all pre- and postsynaptic elements develop nearly simultaneously. As a consequence, it is extremely difficult to determine which factors among those governing synaptogenesis are strictly dependent on inherent properties of each category of neurons and to separate them from those emerging as a result of cellular interactions between the various growing neuronal elements. The obvious way to solve this problem is to simplify the circuitry in a very specific manner, for instance, by eliminating a given category of neurons, and to determine the consequences of this change in the cellular milieu in the final moulding of the cerebellar circuitry. One model is well fitted for this kind of study, that of the granuloprival cerebellum, in which Purkinje cells must grow and make synaptic connections in the absence of their main afferent fibers. In this paper, I will summarize some of the results obtained in our laboratory on synaptic remodeling in granuloprival conditions.

Three etiologically different agranular cerebella were analyzed. Two of them resulted from spontaneous mutations affecting the cerebellum of the mouse (the *weaver* and the *reeler* mutants [38] and the third was experimentally obtained in the rat by early postnatal X-irradiation. *Weaver* is an autosomal incomplete dominant mutation in which, despite the normal mitotic activity of the germinative cells of the external granular layer, almost the complete population of postmitotic granule cells fails to migrate and dies at the interface of the external granular layer and the molecular layer. The result is an agranular cerebellum, in which parallel fibers are never formed. The inbred B 6/CBA/51-wv/wv mice that we have studied usually survive less than 1 month, and therefore our analysis was obtained from mice aged 20–29 days [40]. *Reeler* is also an autosomal recessive mutation which occurs in a different chromosome from that in *weaver* [22]. Unlike *weaver*, this mutation not only causes extensive perturbations in the development of the cerebellar cortex, but also affects the neocortex and the hippocampal formation and leads to a malposition of different

Experimental Brain Research, Suppl. 6

neuronal classes in these cortical structures. In the cerebellum, Purkinje cells are only rarely located at their normal position; usually they are dispersed throughout the granular layer and the white matter. This situation gives rise to a rather unique organization in which the cerebellum is composed of two distinct regions: a very reduced quasi-normal cerebellar cortex, which encloses a central mass consisting mostly of Purkinje cells, some stellate interneurons and deep cerebellar nuclei. The mutation, which was originally described in inbred C 57 BL/6 J mice, also appeared in the Balb/C strain from the laboratory of the C.N.R.S., Orléans La Source. Balb/C – rl/rl animals are fertile and much more resistant than those originating from other strains of mice. Our study concerned mice ranging in age from 1 month to 1 year [27]. The rat granuloprival cerebella were obtained by X-irradiation of newborn rats, according to the schedule proposed by Altman and Anderson [5], consisting of 1,300 rad distributed in seven successive exposures during the first 14 postnatal days. The morphological study was done on rats aged between 6 and 12 months.

The common alteration in these three types of cerebellum is the massive reduction in granule cells. However, the cellular environment slightly differs from one type to another. Thus in *weaver* only granule cells are affected, but stellate and basket cells survive in apparently normal numbers. In the central cerebellar mass of the *reeler*, granule and basket cells are practically absent, but stellate-like cells are intermingled with the malpositioned Purkinje cells. Finally, in the X-irradiated rat cerebellum and in folia in which the external granular layer was completely destroyed, granule cells as well as stellate and basket cells have disappeared. These slight differences in the cellular milieu are responsible for the diversity of synaptic patterns observed in these cerebella.

Autonomous Development of Postsynaptic Elements

In the normal cerebellum, the axons of the granule cells establish synaptic contacts with all the other cortical neurons (the parallel fiber-omnicellular system), although Purkinje cells are their main postsynaptic targets. Parallel fibers account for almost 95% of the inputs reaching Purkinje cells. The absence of the parallel fibers provides, therefore, an optimal situation in which to study the development of Purkinje cells in extreme conditions of deafferentation. In the *weaver* and in X-irradiated cerebella, Purkinje cells are not aligned in a single row, but dispersed in two to four irregular rows which occupy most of the cortical area. The dendritic trees of these neurons, similar to those in the central cerebellar mass of the *reeler* mouse, are oriented at random instead of being arranged in the sagittal plane. In some cells, the dendrites do not arise from a single stem but from several, up to four or five; these cells appear multipolar. Furthermore, spiny branchlets are practically absent and therefore the total length of the tree is reduced. In spite of all these important changes, Purkinje cells are easily recognizable because they develop their own intrinsic features, mainly the peculiar disposition of the agranular reticulum, including the hypolemmal cisterna [31]. The most striking feature of these neurons is the presence of innumerable spines emerging from all their dendritic segments (Fig. 1)

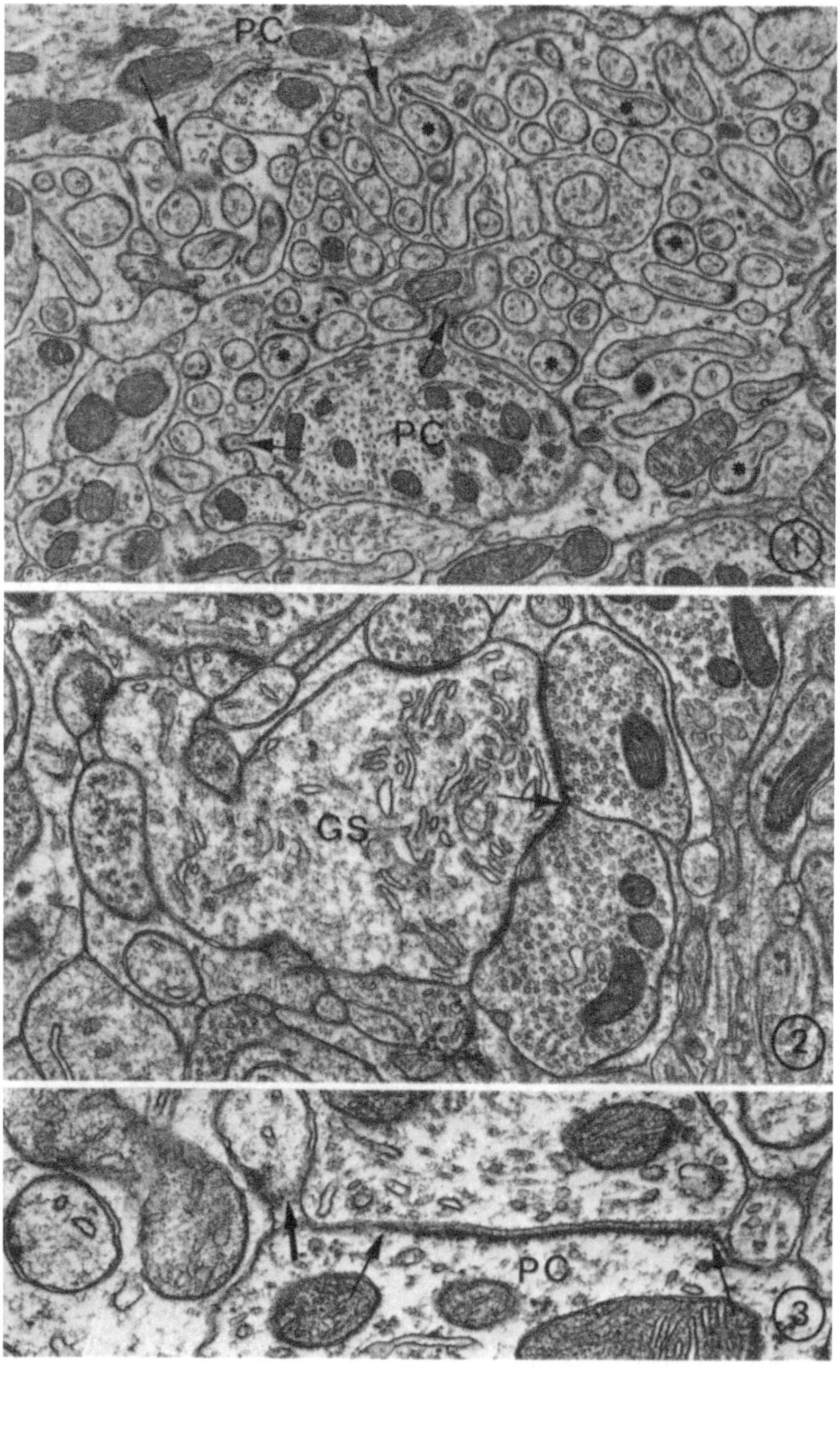
PC
PC
1
GS
2
PC
3

[18, 36, 39]. The large majority of them are similar to the normal branchlet spines, but in the granuloprival cerebella they are devoid of their presynaptic partners. Judging from extended morphological analyses, such as the use of special staining methods to bring out paramembranous differentiations (ethanolic phosphotungstic acid [18] and especially the study of the internal organization of the membranes with the freeze-fracture technique [17, 21], the asynaptic spines have the same morphology as normally innervated spines in control animals.

Asynaptic branchlet spines, together with spines exhibiting a shorter stalk and a more rounded head and occupied by climbing fibers, as in control animals, are not the only kind of postsynaptic differentiation characterizing Purkinje cells in agranular cerebella. Branching and hypertrophic spines are also present. In *weaver* and in *reeler* cerebella some of the hypertrophic spines attain a gigantic size, measuring up to 6 µm in diameter [27]. They contain an electronlucent fine granular matrix, in which numerous cisterns of the smooth endoplasmic reticulum are suspended. Their inner surfaces are undercoated by a long, almost continuous, band of postsynaptic dense material. Their outer surfaces can be free of innervation or occupied by numerous axon terminals, which establish synaptic contacts with them (Fig. 2). In addition, Purkinje cell dendrites bear postsynaptic differentiations, undercoated segments of variable length, on their shafts (Fig. 3). These receptor sites can face glial elements, naked spines, and/or axon terminals. In this last instance, the axon terminals do not develop "active zones" at the level of the postsynaptic differentiation (Fig. 3). All the above-mentioned results point not only to the capacity of Purkinje cells to develop receptor surfaces in an autonomous manner, but also to the possibility exhibited by these neurons for determining the number of acceptable synaptic inputs, by elaborating an almost rigid amount of postsynaptic receptive surface. In fact, there is a reduction in the size of the dendritic tree of Purkinje cells in granuloprival cerebella [12] which will result in a decrease of the total number of dendritic spines. The presence of hypertrophic spines and long postsynaptic differentiations on the dendritic shafts could compensate for this reduction, so that the total amount of receptive membrane, marked by the postsynaptic differentiations, will be the same for all Purkinje cells, independent of their growth in a normal or in an agranular cellular milieu. The recent morphometric work of Hillman and Chen has provided evidence in favor of a constancy in the

Plate I (Figs. 1–3). Electron micrographs of the weaver cerebellar cortex

Fig. 1. Two dendritic profiles of Purkinje cells (*PC*) give off several spines (*arrows*). Numerous "asynaptic" spines, resembling branchlet spines, are engulfed in astrocytic processes. Note the postsynaptic differentiations in these spines (*asterisks*). ×18 000

Fig. 2. Gigantic spine (*GS*) containing abundant canaliculi of the agranular reticulum suspended in a floccular light matrix. A long postsynaptic differentiation is shared by two presynaptic axon terminals (*arrow*). ×23 000

Fig. 3. Postsynaptic differentiation (*thin arrows*) undercoating the shaft of a Purkinje cell dendrite (*PC*). A spine (*thick arrow*) emerges from the dendrite. The postsynaptic differentiation faces an axon terminal belonging to a stellate cell. Note the absence of "active zones" in the terminal. ×46 000

amount of Purkinje cell membrane area undercoated with postsynaptic – like material, in 3 different experimental situations. These results are determinant in considering that the amount of receptive membrane is intrinsically programmed in this category of neurons.

Synaptic Remodeling: Local Circuit Neurons as Presynaptic Elements

The main difference between the *weaver* cerebellum and that obtained in the rat after postnatal X-irradiation is the almost complete absence, in the latter, of stellate and basket cells. This difference results in obvious distinctions between the cerebellar cortical circuitry in the two situations.

In the *weaver* cerebellum, Purkinje cell perikarya are invested by pericellular basket profiles, as well as by smaller boutons containing flattened vesicles which probably represent the endings of the recurrent collaterals from Purkinje cell axons. However, although basket fiber profiles are often in the vicinity of the initial segment of the Purkinje cell axon and occasionally one of them can establish a synaptic contact with it, neither the typical basket formation around the axon hillock nor the pinceau around the initial segment is fully developed [40]. In the X-irradiated cerebellum Purkinje cells are devoid of pericellular baskets. The axon hillock, which normally emerges from one pole of the perikaryon, and the initial segment are almost completely covered by thin astrocytic processes. More aberrant situations have also been observed. Thus, the axon can emerge from a thick dendritic trunk, as illustrated in Fig. 4. In this case, the hillock, identified by the presence of the characteristic fasciculated microtubules, as well as the neighboring dendritic zones, is covered by glia. These Purkinje cells have therefore completely lost their characteristic morphological polarity.

In the hemispheres of the *weaver* cerebellum and in some folia of the X-irradiated rat some granule cells can survive. They give rise to axons, which, although they do not attain the geometrical pattern of normal parallel fibers, can establish synaptic contacts with their appropriate partners, mainly the branchlet spines of Purkinje cells. The varicosities formed by the remaining parallel fibers are larger than in control animals; their diameters can even be twice as large as those in the latter. Each varicosity, instead of contacting, in random sections, one or occasionally two spines, can establish synaptic contacts with two to five spines (Fig. 5). The increase in number of synaptic contacts is an indication of axonal remodeling as defined by Raisman and Field [32] in their concept of multiple synaptic index. These observations further support the

Plate II (Figs. 4, 5). Electron micrographs of the cerebellar cortex of an X-irradiated rat

Fig. 4. A large trunk of a Purkinje cell dendrite (*PC*) is at the origin of the axon hillock (*AH*), identified by the fasciculated microtubules. Note the absence of basket axons around the hillock of the Purkinje cell axon. ×14 000

Fig. 5. Enlarged varicosity of a parallel fiber (*PF*) arising from a granule cell which escaped X-irradiation. The terminal is surrounded by spines of Purkinje cell dendrites. Three of these spines are postsynaptic to the parallel fiber (*arrows*). ×25 000

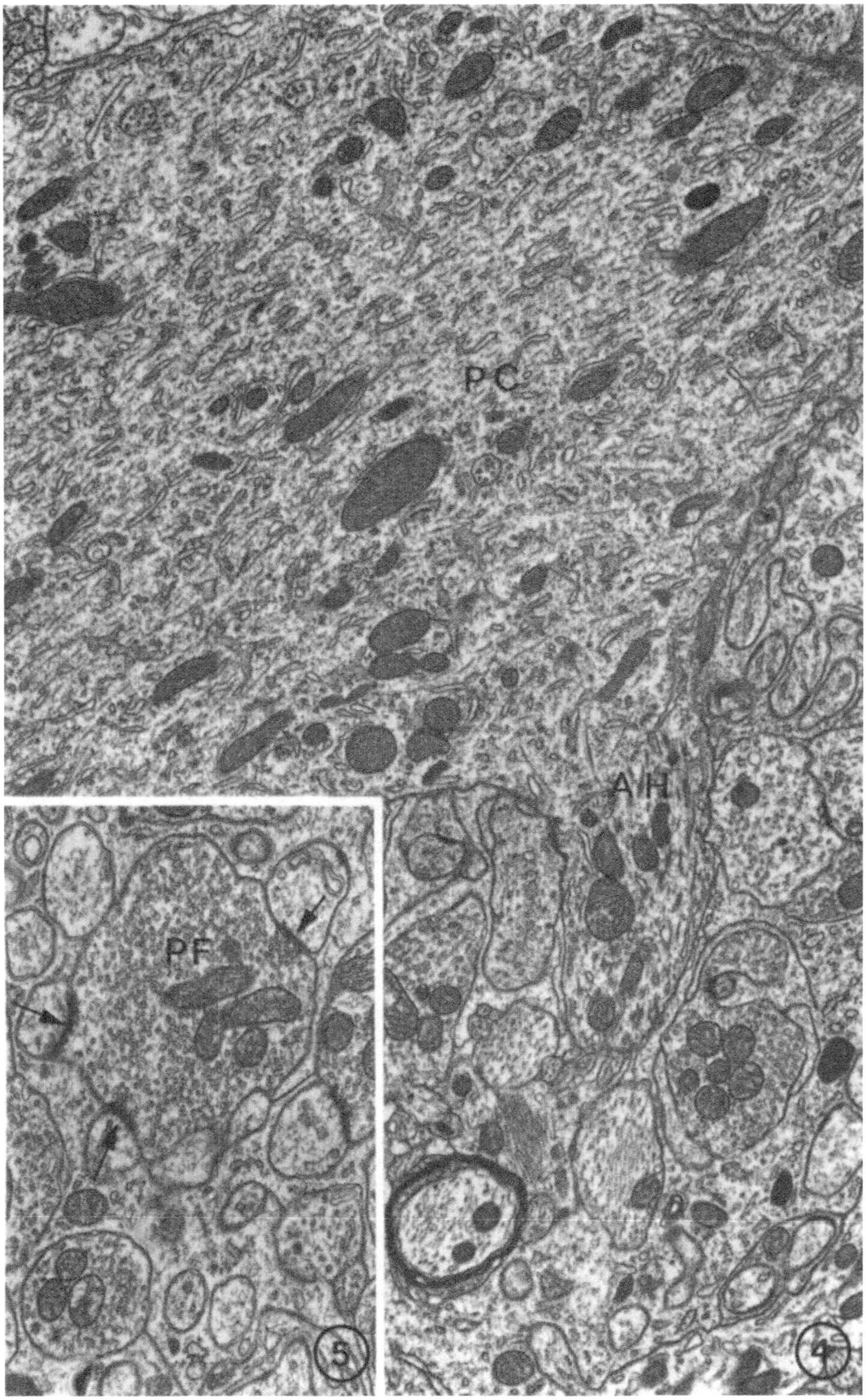
PC
A H
PF
5
4

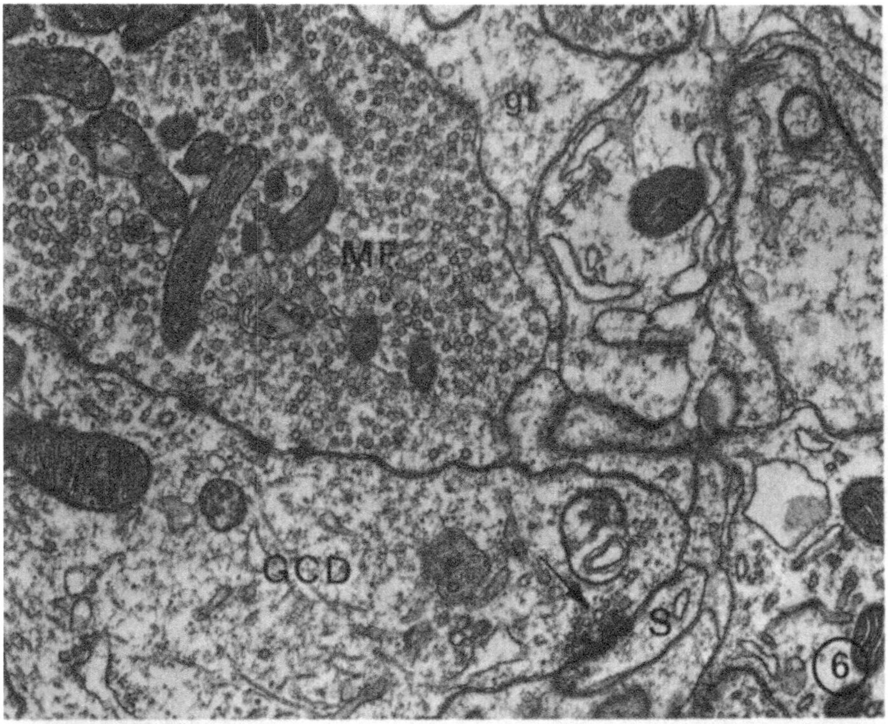
gl
MF
GCD
S
6

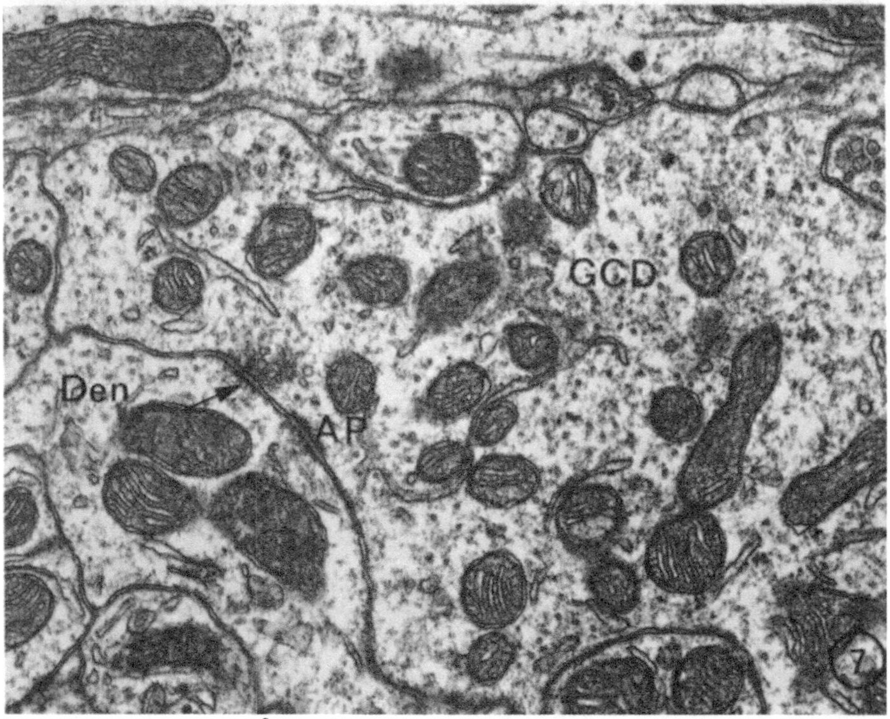
GCD
Den
AP
7

hypothesis that Purkinje cells possess the inherent property to determine the maximum number of synaptic contacts they can receive, since presynaptic afferents, such as parallel fibers, can increase their number of synaptic junctions when postsynaptic space is available.

The main difference between the cortical circuitry of the *weaver* and that of the X-irradiated rat cerebella concerns Golgi cells. In the irradiated cerebellum, as stated above, the only inhibitory interneurons which escape the lethal action of the X-rays are the Golgi cells. Under these conditions, in a relatively important proportion of Golgi dendrites and perikarya, clusters of synaptic vesicle-like profiles are suspended in the cytoplasmic matrix (Figs. 6, 7). These clusters are located at the periphery of the neuronal profile in association with a small region of the plasmalemma, where they form typical presynaptic vesicular grids. The most common postsynaptic partners in these heterologous-ectopic synapses (according to the nomenclature previously defined [41]) are branchlet spines (Fig. 6).

Occasionally, the postsynaptic elements are the actual shafts of Purkinje cell dendrites or other dendritic profiles probably belonging to remaining interneurons (Fig. 7). These observations demonstrate that, in the absence of neurons derived from the external granular layer, Golgi cells can change their functional polarity and transfer synaptic information not only through their axons, as in the normal cerebellum, but also through their perikarya and dendrites. The existence of such unconventional synapses appears to be a fundamental feature of neuronal networks in many other regions of the central nervous system, especially in sensory thalamic nuclei (see, for example, ref. 35). Their presence in some regions and their absence in others raises the question of whether (a) there are two distinct categories of local circuit neurons, or whether (b) all these interneurons have the intrinsic potential of transmitting through axons and dendrites. Our results favor the second interpretation. Golgi cells in the cerebellum seem to possess this potentiality, but it is only expressed if certain specific cellular interactions occur during the establishment of the cerebellar network. Since these heterologous-ectopic synapses have not been observed in the *weaver* cerebellum, it could be concluded that the lack of basket and stellate cells is the major factor determining the expression of the change of polarity by Golgi cells.

In the thin cortical region covering the central cerebellar mass of the *reeler* mouse, malpositioned Purkinje cells are dispersed through the granular layer [27]. The peculiarity in this layer is the presence of vertical septa of neuropil

Plate III (Figs. 6, 7). Electron micrographs of the cerebellar cortex of a X-irradiated rat

Fig. 6. A mossy fiber (*MF*), partially covered by glia (*gl*) is in synaptic contact with a large dendrite of a Golgi cell (*GCD*). An active zone (*arrow*) is present at the periphery of this dendrite. The active zone forms a synaptic contact with a spine (*S*) belonging to a Purkinje cell dendrite. ×28 000

Fig. 7. Large dendritic profile of a Golgi cell (*GCD*) directly apposed to a medium-sized dendrite of a cerebellar interneuron (*Den*). At the interface between the two dendrites an attachment plate (*AP*) and a synaptic complex (*arrow*) are present, the Golgi cell dendrite being presynaptic. ×32 000

distributed among clusters of granule cells. The ascending dendrites of the Purkinje cells occupy the large majority of the volume of the septa, providing a unique cellular milieu, different from those characterizing the *weaver* and the X-irradiated cerebella. In this milieu, Purkinje cell dendrites, contacted by climbing and parallel fibers but still bearing naked spines, ascend across the granular layer directly apposed to neuronal elements belonging to this layer, mostly the cerebellar glomeruli. Golgi axons, located at the periphery of the glomeruli are able, under these conditions, to synapse not only on granule cell dendrites, but also on spines of the ascending Purkinje cell dendrites (Fig. 8). This new type of heterologous synapse [44] provides new evidence of the important role played by the local cellular milieu in regulating the specificity of synapse formation.

Synaptic Remodeling: The Mossy Fiber System

In the three examples of granuloprival cerebellum considered here, the large majority of the postsynaptic targets for mossy fibers, the granule cell digits, do not exist. However, this system of afferents succeeds in forming some peculiar glomerular arrangements, in which the central mossy rosette is surrounded by Golgi cell dendrites (Fig. 6). Furthermore, these rosettes can be in synaptic contact exclusively with the dendritic spines of the Purkinje cells or more often a portion of the rosette membrane synapses on Golgi cell dendrites and the other portion on Purkinje spines [5, 26, 39, 40]. Although these heterologous synapses are undoubtedly present in the three examples of agranular cerebellum, they are more numerous in the irradiated rat and in the *reeler* than in the *weaver*, probably because in the latter the density of mossy rosettes is less than in the other two.

In the *reeler* cerebellum heterologous synapses between mossy rosettes and spines of Purkinje cell dendrites are present in the granular layer (Fig. 8) and in the central cerebellar mass (Fig. 9). In the former the mossy rosettes are generally smaller than in normal glomeruli. Within the plane of the section each of these mossy profiles synapses on three to five granule cell dendrites and one to two Purkinje cell spines (Fig. 8). In the central cerebellar mass large axon terminals resembling mossy rosettes are rare [27]. However, there are numerous smaller terminals sharing the intrinsic cytological features of mossy fibers and emerging from myelinated fibers (Fig. 9). These terminals, identified as be-

Plate IV (Figs. 8, 9). Electron micrographs of the *reeler* cerebellum

Fig. 8. Glomerular arrangement in the granular layer. A central mossy rosette (*MF*) establishes synaptic contacts with granule cell dendrites (*asterisks*) as well as with spines of the Purkinje cell dendrites (*S*). At the periphery of the glomerulus a Golgi cell axon (*GCA*) synapses not only on a granule cell dendrite (*arrowhead*) but also on a Purkinje cell spine (*arrow*). ×36 000

Fig. 9. Central cerebellar mass. A medium-sized axon terminal, containing rounded synaptic vesicles, emerges from a myelinated fiber (*My*). The terminal, identified as a mossy fiber (*MF*), synapses on a hypertrophic spine (*HS*) arising from a Purkinje cell dendrite (*PC, arrow*). ×23 000

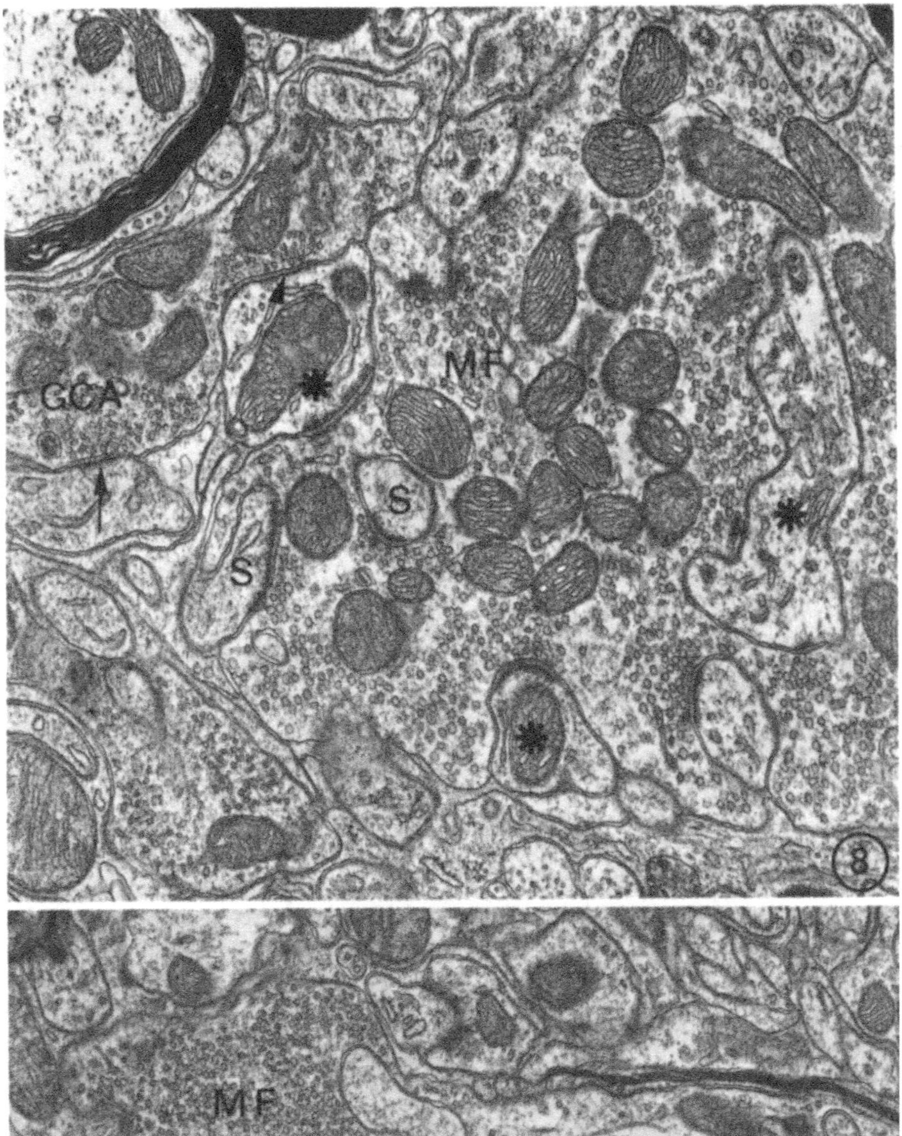
GCA
MF
S
S
8

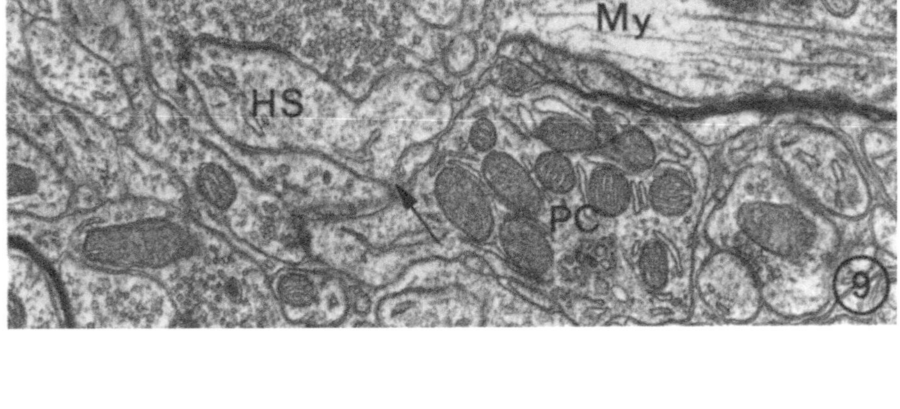
MF
My
HS
PC
9

longing to the mossy afferent system, are often in synaptic contact with spines of the Purkinje cell dendrites (Fig. 9). Therefore, these heterologous synapses are not "rare but unequivocally present," as I have described them before [27], but are a common feature of the *reeler* cerebellum. Collaborative electrophysiological work done by Mariani and Crepel [27] has shown that these synapses are functional.

Synaptic Remodeling: The Serotonin Afferent System

In collaboration with Dr. Alain Beaudet we have analyzed the influence of the granuloprival condition on the synaptic modeling of a cerebellar input of known neurotransmitter content [7, 43]. The serotonin projection [11, 13, 15, 20] appeared as a particularly suitable model, since 5-HT neurons have been shown to possess remarkable adaptative properties [6, 10] and are thought to exert an important regulatory role upon the onset of differentiation of their future target neurons [24, 25].

On account of regional variations in the 5-HT projection to the rat cerebellar cortex [13], we have confined our analysis to the posterior vermis, lobes VII–IX. In normal vermis, according to the cytological features of axonal varicosities labeled by the uptake of tritiated serotonin, two different systems of cerebellar serotonin-containing afferents could be described: (a) a small contingent belongs to typical mossy fibers, sparsely distributed through the granular layer (Fig. 10); (b) the large majority are fine beaded axons, dispersed through all layers (Fig. 11), forming a "diffuse system." Labeled mossy fibers share their cytological characteristics with unlabeled ones: an electron-light axoplasmic matrix containing a mitochondrial core surrounded by numerous clear and round synaptic vesicles and some rare large granular vesicles (LGV) (Fig. 10). Most of these reactive rosettes are directly apposed to granule cell dendrites, on which they establish several Gray's type 1 synapses (Fig. 10). Similar labeled mossy fibers have been previously reported [11, 13]. The "diffuse system" consists of small axonal enlargements (mean diameter: 0.57 μm), filled with minute, round or flattened agranular vesicles, often associated with short tubular organelles (Fig. 11). Most varicosities also contain one to five

Plate V (Figs. 10, 11). Electron microscope radioautographs of the cerebellar cortex of a normal rat after 3 h superfusion with 10^{-4} *M* ^{3}H-5-HT combined with 10^{-3} *M* nonradioactive noradrenaline. Monoamine oxidase inhibited

Fig. 10. Cerebellar glomerulus formed by labeled central mossy rosettes (*MF*) surrounded by granule cell dendrites. The cytological features of the labeled mossy terminals are similar to those exhibited by the majority of the mossy fiber system. The labeled terminals establish Gray's type 1 synapses with the granule cell dendrites (*arrows*). ×28 000

Fig. 11. Labeled varicosity in the molecular layer. This axon terminal exhibits the cytological features characteristic of the "diffuse system" of 5-HT afferents. Numerous elongated vesicles, a large granulated vesicle (*arrow*) and short tubular organelles are suspended in a moderate electron-dense axoplasmic matrix. Note the absence of synaptic differentiation between the labeled terminal and the surrounding neuronal elements. The nearby parallel fiber varicosity (*PF*) synapses on a spine (*S*) of a Purkinje cell dendrite. ×41 000

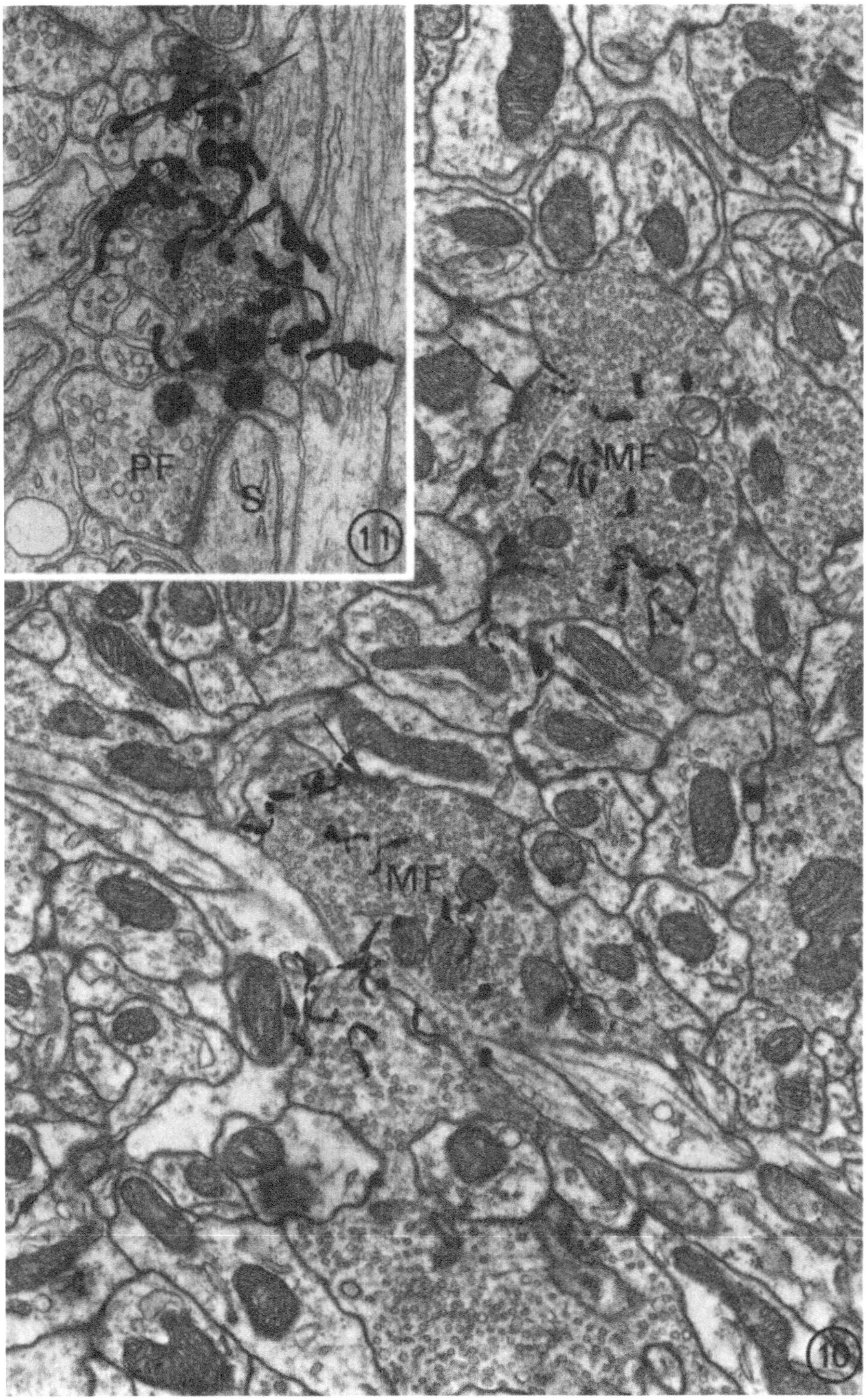
PF
S
11
MF
MF
10

LGVs and exhibit a moderately dense axoplasmic matrix. Axons belonging to this system were also previously reported [13]. In random sections, the labeled axon terminals of the diffuse system are directly apposed to neuronal elements (Fig. 11) or occasionally to glia, but only about 3% of the studied terminals (4 out of 125) establish synaptic contacts, in two cases with Purkinje cell branchlet spines and in the two others with Golgi cell dendrites. Mathematical calculations [7] have made it possible to determine that less than 9% of the axonal varicosities belonging to the "diffuse system" are actually engaged in junctional synaptic relationships. The existence in normal cerebellum of these two different systems of axon terminals, both possessing a high affinity uptake mechanism for 5-HT, raises the question of whether both systems are actually serotonergic; that is to say, whether the two categories of varicosities originate from the same or from different 5-HT neurons of the raphe nuclei, and whether both of them are able to synthetize and release serotonin. This question becomes crucial when it is known that serotonin microiontophoretically applied to the Purkinje cell produces inhibition [19] and that high affinity uptake is not "per se" a reliable criterion to define the neurotransmitter. Thus, supra- and subependymal nerve fibers in the rat, which are serotonergic [14], are also able to selectively accumulate exogenous GABA [8]. Furthermore, if there is endogenous 5-HT in some mossy rosettes, it is not sufficient to permit them to be visualized by means of the classic histofluorescence histochemistry.

Indolamine-accumulating mossy fibers were reported by Hökfelt and Fuxe [20], but only after incubation of cerebellar slices with 6-hydroxytryptamine. More direct evidence for the existence of endogenous 5-HT is needed before accepting the serotonergic nature of these mossy fibers. The 5-HT innervation of the agranular cerebellar cortex exhibits two major differences from that of the normal cerebellum: (a) a complete disappearance of the mossy fiber contingent and (b) a tremendous increase in the overall density of the "diffuse system". However, the absolute number of 5-HT varicosities is not significantly different from that of the controls due to the large reduction in the volume of the granuloprival cerebellum. Most of the labeled varicosities share their cytological features with those of the "diffuse system" in normal cerebellum. They have almost the same average diameter (0.63 μm) and contain a similar array of tiny, round or flattened agranular vesicles and short canaliculi associated with a variable number of LGVs (Figs. 12, 13). Although a large proportion of these ter-

Plate VI (Figs. 12, 13). Electron microscope radioautographs of the agranular cerebellar cortex of an X-irradiated rat treated as the one illustrated in Figs. 10 and 11

Fig. 12. A small labeled axonal varicosity contains in addition to the organelles characterizing the "diffuse system" of 5-HT afferents, some small granulated vesicles (*arrow*). The labeled profile does not establish synaptic contact. Note the large number of "asynaptic" Purkinje cell spines (*S*) in this agranular cerebellar cortex. ×35 000

Fig. 13. Labeled axonal varicosity exhibiting the cytological features of the "diffuse system" of 5-HT afferents. This axon is directly apposed to two spines (*S*) belonging to a Purkinje cell dendrite. A synaptic complex (*arrow*) is present between the labeled terminal and one of the spines. ×35 000

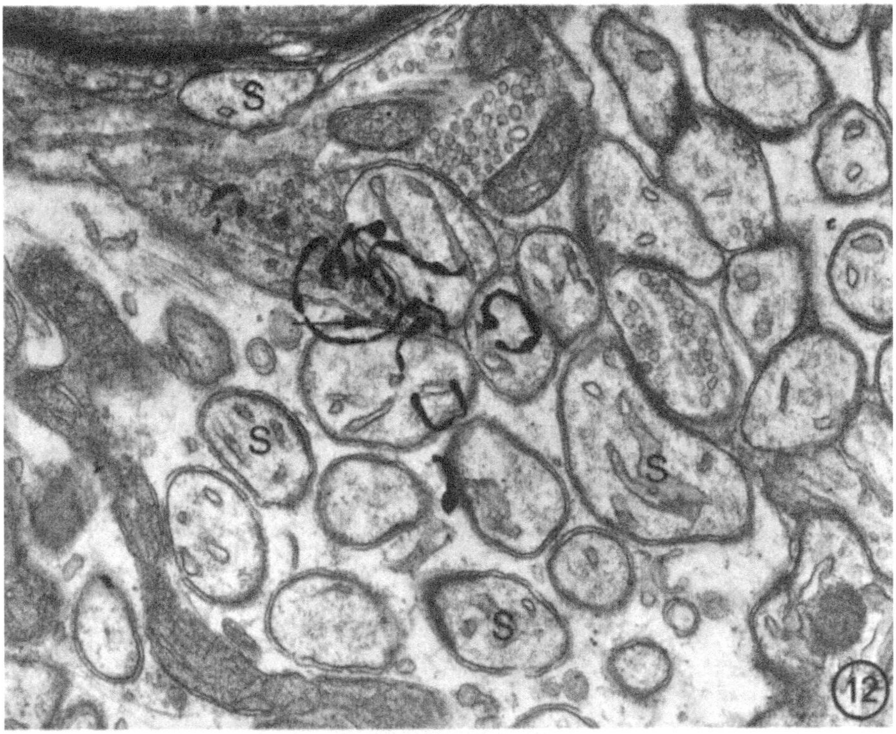
S
S
S
S
12

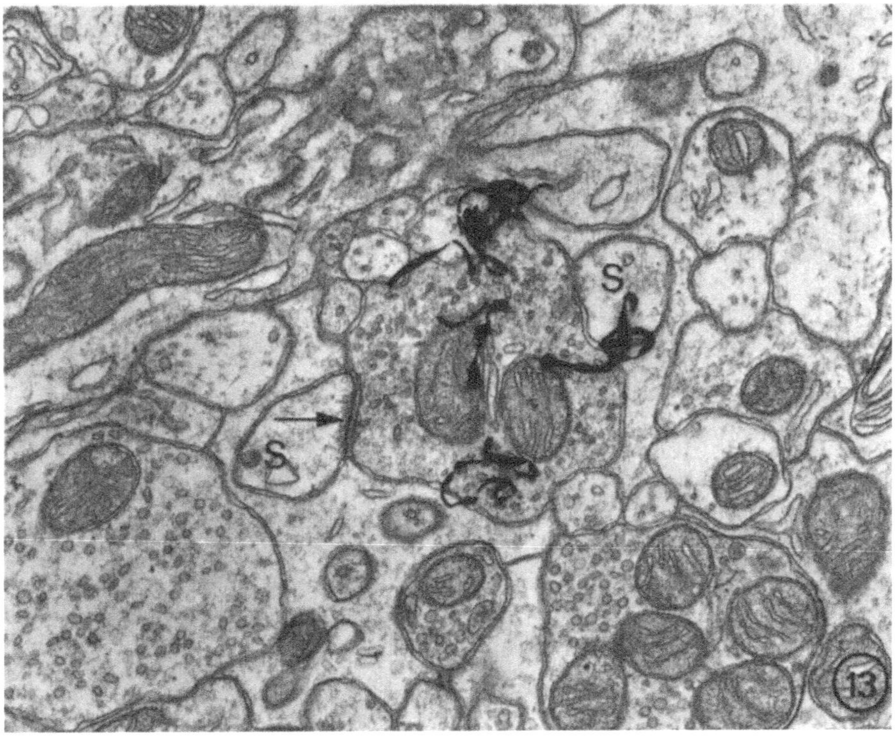
S
S
13

minal profiles do not establish synaptic contacts with nearby neuronal elements (Fig. 12), the major qualitative difference in the innervation pattern is that in the agranular condition 35% of them, instead of 3%, are in synaptic contact. The vast majority of these contacts are Gray's type I synapses on the branchlet spines of Purkinje cell dendrites (Fig. 13), and only occasionally do they synapse on the perikarya and/or the dendrites of the inhibitory interneurons which have survived the X-irradiation.

That 35% of the labeled profiles in random sections bear a junctional synaptic complex indicates that all of the 5-HT varicosities detected are actually engaged in synaptic relationships *sensu stricto* [7]. Thus, in the absence of granule cells, the 5-HT innervation of rat cerebellar cortex evolves from a mostly "non-junctional" into a completely "junctional" input. This result indicates that the territory of innervation can exert a determinant influence on the synaptic modeling of incoming 5-HT afferents.

General Conclusions

In the three examples of cerebellar cortices reviewed here, most of the aberrant connectivity patterns are common to all of them. In view of the different etiological factors involved, these common defects can only be attributed to the common abnormality in the cellular environment, namely the absence of granule cells. Therefore, the results summarized above disclose the role played by interactions between granule cells and the other cerebellar components in the formation of the cerebellar circuitry. This "sociocytological" analysis has once more emphasized that genetic factors are particularly important in synapse formation. For Purkinje cells, the random growth of their dendrites and the formation of postsynaptic receptor sites depend on inherent properties of these neurons. Furthermore, the number of presynaptic inputs allowed to impinge on Purkinje cells during normal development seems also to be regulated by their intrinsic program. However, epigenetic factors, through local functional interactions between the growing neurons, can partially modulate the genetic program to achieve the selectivity of connections. In fact, the existence of several kinds of heterologous synapses, each one related to a specific cellular environment, indicates that the intrinsic specificity for afferent-efferent coupling during the formation of the cerebellar circuitry can be overridden, to a certain extent, by the local cellular milieu.

References

1. Altman J (1969) Autoradiographic and histological studies of postnatal neurogenesis. III. Dating the time of production and onset of differentiation of cerebellar microneurons in rats. J Comp Neurol 136:269–294
2. Altman J (1972) Postnatal development of the cerebellar cortex in the rat. I. The external germinal layer and the transitional molecular layer. J Comp Neurol 145:353–398
3. Altman J (1972) Postnatal development of the cerebellar cortex in the rat. III. Maturation of the components of the granular layer. J Comp Neurol 145:465–514

4. Altman J (1976) Experimental reorganization of the cerebellar cortex. VII. Effects of late X-irradiation schedules that interfere with cell acquisition after stellate cells are formed. J Comp Neurol 164:65–76
5. Altman J, Anderson WJ (1972) Experimental reorganization of the cerebellar cortex. I. Morphological effects of elimination of all microneurons with prolonged X-irradiation started at birth. J Comp Neurol 146:355–406
6. Azmitia EC, Buchan AM, Williams JH (1978) Structural and functional restoration by collateral sprouting of hippocampal 5-HT axons. Nature 284:374–376
7. Beaudet A, Sotelo C (1981) Synaptic remodeling of serotonin axon terminals in rat agranular cerebellum. Brain Res 206:305–329
8. Belin MF, Gamrani H, Aguera M, Calas A, Pujol JF (1980) Selective uptake of ^{3}H γ-aminobutyrate by rat supra- and subependymal nerve fibers, histological and high resolution radioautographic studies. Neuroscience 5:241–254
9. Berry M, Bradley P (1976) The growth of the dendritic trees of Purkinje cells in the cerebellum of the rat. Brain Res 112:1–35
10. Björklund A, Katsman R, Stenevi U, West KA (1971) Development and growth of axonal sprouts for noradrenaline and 5-hydroxy-tryptamine neurons in the rat spinal cord. Brain Res 31:21–33
11. Bloom FE, Hoffer BJ, Siggins GR, Barker JL, Nicoll RA (1972) Effects of serotonin on central neurons: microiontophoretic administration. Fed Proc 31:97–106
12. Bradley P, Berry M (1976) The effects of reduced climbing and parallel fiber input on Purkinje cell dendritic growth. Brain Res 109:133–151
13. Chan-Palay V (1975) Fine structure of labeled axons in the cerebellar cortex and nuclei of rodents and primates after intraventricular infusions with tritiated serotonin. Anat Embryol (Berl) 148:235–265
14. Chan-Palay V (1976) Serotonin axons in the supra- and subependymal plexuses and in the leptomeninges; their roles in local alterations of cerebrospinal fluid and vasomotor activity. Brain Res 102:103–130
15. Chan-Palay V (1977) Cerebellar dentate nucleus. Springer, Berlin Heidelberg New York, pp 390–433
16. Fujita S (1967) Quantitative analysis of cell proliferation and differentiation in the cortex of the postnatal mouse cerebellum. J Cell Biol 32:277–288
17. Hanna RB, Hirano A, Pappas GD (1976) Membrane specializations of dendritic spines and glia in the *weaver* mouse cerebellum: a freeze-fracture study. J Cell Biol 68:403–410
18. Hirano A, Dembitzer HM (1973) Cerebellar alterations in the *weaver* mouse. J Cell Biol 56:478–486
19. Hoffer BJ, Siggins GR, Bloom FE (1968) Responsiveness of rat cerebellar Purkinje cells to microelectrophoresis of possible transmitter substances. Fed Proc 29:443
20. Hökfelt T, Fuxe K (1969) Cerebellar monoamine nerve terminals, a new type of afferent fibers to the cortex cerebelli. Exp Brain Res 9:63–72
21. Landis DMD, Reese TS (1977) Structure of the Purkinje cell membrane in *staggerer* and *weaver* mutant mice. J Comp Neurol 171:247–260
22. Lane PW, Sweet HO (1974) Linkage data. Mouse Lett 50:44
23. Larramendi LMH (1969) Analysis of synaptogenesis in the cerebellum of the mouse. In: Llinás R (ed) Neurobiology of cerebellar evolution and development. Amer Med Ass, Chicago, pp 803–843
24. Lauder JM, Bloom FE (1974) Ontogeny of monoamine neurons in the locus coeruleus, raphe nuclei, and substantia nigra of the rat. I. Cell differentiation. J Comp Neurol 155:469–481
25. Lauder JM, Krebs H (1976) Effects of p-chlorophenylalanine on time of neuronal origin during embryogenesis in the rat. Brain Res 198:638–644
26. Llinás R, Hillman DE, Precht W (1973) Neuronal circuit organization in mammalian agranular cerebellar cortex. J Neurobiol 4:69–94
27. Mariani J, Crepel F, Mikoshiba K, Changeux JP, Sotelo C (1977) Anatomical, physiological and biochemical studies of the cerebellum from *reeler* mutant mouse. Philos Trans R Soc Lond [Biol] 271:1–28
28. Miale IL, Sidman RL (1961) An autoradiographic analysis of histogenesis in the mouse cerebellum. Exp Neurol 4:277–296

29. Mugnaini E (1969) Ultrastructural studies on the cerebellar histogenesis. II. Maturation of nerve cell populations and establishment of synaptic connections in the cerebellar cortex of the chick. JAMA 749–782
30. Mugnaini E, Forstrønen PF (1967) Ultrastructural studies on the cerebellar histogenesis. I. Differentiation of granule cells and development of glomeruli in the chick embryo. Z Zellforsch Mikrosk Anat 77:115–143
31. Palay SL, Chan-Palay V (1974) Cerebellar cortex. Cytology and organization. Springer, Berlin Heidelberg New York, pp 28–29
32. Raisman G, Field PM (1973) A quantitative investigation of the development of collateral reinnervation after partial deafferentation of the septal nuclei. Brain Res 50:241–264
33. Rakic P (1971) Neuron-glia relationship during granule cell migration in developing cerebellar cortex. A Golgi and electron-microscopic study in *Macacus rhesus*. J Comp Neurol 141:283–312
34. Rakic P (1972) Extrinsic cytological determinants of basket and stellate cell dendritic pattern in the cerebellar molecular layer. J Comp Neurol 146:335–354
35. Rakic P (1975) Local circuit neurons. Neurosci Res Program Bull 13:291–446
36. Rakic P, Sidman RL (1973) Organization of cerebellar cortex secondary to deficit of granule cells in *weaver* mutant mice. J Comp Neurol 152:133–162
37. Ramón y Cajal S (1911) Histologie du Système Nerveux de l'Homme et des Vertébrés. Maloine, Paris. Translated by L Azoulay, Vol. II
38. Sidman RL, Green MC, Appel SH (1965) Catalog of the neurological mutants of the mouse. Harvard University Press, Cambridge, Mass
39. Sotelo C (1973) Permanence and fate of paramembranous synaptic specializations in mutants and experimental animals. Brain Res 62:345–351
40. Sotelo C (1975) Anatomical, physiological, and biochemical studies of the cerebellum from mutant mice. II. Morphological study of cerebellar cortical neurons and circuits in the *weaver* mouse. Brain Res 94:19–44
41. Sotelo C (1977) Formation of presynaptic dendrites in the rat cerebellum following neonatal X-irradiation. Neuroscience 2:275–283
42. Sotelo C (1978) Purkinje cell ontogeny: Formation and maintenance of spines. Prog Brain Res 48:149–170
43. Sotelo C, Beaudet A (1979) Influence of experimentally induced agranularity on the synaptogenesis of serotonin nerve terminals in rat cerebellar cortex. Proc R Soc Lond [Biol] 206:133–138
44. Wilson L, Sotelo C, Caviness VS (1981) Heterologous synapses upon Purkinje cells in the cerebellum of the *reeler* mutant mouse: An experimental light and electron microscopic study. Brain Res 213:63–82
45. Hillman DE, Chen S (1980) Plasticity of synaptic size with constancy of total synaptic contact area on Purkinje cells in the cerebellum. XIth International Congress of Anatomy, Abstract book, pp 308–309, Mexico

Discussion

Dr. Altman pointed out that in view of the fact that the Purkinje cells in the cerebellum of the mutant animals remained near the neuroepithelium and failed to migrate toward the pial surface, one must conclude that there is some interference in the very early step of cell migration and that there is some abnormality in the Purkinje cells to start with.

Dr. Krnjevic raised the possibility that the varicosities described by Dr. Sotelo may be some other types of synapse which do not normally take up serotonin but do so in the agranular cerebellum. Indicating that this was unlikely,

Dr. Sotelo emphasized that the intrinsic cytological features of these serotonin-labelled varicosities, e.g., the microtubular structures, small pleomorphic vesicles, electron-dense cytoplasm, etc., are exactly the same as in the normal cerebellum.

Dr. Korn asked if there was any evidence to indicate that these heterologous synapses are functional. Dr. Sotelo made several comments in answering this question. First, he cited the work of Llinás et al. [1] on the virus-infected ferret where it was found that mossy fibers can monosynaptically activate Purkinje cells. He also indicated that his own collaborative work [2] on the *reeler* cerebellum gave the same results. He then pointed out that no functional study has been done on the effects of stimulating serotonin axons. Most of the serotonin axons in the agranular cerebellum synapse on the branchlet spines, which in the normal cerebellum are contacted by parallel fibers. The parallel fibers, it should be noted, are believed to use glutamate as the neurotransmitter. Thus, the serotonin fibers appear to synapse on receptor sites prepared to receive glutamate-releasing axons. Dr. Sotelo concluded that a matching between the neurotransmitter and receptor is needed under these circumstances in order to have functional synaptic transmission between serotoninergic fibers and Purkinje cell spines.

Dr. Oster-Granite pointed out that in the *reeler* mutant, ectopic neurons do not necessarily represent the only locus of action of the mutant gene. In *reeler-normal* chimeras, Mullen [3] found mutant as well as normal cells in both the ectopic loci and in the regions of the cerebellar cortex showing a more normal organization. It would therefore appear that the *reeler* mutation does not act intrinsically in large migratory cell populations. Rather, it may act extrinsically; cells located in an abnormal ("mutant") environment fail to migrate normally and form ectopic nests of cells. In the absence of a cell marker which can distinguish the nature of the cellular environment in such chimeras, it would be difficult to state unequivocally that the locus of action of the *reeler* mutant is only within the large migratory cell populations.

There was a lengthy discussion on the differences in the observations of Dr. Sotelo and of Dr. Chan-Palay. These differences included: (a) serotoninergic fiber synapses on Purkinje cells seen in Dr. Sotelo's work but not in Dr. Chan-Palay's work, (b) synapses with interneurons in the molecular layer, however, were seen by Dr. Chan-Palay but not by Dr. Sotelo, and (c) higher density in the granular layer than in the molecular layer observed by Dr. Sotelo, the reverse being seen in Dr. Chan-Palay's studies. After much discussion, it became apparent that these discrepancies were due to the regional differences in the organization of the cerebellum, rather than due to any differences in the sampling procedure. All of Dr. Sotelo's observations involved lobes 7, 8, and 9 in the medial part of the posterior vermis, whereas Dr. Chan-Palay focussed her attention on the lateral lobes of the cerebellum, i.e., the hemispheres. The possibility of the varicosities being of different kinds including synaptic, nonsynaptic, and transitional forms was raised by Dr. Chan-Palay. But both Dr. Sotelo and Dr. Chan-Palay agreed on the interpretation that the absence or paucity of the granule cells imposed a modulating influence, in that the serotonin fiber system partially compensated for the lack of parallel fiber synapses on Purkinje cell dendrites. Dr. Sotelo summed up saying that in the normal cerebellum there seems to be a diffuse system, mainly asynaptic and releasing the transmitter far from the receptors, whereas in the agranular cerebellum this situation is changed dramatically with morphologically conventional synapses (with postsynaptic elements). He could not speculate on the physiological significance of these observations.

In response to a question from Dr. Balázs, Dr. Sotelo expressed his view that the mossy fiber system selectively picks up serotonin, but does not appear to contain endogenous serotonin.

Dr. Chan-Palay revealed, however, that she does have immunohistochemical evidence showing that the mossy fiber system does produce serotonin. Dr. Balázs, on the other hand, indicated that his work with glomerular fractions does not corroborate Dr. Chan-Palay's evidence.

References

1. Llinás R, Hillman DE, Precht W (1973) Neuronal circuit reorganization in mammalian agranular cerebellar cortex. J Neurobiol 4:69–94
2. Mariani J, Crepel F, Mikoshiba K, Changeux J-P, Sotelo C (1977) Anatomical, physiological and biochemical studies of the cerebellum from *reeler* mutant mouse. Philos Trans R Soc Lond [Biol] 281:1–28
3. Mullen RJ (1977) Site of pcd gene action and Purkinje cell mosaicism in cerebella of chimeric mice. Nature 272:245–247

Morphophysiological Studies of a Culture Model of the Cerebellum

K. C. Marshall and W. J. Hendelman

Introduction

We have recently been studying the morphological and electrophysiological characteristics of an experimental model of the cerebellum, i.e., cultured explants of cerebellar tissue. An interesting property of such cultures is the absence of extracerebellar nuclei which normally provide sources of afferents and targets for efferent fibers of the cerebellum. The explants are taken from newborn mice and develop and mature in Maximow chambers in about 3 weeks (e.g., [3, 9]). This technique permits maximal retention of organizational features of the tissue, and the resulting cultures have been called "organotypic." During the culture period there is thinning of the explants and some can be selected in which there is a clear separation of the cortical and deep nuclear regions; this occurs particularly with explants taken from the parapeduncular zone (Fig. 1).

An important property of the explants for physiological studies is that the somata of individual neurons can be distinguished in the living state. The large neurons of the cortical region are round, about 18–20 μm in diameter, and are often arranged in clusters or in extended arrays (Fig. 2A). In experiments using intracellular injections of horseradish peroxidase (HRP), we have found that almost all such cells have morphological characteristics appropriate for Purkinje neurons. Cells in the deep nuclear (DN) region are somewhat larger (20–25 μm) and are embedded in a reticular meshwork of myelinated fibers (Fig. 2B). Axons of these neurons stained with HRP have characteristics that are clearly different from those of the cortical neurons [5]. Coursing between the two regions can be seen heavy bands of myelinated fibers, most of which are thought to be axons of Purkinje neurons.

Electrophysiological studies and intracellular injections of HRP are carried out with the explant in a chamber mounted on the stage of an inverted microscope. By means of discrete electrical stimuli (maximally 15 μA), neurons within 50–100 μm radius of the stimulating electrode can be activated, while extra- or intracellular recordings can be made from cells in relatively distant parts of the culture (over 400 μm).

* This work was supported by the Medical Research Council of Canada

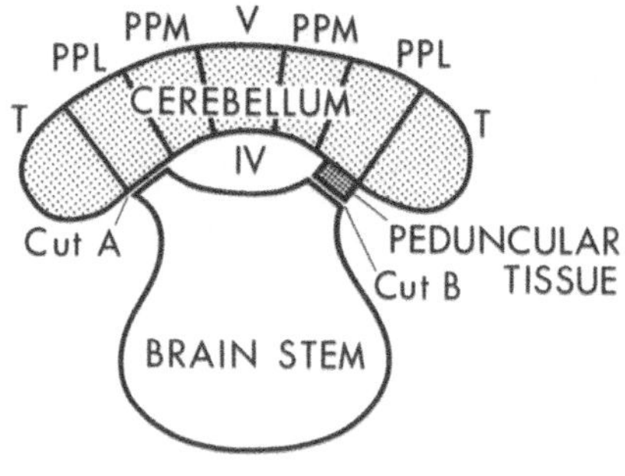

Fig. 1. Schematic diagram of the cerebellum and brain stem of the newborn mouse, in the transverse plane. The cerebellum is detached from the brain stem as indicated (*cut A*) and divided into seven pieces; *V*, vermis; *PPM*, *PPL*, parapeduncular, medial and lateral; *T*, tip. An area of the brain stem can be dissected (*cut B*) and this peduncular tissue is then explanted either attached to the cerebellum or alone. *IV*, fourth ventricle

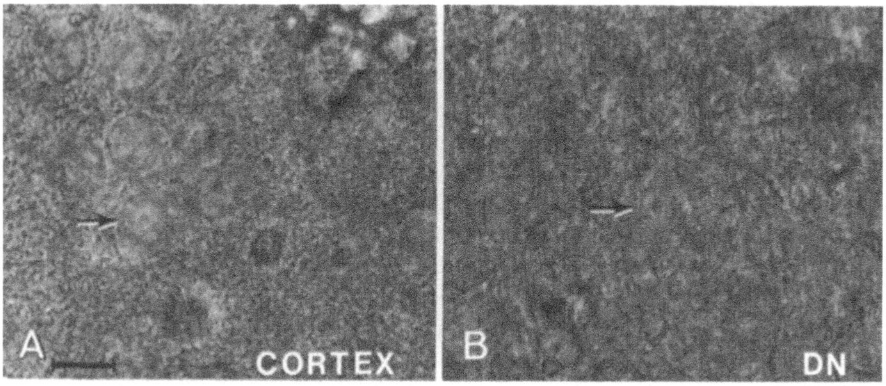

Fig. 2A,B. Cells in the living cultures. **A** Cortical region. The Purkinje neurons generally have a rounded soma (*arrow*) and are dispersed throughout the cortical region. **B** Deep nuclear region. The DN neurons (*arrow*) are situated within a meshwork of myelinated fibers and are usually more difficult to visualize. Calibration bar = 20 μm

The Pathway from Cortex to Deep Nucleus

Stimulation within the cortical region consistently evokes an inhibition in neurons of the DN area. With intracellular recording it can be seen that the inhibition is caused by inhibitory postsynaptic potentials having the characteristics of monosynaptic transmission, i.e., constant latency and high frequency following (Fig. 3). Convergence of inhibitory activity from several cells is indicated by the demonstration of graded inhibitory strength with graded stimulation intensity and by inhibition of the same DN neuron following microstimulation of widely separated cortical areas [7]. A morphological corroboration of this projection has been demonstrated by HRP injections of single cortical neurons. The axons of most of these cells project in a rather direct course toward the DN region and then branch repeatedly, giving numrous bouton-like swellings in that area [5]. The inhibition of DN cells is usually blocked selectively by bicuculline or picrotoxin in low concentrations in the perfusing solution, thus indicating its mediation by γ-aminobutyric acid [8].

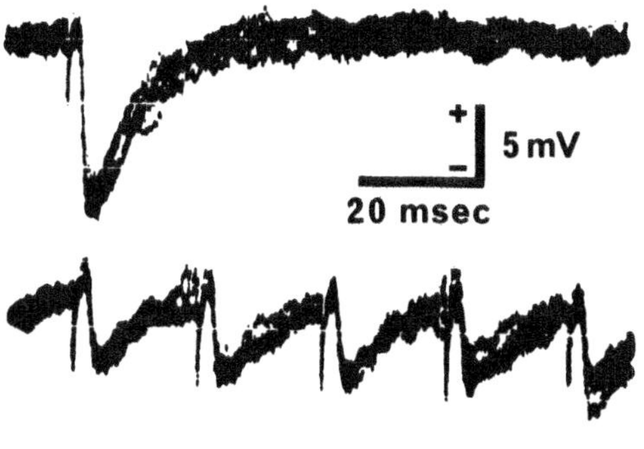

Fig. 3. Inhibitory PSP evoked in DN neuron following stimulation of the cortical region (superimposed oscilloscope traces). The upper record shows constant latency of the evoked potential at 5/s stimulation rate. The lower record shows the same at 50/s stimulation. Marshall et al. [7]

Thus both the "pathway" from Purkinje neurons to DN cells and the appropriate neurotransmitter system appear to develop in this culture model.

The Pathway from Deep Nucleus to Cortex

For the physiological study of projections from the DN neurons, the cultures offer a clear advantage over animal studies. In vivo, the deep nuclei are closely apposed to numerous afferent fibers from extracerebellar sources, so that electrical stimulation is likely to activate climbing fibers and mossy fibers as well as the DN neurons. In explants which do not include the peduncular region, there is no extracerebellar tissue, and stimulation of the DN region should give responses in the cortex that are mediated only by processes that interconnect the two regions.

Either excitatory or inhibitory effects or both can be observed in cortical neurons following stimulation of the DN region. In Fig. 4, intracellularly recorded responses from two different cortical neurons are shown. At stimulus intensity just above threshold, a hyperpolarizing response was evoked in one cell (Fig. 4A), but a depolarization was evoked in the other (Fig. 4B). Stronger stimuli evoked phasic depolarizations in both cells, with prominent hyperpolarizations commencing 1–2 ms later. Such biphasic depolarizing/hyperpolarizing responses were observed in two-thirds of the 30 cortical neurons recorded intracellularly. About half of the depolarizing potentials were consistently evoked, even at stimulus frequencies of 30–40/s (Fig. 4), though the others were not. It can be seen that the hyperpolarizing components did not follow the high frequency stimulation. In the cortical neurons not showing these biphasic responses, simple hyperpolarizations were usually evoked by DN stimulation. About one-half of these also followed stimulation at 40/s.

Horseradish peroxidase injections into DN cells have demonstrated that the axons of these neurons divide into several branches and project, often by a long circuitous route, to the cortical region. Some terminal enlargements are seen in the cortical area, but they are much less numerous than are those of axons of cortical cells terminating in the DN region. Morphological studies of the nucleocortical projection in animals indicate that the DN axons terminate as mossy fibers in the granular layer of the cortex (this volume, Chap. 13).

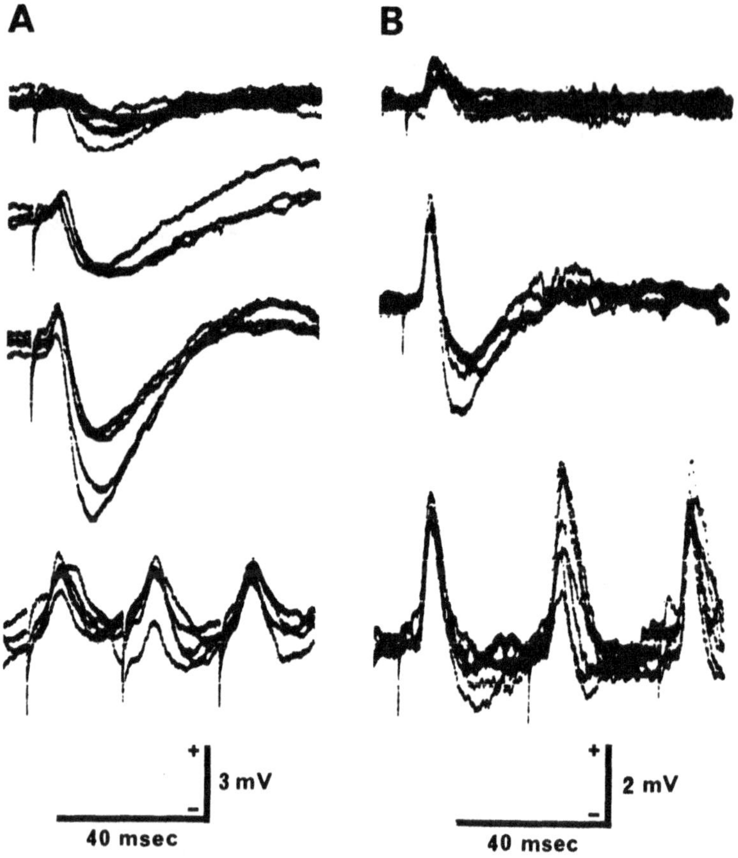

Fig. 4A,B. Synaptic potentials recorded from cortical neurons following stimulation of the DN region; intracellular recording, superimposed traces. **A** Near threshold stimulation (8 μA) evokes an inhibitory PSP (IPSP) in the upper record, while stronger stimuli give EPSP/IPSP complexes of increasing amplitude (second trace, 10 μA; third trace, 15 μA). The EPSP is evoked with constant latency at 40/s repetition rate. **B** Another cortical neuron in which an EPSP is evoked at perithreshold stimulus intensity (4 μA). With stronger stimulation (7 μA), an EPSP/IPSP complex is evoked (middle record). The EPSP was evoked with constant latency at 30/s (lower record) and 50/s (not illustrated) repetition rates. Marshall et al. [7]

The biphasic depolarizing/hyperpolarizing potentials elicited by DN stimulation are similar to those evoked in Purkinje cells by the mossy fiber-granule cell path in vivo. Since about one-half of the excitatory postsynaptic potentials (EPSPs) did not follow high-frequency stimulation, they are probably not monosynaptically mediated and could be generated by granule cells which are activated by DN axons. The EPSPs that *do* follow stimulation at 40/s might result from direct termination of DN axons on the cortical cells. Mossy fibers have been shown to terminate directly on Purkinje cells in animal models of agranular cerebellum (e.g., [6]). However, mossy fiber-granule cell activation of Purkinje cells is also capable of following high-frequency stimulation [2], so that it is not possible to determine whether the responses are mono- or disynaptic from our physiological evidence.

Electron microscopic studies of the cortical region of cerebellar explants [1] have revealed large terminals which contact multiple spines of Purkinje cells. These are thought to be hypertrophic terminals of granule cell axons. Mossy-fiber-like terminals were also observed, and on rare occasions they terminated directly on spines of Purkinje neurons. Thus the results of the electron microscopic studies favor the interpretation that most but not all of the excitation of cortical neurons after stimulation of the DN region is mediated by a mossy fiber to granule cell to Purkinje cell path. Though the number of granule cells is reduced in the explants, the hypertrophic terminals might compensate for this by increasing the synaptic strength of each terminal.

The inhibitory PSPs in cortical neurons are probably mediated by axons of DN cells via cortical interneurons in those cases in which they did not follow high-frequency stimulation. For those which did follow, a more likely route for the inhibitory potentials is via recurrent collaterals of antidromically activated Purkinje axons. Such recurrent collaterals in explant cultures have been observed to terminate on Purkinje neurons [1, 4]. The possibility that some of these "secure" inhibitions may be disynaptic via strongly activated inhibitory cortical interneurons cannot, however, be discounted.

It is our impression, therefore, that considerable synaptic specificity has been retained in these explant cultures, and that that there is a rich degree of synaptic connectivity between the neurons. Our continuing studies include the use of explants from the peduncular region (PPL in Fig. 1). Catecholamine fluorescence has been demonstrated in fibers of such cultures, and it is likely that they originate from cells of locus coeruleus that are included in the explant. In this way a possible locus coeruleus-to-cerebellar cortex pathway has been added to our model, and it should provide an interesting substrate for further combined anatomical and electrophysiological studies.

References

1. Aggerwal AS, Hendelman WJ (1980) The Purkinje neuron II: Electron microscopic analysis of the mature Purkinje neuron in organotypic culture. J Comp Neurol 193:1081–1096
2. Allen GI, Azzena GB, Ohno T (1974) Cerebellar Purkinje cell responses to inputs from sensorimotor cortex. Exp Brain Res 20:239–254
3. Allerand CD (1971) Pattern of neuronal differentiation in developing cultures of neonatal mouse cerebellum: A living and silver impregnation study. J Comp Neurol 142:167–204
4. Calvet M-C, Calvet J (1979) Horseradish peroxidase iontophoretic intracellular labelling of cultured Purkinje cells. Brain Res 173:527–531
5. Hendelman WJ, Marshall KC (1980) Axonal projection patterns visualized with horseradish peroxidase in organized cultures of cerebellum. Neuroscience 5:1833–1846
6. Llinás R, Hillman DE, Precht W (1973) Neuronal circuit reorganization in mammalian agranular cerebellar cortex. J Neurobiol 4:69–94
7. Marshall KC, Wojtowicz JM, Hendelman WJ (1980) Patterns of functional synaptic connections in organized cultures of cerebellum. Neuroscience 5:1847–1857
8. Wojtowicz JM, Marshall KC, Hendelman WJ (1978) Electrophysiological and pharmacological studies of the inhibitory projection from the cerebellar cortex to the deep cerebellar nuclei in tissue culture. Neuroscience 3:607–618
9. Wolf MK (1964) Differentiation of neuronal types and synapses in myelinating cultures of mouse cerebellum. J Cell Biol 22:259–279

Discussion

Llinás: Given the suggestion by Dr. Ito [1] that in order for Purkinje cells to release transmitter (i.e., to be inhibitory) these cells must receive a climbing fiber input. I noticed that you have no climbing fiber input in your culture, and yet you showed clear inhibition by Purkinje cells on nuclear neurons. I wonder whether you would like to comment on this discrepancy.

Marshall: I can confirm that there is no inclusion of inferior olive in these culture explants, and that the cortex-to-deep nuclei inhibition is strong, as seen in extracellular recordings [2]. So there is indeed an apparent contradiction between Dr. Ito's results and ours. However, there are other differences which should be taken into consideration. Dr. Ito's evidence is from the cortex-to-Deiters nucleus projection, and is from animals in which an active olivo-cerebellar influence has been removed, whereas ours is from a cortex-to-deep nuclei path that has not previously been under the control of the inferior olive.

References

1. Ito M, Orlov I, Shimoyama I (1978) Reduction of the cerebellar stimulus effect on rat Deiters neurons after chemical destruction of the inferior olive. Exp Brain Res 33:143–145
2. Wojtowicz JM, Marshall KC, Hendelman WJ (1978) Electrophysiological and pharmacological studies of the inhibitory projection from the cerebellar cortex to the deep cerebellar nuclei in tissue culture. Neuroscience 3:607–618

Cell Lineage Analyses of Purkinje Cells in Murine Chimeras

M. L. Oster-Granite and J. Gearhart

Introduction

Neuroscientists have refined and extended the analysis of the basic events of cerebellar development described almost 100 years ago by Cajal [62, 63]. Studies of normal cerebellar development have provided us with a static picture of cells and their relationships at various developmental periods [2, 11, 12, 24, 36, 43, 53, 56, 58, 61, 62, 63, 66, 71, 72, and this volume, Chap. 2]. Several experimental approaches have been used to examine cellular interactions and mechanisms of development which give rise to these static pictures. Experimental neurobiologists have utilized selective developmental perturbations that arise from intrinsic alterations, such as genetic mutations [7, 26, 30, 69, and this volume, Chap. 3], or from extrinsic alterations, such as surgical extirpation [5, 53, 69, and this volume, Chap. 3], drugs [39, 53, 59, 80], neurotropic viruses [33, 53, 57], or X-irradiation [9 and this volume, Chap. 2]. Ectopic transplantations of the developing cerebellum have been studied to better define the extent of structural and synaptic plasticity that may occur [10, 34, 79].

From these studies of cerebellar development, several generalizations can be made. First, there is a definite temporal sequence of reciprocating cellular interactions between cell populations (like Purkinje cells and granule cells) that is requisite for normal development to proceed [53]. Second, perturbations occurring at younger ages tend to produce a cascade of effects, which confounds the retrospective interpretation of the events, their sequence, and their contribution to the development of the normal individual [53, 69]. Third, there is a basic scheme of intrinsic connectivity that is established among the cell populations whether they develop in an ectopic site, in a cytoarchitectonically disrupted environment, or in the normal environment.

Although such studies have helped to create a more dynamic view of cellular interactions during development, they have not permitted the prospective elucidation of the mechanisms which underlie observed features of early cerebellum development. To do this, one must have a means to identify and follow the cell populations present and their progeny at early developmental periods. Recently, mammalian chimeras (or mosaics) have been used to provide such a means to probe the underlying organization of the cerebellum and its development. Chimeras represent a powerful approach for the prospective as well as retrospective analyses of early developmental events.

Experimental Brain Research, Suppl. 6

Mammalian Chimeras

Mammalian chimeras (allophenics, tetraparentals) are composed of two (or more) populations of genotypically different cells [42, 44]. Murine chimeras are produced by aggregation [44] or injection [20] procedures (Fig. 1). Aggregation chimeras are produced by placing together in a culture dish, zona-pellucida-free, 8–12-cell mouse embryos of different genotypes. Injection chimeras are produced following the injection of an isolated blastomere(s) or inner cell mass cell(s) into the blastocyst cavity adjacent to the inner cell mass. The composite embryos formed by either procedure are transferred to the uterus of a pseudopregnant mouse where they implant and are carried to term. If cells of both genotypes are among the limited number of inner-cell-mass cells that give rise to the embryo proper [41], the result is a chimeric embryo. If appropriate coat pigmentation markers are used, the results of either method are normal-sized 'striped' mice, whose other tissues, like their coats, have variable proportions of the cells of both genotypes [20, 42, 44, 45, 51].

Mammalian chimeras can be used to follow the progeny of genetically marked cells throughout the development of the cerebellum, i.e., to analyze cell lineage of cell populations. These genetically marked cells may be derived from normal, or wild-type (+/+) animals, or from animals expressing neurological abnormalities resulting from genetic mutations. By combining embryos of normal

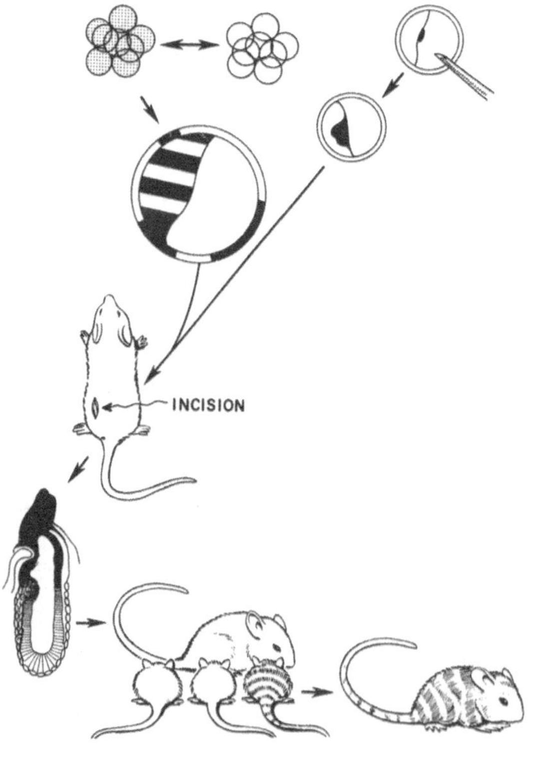

Fig. 1. Production of chimeric mice by aggregation and injection techniques. See text for explanation

and neurologically mutant mice, a chimeric nervous system with a unique mixture of cells results, which may provide the means to determine the site of action of the neurologically mutant genes. Of the 800 or more genetic loci that have been defined in the mouse genome, about 150 have alleles that produce behavioral or structural alterations in the nervous or neuromuscular systems. Fifteen to 20 of these affect the development or organization of the cerebellum directly [6, 48]. In a chimera in which normal and mutant cells have an opportunity to interact with one another, one can separate intrinsic defects, which result in the loss or maldevelopment of a particular cell population, from extrinsic or environmental effects, which cause the cell population to express the mutant phenotype indirectly.

Chimeras and Cell Lineage Analysis

Cell lineage studies have been carried out in the developing nervous systems of invertebrates [6, 16, 31, 32, 52, 75], amphibians [16, 28, 31, 32], and avians [32, 38], utilizing classic experimental embryological approaches, such as vital-dye staining [32], carbon-particle marking [32], intracellular injections of horseradish peroxidase [28, 52, 75], selective ablation [32], genetic mosaics [6, 16, 32], and xenoplastic transplantation chimeras [16, 32, 38].

There are several reasons why the mammalian cerebellum has been refractory to many such classic and more contemporary experimental embryologic approaches. First, mammals are viviparous. The embryo or fetus is not accessible to direct experimental manipulation during the earliest periods of cerebellar development. Second, the cells of the early mammalian embryo are significantly smaller than those of invertebrates or amphibians. Thus they are technically more difficult to mark and follow through their many successive generations than cells from a similar staged invertebrate or amphibian embryo. Finally, mammalian studies have also been precluded by the paucity of intrinsic cell marker systems which can be used to identify unequivocally the populations of cells throughout development.

Murine chimeras can be used to circumvent the problems associated with viviparity. By their use, early stages of cerebellar development become directly accessible to study. They have only recently begun to be utilized in studies of the developing cerebellum for several reasons. First, very few laboratories have the facilities or resources necessary to produce large numbers of chimeras of particular strain combinations to yield statistically significant results. Second, neurologically mutant $\leftrightarrow$ normal chimeras are difficult to obtain, often because of the pleiotrophic effects of the mutant gene on fertility, fecundity, or both. Only a few neurological mutant colonies can be maintained by mating homozygous animals [6, 48]. Even with the successful mating of homozygotes, progeny may not survive if the females are unable to carry pregnancy to term or if survival is compromised in the neonatal period by behavioral or coordination problems. If homozygous mutant matings are impractical, one must rely on using one or two heterozygous parents. One cannot distinguish which embryos from such a combination are homozygous or heterozygous when chimeras are formed. As a result one must attempt to distinguish mutant ↔ normal animals by overt mutant behavioral phenotype, or rely upon breeding data to identify the components present in the germ cell line and thus to reveal those chimeras formed between neurologically mutant ↔ normal embryos. This precludes the study of very young chimeras of many such strain combinations [6, 48]. Most importantly, many experimental embryologists who routinely study chimeras have avoided the nervous system because the limitations imposed by the available marker systems make it difficult to score many of the cell populations present in such a complex tissue [42, 55].

Unanswered Questions About Cerebellar Development That Chimeras May Help to Answer

Both normal ↔ normal and neurologically mutant ↔ normal murine chimeras could be used to probe very early periods of cerebellar development. Thus, they could perhaps help us to understand at what time the rhombic lip cells that give rise to the mammalian cerebellum originate, how the cells of the cerebellum attain their final cell positions, and perhaps how they establish their patterns of intrinsic and extrinsic circuitry. Such analyses could also help to develop a more unified concept of the regulative and determinate mechanisms which operate to influence and control cerebellar development. When used in conjunction with genetic mutations, such analyses could help to us understand how, when, and where certain genes exert their effects on cerebellar development.

Several observations that have been made concerning cerebellar developmental organization could be explained more readily if the interconnected cells shared a common or clonal origin. Murine chimeras can be used to assess the mosaicism present in the various chimeric components and thus to visualize clones of cells that may be present or persist [6, 31]. Cell populations in the cerebellar cortex migrate from a unique portion of the rhombencephalon called the rhombic lip. Cells are generated in two locations, a ventricular neuroepithelium and a unique germinative zone, the external germinal layer.

The continuous proliferation of these germinative zones produces clones of cells, which migrate from the origin into the cerebellar anlage or developing cerebellar cortex. Such clones of cells might maintain a contiguous relationship during their early migratory and developmental history, giving rise to clusters or 'patches' of cells in the anlage. As foliation ensues, four factors disrupt such 'patches' of cells: cell migration, cell intermingling, cell selection, and cell death. One or more of these factors acting in concert could produce a complete randomization of cells [6 and this volume, Chap. 2].

However, it is difficult to believe that the anatomic and physiologic properties we study result from a random distribution of cells of a given cell population, particularly in a structure so exquisitely organized as the cerebellar cortex. For example, the Purkinje cells form a single linear array in the adult cerebellar cortex. Functionally, small groups of these cells are activated by 'columns' of parallel fiber axons when stimulated through the mossy fiber system. During early embryogenesis, cell 'clusters' containing cells destined to be the Purkinje cells are observed in the cerebellar anlage of many species (this volume, Chap. 2). As development proceeds and foliation ensues, the multiple layers of Purkinje cells spread into a single layer, and the 'clusters' disappear [53, 56, and this volume, Chap. 2]. This sequence of events raises questions as to whether contiguous Purkinje cells in the adult represent patches of cells which had originated from a common ventricular neuroepithelial cell, or whether sister cells become randomly arranged during the cell migration that occurs during the process of foliation. Does cell intermingling occur as the cells are formed in the ventricular neureopithelium? Do neurons and glia have the same progenitor cell in the ventricular neuroepithelium? Does the columnar functional unit which is observed between Purkinje cells and granule cells in physiologic studies have an anatomic basis in a population of granule cells which arise from the same progenitor cells in the external germinal layer? Is the patch of Purkinje cells activated by that functional unit of granule cells derived from a common precursor cell?

By utilizing a cell marker system to distinguish the two chimeric components, mammalian chimeras provide an ideal experimental system in which to address these questions about cerebellar cell lineage.

Available Cell Markers for Lineage Studies

To date, the greatest limitations to the use of mammalian chimeras for cell lineage studies have been problems inherent in the cell markers that are available to distinguish the cells of the two genotypes [12]. To study cell lineage in the mammalian cerebellum (as well as in other tissues), one would need a genotype-specific cell marker that meets the following criteria [18, 42].

The marker should exist in variant forms that are (a) cell localized, not secreted into the external milieu; (b) cell autonomous, not transferred among cells; (c) selectively neutral, exerting no effect on the basic process of neurogenesis; (d) distinguishable in histologic sections; and (e) present and detectable in *all* cells of the cerebellum throughout its development, in neurons as well as glia, in small as well as large cell populations.

A variety of proteins have been isolated and purified from the CNS of mammals. These include surface receptors, neurotransmitters, enzymes involved in neurotransmitter synthesis or degradation, structural proteins, and cell specific enzymes which have been used to identify and classify CNS cells during development [3, 29, 35, 60, 68, and this volume, Chaps. 15 and 26]. Unfortunately, many of these cell markers fail to satisfy one or more of the above ideal requirements. Some can be used to score only a limited number of cell populations (such as certain populations of neurons or glia). Many are not expressed before differentiation begins. Other, more conventional labeling methods, such as radiolabeling [77], or direct injection of horseradish peroxidase [28] have thus far proven inadequate for these types of cell lineage studies for two reasons. First, the label may not be detectable if introduced during early developmental stages because too much dilution of label may occur during extensive cell division in the mammal. Second, there are technical difficulties in administering the label to the developing cerebellum at very early developmental stages.

Three types of markers have been used in studies of the nervous system of murine chimeras. Variants in nuclear or cytoplasmic morphology have been distinguished by light and electron microscopy [6]. Histocompatibility antigen differences have been distinguished by immunofluorescence techniques [13]. Variants in the activity or electrophoretic mobility of enzymes have been distinguished by histochemical, immunocytochemical, and biochemical techniques [6, 13, 15, 17, 18, 19, 22, 25, 26, 27, 47, 48, 55].

The use of nuclear or cytoplasmic morphologic markers has been explored because such markers are utilized to great advantage in analysis of cell lineage in the nervous system of chick-quail (xenoplastic transplantation) chimeras [38]. Mullen has used the nuclear heterochromatin pattern differences present in certain cell populations of the mouse mutant *ichthyosis* (*ic*) to score mosaicism in small cell populations, like the cerebellar granule cells [6]. He has also utilized cytoplasmic structural markers, such as lysosomal accumulations found in certain cell populations of the mouse mutant *beige* (bg^J) [6]. There are few cell populations in the cerebellum that can be scored with either of these markers. To complicate matters, scoring within a population may be equivocal, since wild type (+/+) cells (especially with the marker *ichthyosis*) may show some features of the structural marker's characteristics. These difficulties restrict the usefulness of these types of cell marker in studies of cell lineage in the developing cerebellum. The pigmentary system has been used to advantage by several groups [37, 46, 50, 65, 74] in their studies of the retina, its development, and the site of neurologically mutant gene action. It cannot be used to score mosaicism in the cerebellum.

Dewey et al. [13] utilized histocompatibility antigen differences that exist at the *H-2* locus in mice as a cell marker. An immunofluorescence staining technique was developed by Gervais [13] by employing allogeneic antibodies to murine lymphocytes. Thus, they could identify the mouse strain from which both Purkinje cells and granule cells were derived in the chimeric combination. On qualitative examination of sections throughout the cerebellum, Dewey et al. [13] found that Purkinje cells of like genotype occurred in short runs while the granule cells were found in clusters of up to 20 cells of like genotype.

Most investigators who have studied chimerism in the mammalian CNS have used variants of enzymes as their cell markers. They have attempted to visualize the location of cells containing the variants of cellular enzymes, whether lysosomal or cytoplasmic, by histochemical, biochemical, or immunocytochemical techniques. Histochemical techniques have been utilized to reveal the location of variants in the activity of the lysosomal enzymes, β-glucuronidase [6, 15, 25, 26, 27, 47, 48] and β-galactosidase [13]. Several inherent problems limit the use of either of these marker systems in extensive analysis of cell populations in the cerebellum. The enzymes are not detectably present in all cells of the cerebellum; enzyme activity is demonstrated consistently by histochemical methods only in a limited number of cell populations, such as the cerebellar Purkinje cells. β-glucuronidase is not cell autonomous, in that low-activity cells may take up enzyme. This uptake creates an intermediate phenotype, thus obscuring the genotype of the cell [15]. To circumvent this, heat inactivation has been used to destroy enzyme uptake by low-activity cells [25]. Even so, with either enzyme marker system, the technical difficulties associated with the histochemical technique have thus far precluded extensive serial section reconstruction and the scoring of the chimeric components throughout a given nuclear region.

Utilizing C3H ↔ C57BL/6J chimeras, Feder [15] examined the mosaicism present in other parts of the CNS (spinal cord). He found that the mosaicism was finely grained with small patches of less than nine cells distributed in no consistent fashion. A similar 'fine-grained' mosaicism was observed by Dewey [14] in cerebellar Purkinje cells. Mullen [6, 47] extended this qualitative observation by quantifying the distribution of Purkinje cell mosaicism. He found their distribution to be random or nearly random in C3H ↔ BL/6 chimeras [47]. Unfortunately, with these enzyme markers one could not detect the extent of mosaicism in other cerebellar cell populations.

In conjunction with β-galactosidase studies of CNS mosaicism, Dewey et al. [13] used the electrophoretic variants of the glycolytic enzyme, glucosephosphate isomerase (GPI, E.C. 5.3.1.9) to compare the extent of cerebellar mosaicism that the two cell markers could detect. This cell marker system, which fulfills more of the ideal criteria than any other, is the most commonly used biochemical marker in studies of murine chimeras [18, 42]. GPI is ubiquitous, cell localized, cell autonomous, and present throughout development [18, 19, 21, 54, 55]. The structural locus *Gpi-1* codes for selectively neutral electrophoretic variants or allozymes. The two most common variants of murine GPI, GPI-1A and GPI-1B, can be distinguished following electrophoresis on starch [17] or cellulose acetate gels [14] by indirect tetrazolium staining [17].

After assaying sections adjacent to those stained for β-galactosidase for the proportions of the GPI variants by starch gel electrophoresis, Dewey et al. [13] found that although there were differences in the proportions of genotypes observed with each of the markers, the proportions were consistent. To attempt to localize the cells containing GPI, and thus to define clearly the cell populations contributing to the electrophoretic ratios observed, Dewey et al. [13] used a standard, indirect histochemical technique. The histochemical technique for GPI cannot distinguish the variant forms [13, 18, 19]. Additionally, the technique Dewey used failed to detect GPI in the cerebellar Purkinje cells – a population that has been found to contain high levels of GPI by both modified histochemical and immunocytochemical methods [18, 19, 54, 55].

Thus, until recently, the greatest disadvantage of GPI as a marker system was that its electrophoretic variants were revealed only following destruction of cells or tissues. Hence, the precise localization and distribution of the variants (and thus the cell genotype) could not be assessed, although their relative proportions could be determined.

This disadvantage was overcome [18, 19, 22] with the adaptation of the GPI marker system. By absorbing xenogeneic antisera containing allozyme-specific antibodies to the GPI-1B variant on allozyme-conjugated Sepharose columns, we obtained anti- GPI-1B specific antibodies [18, 22]. These antibodies could

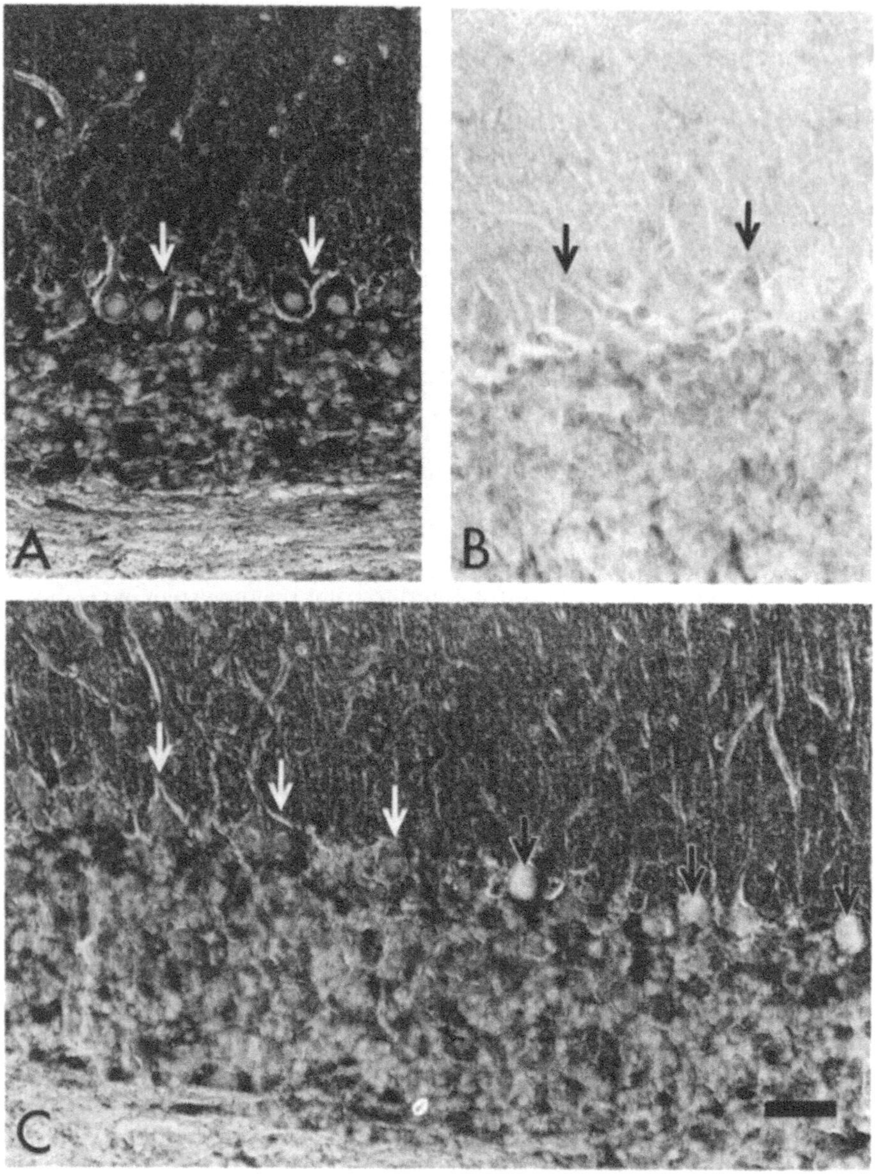

Fig. 2A–C. Sections of cerebellar cortex stained with purified anti-GPI-1B antisera in PAP staining procedure. No counterstain was used on these sections. *Bar*, 50 μ. **A** C57BL/6J control. Note that all the Purkinje cells are stained (*white arrows*), as are all other cells in the cerebellar cortex. Nuclei are unstained. **B** BALB/cBy[J] control. Note that the cells present are not stained by the anti-GPI-1B antisera. Purkinje cells, *black arrows*. **C** Chimera 1 cerebellar cortex. The cerebellum of chimera 1 (Table 1) was fixed with 96% ethanol, 1% acetic acid [18]. Note that stained (*white arrows*) and unstained (*black arrows*) Purkinje cells are present in this section. Unstained Purkinje cells in an adjacent 5-μ section were stained by immunoreactivity with control sera, indicating that these cells were of the GPI-1A genotype

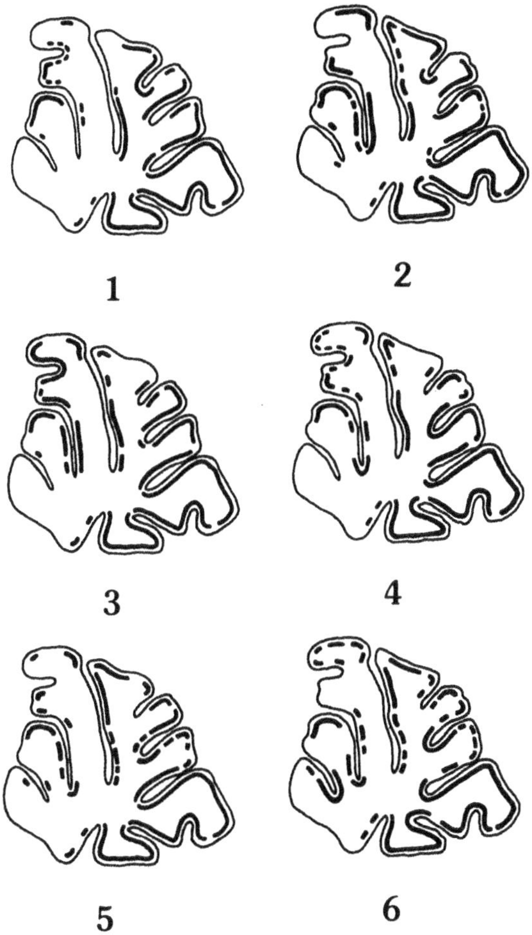

Fig. 3. 15-μ alternating step reconstructions were made of sections from the cerebellum of chimera 1 (Table 1). The distribution of Purkinje cells stained by anti-GPI-1B antisera is indicated in black, unstained Purkinje cells in gray. ×10

then be used in immunofluorescence or immunoperoxidase (PAP) staining techniques to distinguish cells of each genotype in chimeric tissues [18, 19, 21, 54, 55]. We utilized sera that reacted equally well with both the GPI-1A and GPI-1B variants as immunoreactivity controls, to ensure that cells unstained by anti-GPI-1B were immunoreactive when stained with anti-GPI. We showed that small as well as large cell populations, neurons as well as glia, could be scored in the brains of chimeric mice [54, 55]. With this adapted cell marker system the location and distribution of the genotypes in various cell populations of the cerebellum, not only Purkinje cells, but the Bergmann glia, basket, stellate, Golgi, and granule cells of the cerebellar cortex as well, can be visualized. Following a quantitative statistical analysis [6, 47, 64, 76] of the cerebellar cortex of four BALB/cByJ ↔ C57BL/6J chimeras [55], we found that the Purkinje cells in this strain combination were not randomly arranged, but tended to exist as small three-to-eight-cell patches of like genotype throughout the cerebellar cortex (Fig. 2). In chimera 1 (Fig. 3) there was a predominance of unstained (GPI-1A) cells in the anterior cerebellar lobules and stained (GPI- 1B) in the

Table 1. Summary of Purkinje cell analyses

Chimera	Proportion	Estimated patch size	Observed patch size
1	0.494	1.98	8.18 ± 1.89
2	0.431	1.76	3.94 ± 0.18
3	0.544	2.19	3.96 ± 0.29
4	0.158	1.19	2.28 ± 0.22

posterior lobules. Twelve hundred and seventy-five Purkinje cells were scored in sections 1 through 4 from this chimera (Fig. 3). Among these, there were 82 patches of stained cells (628 cells) with an observed patch size (cells of like genotype) of about eight cells/patch (Table 1). Had the Purkinje cells been randomly arranged in this chimera, the expected patch size would have been about two cells/patch (Table 1). This expected patch size is calculated by the formula $1/1-p$ [64, 76] where p is the proportion of stained cells present throughout the population being scored. Similar analyses were carried out on the other three chimeras as well (Table 1) [55]. General inspection showed that the granule cell population was arranged in patches of as many as eight cells/5 μ-section in each of these four animals.

Comparison of Results of Mammalian Cell Lineage Studies

To date, several groups of investigators have attempted to analyze cell lineages in the mammalian CNS with the intent of detecting the distribution of cells

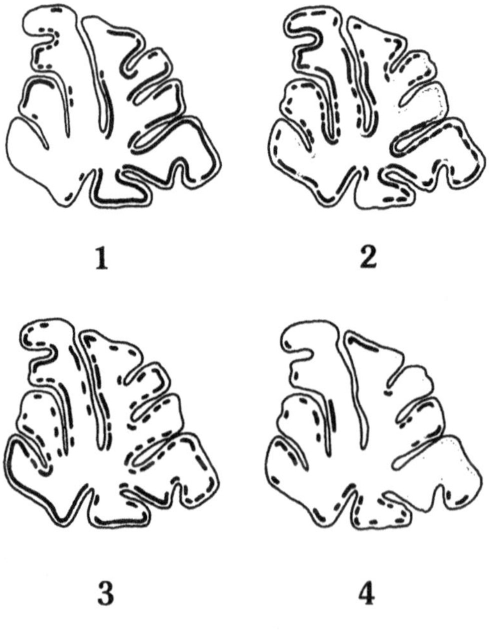

Fig. 4. Representative 15-μ reconstruction sections from cerebellar cortex of chimeras *1 – 4*. Note that although the proportion of stained cells is nearly equal in chimeras *1 – 3* (Table 1), the distribution of the patches is quite different. Even chimera *4*, with a preponderance of cells that were unstained (GPI-1A), had a distribution significantly different from that expected in a random array (Table 1)

with like genotype [6, 13, 15, 18, 27, 47–50, 54, 55, 65, 74]. They have focused their attention primarily upon the cerebellum, the spinal cord, and the retina. Several have been concerned simply with the demonstration of chimerism in various cell populations [6, 13, 15, 27, 55, 65, 74], but a few have quantified the extent or distribution of the chimeric components [6, 46, 47, 55]. Cerebella of limited numbers of animals or portions of the cerebellum of one animal have been analyzed [6, 13, 27, 47, 55]. In some instances, the reason for the limited numbers of animals is obvious because neurologically mutant ↔ normal animals are involved.

To the casual observer, the distribution of the chimeric components described by each of these groups is "fine grained" [13, 15], with small clusters or short runs of cells of like genotype. Whether such a distribution is random or nonrandom is unresolved. For example, both Feder [15] and Dewey et al. [13] observed small patches (in Feder's case less than nine cells/patch) of stained cells in various portions of the CNS. Mullen [6, 47] and Oster-Granite and Gearhart [55] carefully analyzed and quantified the distribution of mosaicism in the cerebella of chimeric mice. In normal ↔ normal chimeras, Mullen found a random or nearly random arrangement of the Purkinje cells following analysis of sagittal sections throughout the lobules of the cerebellar cortex. In his analysis of one lobule from a neurologically mutant ↔ normal chimera, in which 75% of the Purkinje cells were missing, he found an apparently random arrangement of the remaining Purkinje cells. Although these surviving cells were of the +/+ genotype, Mullen could not determine whether *only* mutant Purkinje cells had died. Statistically, he observed many patches which contained only one cell. As Feder [15] points out, a patch size of one means that either the two sister cells became separated during migration or that one of them died. In neurologically mutant ↔ normal combinations the loss of normal cells contiguous to patches of degenerating mutant cells could give rise to randomness by reducing patch size to one or two cells. Certainly the Purkinje cell patch size observed by Oster-Granite and Gearhart [55] was not large (three to eight cells) but was consistent and nonrandom.

Given the small numbers of animals that have been analyzed rigorously for the distribution and location of the genotypes in the grain of chimeras, it is not possible at present to explain readily the differences observed amongst the various groups. The analysis of the nervous system of murine chimeras is just beginning. With the GPI marker available now to score diverse populations, the discrepancies in observations that have been noted probably will be resolved in the near future.

There are several things that one must continuously keep in mind when reading or evaluating chimera literature.

At present, the marker systems available dictate the type and variety of strain combinations that can be made. For example, the majority of studies have utilized the C3H ↔ C57BL/6 strain combination (Table 2). Although they differ at the structural loci coding for the enzymes β-glucuronidase (*Gus*) and β-galactosidase (*Bgs*) both strains have the *Gpi-1*^{b} allele and express the GPI-1B variant (Table 2). In the absence of a congenic C3H or BL/6 strain with the *Gpi-1*^{a} allele, the GPI marker cannot be used in this strain combination. Simi-

Table 2. Strain combinations used in murine chimeras

Strain	Genotype			
C3H	*Gus* ^{h}	*Bgs* ^{h}	*Gpi-1* ^{b}	*H-2* ^{k}
C57BL/6J	*Gus* ^{b}	*Bgs* ^{d}	*Gpi-1* ^{b}	*H-2* ^{b}
BALB/c	*Gus* ^{b}	*Bgs* ^{d}	*Gpi-1* ^{a}	
AKR/J	*Gus* ^{h}	*Bgs* ^{h}	*Gpi-1* ^{a}	

Combinations
C3H ↔ C57BL/6 [13, 15, 47]
C3H ↔ BALB/cWt [13, 15]
AKR/J ↔ C57BL/6J [13, 15]
AKR/J ↔ BALB/c [15]
BALB/cBy^{J} ↔ C57BL/6J [55]

larly, the BALB/c ↔ BL/6 combination cannot be scored with the β-glucuronidase or β-galactosidase markers (Table 2). An ideal strain combination at present might be AKR/J ↔ BL/6 since these strains differ at all three loci. Unfortunately, no quantitative studies have been done on this strain combination. Strain- specific differences could contribute to the differences that have been observed. Strain-specific differences have been observed in the rate, timing, and extent of cell selection and death in the murine CNS [4, 23, 67, 73, 78]. Previous studies of murine chimeras have shown that there are strain-specific influences exerted upon the development of various organ systems [20, 42, 45]. Age-related, strain- specific effects also have been observed in the coat, hematopoietic system, and germ cells of chimeras of various strain combinations [20, 42, 45, 51]. As the numbers of normal ↔ normal and neurologically mutant ↔ normal chimeras that are studied increase, the contributions that the strain combination makes to the location and distribution of chimerism will become apparent. Ideally, such problems would be circumvented by the future development of the appropriate congenic strains of mice.

It is quite conceivable that as more mutant ↔ normal combinations are studied, factors other than strain differences could be shown to affect the apparent randomness that some have observed. At the present time, it is difficult to assess how much randomness arises from differences in the numbers of cells generated originally, in the rate that cells gain access into the anlage, and in the cell interactions (such as extensive cell death in mutants) that occur during development. That these factors may affect the patterns seen has been shown by Herrup and Mullen's recent description of significant alterations in the numbers of both normal and mutant cell populations in the cerebella of *staggerer* ↔ normal chimeras [26, 27].

If randomness is not the norm in the cerebellum, what might one expect to see when progressively younger developmental stages are analyzed? If, as our results with the BALB/c ↔ BL/6 strain combination indicate, there are small patches of like genotype that persist in the adult, there may well be a basis for the patterns of functional and anatomic connectivity that Miale and Sidman

[43] and Jacobson [32] have previously suggested. Larger, more coherent patches of Purkinje cells may exist in the anlage before foliation occurs, and thus may contribute to the clusters others have observed. Although cell death and the spread of such patches might occur, the patches would merely be distorted, but not eliminated as foliation proceeds. Granule cell precursors may become contiguous to such patches as the external germinal layer forms. As the cortex expands during foliation, they may funnel between groups of Purkinje cells with which they will later interconnect. Although the association with Bergmann glial fibers during development may be merely a fortuitous rather than a requisite one [36, 56, 57, 61, 66], the glial pillars could provide the necessary avenue for passage of clones of granule cells between the forming hexagonal array of Purkinje cells. If the Bergmann glia shared a common origin with the patch of Purkinje cells, they might well provide a basis for the connectivity that results. Evidence from three groups certainly suggests that the granule cells do exist as patches of up to as many as 20 cells of like genotype in these chimeras, which corresponds well to the functional unit size (11–15 cells) that has been observed.

From autoradiographic studies it is obvious that the general migratory pattern in the cerebellum is radial [7, 61, 66], regardless of its direction, i.e., inside-out or outside-in. Because of this common orientation it is possible that sister cells would go out into the anlage in tandem rather than become diffusely separated. Since the cells do go out as waves, presumably at the same rate, it seems more likely that they do so by the shortest route possible to the surface, rather than by mingling extensively as they migrate through the anlage. Thus, one might speculate that as the clusters of the anlage are formed, cells of like genotype might occur in tandem whether associated with glial guides or not.

These speculations await the direct analysis of fetal or newborn chimeras to determine whether or not clones of cells give rise to the patches observed in the adult. With the adaptation of the GPI cell marker system, we now have a means to analyze prospectively as well as retrospectively very early stages of cerebellar development and thus to determine the interactions of cell populations at these times. Only direct examination will enable us to determine how much randomization of Purkinje and other cell populations does occur due to cell migration and intermingling, cell selection, and cell death in the developing cerebellar cortex, and whether the anatomic and functional units we observe are derived from clones of cells.

Acknowledgments. The authors thank Betsy Buell and James Musser for their technical assistance. Ms. Ilene Ferguson typed and proofread the manuscript. This research was supported by the NIH (HD 12685), the NSF (PCM 16763), the March of Dimes-Birth Defects Foundation, and the Paralyzed Veterans of America. MLO-G is an Alfred Sloan Foundation Fellow. JG is the recipient of a Basil O'Connor Starter Grant from the March of Dimes-Birth Defects Foundation.

References

1. Deleted in production
2. Altman J, Bayer SA (1978) Prenatal development of the cerebellar system in the rat. I. Cytogenesis and histogenesis in the deep nuclei and the cortex of the cerebellum. J Comp Neurol 179:23–48
2. Barclay AN (1979) Localization of the Thy-1 antigen in the cerebellar cortex of the rat brain by immunofluorescence during postnatal development. J Neurochem 32:1249–1257
4. Berger B, Herve D, Dolphin A, Barthelemy C, Gay M, Tassig JP (1979) Genetically determined differences in noradrenergic input to the brain cortex: a histochemical and biochemical study in two inbred strains of mice. Neuroscience 4:877–888
5. Brand S, Mugnaini E (1976) Fulminant Purkinje cell death following axotomy and its use for analysis of the dendritic arborization. Exp Brain Res 26:105–119
6. Breakefield XO (ed) (1979) Neurogenetics: Genetic Approaches to the Nervous System. Elsevier, New York
7. Caviness VS Jr, Rakic P (1978) Mechanisms of cortical development: a view from mutations in mice. Ann Rev Neurosci 1:297–326
8. Deleted in production
9. Das GD (1978) Premature death of Purkinje cells following low-level X-ray irradiation during embryonic development. Acta Anat (Basel) 101:225–233
10. Das GD (1980) Growth of neural transplants from embryos of different ages. Anat Rec 196:41 A
11. Del Cerro MP, Snider RS (1968) Studies on the developing cerebellum. Ultrastructure of the growth cones. J Comp Neurol 133:341–362
12. Del Cerro MP, Snider RS (1972) Axosomatic and axodendritic synapses in the cerebellum of the newborn rat. Brain Res 43:581–587
13. Dewey MJ, Gervais AG, Mintz B (1976) Brain and ganglion development from two genotypic classes of cells in allophenic mice. Dev Biol 50:68–81
14. Eicher E, Washburn LL (1978) Assignment of genes to regions of mouse chromosomes. Proc Natl Acad Sci USA 75:946–950
15. Feder N (1976) Solitary cells and enzyme exchange in tetraparental mice. Nature 263:67–69
16. Ferrendelli JA, Gurvitch G (eds) (1979) Aspects of Developmental Neurobiology. Soc Neurosci Symp 4. Soc Neurosci, Bethesda
17. Gearhart J, Mintz B (1972) Clonal origin of somites and their muscle derivatives. Evidence from allophenic mice. Dev Biol 29:27–37
18. Gearhart J, Oster-Granite ML (1978) Antibodies to allozymes as potential cell markers for chimeric mouse studies. In: Russell LB (ed) Genetic Mosaics and Chimeras in Mammals. Plenum, New York, pp 111–121
19. Gearhart J, Oster-Granite ML (1980) An immunofluorescence procedure for the tissue localization of glucosephosphate isomerase. J Histochem Cytochem 28:245–249
20. Gearhart J, Oster-Granite ML (1981) Age related changes in coat pigmentation of allophenic mice. J Hered 72:2–5
21. Gearhart J, Oster-Granite ML (1980) Distribution of glucosephosphate isomerase in ovarian follicles and early embryonic stages of the mouse. Biol Reprod 23:837–845
22. Gearhart J, Oster-Granite ML, Musser J (1981) Allozymes of murine glucosephosphate isomerase. Isolation, purification, and immunoreactivity. Biochem Genet 19:445–455
23. Hegmann JP (1979) Gene influences timing the development of size and nervous system functional differences. Behav Neural Biol 25:510–522
24. Heinsen H (1977) Quantitative anatomical studies on the postnatal development of the cerebellum of the albino rat. Anat Embryol 151:201–218
25. Herrup K, Mullen RJ (1977) Biochemical and genetic factors in the heat inactivation of murine β-glucuronidase. Biochem Genet 15:641–643
26. Herrup K, Mullen RJ (1979) Regional variation and absence of large neurons in the cerebellum of the *staggerer* mouse. Brain Res 172:1–12
27. Herrup K, Mullen RJ (1979) *Staggerer* chimeras: intrinsic nature of Purkinje cell defects and implications for normal cerebellar development. Brain Res 178:443–457

28. Hirose G, Jacobson M (1979) Clonal organization of the central nervous system of the frog. I. Clones stemming from individual blastomeres of the 16 cell or earlier stages. Dev Biol 71:191–202
29. Hooghe-Peters EL, Fowhles BJ, Hooghe RJ (1979) A new neuronal marker identified by phosphorylcholine binding myeloma proteins. Nature 281:376–378
30. Ide C (1978) Genetic dissection of cerebellar development: mutations affecting cell position. Am Zool 18:281–287
31. Jacobson M (1978) Clonal origins of the central nervous system: towards a developmental neuroanatomy. In: Jacobson CO, Ebendal T (eds) Formshaping Movements in Neurogenesis. Almqvist & Winsell, Stockholm, pp 149–156
32. Jacobson M (1978) Developmental neurobiology. Plenum, New York
33. Johnson RT (1977) Viral infections and brain development. In: Berenberg SR (ed) Brain: Fetal and Infant. Current Research on Normal and Abnormal Development. Martinus Nijhoff Med Div, The Hague, pp 213–223
34. Kromer LF, Bjorklund A, Stenevi U (1979) Intracephalic implants: a technique for studying neuronal interactions. Science 204:1117–1119
35. Lagenaur C, Sommer I, Schachner M (1979) Glial cell antigens detected by monoclonal antibodies (Abstr). Soc Neurosci 5:102
36. Lapham LW, Bignami A, Del Cerro MP, Mugnaini E, Rakic P (1977) Astrogliogenesis and neuronal-glial interactions during development. BIS Conf Rep 46:79–97
37. LaVail MM, Mullen RJ (1976) Role of the pigment epithelium in inherited retinal degeneration analyzed in experimental mouse chimeras. Exp Eye Res 23:227–245
38. LeDouarin N, LeLievre C (1978) Cell migration during embryogenesis. An experimental analysis of neural crest evolution by using the quail-chick marker system. Birth Defects 342:141–153
39. Lovell KL, Jones MZ (1979) Kianic acid neurotoxicity in the mouse cerebellum (Abstr). Soc Neurosci 5:104
40. Deleted in production
41. Markert CL, Petters RM (1978) Manufactured hexaparental mice show that adults are derived from three embryonic cells. Science 202:56–58
42. McLaren A (1976) Mammalian Chimeras. Cambridge University Press, Cambridge
43. Miale IL, Sidman RL (1961) An autoradiographic analysis of histogenesis in the mouse cerebellum. Exp Neurol 4:277–296
44. Mintz B (1971) Allophenic mice of multiembryo origin. In: Daniel J Jr (ed) Methods in mammalian embryology. Freeman, San Francisco, pp 186–214
45. Mintz B (1974) Gene control in mammalian differentiation. Annu Rev Genet 8:411–470
46. Mintz B, Sanyal S (1970) Clonal origin of mouse visual retina mapped from genetically mosaic eyes. Genetics 64:43–44
47. Mullen RJ (1977) Site of *pcd* gene action and Purkinje cell mosaicism in cerebella of chimeric mice. Nature 272:245–247
48. Mullen RJ (1978) Genetic dissection of the CNS with mutant – normal mouse chimeras. In: Cowan WM, Ferrendelli JA (eds) Soc Neurosci Symp 2:47–65
49. Mullen RJ, LaVail MM (1975) Two new types of retinal degeneration in cerebellar mutant mice. Nature 258:528–530
50. Mullen RJ, LaVail MM (1976) Inherited retinal dystrophy: primary defect in pigment epithelium determined in experimental rat chimeras. Science 192:799–801
51. Mullen RJ, Whitten WK (1971) Relationship of genotype and degree of chimerism in coat color and gametogenesis in chimeric mice. J Exp Zool 178:165–176
52. Muller KJ, McMahan UJ (1976) The shapes of sensory and motor neurons and the distribution of their synapses in ganglia of the leech: A study using intracellular injection of horseradish peroxidase. Proc R Soc Lond [Biol] 194:481–499
53. Oster-Granite ML (1974) The pathogenesis of rat virus induced cerebellar hypoplasia in the Syrian hamster, *Mesocricetus auratus*. A light, Golgi, and electron microscopic study. PhD Thesis, Johns Hopkins University, Baltimore
54. Oster-Granite ML, Gearhart J (1980) Immunofluorescence and histochemical localization of glucosephosphate isomerase in neural tissue. J Histochem Cytochem 28:250–254
55. Oster-Granite ML, Gearhart J (1981) Cell lineage analysis of cerebellar Purkinje cells in mouse chimeras. Devel Biol 85:199–208

56. Oster-Granite ML, Herndon RM (1976) The development of the cerebellar cortex of the Syrian hamster, *Mesocricetus auratus*. Foliation, cytoarchitectonic, Golgi, and electron microscopic studies. J Comp Neurol 169:433–480
57. Oster-Granite ML, Herndon RM (1976) The pathogenesis of parvovirus-induced cerebellar hypoplasia in the Syrian hamster, *Mesocricetus auratus*. Fluorescent antibody, foliation, cytoarchitectonic, Golgi and electron microscopic studies. J Comp Neurol 169:481–532
58. Palay S, Chan-Palay V (1974) The Cerebellar Cortex: Cytology and Organization. Springer, Berlin Heidelberg New York
59. Press MF (1977) Neuronal development in the cerebellum of lead poisoned neonatal rats. Acta Neuropathol (Berl) 40:259–268
60. Raff MC, Fields KL, Hakomori SI, Mirsky R, Pruss RM, Winter J (1979) Cell type specific markers for distinguishing and studying neurons and the major classes of glial cells in culture. Brain Res 174:283–308
61. Rakic P (1971) Neuroglial relations during granule cell migration in developing cerebellar cortex. A Golgi and EM study in *Macaca rhesus*. J Comp Neurol 141:283–312
62. Ramon y Cajal S (1911) Histologie du System Nerveux de l'Homme et des Vertébrés, vol 2. Malolne, Paris. Translated by L Azoulay. (Reprinted 1952, Consejo Superior de Investigaciones Cientificas, Madrid)
63. Ramon y Cajal S (1929) Studies in Vertebrate Neurogenesis. Thomas, Springfield. Translated by L Guth
64. Roach SA (1968) The Theory of Random Clumping. Methuen, London
65. Sanyal S, Zeilmaker GH (1976) Comparative analysis of cell distribution in the pigment epithelium and visual cell layer of chimeric mice. J Embryol Exp Morphol 36:425–430
66. Sidman RL, Rakic P (1973) Neuronal migration: with special reference to the developing human brain. A review. Brain Res 62:1–35
67. Silver J (1979) Cell death during development of the nervous system. In: Jacobson M (ed) Development of Sensory Systems. Springer, Berlin Heidelberg New York (Handbook of sensory physiology, vol 9, pp 419–436)
68. Slotkin TA (1979) Ornithine decarboxylase as a tool in developmental neurobiology. Life Sci 24:1623–1630
69. Sotelo C (1978) Purkinje cell ontogeny: the formation and maintenance of spines. In: Corner MA, Baker RE, Van de Pol NE, Swaab DF, Uylings HBM (eds) Maturation of the Nervous System. Prog Brain Res 48:149–170
70. Deleted in production
71. Swarz JR (1977) A light, Golgi, and electron microscopic study of the external granular layer in prenatal and postnatal mouse cerebellum. PhD Thesis, Univ Rochester, Rochester
72. Swarz JR, Oster-Granite ML (1978) Presence of radial glia in foetal mouse cerebellum. J Neurocytol 7:301–312
73. Vaughan JE, Hendrickson CK, Chernow CR, Grieshaber JA, Wimer CC (1974) Genetically associated variations in the development of reflex movements and synaptic junctions within an early reflex pathway of mouse spinal cord. J Comp Neurol 161:541–554
74. Wegmann TG, LaVail MM, Sidman RL (1971) Patchy retinal degeneration in tetraparental mice. Nature 230:333–334
75. Weisblat DA, Sawyer RT, Stent GS (1978) Cell lineage analysis by intracellular injection of a tracer enzyme. Science 202:1295–1297
76. West JD (1975) A theoretical approach to the relation between patch size and clone size in chimaeric tissue. J Theor Biol 50:153–160
77. Weston JA (1963) An autoradiographic analysis of the migration and localization of the trunk neural crest in the chick. Dev Biol 6:279–310
78. White JE, Hegmann JP (1974) Development of nervous system function in mice: Normative data and gene effects. Behav Biol 11:83–88
79. Woodward DJ, Seiger A, Olson L, Hoffer BJ (1978) Intrinsic and extrinsic determinants of dendritic development as revealed by Golgi studies of cerebellar and hippocampal transplants in oculo. Exp Neurol 57:984–998
80. Yu WHA (1977) The effect of 5-bromodeoxyuridine on the postnatal development of the rat cerebellum: morphologic and radioautographic studies. Am J Anat 150:89–108

Discussion

In response to a question from Dr. Balázs on the success rate in the yield of chimeras, Dr. Oster-Granite replied that the figure was about 75% in their method of producing aggregation chimeras. She also added that, when one attempts to produce injection chimeras, the recovery of chimeras drops to about 15%. This sharp decrease is due to the fact that only three cells of the approximately 100 mouse blastocyst cells contribute to the embryo proper, and therefore there is a much lower probability that the progeny of the injected cell would be among those three cells.

Comenting on the extent of variability in the experimentally produced chimeras, Dr. Balázs asked about any possible correlation between coat mosaicism and cerebellar mosaicism. Dr. Oster-Granite gave the following details: Although coat mosaicism does not directly correspond to brain mosaicism, in general, when the coat is mosaic most other organs, including the brain, are mosaic as well. The proportions of two genotypes found depend upon the strain combination, and vary amongst different organs. Furthermore, even within a given strain combination, the proportion of mosaicism varies for each organ, each chimera being different from all others. Age superimposes yet another variable. Age-related changes occur in the distribution and proportions of mosaicism in the coat, hematopoietic system, and the germ cells, indicating a continuous cell selection throughout life.

Dr. Altman commented that, in a related study involving ^{3}H-thymidine injection of pregnant rats on embryonic day 16, they found that a small number of Purkinje cells were labelled which were randomly distributed, and not in clusters as in Dr. Oster-Granite's study. Dr. Oster-Granite responded as follows: The radial spread of radioactively labeled cells distributes the cells formed on different days into the anlage. A single ventricular neuroepithelial cell may give rise to a series of Purkinje (or other) cell progeny over several days. Sister cells may then migrate into the anlage in tandem and thus come to be contiguous in the anlage. As the cells spread during foliation, such contiguous cells may then remain together as patches, although they may have formed at different times.

Dr. Sotelo also commented on the nonrandom distribution of Purkinje cells in Dr. Oster-Granite's studies saying that these results were in complete contradiction to those of Mullen [1]. Dr. Oster-Granite pointed out, however, that Mullen's results were based on an inadequate sample of chimeras.

In response to Dr. Chan-Palay's question on the peroxidase antiperoxidase (PAP) technique, Dr. Oster-Granite gave the following outline: The PAP technique used was a conventional one. Solutions containing normal serum (depending upon the source of the primary antibody) were utilized throughout the procedure. Preincubation with methanol and hydrogen peroxide was routinely done to remove any endogenous activity. The primary antibody (anti GPI-1B) was used at a dilution of 1:200 to 1:500 for a very short (30 min) incubation time. Counterstaining with thionin permitted more accurate scoring of the distribution of cells, but there was a tendency to obscure the distinction between the cell populations with and without PAP staining in the photographs, which prompted Dr. Chan-Palay's question on their technique.

Dr. Oster-Granite added a few other details about their methodology. They studied the effects of a variety of alcohol-based, aldehyde-based and double aldehyde fixatives. The antigenicity of the enzyme proved to be remarkably stable, the molecule remaining immunoreactive throughout the conventional paraffin embedding procedure. As a result, they did not have to use vibratome sections. Furthermore, both histochemical and immunocytochemical staining of the enzyme in unfixed frozen sections produced the same distribution of staining. Thus, *serial* reconstructions of the genotype distribution could be prepared throughout the brains of their animals.

Reference

1. Mullen RJ (1977) Site of *pcd* gene action and Purkinje cell mosaicism in cerebella of chimeric mice. Nature 272:245–247

Regional Differences in the Cytoarchitecture of the Cerebellar Cortex

W. Lange

From many embryological studies on the cerebellar cortex, especially those of Hochstetter [6], Larsell [16–18], and Korneliussen [7], we know that parts of the human cerebellar cortex can be distinguished that mature at different times during ontogenesis. These various parts of the cerebellum are of different sizes in species with different degrees of cerebralization. As a result of the phase differences during embryonic development, phylogenetically older and younger parts can be distinguished in the cerebellum.

Similar developmental and maturing processes can also be observed in the telencephalon. However, in the cerebral cortex they are normally linked with the formation of different cortical types, which allow the distinction of phylogenetically younger from older parts, on the basis of the layering of the cerebral cortex. Furthermore, there is also a strongly varying arrangement of the different layers of the same cortical type in various telencephalic regions. Consequently, we can differentiate regional variations in the cytoarchitectonics of the cerebral cortex by means of the simple Nissl method, documented in the detailed cytoarchitectonic maps of Brodmann [1].

Such regional differences in the cytoarchitecture of the cortex could not, until recently, be safely established for the cerebellum, because the monotonous cortical structure extends through all its parts.

In spite of this, many investigators came to the conclusion, resulting from highly subjective, unverifiable impressions, that regional differences do exist in the cytoarchitecture of the cerebellum. Landau [8–12], for example, as a result of his studies on the arrangement of granule cells, stated that regional differences in the cytoarchitecture of the cerebellar cortex must undoubtedly exist. Subsequently, similar statements were frequently published without ever being verified by other authors.

These attempts to differentiate the cerebellar cortex into different parts have in common that they consider only one part of the definition of C. and O. Vogt [20] about the architectonics of a cortical area. Besides regional variations in the arrangement of nerve cells, C. and O. Vogt [20] included the number and rough form of the elements among the criteria for cytoarchitectonic units. Although the arrangement of particular cell types is often highly characteristic, it is rarely proof for cytoarchitectonic differences when considering a cortex like that in the cerebellum.

But on the other hand, unequivocal proof for regional differences in the cerebellar cortex of mammals can be obtained from the rough shape and the num-

Experimental Brain Research, Suppl. 6

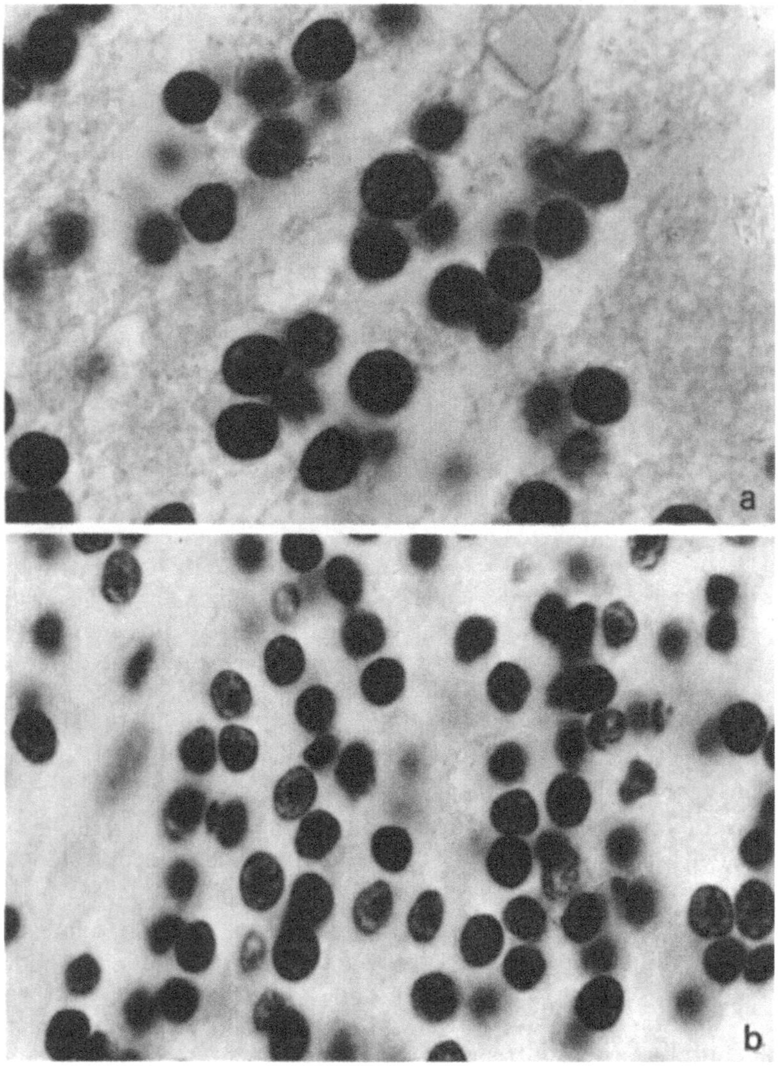

Fig. 1. a Granule cell nuclei from the nodulus (man). **b** Granule cell nuclei from the flocculus (man). ×1550

ber of the individual cellular elements; variations in shape are obviously also understood as differences in size and form of the perikaryon.

A first comparison of the granule cells from various parts of the cerebellum shows that their nuclei vary in size. Only these are visible in preparations using the Nissl techniques.

Figure 1 shows granule cells from the nodulus, a phylogenetic old vermal part (Fig. 1a), and from the paraflocculus ventralis, a young hemispherical part (Fig. 1b). These differences are always demonstrable when comparing systematically younger and older cortical parts from all three cerebellar lobes. Larger cells are always found in the vermal parts rather than in the associated lobes of the hemisphere (Fig. 2). The cell size of 5.1 μm is largest in the nodulus, showing a difference of 0.5 μm compared to those in the flocculus, the associated hemispherical part. This difference of about 10%, obtained by statistical examination of 2000 measured cells in every lobe, is statistically significant ($p < 0.01$). The difference in size of the granule cells between the vermis and the hemisphere is likely to be somewhat larger in the posterior lobe of the cerebellum and somewhat smaller in the anterior lobe. However, it is statistically significant in all parts.

The fact that such significant differences between the younger and older parts of the cerebellar cortex can be demonstrated in such a small cell type as the granule cell suggests the question of whether these differences can be also established with the same regularity among other cell types of the cerebellar cortex. The graph in Fig. 3 shows that the Purkinje cells in the vermal parts of the three cerebellar lobes are always larger than those in the corresponding parts of the hemispheres. Furthermore, differences occur in the cerebellar vermis, as the cells in the nodulus are always somewhat larger than those in the remaining vermal parts. Once more, from measurements of 400 cells of each part, significant differences in size are obtained with 99% probability. This means, apart

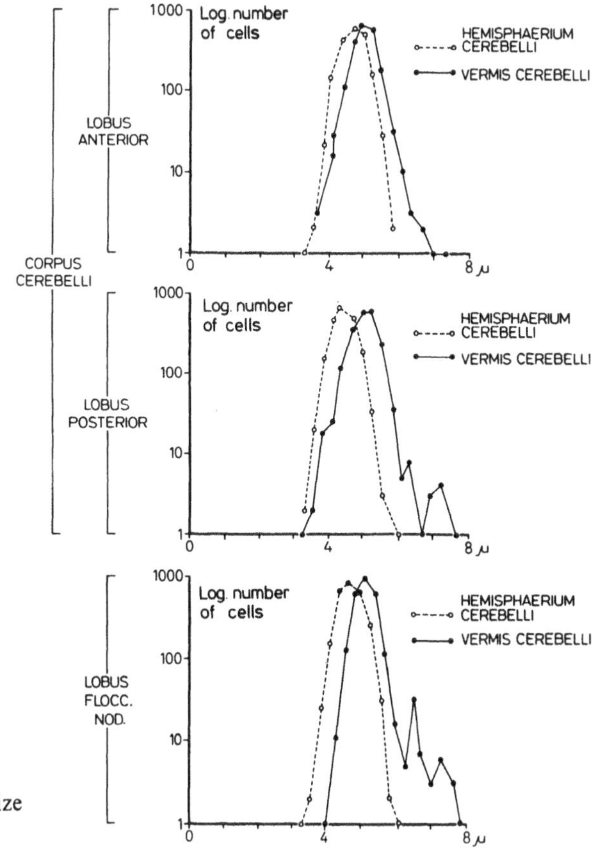

Fig. 2. Distribution of the cell size of granule cells (cat)

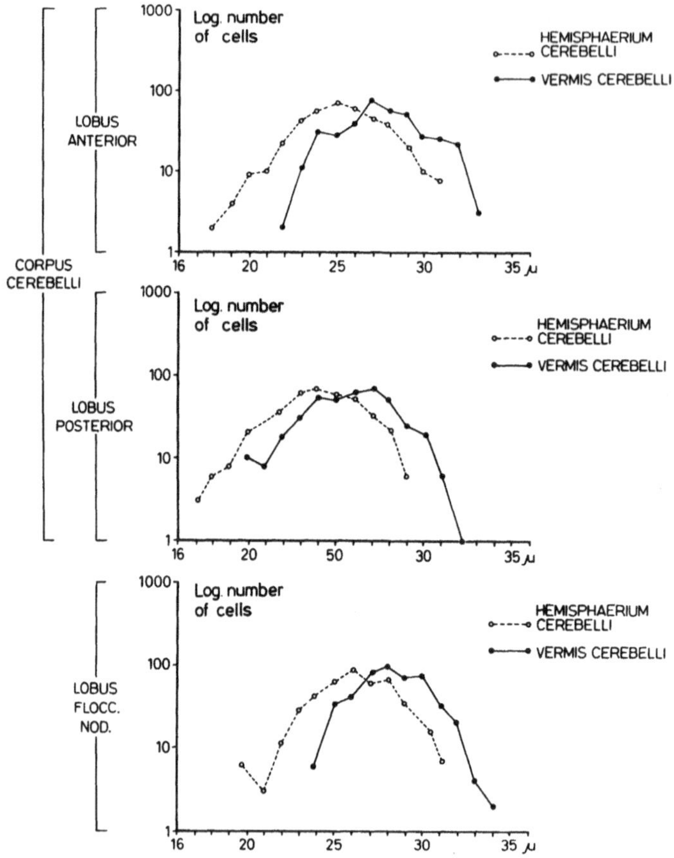

Fig. 3. Distribution of the cell size of Purkinje cells (cat)

from the granule cells, a second cell type, namely the Purkinje cells, shows different cell sizes, which is, according to C. and O. Vogt, an important criterion for regional differences in cytoarchitectonics.

According to C. and O. Vogt [20], a further characteristic for regional differences in cytoarchitectonics is the cell density, i.e., the number of cells per unit volume. It is known that the cell density in the phylogenetically older parts of the cortex cerebri is lower than in the younger ones [5]. On closer examination, a similar principle can be demonstrated in all three layers of the cerebellar cortex. Whereas the cell density in the granular layer is disproportionately higher than in all the other cortical layers of the brain, a comparison distinctly shows that the granule cells in the nodulus are less numerous but larger (Fig. 1). In the flocculus, its lateral continuation in the hemispheres, the cells are considerably more numerous but also a little smaller. On calculating the number of granule cells, which are found in a cube with a side of 0.1 mm, the following proportions are obtained: A cube of that size in the nodulus, the oldest cortical part of the cerebellum, contains 1070 granule cells, whereas in the vermal parts of the anterior and posterior lobes the corresponding number is 1550. Besides these differences in the vermal parts, there are also distinct differences between the vermis and the hemispheres. The number of granule cells per unit volume in the hemispheres is always greater than in the vermis, as is to be seen in Fig. 1.

The differences in cell density between the vermal parts and the hemispheres are similarly developed in the other cortical layers, namely the Purkinje cell layer and the molecular layer. However, the number of cells per 0.001 mm^3 is much lower than in the granular layer: 600 Purkinje cells and 200 interneurones are found per 0.001 mm^3 in the Purkinje cell layer of the nodulus, whereas in the other vermal parts the number of Purkinje cells and interneurones is slightly higher. The differences are statistically significant in all cases. Even in the molecular layer, where cytoarchitectural differences are not so easily detectable because of the low cell density, a similar architectonic principle is retained. Again the cell density in the hemispheres of the cerebellum is higher than in the vermal parts and is lowest in the nodulus, the oldest vermal lobe. The following conclusions on regional differences in the cytoarchitectonics of the cerebellar cortex can be drawn from the previous brief statements.

(a) In the younger parts of the cerebellar cortex a diminution principle, which Haug has already referred to in 1967 as the granulating principle of the cortex cerebri, can be demonstrated in all three layers of the cerebellar cortex. Cells in the younger parts diminish in size where granular layers occur, such as in the stratum granulosum of the cerebellum. These findings are not restricted to man, they are also demonstrable in the rhesus monkey and cat as well and represent a structural principle in all mammals.

(b) Simultaneously, the increase in number of all cell types in the younger parts of the cerebellum is a basic structural principle of the cerebellar cortex. Diminishing size and increasing numbers of cells probably raise the possible number of connections between the individual cellular elements and thus significantly raise the effectiveness of the cortex as an integrating organ.

Hence, considerable differences in the cytoarchitectonics of the cerebellum of mammals can be detected after a quantitative analysis. This is stated in two rarely considered criteria of Vogt's definition of a cytoarchitectural unit: Namely the number and size of cells.

At this stage, I would like to present some results obtained by my co-worker Dr. Heinsen, that reinforce the idea of a regional cytoarchitecture of the cerebellar cortex. From the onset of histology, the Purkinje cells were considered to be lipophobic without a detectable trace of lipopigments. Once again this statement was emphatically confirmed by Friede [4]. Possibly this assumption is based on the fact that animals used for laboratory investigations were too young. My co-worker Dr. Heinsen has been able to detect considerable amounts of lipopigments in the Purkinje cells of three-year-old senescent rats (Fig. 4). This lipopigment exhibits fluorescence when stimulated by UV light. A quantitative evaluation of the amount of lipofuscin in Purkinje cells in various parts of the cerebellum proves that the lipofuscin occupies approximately 4% of the total volume of the perikaryon in the vermal part of the lobus nodulofloccularis, whereas in the vermal parts of lobule V it amounts to approximately 12.5% of the volume of the perikaryon. These results, obtained from

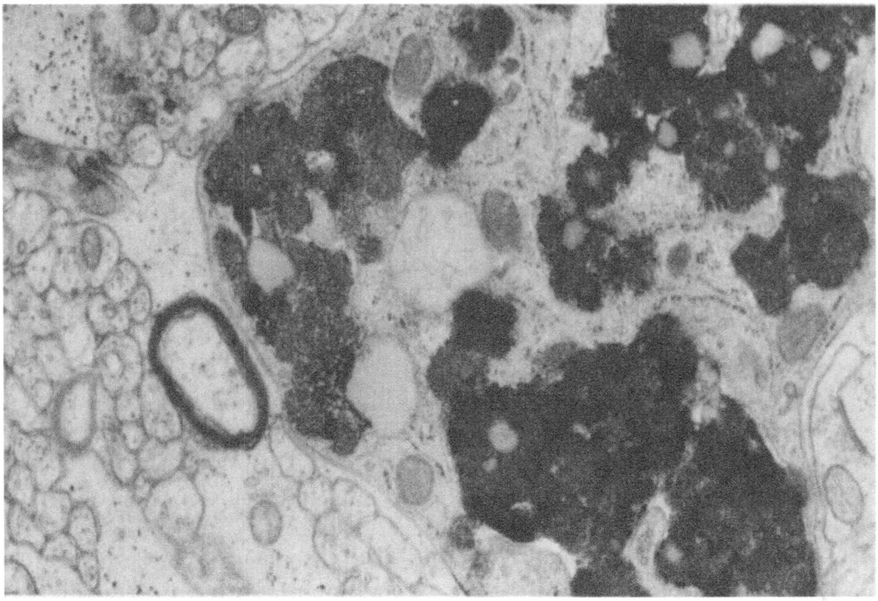

Fig. 4. Lipofuscin in a Purkinje cell of a 3-year-old senescent rat. ×13 600

light microscopic investigations, indicate that, at least the amount and the intracytoplasmatic distribution of lipofuscin in Purkinje cells of different lobules vary considerably. Furthermore an ultrastructural analysis of the pigment in the previously mentioned parts of the cerebellum shows that it can be differentiated in various parts of the cerebellum. The lipofuscin of the Purkinje cells in lobule V shows considerably larger vacuoles which, apart from the not very electron-dense matrix, seem to contain some other substances obviously extracted during preparation. The reason for the varying accumulation of this pigment in different parts of the cerebellar cortex so far is unknown. However, in this context I would like to point out that research into regional peculiarities of metabolism within the cerebellum is only beginning and further evidence probably may lead to a classification of the cerebellar cortex in the future.

The differences in the cytoarchitectonics and pigmentarchitectonics of Purkinje cells, that have been described so far, are not yet sufficient to subdivide the cerebellar cortex according to function. It seems to be necessary to take into consideration not only the differences in the number of granule cells and Purkinje cells but also the distribution of real interneurones such as the Golgi cells, the function of which in the intracortical circuit has been understood in principle since Cajal [2], and in detail since the investigations of Palay and Chan-Palay [19] and Eccles et al. [3].

The Golgi cell axons end with inhibitory synapses on the granule cells. The recurrent collaterals of the Purkinje cells end on the Golgi cells with inhibitory synapses, whereas mossy fibres, climbing fibres, and granule cell axons end on the Golgi cells with excitatory synapses. In this way they are connected with the afferent arc of the mossy and climbing fibres and can modulate the intracortical circuit in many ways. The Golgi cell is a cell type with six to eight dendrites and one axon. In normal Golgi preparations (Fig. 5a), the dendrites appear smooth over large distances; at some points swellings are visible, but in the silver impregnations it cannot be decided whether these are glial sheets or, as is more likely, synaptic swellings. The dendritic arborization is very wide ranging and overlapping between two Golgi cell territories often occurs.

Golgi cells can be distinguished in semi-thin sections (Fig. 5b) from karyochromic granule cells by their pale nucleus and the finely folded nuclear membrane. This large type of Golgi cell, mainly found in the granular layer, below the Purkinje cell layer, does not seem to be the only representative of this cell type. Golgi cells, far smaller than those shown here and with unpleated nuclear membranes, are found in the medullary regions of the granular layer as well as in the Purkinje cell layer. The processes of these Golgi cells are not very long and mostly end in the molecular layer.

Elsewhere Golgi cells are found in the central medullary rays of the folia (Fig. 5c). They are very similar to the Golgi cells in the granular layer. In silver-stained material processes often extend from one folium to another. They are probably identical to the synarmotic cells, described by Landau [13].

In the electron microscope (Fig. 5d), Golgi cells also have a characteristic form. The indentations of the nuclear membrane, that lead readily to identification under the electron microscope, are even more obvious. The cytoplasm is not very electron dense, the Golgi apparatus is very distinct, and the ergastoplasm is lightly distributed over the whole cell body. Occasionally lipofuscin granules can be observed.

A comparison of the size of granule cells in different vermal and hemispherical parts of the three cerebellar lobes (Fig. 2) shows a number of larger cell nuclei especially in the vermis of the lobus noduloflocculáris, marked by a solid line in this illustration.

The diameter of these cell nuclei varies considerably from that of the granule cells and is identical to that of the Golgi cells.

The size distribution diagram of the granule cells in the corresponding hemispherical part, the broken line in the diagram, shows no such appendix. This finding is not restricted to the lobus noduloflocculáris, but is also true for the posterior lobe, where a number of larger cell nuclei, identical to those of the Golgi cells, are found in the vermal part as well. Only the size distribution diagram for the anterior lobe shows no such appendix, the absence of which would suggest the occurrence of only a small number of Golgi cells.

Systematic counts in the vermal and hemispherical parts show the presence of approximately 700 Golgi cells per 0.001 mm^3 in the vermal parts of the posterior lobe, but only about half that number in the corresponding hemispherical part. In the vermal part of the anterior lobe, about 550 Golgi cells per 0.001 mm^3 are found with only 350 cells per 0.001 mm^3 in the corresponding hemispherical parts. Thus, a distinct difference exists between the vermis and hemispheres in all cerebellar lobes. The schematic diagram in Fig. 6 shows these quantitative relationships in the distribution of Golgi cells even more distinctly.

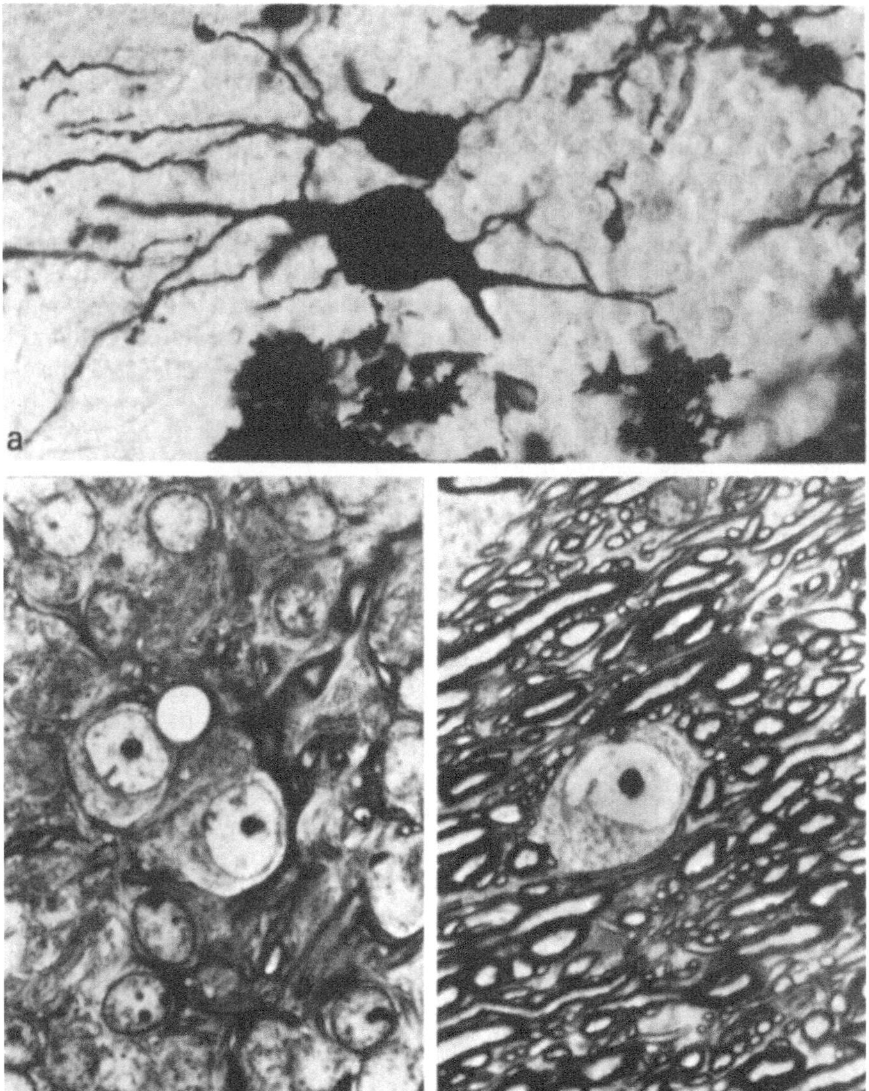

Fig. 5. **a** Golgi cell in the granule layer of the cat. Golgi-Bubenaite impregnation. ×800. **b** Golgi cell in the cerebellar cortex of the cat. The infoldings of the nuclear membrane are visible. ×1300. **c** Golgi cell in the central medullary ray of the nodulus. ×1300

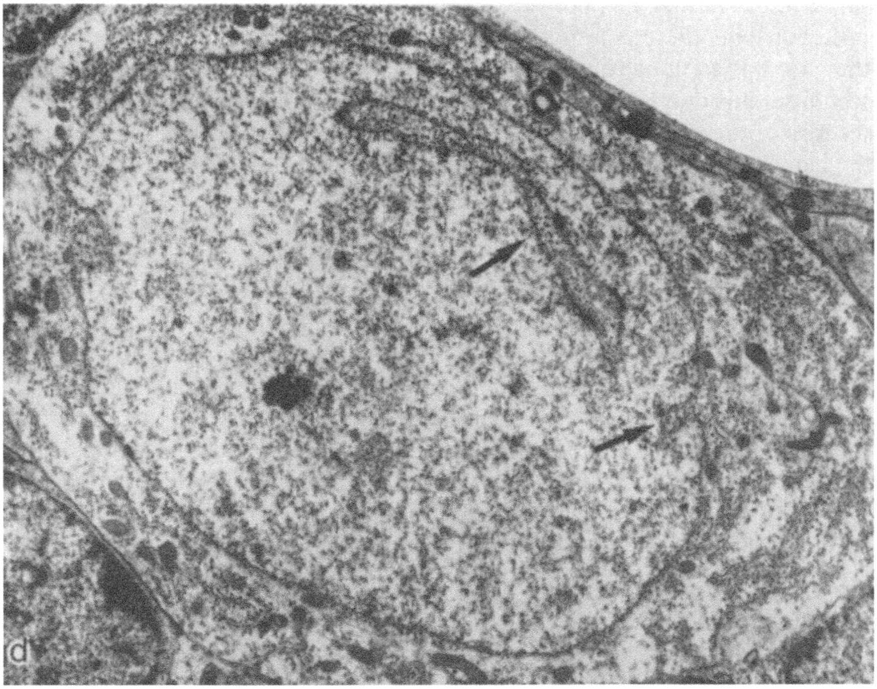

Fig. 5. d Golgi cell in the cerebellar cortex of the rat. The *arrows* indicate the infoldings of the nuclear membrane. ×6300

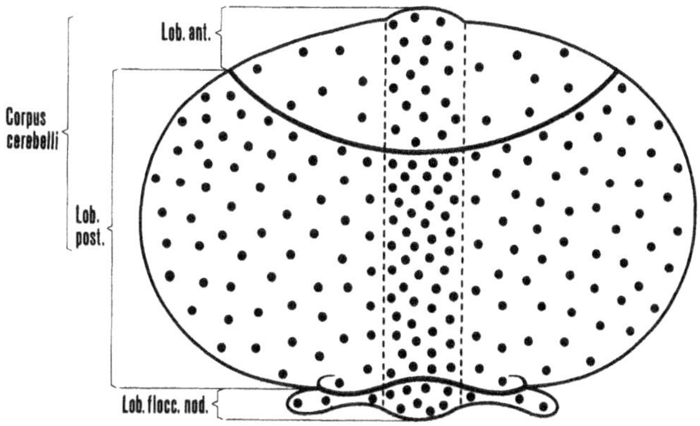

Fig. 6. Schematic diagram showing the distribution of Golgi cells in the mammalian cerebellar cortex. Note the high number of Golgi cells in the inferior vermal parts and the lower cell density in the vermal parts of the anterior lobe and in the hemispheres

In the lower vermis, i.e., the vermal part of the lobus noduloflocculàris and the posterior lobe, there is a high number of Golgi cells in the granular layer, but they are not as numerous in the upper vermal lobes. Furthermore, it can be seen from this diagram that statistically significant differences exist between all sections of the vermis and the hemispheres. Thus, the number of Golgi cells in the hemisphere of the lobus noduloflocculàris and the posterior lobe is greater than in the hemispherical part of the anterior lobe.

At this point I would like to digress slightly. It is necessary to state that the relationships described up to now are mainly based on the human cerebellum. Beginning from Goethe's and also Oken's idealistic morphology, comparative anatomy and especially comparative neuroanatomy has not lost any actuality because it has highly influenced and enriched the theory of descent. This train of thought probably led Immanuel Kant to describe the human being as a "being in itself", which is not comparable to anything else. The neuroanatomist, especially the comparative neuroanatomist, is forced in the interest of human self-understanding to describe and understand the reasons or structural changes during phylogenesis, which make the human brain a "being in itself", according to Oken perhaps the most perfect form occurring in the natural world. Solely studying the human brain obstructs the view of the special evolutionary result, which human brain development has achieved in the history of mammalian phylogenesis.

For this reason, I would like to describe shortly a few other results which in my view show the unique structure of the cerebellum and which will be a warning against generalizing interspecifically from intraspecific results without other considerations.

Studying the ratio of Purkinje cells to granule cells in 20 different mammals, we obtained the following relationships as seen in Table 1. In humans, approxi-

Table 1. Ratio of Purkinje cells to granule cells in man and some other mammals

Man (*Homo sapiens*)	1 : 2991
Vervet monkey (*Cercopithecus aethiops*)	1 : 2128
Rhesus monkey (*Macaca mulatta*)	1 : 1896
Elephant (*Loxodonta africana*)	1 : 1866
Squirrel monkey (*Saimiri sciureus*)	1 : 1864
Bottle-nose dolphin (*Tursiops truncatus*)	1 : 1812
Pilot whale (*Globicephala macrorhyncha*)	1 : 1790
Common porpoise (*Phocaena phocaena*)	1 : 1762
Fox (*Vulpes vulpes*)	1 : 1739
Horse (*Equus caballus*)	1 : 1612
Cat (*Felis domestica*)	1 : 1580
Sheep (*Ovis aries*)	1 : 1568
Bull (*Bos taurus*)	1 : 1508
Guinea pig (*Cavia cabava*)	1 : 959
Opossum (*Didelphys virginiana*)	1 : 952
Rabbit (*Oryctolagus cuniculus*)	1 : 931
Rat (*Rattus norvegicus*)	1 : 897
Mouse (*Mus musculus domesticus*)	1 : 778
Mole (*Talpa europaea*)	1 : 706
Hedgehog (*Erinaceus europaeus*)	1 : 609

mately 3000 granule cells are found for each Purkinje cell, whereas in all other species studied, the ratio is in favour of the Purkinje cells. At best, ratios comparable to those found in humans occur in monkeys and aquatic mammals. Thus, during evolution, the number of interneurons, and granule cells may be considered as such, has increased and enabled differentiated propagation of stimuli in the cortex. With increasing degree of brain organization, the same principle can be detected using a different cell type, namely the Golgi cell. Whereas in the mole and hedgehog six Purkinje cells occur for each Golgi cell, there are only three in rhesus monkeys and cats, and only two Purkinje cells occur for each Golgi cell in the human. The intracortical circuit in less evolved species is possibly not so finely modulated as in the rhesus monkey, the cat or human being because of the poor ratio of Purkinje cells to Golgi cells.

From these two examples we can see that the unique structure of the human brain can nowadays well be attributed to quantitative cytological conditions, allowing us an insight into the degree of organization in the human brain. This very narrow insight, however, still does not answer the question which every comparative neuroanatomist always asks himself, when studying identical brain parts from different species under the microscope: Whence has the human being come and where will it lead? The daily comparative efforts contribute to better self-understanding and fans the flame of curiosity to search for answers to these questions.

I shall now describe briefly another cell population. In considering the cerebellar cortex, the nerve cells are usually given preference, whereas the glial cells are rarely included in research about regional varieties. An exact analysis of the myeloarchitectonics, and an assessment of the oligodendroglia can only be developed by this method, shows that the plexus supraganglionaris in various parts of the cerebellum is dissimilarly developed. In 1967 Eccles et al. [3] still assumed that the plexus supraganglionaris consisted only of one fibre population, namely the recurrent collaterals of the Purkinje cells because there are no other myelinated fibres, except the Cajal-Smirnov fibres, in the molecular layer.

My own research in the past few years has shown [14, 15] in contrast to this assumption, that the plexus supraganglionaris is almost exclusively composed of myelinated parallel fibres (Fig. 7 a, b), whereas recurrent collaterals represent only a minority in this plexus. But a myelinated fibre population can only be built up if the number of oligodendrocytes is sufficiently increased during the corresponding maturing process. It seemed logical to determine the number of oligodendrocytes in various areas of the cerebellum in the lower third of the molecular layer. It was soon obvious, that few oligodendrocytes are found in parts such as the nodulus, where the plexus supraganglionaris is sparsely developed, whereas this cell type is very numerous in the vermis and hemispherical parts of the anterior lobe. These differences were significant in all three species examined, namely humans, rhesus monkeys, and cats. In this context, I would like to point out that this outline of a regional glia architecture of the cerebellar cortex cannot be generalized or taken as a general structural principle. I can only reemphasize the statement made by Cajal [2] that the plexus supraganglionaris shows very strong interspecific differences, unlike any other structure

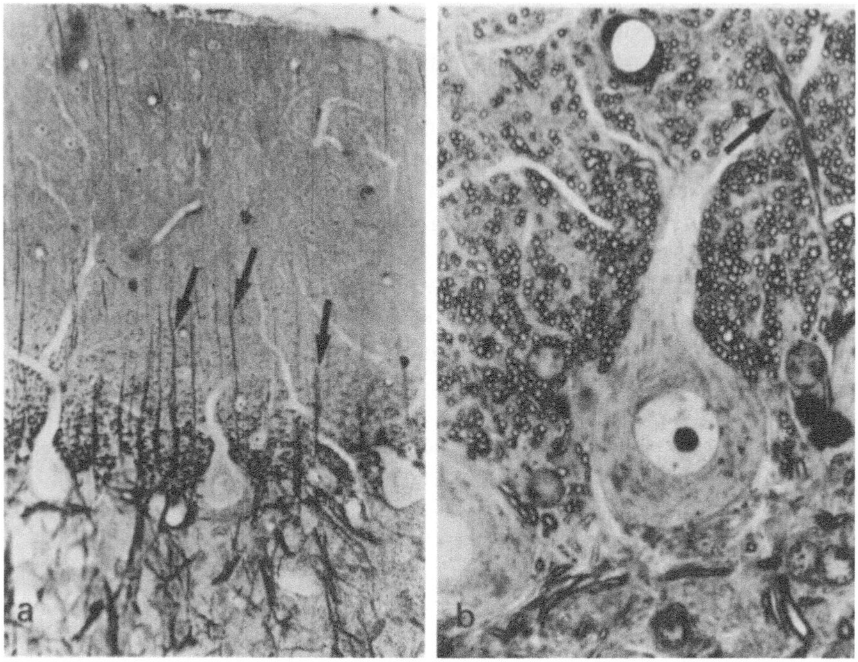

Fig. 7. **a** Cerebellar cortex of the rhesus monkey, vermal part of lobule VIII. The supraganglionic plexus is well developed. Note the bundles (*arrow*) of myelinated granule cell axons, which traverse the plexus to the molecular layer. ×380. **b** The supraganglionic plexus consists of fibers of nearly equal diameter. Note the ascending myelinated fiber (*arrow*). ×2300

in the cerebellar cortex. For this reason, the prospects for further progress on the subject of a regional classification of oligodendroglia are not very promising.

On the other hand, some new results on astroglia from my co-worker Dr. Heinsen, justify new expectations.

Bergmann cells, which according to ultrastructural results can be classified as astroglia, show some peculiarities in the nodulus and the adjoining folium of the uvula. Regular inclusions of pigment particles in the astroglia of these parts can be detected with a phase contrast microscope, whereas they have not been detected in other parts of the cerebellum. Unfortunately the chemical analysis of these pigments is still lacking. This result, however, can be generalized as these inclusions have been observed on very fresh human material. This survey of the regional cytoarchitectonic classification of the cerebellar cortex may be, compared to the very detailed mapping of the telencephalic cortex worked out by Brodmann, rated as a modest attempt to establish a regional differentiation of the cerebellar cortex that is justified by physiological evidence.

References

1. Brodmann K (1909) Vergleichende Lokalisationslehre der Großhirnrinde. Barth, Leipzig
2. Cajal SRY (1911) Histologie du système nerveux de l'Homme et des Vertébrés vols I and II. Maloine, Paris. Translated by L Azoulay
3. Eccles J, Ito M, Szentagothai J (1967) The cerebellum as a neuronal machine. Springer, Berlin Heidelberg New York
4. Friede RL (1962) The relation of the formation of lipofuscin to the distribution of the oxidative enzymes in the human brain. Acta Neuropathol (Berl) 2:113–125
5. Haug H (1967) Zytoarchitektonische Untersuchungen an der Hirnrinde des Elefanten. Anat Anz 120:331–337
6. Hochstetter F (1929) Beiträge zur Entwicklungsgeschichte des menschlichen Gehirns. Deuticke, Vienna Leipzig
7. Korneliussen HK (1968) On the ontogenetic development of the cerebellum (nuclei, fissures and cortex) of the rat, with special reference to regional variations in corticogenesis. J Hirnforsch 10:379–413
8. Landau E (1927) Beitrag zur Kenntnis der Körnerschicht des Kleinhirns. Vorläufige Mitteilung. Anat Anz 62:391–398
9. Landau E (1928) Zweiter Beitrag zur Kenntnis der Körnerschicht des Kleinhirns. Anat Anz 65:89–93
10. Landau E (1928) Über cytoarchitektonische Bauunterschiede in der Körnerschicht des Kleinhirns. Z Anat Entwicklungsgesch 87:551–557
11. Landau E (1929) Einige Worte über die Nervenzellen der Körnerschicht des Kleinhirns. Z Gesamte Neurol Psychiat 122:450–451
12. Landau E (1952) Zur Cytoarchitektonik des Kleinhirns. Dtsch Z Nervenheilkd 124:182–184
13. Landau E (1933) La cellule synarmotique dans le cervelet humain. Arch Anat 17:273–285
14. Lange W (1972) Über regionale Unterschiede in der Myeloarchitektonik der Kleinhirnrinde. Z Zellforsch 134:129–142
15. Lange W (1976) The myelinated parallel fibers of the cerebellar cortex and their regional distribution. Cell Tissue Res 166:489–496
16. Larsell O (1934) Morphogenesis and evolution of the cerebellum. Arch Neurol 31:373–395
17. Larsell O (1947) The development of the cerebellum in man in relation to its comparative anatomy. J comp Neurol 87:85–130
18. Larsell O (1954) The development of the cerebellum of the pig. Anat Rec 118:73–108
19. Palay S, Chan-Palay V (1974) Cerebellar Cortex. Cytology and Organization. Springer, Berlin Heidelberg New York
20. Vogt C, Vogt O (1928) Die Grundlagen und die Teildisziplinen der mirkoskopischen Anatomie des Zentralnervensystems. In: Nervensystem. Springer, Berlin Heidelberg New York (Handbuch der mikroskopischen Anatomie des Menschen, vol 4/1, pp 448–477)

Discussion

Balazs: Do you have any indication that there are different populations or kinds of Golgi cells?

Lange: These are best described in the atlas of Drs. Palay and Chan-Palay as large and small cells.

Balazs: Yes, but is there any indication that there are differences in the distribution of either type in different parts of the cerebellum?

Lange: No, I counted the number of Golgi cells per unit volume, but they were not separated into two types.

Gould: Some people have described rather large interstitial cells in the central white matter. Do these correspond to your displaced Golgi cells? They are AChE-positive.
Lange: There are species differences. They are large and numerous in the opossum and although present in the monkey, they are smaller. In silver impregnations their processes cross between the medullary rays.
Gould: Are these Golgi cells?
Lange: Yes, I think so.
Voogd: There is an old paper by Ogawa on aquatic mammals in which there is a layer of cells below the granular layer. I thought they were more related to the central nuclei rather than to the Golgi cell.
Lange: In my material (whales and dolphins) I could not see these cells. Perhaps they are present in sea lions as described by Ogawa, but they are not present in my material.
Voogd: Then I wanted to make a remark regarding the difference in sizes of the axons of Purkinje cells. There is a certain medial-lateral transition from large ones to small ones, then large again within the hemisphere. Could you see differences within the hemispheres?
Lange: No, I did not measure these. I only measured the most lateral part of the hemisphere and compared them to the medial vermal zones.
Simpson: In your talk you equated the vermal part of the cerebellum with the paleocerebellum and the lateral part with the neocerebellum. But, there seems to be a problem regarding the flocculus. That is a phylogenetically old part of the cerebellum, but it is really more like the neocerebellum in terms of cell density.
Lange: I never thought that the flocculus would be a phylogenetic young part of the cerebellum, but as you say this is true based on cell density.
Ito: I am curious about the functional implications of the myelinated parallel fibers. Do you find any special distribution of them?
Lange: In the vermal parts of the anterior lobe, this plexus is very dense. It is sparsely developed in the nodulus and the posterior lobe.
Ito: Are these related to spinal inputs?
Lange: I don't know.
Voogd: Why, the question?
Mugnaini: Because they come from granule cells.
Voogd: But, why spinal?
Ito: I am recalling Dr. Altman's slide in which he indicated that spinal afferents project to the deep granule cell layer.
Voogd: But spinal cerebellar fibers terminate throughout the granular layer from deep to superficial, so it can not be true.
Palay: Some years ago, W. J. Brown and I found a differential distribution of AChE in the cerebellum. No specific function could be attributed to this observation. However, there is much more in the posterior lobe than the anterior lobe and much less in the hemisphere than in the vermis. In addition to this comment, I would like to emphasize the differences in the number and sizes of cells which suggest differences in the number of terminals and lengths of axons. These data provide the basis for a word of caution to people who are making

measurements in the cerebellum and then constructing models of how the cerebellar circuitry should be conceived. Such models have to be quite restricted to a single lobe or perhaps a specific cubic millimeter of tissue in a particular species.

Lange: This is true. For example the ratio of P cells to granular cells and Golgi cells varies from mammal to mammal and inhibition in the higher developed brains is stronger. So such findings cannot be generalized.

Palay: Just to follow up on that, when you go through the literature and try to collect numbers such as the ratio of P cells to granule cells or even the number of granule cells, tremendous and unexplained discrepancies exist between different authors even using the same species. I wonder if this could be due to the fact that not everyone is looking at the corresponding spots in the cerebellar cortex.

Lange: Probably that and there are different methods of counting cells and various methods of histological preparation as well as different factors used for correcting the numbered sample. Most of these differences in the literature, however, can be corrected when these factors are properly considered.

Llinas: Before casting any big doubts on these generalizations, it would be nice to have more information on the cytology of these cells. Basically what I have heard is that the numbers of nuclei are different. Do you have any measurements of the telodendria of Golgi cell axons in different parts of the cortex or the length of the parallel fibers. These may be even more important to the physiology than the actual numbers.

Lange: Not yet.

Altman: Some 20 years ago Brodal showed different kinds of mossy fibers in the vestibulocerebellum. This could make a difference in the packing density.

Mugnaini: I would like to comment on the length of parallel fibers in the cat. We have measured parallel fibers in the anterior lobe, posterior lobe, and paramedian lobule. There are conspicuous differences in the length and pattern of distribution in parallel fibers. In the paramedian lobules, for example, they were much shorter.

Altman: Dr. Lange, was your implication that as we ascend in the phylogenetic scale there is an increase in the proportion of interneurons? You would probably also predict that the dendritic arbor becomes more complex.

Lange: Yes, this is true.

The Cerebropontocerebellar Pathway: Salient Features of Its Organization

P. Brodal

Introduction

Among the various afferent pathways to the cerebellum, the one arising in the pontine nuclei is particularly prominent in higher mammals. The size of the pontine nuclei furthermore undergoes a dramatic absolute and relative increase in parallel with the growth of the cerebellar hemispheres during evolution. The vast majority of *afferents to the pontine nuclei* arise in the cerebral cortex; only minor contingents come from other sources such as the colliculi and the intracerebellar nuclei. Also, from the point of view of the cerebellar role in motor control, the connections from the cerebral cortex are of particular interest. In order to understand the kind of information conveyed from the cerebral cortex to the cerebellum, a detailed knowledge of the anatomy of the corticopontocerebellar pathway seems essential; only against such a background can physiological data be soundly interpreted. Other pathways from the cerebral cortex to the cerebellum, synaptically interrupted in the reticular tegmental nucleus of Bechterew, the lateral reticular nucleus, and certain other cell groups, are quantitatively less important. These nuclei also differ anatomically from the pontine nuclei in several respects, for example, in the types of dendritic arborizations and in that only the pontine nuclei receive their main inputs from the cerebral cortex.

During the last decade a large number of anatomical studies have been devoted to the corticopontocerebellar pathway in several species. Most of these studies have dealt with the first link in the pathway, the corticopontine projection, mainly with the use of degeneration techniques, but to some extent also with anterograde axonal transport of radioactively labeled amino acids. Only recently, with the use of retrograde axonal transport of horseradish peroxidase (HRP) has it become possible to study the pontocerebellar projection in comparable detail. Such studies are presently pursued in several laboratories, partly in conjunction with studies of the corticopontine projection in the same animals. New information concerning the intrinsic organization of the pontine nuclei has also been provided by Golgi studies and electron microscopic investigations during the last 10–15 years. The following account will be limited to recent anatomical results, particularly such that indicate general principles of organization; it does not pretend to give a complete review of the subject. Furthermore, the emphasis will be on conditions in primates, as far as such data are available, and the illustrations will be from my own research in the cat and monkey. For reviews dealing with the cerebropontocerebellar pathway see refs. 3, 7, 44, and 63.

Experimental Brain Research, Suppl. 6

Origin of the Corticopontine Projection

It has been customary to say that the corticopontine projection arises in most parts of the cerebral cortex, that is, in all sensory receiving areas, in the motor cortex, and in the "association areas". Furthermore, it is usually tacitly assumed that projections from these various regions are quantitatively of about equal importance. This notion probably stems from older studies with the Marchi method and of human pathological material; such methods give only limited quantitative information and the emphasis was therefore mainly on the question of whether or not a certain part of the cortex projects to the pontine nuclei. However, the use of more sensitive methods has revealed that only relatively minor parts of the cortex project *heavily* onto the pontine nuclei (Fig. 1). Although not all parts of the cortex have been explored it seems safe to say that *in the monkey* the majority of fibers arise in the pericentral cortex, that is Brodman's areas 6, 4, 3, 1, 2, and 5. Among these, the motor and somatosensory areas clearly contribute most [18, 27, 64]. A heavy projection also arises in parts of the visual cortex [18], while a more modest contribution comes from the second somatosensory area [64]. Only relatively scant projections arise in the prefrontal cortex, area 7 and the temporal lobe. Conditions are similar in the cat [10–16, 24, 50, 58], although it appears that a relatively larger proportion of fibers arise in parietal association areas and regions surrounding the visual cortex than is the case in the monkey [15, 50]. In fact, the scarcity in primates of pontine projections from what are usually called association areas calls for revision of some concepts of cerebrocerebellar cooperation [see ref. 63]. Thus, the available evidence indicates that among association areas, only area 5 has a substantial pontine projection [18]. (If area 6 is grouped with association areas, its pontine projection appears to be slightly less heavy than that from area 5.) Even from subdivisions of one functional region, such as the somatosensory, the visual, and the auditory cortices, the intensity of projection varies considerably. Thus, the pontine projection is more intense from the motor cortex than from the somatosensory cortex in the monkey (Fig. 1A), and the same is true in the cat for the projection from the posterior part of the sensorimotor cortex (posterior to the postcruciate dimple, Fig. 1B). Furthermore, the pontine projection from the part of the cat sensorimotor cortex representing the face (coronal gyrus) is much less than from the parts representing the forelimb and hindlimb (Fig. 1B). The pontine projection from the cat visual cortex also emanates preponderantly only from certain parts (Fig. 1C). Lesions or injections of tritiated leucine of central parts of areas 17, 18, and most likely area 19 reveal consistently sparse or no pontine termination while lesions or injections affecting regions representing peripheral parts of the visual field show heavy pontine termination [14, 15, 58]. An electrophysiological study by Albus and Donate-Oliver [2] supports the finding that few pontine fibers emanate from central parts of area 17.

In the monkey, the relative density of pontine projections from different parts of the visual cortex has not been worked out in comparable detail. However, in the macaque large lesions of the parts of areas 17 and 18 situated on the convexity, that is, representing central parts of the visual field, produced only sparse pontine degeneration, while a small lesion of area 19 on the medial surface of the hemisphere (presumably representing peripheral parts of the visual field) gave heavy degeneration [18]. Nyby and Jansen [52] found with the Marchi method heavy pontine degeneration following a lesion affecting mainly area 18 on the medial wall. Thus, it seems likely that also in the monkey pontine fibers from the visual cortex arise predominantly from parts representing peripheral parts of the visual field. However, this question deserves further study. As a final example of quantitative differences, pontine projections from the cat's auditory cortex arise mainly in area AII, while very few fibers emanate from areas AI and Ep [16, 42].

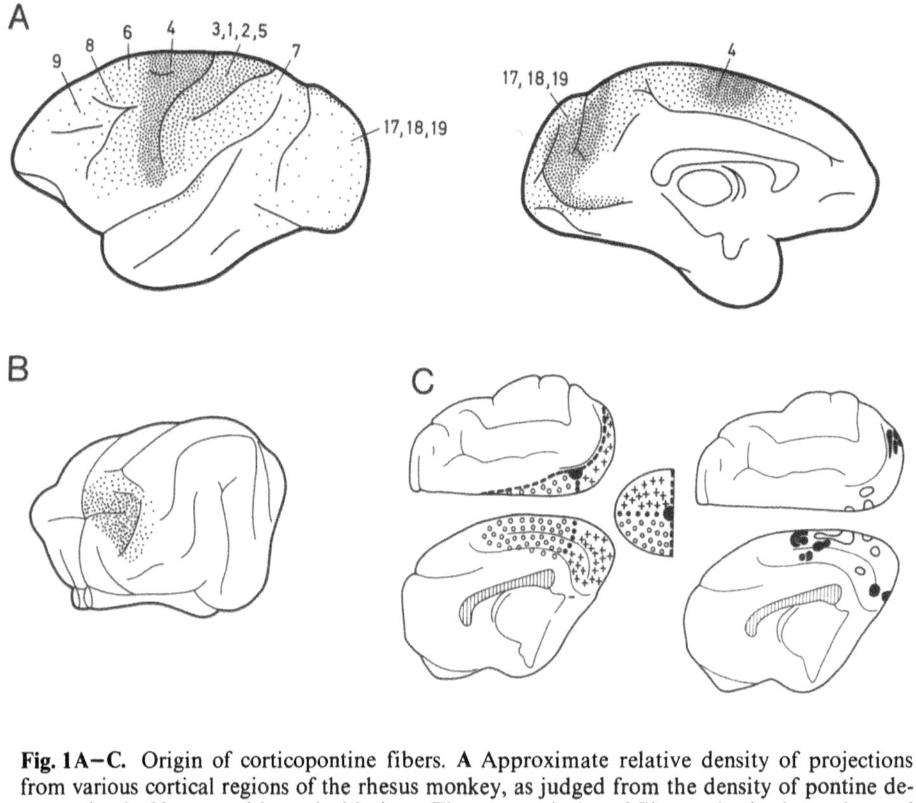

Fig. 1A–C. Origin of corticopontine fibers. **A** Approximate relative density of projections from various cortical regions of the rhesus monkey, as judged from the density of pontine degeneration in 38 cases with cortical lesions. The vast majority of fibers arise in the pericentral region, including the premotor cortex (area 6) and area 5. Note that among the association areas only area 5 has a substantial pontine projection. A dense projection also arises in parts of the visual cortex, cf. text. Brodal [18]. **B** The relative density of projections from various parts of the cat's sensorimotor cortex. The posterior part (posterior to the postcruciate dimple) has a less dense projection than anterior parts (compare with similar difference between projections from pre- and postcentral gyri in Fig. 1A.) The projection from the face region (coronal gyrus) is less intense than that arising in the regions representing the extremities. Brodal [10]. **C** The relative density of corticopontine fibers from various parts of the cat's striate area (area 17). Lesions shown in *black* gave rise to dense pontine degeneration while lesions shown in *outline* produced only sparse degeneration. Note the correspondence between the representation of the peripheral visual field and location of lesions in *black* (cf. text). Brodal [14]

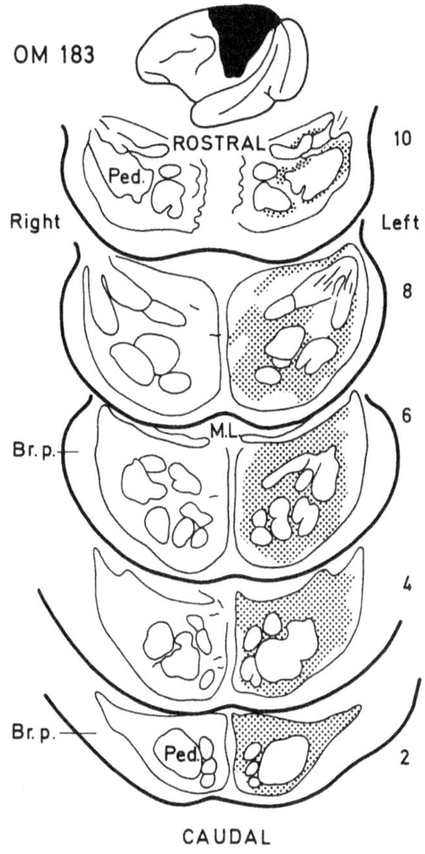

Fig. 2. The distribution of pontine degeneration after a unilateral lesion (*black*) mainly comprising the sensorimotor cortex and area 5 of a rhesus monkey. The premotor cortex is not involved. The degeneration is entered as *dots* in drawings of coronal sections through the pons. Note that only minor parts of the pontine nuclei are free from degeneration. The free parts receive fibers mainly from regions in front of the lesion and from the occipital lobe, see Fig. 5. Brodal [18]

The quantitative differences discussed above suggest that the types of information sent from the cerebral cortex to the cerebellum might be less diverse than previously held. Particularly in the monkey, the preponderance of projections from the central region, which also gives origin to the bulk of corticospinal fibers, is conspicuous. Figure 2 illustrates that only minor parts of the pontine nuclei are free from degeneration after a lesion comprising large parts of the motor and somatosensory areas and area 5. It seems likely – and perhaps self-evident – that mainly cortical neurons related to aspects of *movement* would project to the pontine nuclei. However, only with regard to the visual cortex has this been proved by recording from single corticopontine cells in area 18 [32]. In area 5 of the monkey, many cells are active immediately before certain types of movements [45, 51], but the properties of neurons in area 5 projecting to the pontine nuclei have apparently not been studied. In the somatosensory cortex, many cells are activated preferentially by moving stimuli on the skin, by joint rotation, and from muscle spindle afferents, but again the properties of cells projecting to the pontine nuclei are not known.

Horseradish peroxidase injections in the pont' nuclei have given further evidence of the nonuniform distribution of corticopontine neurons [41, 42]. Thus,

A

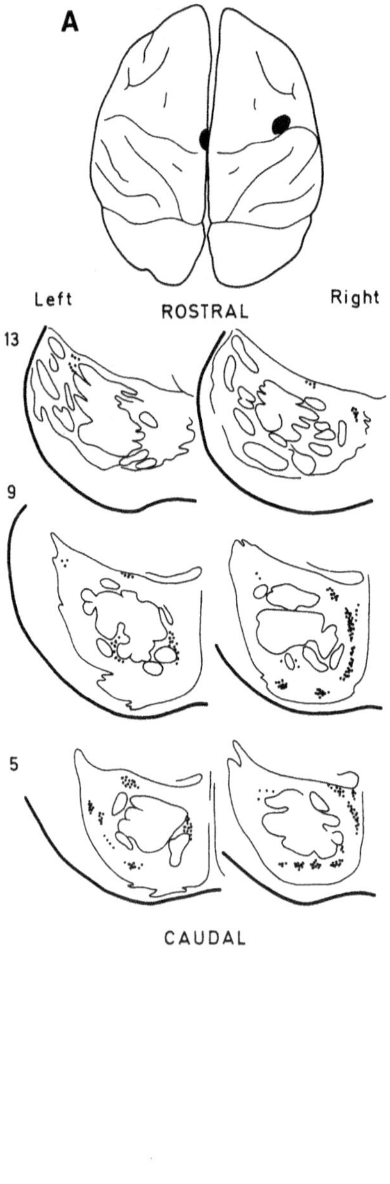

Fig. 3. **A** A case with small, bilateral lesions of the motor cortex which illustrates several typical features of the corticipontine projection. The degeneration is entered as *dots* in drawings of transverse sections of the pons. The drawings of the right halves of the pons have been turned around to facilitate comparisons of the two sides. Note the patchy distribution of degeneration, the tendency to form bands (lamellae), and the different distribution on the two sides, showing the somatotopical pattern. Brodal [18]

Fig. 3 B–D. Photomicrographs of patches and bands of degeneration from the experiment illustrated in **A**. Note the high density of degeneration and the sharp borders towards normal neuropile. The *bar* in each photomicrograph represents 100 μm. Wiitanen [65] method. Survival time 6 days

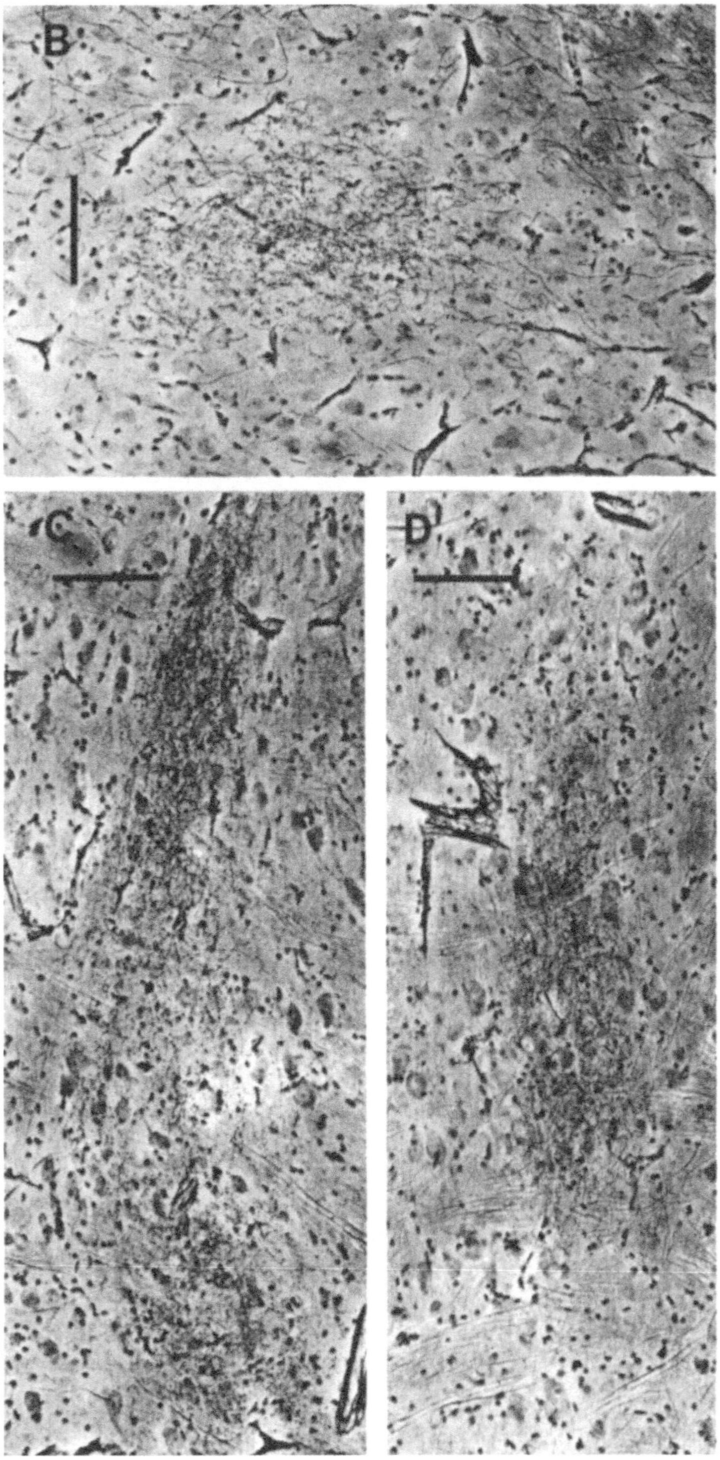
B
C
D

after a small pontine injection in the monkey, labeled cells tended to occur in several narrow bands (0.5–1 mm) extending mediolaterally [41]. The functional significance of this arrangement, which is found also in other cortical efferent connections, is not clear. Nevertheless, it seems compatible with the notion that only cells with certain functional characteristics send information to the cerebellum via the pontine nuclei, as is also the observation that, on the whole, different populations of cortical neurons project to various subcortical structures, such as the thalamus, basal ganglia, and the pontine nuclei [41]. Furthermore, only for a few (15%) of the pontine neurons excited by stimulation of the sensorimotor cortex did this appear to occur by way of collaterals of corticospinal neurons [56].

From a simple quantitative point of view, it is obvious that only a tiny fraction of afferents to the pontine nuclei can be collaterals of corticospinal fibers: In man, the number of corticospinal fibers on one side is approximately 1 million, while there are probably about 18 million corticopontine fibers [62].

Principles of Termination of Corticopontine Fibers

A number of studies with degeneration techniques and autoradiographic tracing methods in the cat [10, 11, 14, 24, 50, 58], rat [23, 48, 66], and monkey [18, 27, 52, 64], have shown that even a very small part of the cortex sends fibers to widely separated parts of the pontine nuclei. For example, a lesion of the cat's sensorimotor cortex less than ½ mm in diameter will give rise to degeneration in several discrete places [10, 16]. Another important feature is the termination in patches, bands or column-like regions, often with remarkably sharp borders (Figs. 3, 4). Obviously, such a pattern poses formidable problems when trying to determine the degree of precision and specificity in the projection. However, anatomical experiments in the cat, monkey, and, to some extent, also in the rat show that projections from major cortical regions, such as sensorimotor, premotor, visual, and auditory areas, terminate in largely different parts of the pontine nuclei (Figs. 4, 5, 6). In the monkey there is a rough mediolateral sequence of termination in the pontine nuclei as one moves from frontal to occipital and temporal parts of the hemisphere (Figs. 5, 6A), and the pontine terminal regions tend to form lamellae. The overall picture seen in transverse sections resembles the skin of an onion, with the sensorimotor cortex represented in a large core (Figs. 5, 6). The scheme presented by Nyby and Jansen [52] and by Wiesendanger et al. [64] for the monkey agrees with the one in Fig. 6A on the main points.

In the cat, the lamella-like pattern is less clear. More important, however, is that the mediolateral topography is much less clear-cut than in the monkey and that certain cortical regions project to strikingly different pontine regions in the cat and monkey (Figs. 4, 5, 7). The corticopontine topography in the rat appears, at least in certain respects, to be more like that in the monkey than in the cat [18, 19].

From what is said above it appears that as a rule, separate populations of pontine cells are acted upon from the premotor, the sensorimotor, the visual, and

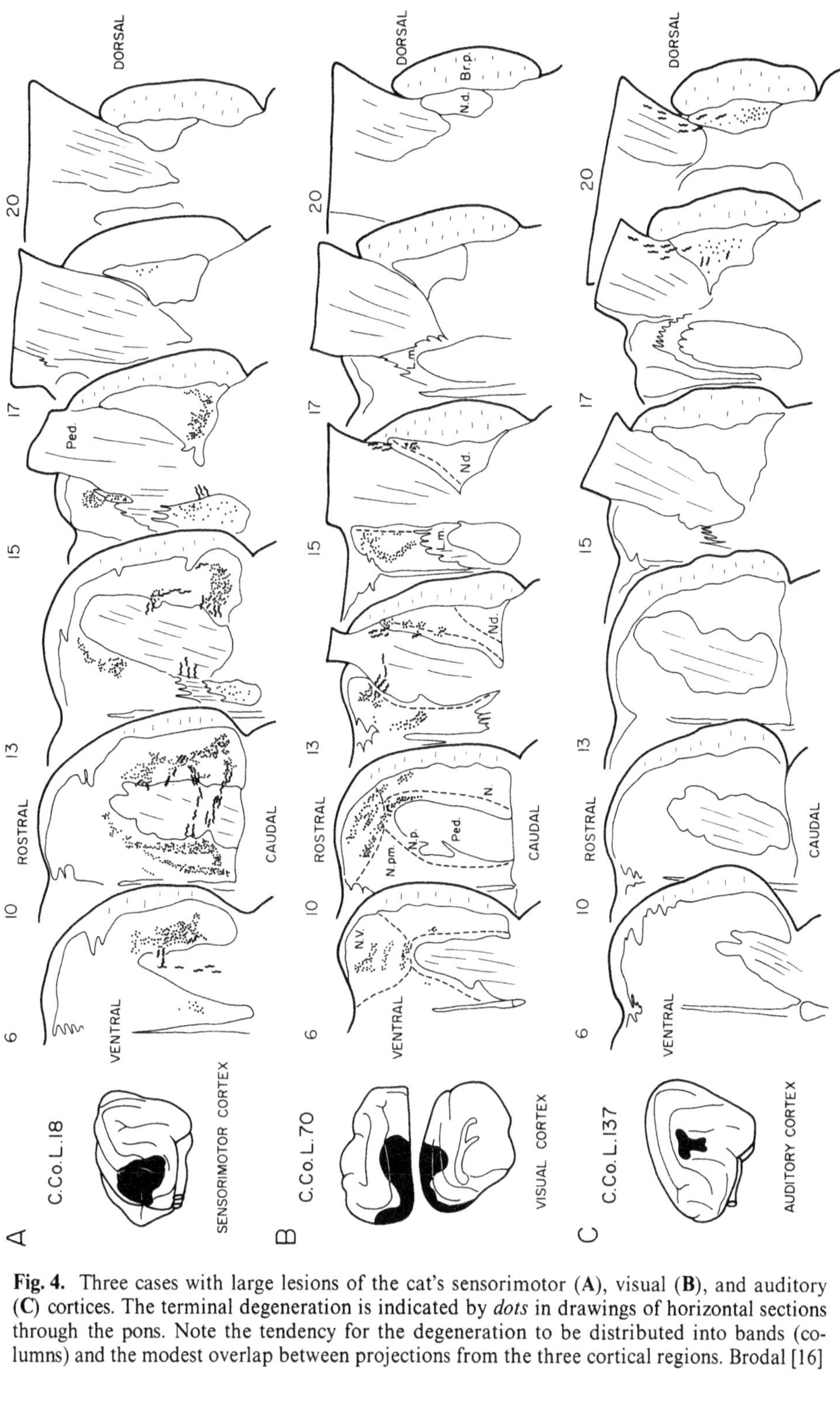

Fig. 4. Three cases with large lesions of the cat's sensorimotor (**A**), visual (**B**), and auditory (**C**) cortices. The terminal degeneration is indicated by *dots* in drawings of horizontal sections through the pons. Note the tendency for the degeneration to be distributed into bands (columns) and the modest overlap between projections from the three cortical regions. Brodal [16]

the auditory cortices. The presence of some degree of overlap between terminal fields of fibers from some of these regions does not invalidate this principle, which is also supported by physiological data. Thus, pontine cells activated by visual stimuli do not respond to somatosensory or auditory stimuli [4] and there appears to be only limited convergence on single pontine cells from sensorimotor and parietal cortical areas in the cat [53].

With regard to termination of projection from *subdivisions* of the major regions of the cortex, there is also evidence of topographical differences. Thus, fibers from the motor and somatosensory areas terminate in partly different regions of the pontine nuclei both in the cat [10] and in the monkey (Fig. 5). Furthermore, the corticopontine projection from the sensorimotor cortex is somatotopically organized in the rat [49], cat [10], and monkey ([18, 27]; Fig. 3).

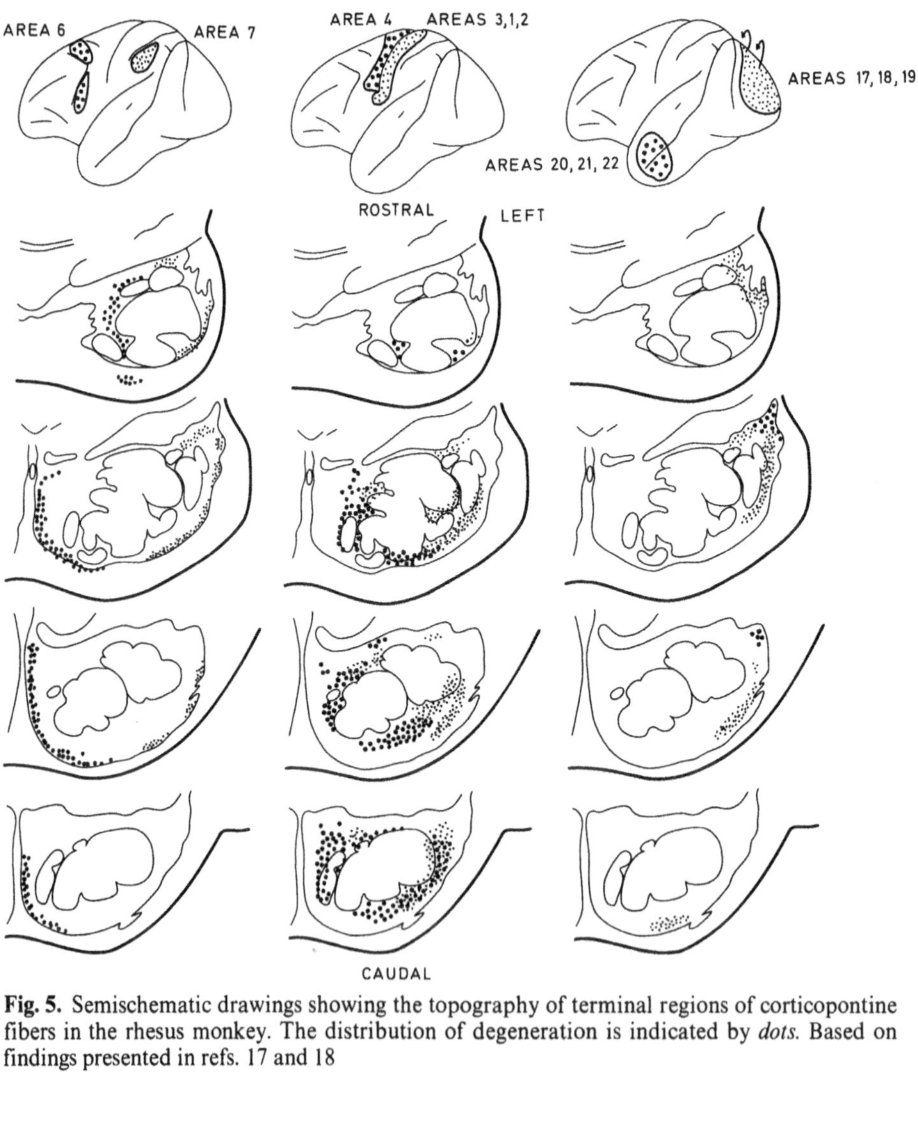

Fig. 5. Semischematic drawings showing the topography of terminal regions of corticopontine fibers in the rhesus monkey. The distribution of degeneration is indicated by *dots*. Based on findings presented in refs. 17 and 18

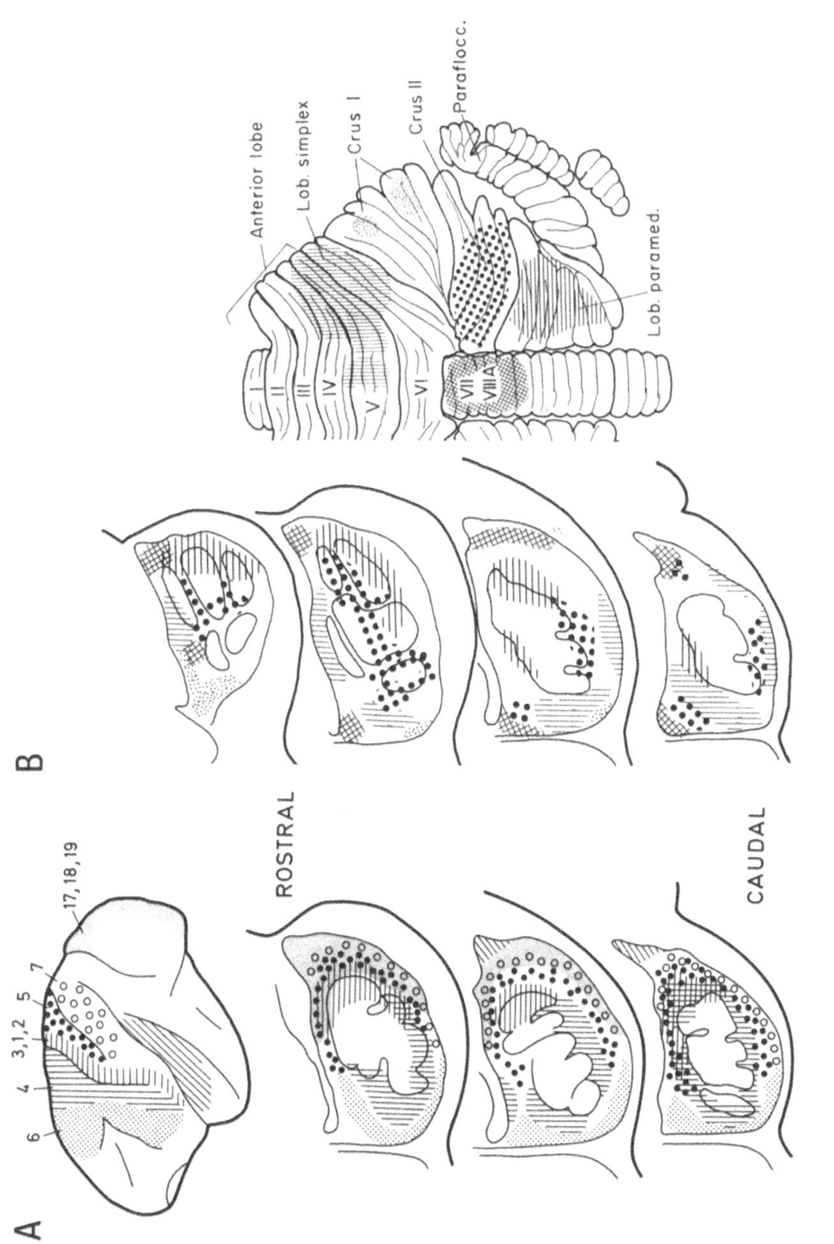

Fig. 6. A Schematic diagram summarizing the termination of corticopontine fibers from major parts of the cortex of the rhesus monkey. Based on findings in 38 monkeys, each with one or two cortical lesions. Note that the motor and somatosensory areas project to a large central core while projections from other cortical regions are added externally, resembling the skins of an onion. Brodal [18]. **B** Schematic diagram summarizing the topography of the pontine projection to main parts of the cerebellar cortex of the rhesus monkey. Based on findings after cerebellar injections of horseradish peroxidase in nine monkeys. Comparison of Figs. 6A and B can yield some information concerning the topography of cerebrocerebellar connections. Brodal [19]

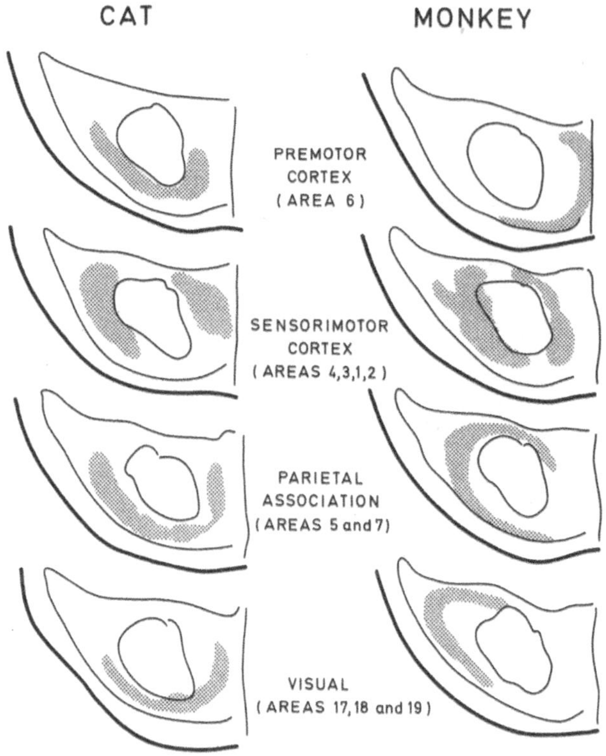

Fig. 7. Schematic diagram showing some major differences between the termination of corticopontine fibers in the cat and monkey. The projections from all cortical regions are shown as terminating in a transverse section at the same rostrocaudal level. Note that projections from the sensorimotor cortex terminate similarly in the two species, while very different patterns are found with regard to projections from other cortical areas. [Based on refs. 10, 14, 15, 18 and 50]. Brodal [18]

In order to further elucidate the degree of spatial separation in the corticopontine system, several authors have placed small lesions or injections of tritiated amino acids in the motor, somatosensory, and visual areas [10, 11, 14, 15, 16, 18, 27, 58, 64]. While some authors tend to emphasize the degree of overlap apparent in such experiments [27, 58, 63, 64], others pay more attention to the evidence of spatial separation [10, 14, 18, 49]. However, because of the patchy and widespread termination of corticopontine fibers it is often impossible to decide whether two patches are truly congruent or only close together. The use of small, differentially placed, bilateral lesions may be of help in this respect [10, 11, 14, 16, 18]. There is evidence from such experiments that some "patches" receiving fibers from one cortical site are situated very close to, without actually overlapping, patches supplied from other sites. Nevertheless, in other places considerably overlap seems to occur.

Physiological data support the conclusion that some pontine cells receive an input from one small part of the cortex only, or predominantly, while others receive converging inputs from several sites [53, 56, 57]. However, such physiological experiments do not give final answers to the questions concerning the degree of specificity and precision in the corticopontine projection. Thus, the results can be interpreted at least in two ways: a) that the degree of overlap between pontine projections from various cortical sites is due to a rather nonspecific or diffuse termination of fibers, the convergence having no special functional significance; or b) that the overlap or convergence is not random, but serves to integrate specific sets of information at a precerebellar level. In my opinion, the anatomical data so far tend to favor the second alternative, although the two alternatives are, of course, not mutually exclusive. For example, the fact that fibers from the leg and arm subdivisions of the motor cortex converge on certain cell groups in the pontine nuclei does not necessarily imply lack of precision. One may imagine that the corticopontine neurons are collected in smaller groups with different functional characteristics, and that such groups of cortical cells may have partly identical and partly different pontine targets. This would resemble the arrangement of corticospinal neurons [39, and others], and be different in principle from a gradual shift of terminal sites corresponding to a gradual shift in the location of the cell bodies in the cortex. One way to approach this problem anatomically is to use in one experiment two different markers for axonal termination applied at adjacent sites in the cortex. A method combining anterograde degeneration and autoradiography has been applied successfully in other regions [5].

Intrinsic Organization of the Pontine Nuclei

During recent years this topic has been studied with the Golgi method [26, 46, 48] and with electron microscopy [25, 38, 47, 48]. Only certain points from these studies will be mentioned here together with some of my own results from an ongoing Golgi study. Of particular interest are whether the pontine nuclei contain interneurons, whether pontocerebellar projection neurons give off recurrent collaterals, and the synaptology of the pontine nuclei.

Cajal described in the pontine nuclei of the human infant a peculiar, apparently very rare, cell type with a short locally branching axon [54]. Cooper and Fox [26], however, found no similar cell type in the adult monkey and were inclined to believe that the "hairy or mossy cell" of Cajal represented an artefact. On the other hand, Cooper and Fox classified a cell type with a small cell body and few dendrites as an intrinsic neuron. Their conclusion appears to be based on its general similarity to intrinsic neurons in certain other nuclei, for example, the presence of special dendritic appendages and sometimes "axon-like processes" emerging from the dendrites. Only in one instance was a locally branching axon seen. Judging from their Figs. 27–30 the identification of this process as an axon does not seem quite certain. Mihailoff and King [48] presented a drawing of a cell from the opposum pontine nuclei with a locally branching axon. My own Golgi studies of the pontine nuclei in the newborn monkey, cat, and adult monkey have so far failed to reveal any neuron with a locally branching axon. The Golgi-Rapid method was employed in all cases, and in some cases the blocks were double- or triple-impregnated. Drawings of neurons were made using a Leitz drawing tube and a magnification of 652 (Figs. 8, 9) or 162 (Fig. 10). A 40 × water objective was used. Some typical examples of presumed projection neurons from the newborn monkey are shown in Fig. 8. The axons are impregnated only for a short distance, presumably to the first node of Ranvier (Fig. 8A, B, C). The large number of spines and other types of dendritic

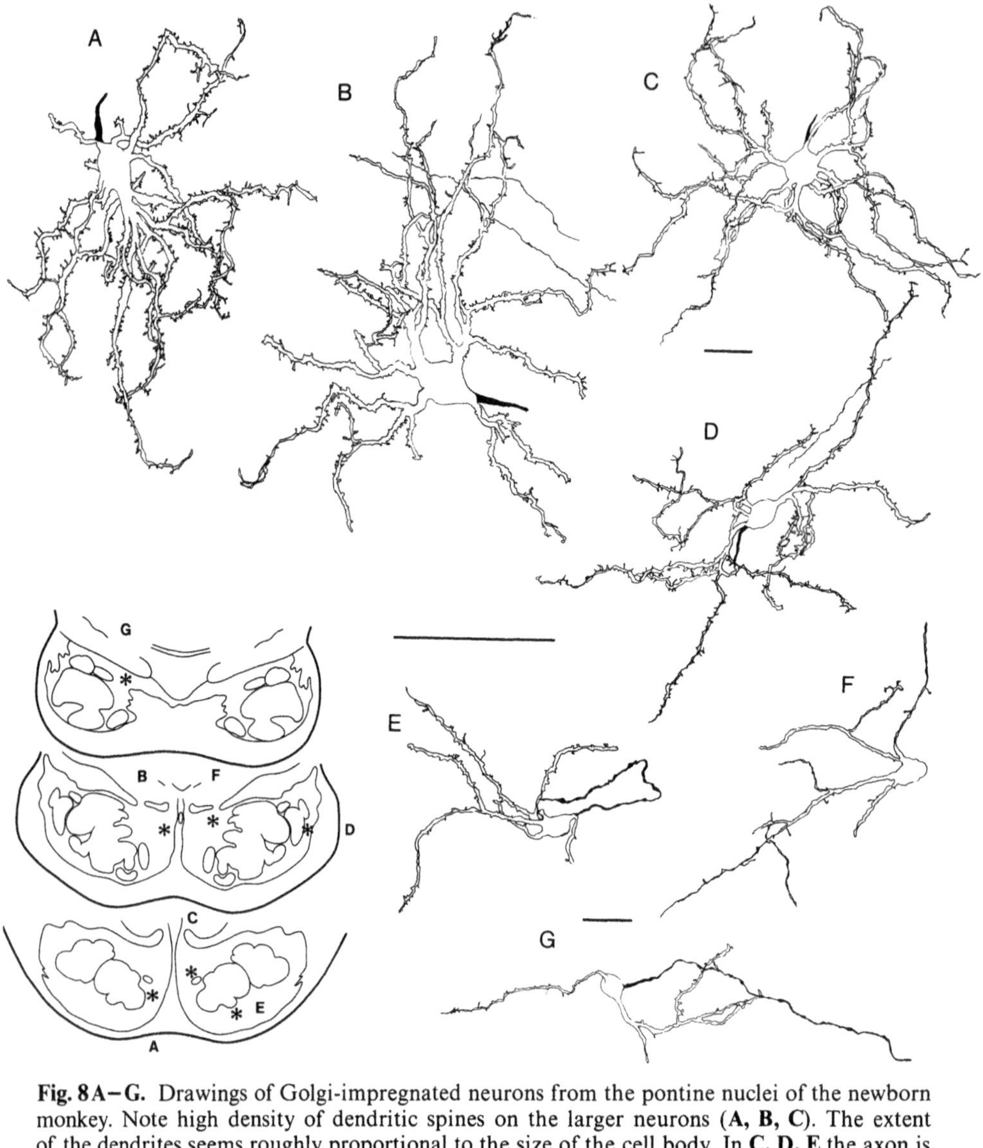

Fig. 8A–G. Drawings of Golgi-impregnated neurons from the pontine nuclei of the newborn monkey. Note high density of dendritic spines on the larger neurons (**A, B, C**). The extent of the dendrites seems roughly proportional to the size of the cell body. In **C, D, E** the axon is traced for some distance, but no branching of the axon has been observed in these and other small neurons. In **F** some dendritic appendages can be seen. The locations of the neurons are indicated to the *lower left* in drawings of transverse sections of the pons, and the neurons are represented in their correct orientation. Golgi-Rapid method. The *long bar* represents 100 μm, the *short bar* 30 μm

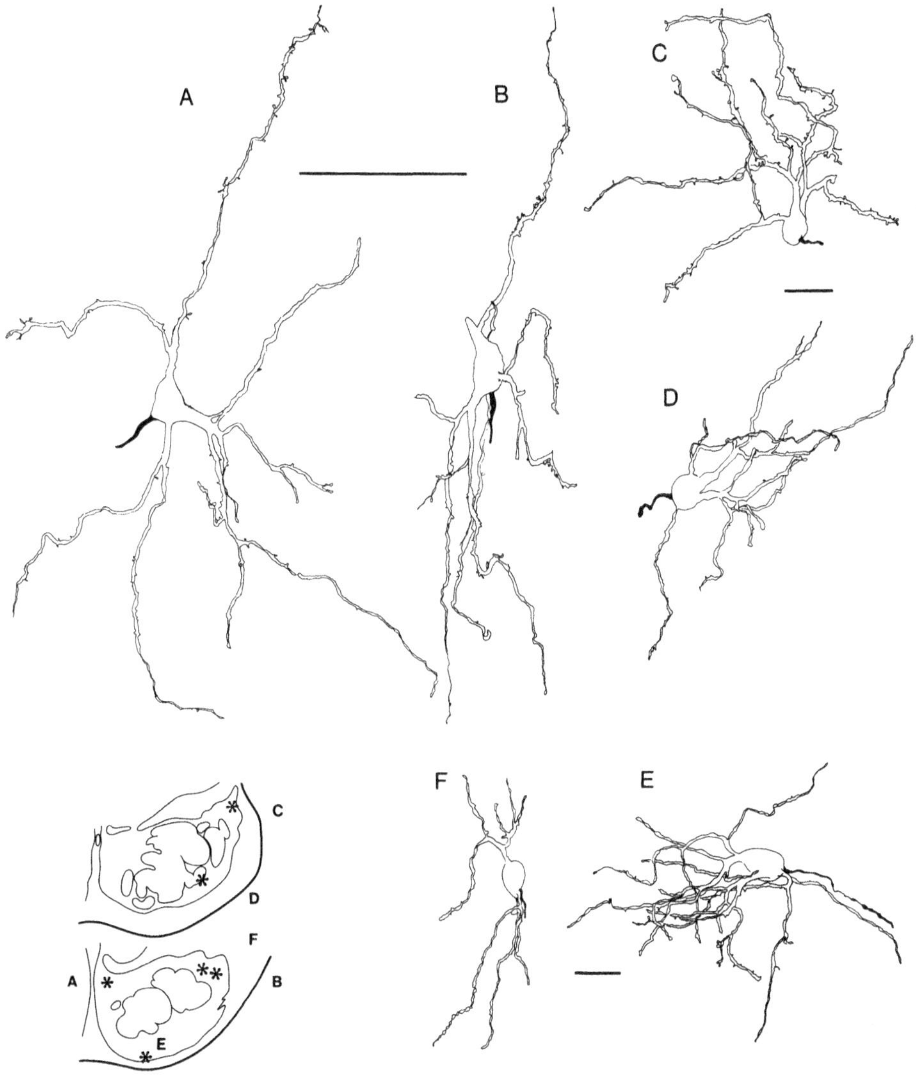

Fig. 9. Drawings of Golgi-impregnated neurons from the pontine nuclei of the adult monkey. Note the scarcity of dendritic spines as compared with the neurons from infant monkeys in Fig. 8. The locations of the neurons are indicated in drawings of transverse sections of the pons. The neurons are represented in their correct orientation. Golgi-Rapid method. *Bars* represent 100 μm and 30 μm, respectively

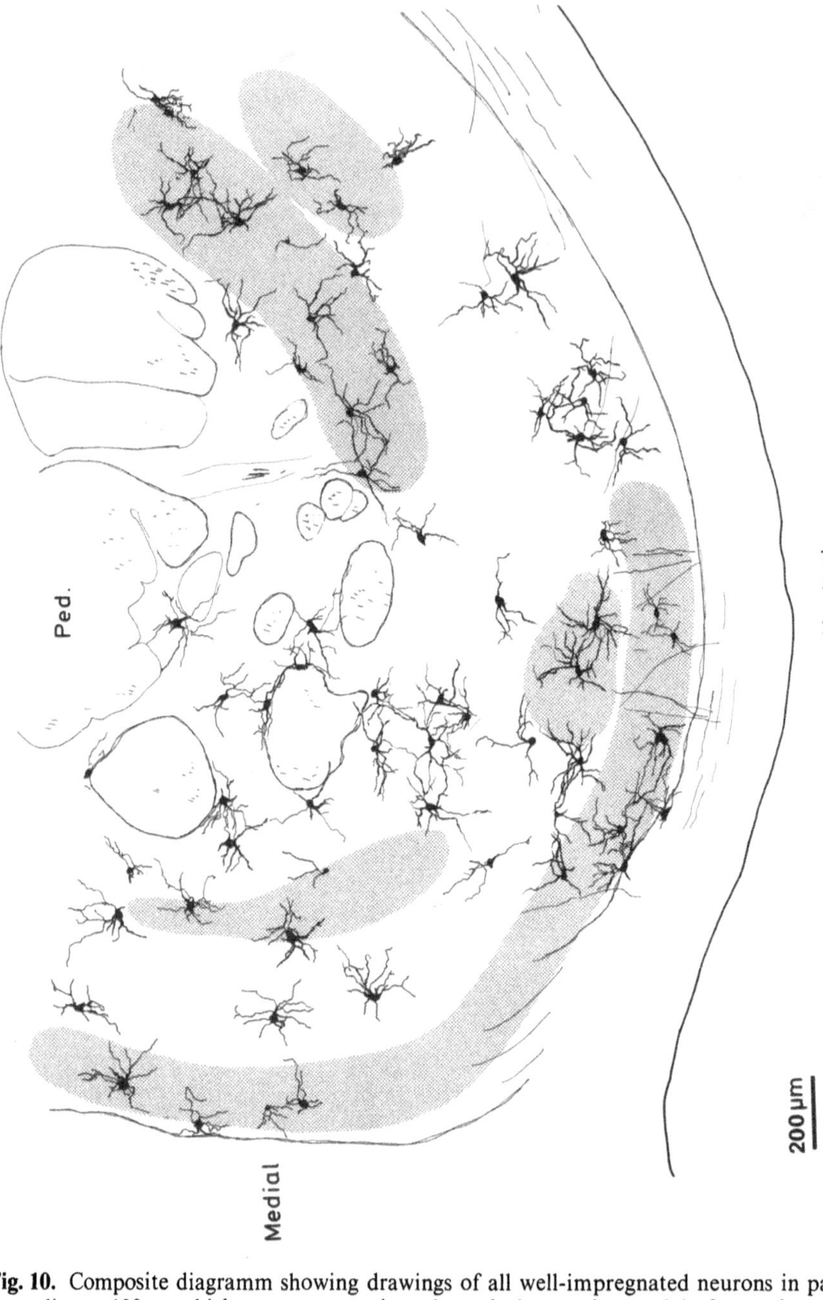

Fig. 10. Composite diagramm showing drawings of all well-impregnated neurons in parts of two adjacent 100-µm thick transverse sections through the pontine nuclei of a newborn monkey. Golgi-Rapid method. The extension of some bands of termination of corticopontine fibers from the motor cortex (see Fig. 3) have been superimposed in *shading* to show their relation to the dendritic fields of the pontine cells. Drawn with a magnification of 162 and subsequently reduced

protrusions is conspicuous and contrasts with the adult pattern where spines are much less frequent (Fig. 9). The axons of cells with small cell bodies are often impregnated for a longer distance, although so far never more than for 200 μm. They often have a beaded appearance, but as a rule follow a fairly straight course and branching has not been observed (Fig. 8D–G). In conclusion, *it still seems to be an open question whether interneurons (in the classical sense of Golgi type II) occur regularly in the pontine nuclei.*

The evidence from Golgi studies of *recurrent collaterals* from pontocerebellar axons is also limited. Cajal [54] found no such collaterals in the several species he studied. In my own Golgi material many, putative pontocerebellar axons coursing transversely through the pontine nuclei, and often seen to enter the brachium pontis, are impregnated for several hundred microns. Only in one instance, in the newborn cat, has such an axon been seen to give off collaterals. Mihailoff [46] illustrated a presumed pontocerebellar axon in the opossum giving off a thin, recurrent branch with further fine branches. He also made cerebellar cortical lesions and looked in the electron microscope for degenerating boutons as evidence of recurrent collaterals. Although certain boutons showed changes suggestive of degeneration, more direct evidence seems needed to prove the regular occurrence of recurrent collaterals from pontocerebellar axons. The application of horseradish peroxidase to minor transected parts of the brachium pontis may be one way of studying the intrapontine course of pontocerebellar axons. Intracellular application of HRP would be another possible approach (see, for example, ref. [21]).

The *extension and orientation of the dendrites* in relation to the incoming corticopontine fibers are of importance for the spatial separation of afferent inputs. My own Golgi material shows no clear-cut differences in the configuration and extension of the dendrites in sections cut in the transverse, sagittal, or horizontal plane, respectively. The average extent of the dendritic tree in the transverse plane was 192 μm for 106 well-impregnated cells from the newborn monkey. In the adult monkey fewer cells have been studied; the average for 25 cells was 220 μm. The variation between the orientation of dendrites of individual cells seems to depend mostly upon whether fibre bundles restrict the available space in certain directions, as described by Cooper and Fox [26]. However, there is a tendency for the dendrites in the transverse plane to be longer in the direction of the lamellae formed by the terminating corticopontine fibers (Fig. 10, see also Figs. 3, 6). Thus, for 50 well-impregnated neurons in the paramedian, ventral, and lateral pontine nuclei of the newborn monkey the mean extent of dendrites along the lamellae was 212 μm, while the extent of dendrites across the lamellae was 170 μm. Figure 10 further shows that the width of the lamellae produced by small lesions of the motor cortex corresponds approximately to the extent of the dendrites. Supposing that the lamellae do not overlap to any appreciable extent, each pontine cell would receive its predominant input from one lamella only, with additional weaker inputs from one or maximally two neighboring lamellae.

The *synaptology of the pontine nuclei* has been studied ultrastructurally in the cat [38], the opposum [47, 48], and the monkey [25]. The overwhelming majority of synapses are axodendritic in all species studied; in the cat and monkey axosomatic synapses are extremely rare. Furthermore, the synaptic density on proximal dendrites is very low and even the distal ones are far from being covered by boutons. In the cat, only 16% of the dendritic surface is covered by boutons [38]. Dendrodendritic synapses have been claimed to be present in the pontine nuclei [47]. A particular type of vesicle-containing profile was assumed to represent dendrites or the dendritic appendages, seen frequently on the smaller pontine cells [25, 48]. Mihailoff [47] shows one electron micrograph where this type of structure appears to be postsynaptic to a bouton and at the same time presynaptic to a dendrite, and a similar serial synapse involving a pale, vesicle-containing profile is illustrated by Cooper and Beal [25] in the monkey. Although further study is needed to verify the dendritic nature of such pale, vesicle-containing profiles, the available evidence suggests the possibility of rather complex interactions between pontine cells.

The Pontocerebellar Projection

Although the gross features of the pontocerebellar projection were revealed by retrograde degeneration techniques [9, 43] it was only after the introduction of the method for tracing connections by retrograde axonal transport that this projection could be studied in as detailed manner as the corticopontine projection.
A number of such studies have now been performed in the rat [22, 23, 29, 30], rabbit [35], cat [8, 20, 34, 36, 37], and monkey [19]. In general, they indicate that the pontocerebellar projection, just like the corticopontine, exhibits a complex pattern of divergence and convergence. Thus, after a single injection of HRP in the cerebellum, several discrete groups of labeled cells occur in the pontine nuclei (Figs. 11, 12). A particular pontine cell group may furthermore be labeled after injections in two or more widely separated parts of the cerebellum. This divergence seems to occur both by branching of pontocerebellar axons and by different cells within one group projecting to different targets, as judged from the distribution of labeled cells after injections of two different retrograde tracer substances (Evans Blue and Bisbenzimide, [55]). Thus, in regions of overlap, cells fluorescing either red (Evans Blue) or green (Bisbenzimide) were seen, and in addition some neurons showed double fluorescence [55].
It is a further conspicuous feature of the pontocerebellar projection that cells projecting to a minor part of the cerebellar cortex are distributed into usually rostrocaudally oriented slab- or column-like regions (Figs. 12, 13B) resembling the terminal regions of corticopontine fibers (Figs. 3–5).
With regard to the topography of the pontocerebellar projection, each major cerebellar region as a rule receives afferents largely from its "own" territory of the pontine nuclei, but to some degree also from regions projecting to other parts of the cerebellum (Figs. 6B, 12, 13B). This appears to hold true, for example, for projections to the anterior lobe [19, 20], crus I and II [19, 22], paramedian lobule [19, 34], the paraflocculus [23, 29, 35], the vermal visual area [19, 37], and the uvula [8, 30], although the exact location of cell groups projecting to a certain cerebellar region differs considerably between species. Such dif-

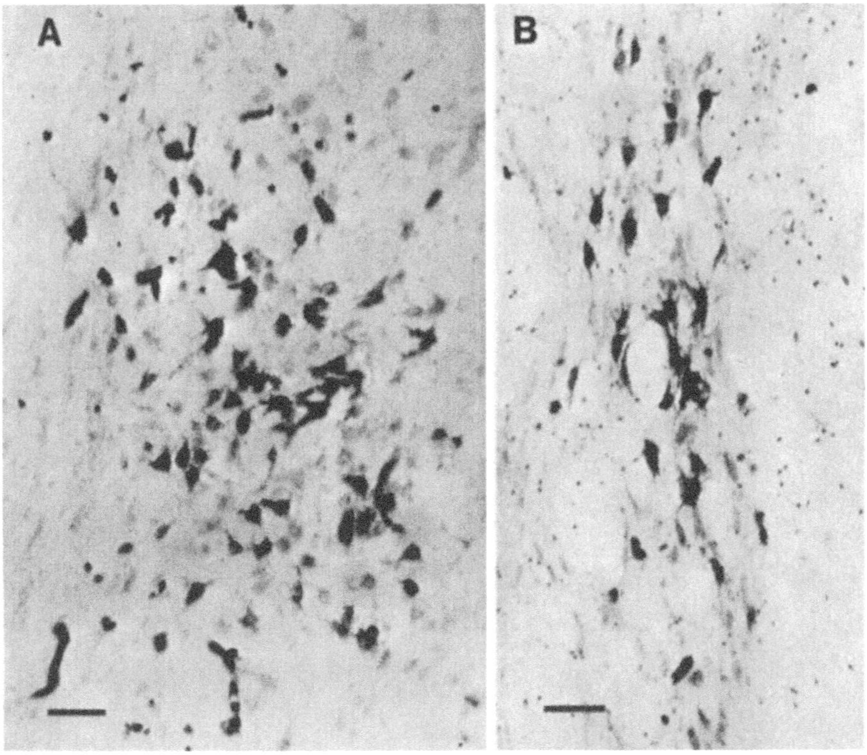

Fig. 11. Photomicrographs showing two well-restricted groups of labeled cells in the monkey's pontine nuclei after injection of horseradish peroxidase in crus II of the cerebellum. This case (OM 335) is also illustrated in Fig. 13B, and is fully described in ref. 19. 0-dianisidin incubation, 2 days survival time. Note the variation in intensity of cell labeling. *Bar* represents 50 μm

ferences seem to be most marked with regard to the hemispheric part of the posterior lobe.

The question of whether there is a more fine-grained topography in the pontocerebellar projection, has been approached in several HRP studies. As one would expect from physiological data and from the anatomical organization of the corticopontine projection, the pontine projection to the anterior lobe shows a fairly clear somatotopical pattern ([20]; Fig. 13A). A less clear-cut somatotopical pattern appears to exist in the projection to the paramedian lobule [34]. There are also certain topographical differences between projections to adjacent vermal lobules, such as VI, VII, and VIII of the cat [37], and lobules VII and VIII of the monkey [19]. Furthermore, the dorsal and ventral paraflocculus receive from slightly different pontine regions in the rat [29] and the rabbit [35]. Finally, the pontine projection to sublobules of the uvula is topographically organized in the rat [30]. On the other hand, no clear-cut differences in distribution of labeled cells were found after microinjections of HRP in the medial and lateral parts, respectively, of the cat's paramedian lobule [34].

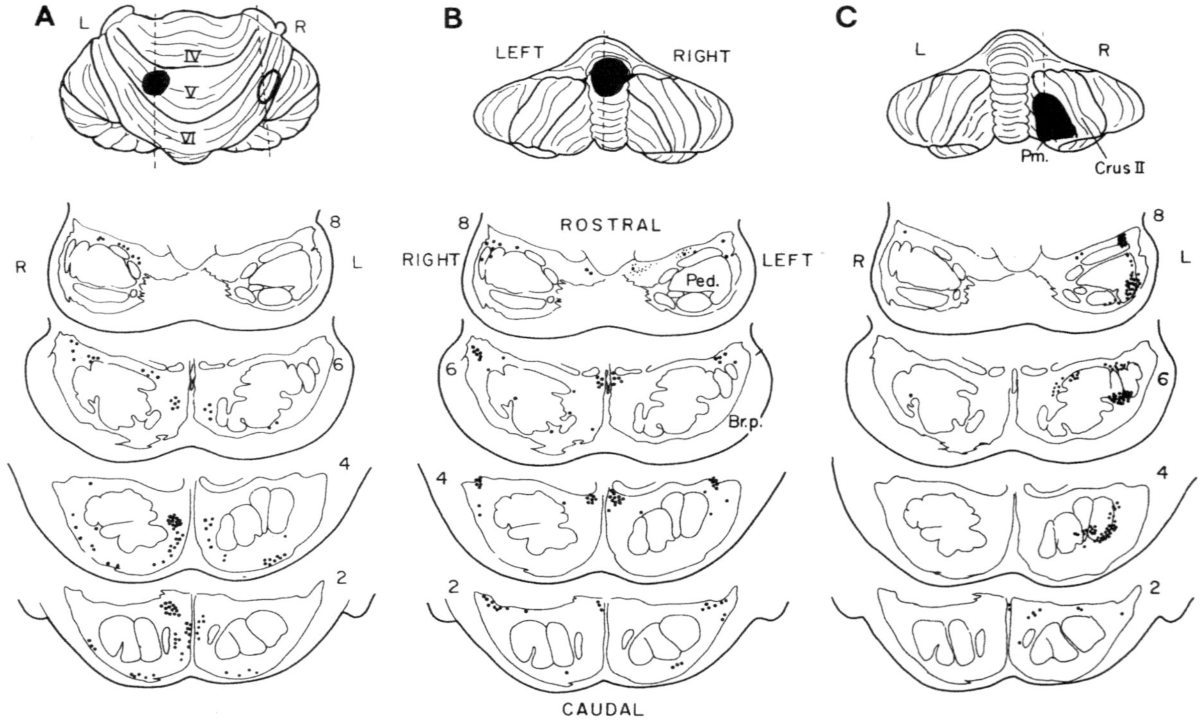

Fig. 12 A–C. Three experiments illustrating some features of the ponto-cerebellar projection in the rhesus monkey. Cerebellar injections of 0.2–0.4 μl of horseradish peroxidase were made 2 days before perfusion of the animals. In **A** the staining shown in *black* involves lobulus V of the anterior lobe; the injection in lobulus VI apparently did not lead to significant uptake and is only shown in outline. In **B** the vermal visual area (lobules VII and VIII A) is stained while in **C** the staining affects mainly the paramedian lobule. Note the tendency for labeled cells (*dots*) to be distributed in bands and patches, and that each cerebellar site receives from several discrete pontine cell groups, often situated far apart. Note also that labeled cells are arranged into rostrocaudally oriented slab or column-like regions (cf. also Fig. 6 B). Brodal [19]

It appears from physiological studies that the cerebellar cortex may consist of a mosaic of small, functionally different parts. For example, Purkinje cells situated fairly close together in the anterior lobe may show rather different activity in relation to movements [33]. Furthermore, Shambes and co-workers [60] described with electrophysiological micromapping methods a fine-grained mosaic of tactile projections in the rat cerebellar hemisphere. Interestingly, the somatotopy was often "fractured", so that two adjacent small groups of granule cells had inputs from different parts of the body, although each received only from a fairly small cutaneous field.

However, one cutaneous field was as a rule represented in several patches. These findings would seem to implicate that each small patch of the mosaic receives a specific set of afferents, different from those of neighbouring patches. It is surely a formidable task to decide anatomically whether the pontocerebellar projection is so organized, but it seems compatible with its complicated pattern of divergence and convergence: It seems indeed likely that afferents from several, maybe many, discrete pontine cell groups would converge onto a given cerebellar "patch". When it is taken into consideration that each pontine cell group is likely to receive convergent inputs from several sites in the cerebral cortex, the nature of the information ultimately reaching a cerebellar "patch" must be extremely difficult to analyze.

Cerebropontocerebellar Topography

The problem of deciding to which parts of the cerebellum individual parts of the cerebral cortex project has been studied electrophysiologically [1, 28, 40, 59, 61, and others]. However, such methods have so far only yielded information on rather gross area-to-area connections. Anatomically, the problem of cerebrocerebellar topography is studied by comparing sites of termination of corticopontine fibers with distribution of pontocerebellar neurons. However, because of the patchy character and complex patterns of divergence and convergence within both systems such comparisons meet with great difficulties [see refs. 18, 19]. In order to obtain more definite answers, one may combine different methods to visualize in the same section the terminations of corticopontine fibers and the distribution of pontocerebellar neurons. Burne, Mihailoff, and Woodward [23] injected tritiated leucine in the rat visual cortex and at the same time injected HRP into the paraflocculus. They were then able to show that of the two pontine cell groups projecting to the paraflocculus, one received a strong projection from the visual cortex while the other did not (at least not from the parts of the visual cortex injected). I am presently using essentially the same approach, but the anterograde degeneration technique is used instead of autoradiography [6]. The sections through the pontine nuclei are first incubated in the ordinary way with diaminobenzidine to visualize HRP granules in the pontine cells, and then treated according to the Fink and Heimer [31] silver impregnation method (Fig. 13A). In this experiment, the correspondence between the termination of corticopontine fibers from the sensorimotor cortex and pontine cells projecting to the anterior lobe is striking, and

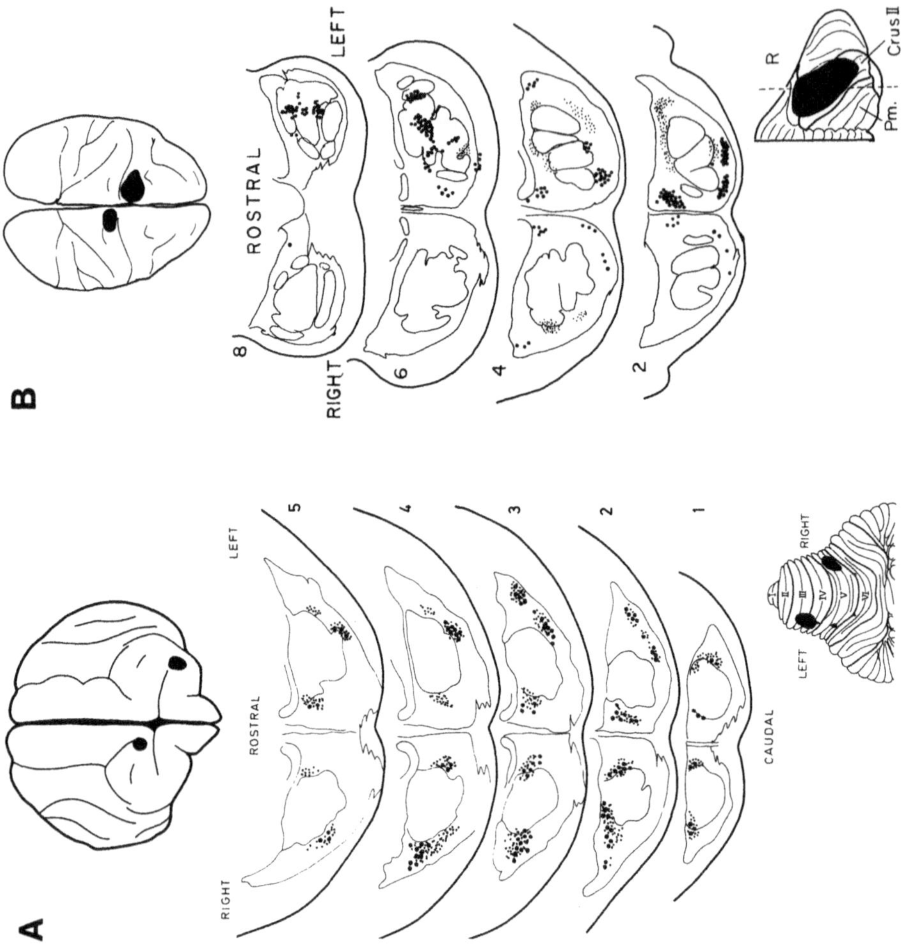

Fig. 13 A, B. Two examples of experiments combining methods for visualizing termination of corticopontine fibers and location of pontocerebellar neurons. **A** Combination of anterograde degeneration technique and retrograde transport of horseradish peroxidase. Two injections of 0.1 μl horseradish peroxidase were placed in the anterior lobe of a cat. Two days survival time. On the *left* side the staining involves the intermediate part of lobulus V ("forelimb region"), on the *right* side lobulus III and IV are stained ("hindlimb region"). Labeled cells are shown with *heavy dots* in drawings of transverse sections through the pons. The pontocerebellar projection to the anterior lobe is mainly crossed [20], and labeled pontine cells are differently located on the two sides. Four days before the injections of HRP, bilateral lesions were made of the sensorimotor cortex, on the left side of the forelimb region, and on the right of the hindlimb region. After perfusion of the animal, frozen sections were incubated with diaminobenzidine and subsequently treated according to the Fink and Heimer method [6]. Terminal degeneration is indicated by *small dots.* Note the close correspondence between termination of fibers from, for example, the sensorimotor forelimb region and the location of pontine cells projecting to the intermediate part of lobulus V. **B** Experiment combining anterograde and retrograde transport of HRP in the monkey. Bilateral injections of 0.5 μl HRP were placed in the pre- and postcentral gyri (leg-trunk representation) and during the same operation an injection of 0.2 μl HRP was placed in the right crus II of the cerebellum. Termination of corticopontine fibers is indicated by *fine stippling,* labeled pontocerebellar neurons with *heavy dots.* Note the lack of overlap between the terminal areas of fibers from the motor leg-trunk region and the cell groups projecting to the crus II. Brodal [19]

the somatotopical patterns within both projections are evident. Experiments combining anterograde and retrograde transport of HRP can also be used (Fig. 13B), although in my experience the anterograde transport is much more capricious than the retrograde transport. The particular experiment illustrated in Fig. 13B shows lack of overlap in regions where termination of corticopontine fibers from the motor leg region comes very close to groups of cells projecting to the crus II.

Such combined experiments clearly demonstrate several of the general principles applicable to the corticoponto-cerebellar pathway, and more significantly provide direct evidence of cerebropontocerebellar connectivity, not obtainable from comparison of individual experiments.

Concluding Remarks

Although the last few years have brought a wealth of information about the corticopontocerebellar pathway, we still do not understand its basic organizational principles, not to mention its functional role in cerebellar operations. Nevertheless, it seems reasonable to expect further progress from future detailed studies combining various anatomical techniques and from combinations of anatomical and physiological methods. From an anatomical point of view, one outstanding problem is to define more clearly, with regard to afferent connections and intrinsic organization, the smallest "subunit" of the pontine nuclei. Another important and cumbersome task will be to find the smallest cerebellar cortical area that can be defined by a specific set of afferents from the pontine nuclei.

References

1. Adrian ED (1943) Afferent areas in the cerebellum connected with the limbs. Brain 66:289–315
2. Albus K, Donate-Oliver F (1977) Cells of origin occipitopontine projection in the cat: functional properties and intracortical location. Exp Brain Res 28:167–174
3. Allen GI, Tsukahara N (1974) Cerebrocerebellar communication systems. Physiol Rev 54:957–1006
4. Baker J, Gibson A, Glickstein M, Stein J (1976) Visual cells in the pontine nuclei of the cat. J Physiol 255:415–434
5. Berkley KJ (1974) Differential labeling of neural pathways converging on the ventrobasal complex of cat thalamus. Brain Res 66:342–348
6. Blomqvist A, Westman J (1975) Combined HRP and Fink-Heimer staining applied on the gracile nucleus in the cat. Brain Res 99:339–342
7. Brodal A (1972) Cerebrocerebellar pathways. Anatomical data and some functional implications. Acta Neurol Scand [Suppl] 51:153–196
8. Brodal A, Hoddevik GH (1978) The pontocerebellar projection to the uvula in the cat. Exp Brain Res 32:105–116
9. Brodal A, Jansen J (1946) The pontocerebellar projection in the rabbit and cat. Experimental investigations. J Comp Neurol 84:31–118
10. Brodal P (1968) The corticopontine projection in the cat-I. Demonstration of a somatotopically organized projection from the primary sensorimotor cortex. Exp Brain Res 5:210–234

11. Brodal P (1968) The corticopontine projection in the cat. Demonstration of somatotopically organized projection from the second somatosensory cortex. Arch Ital Biol 106:310–332
12. Brodal P (1971) The corticopontine projection in the cat. I. The projection from the proreate gyrus. J Comp Neurol 142:127–140
13. Brodal P (1971) The corticopontine projection in the cat. II. The projection from the orbital gyrus. J Comp Neurol 142:141–152
14. Brodal P (1972) The corticopontine projection from the visual cortex in the cat. I. The total projection and the projection from area 17. Brain Res 39:297–317
15. Brodal P (1972) The corticopontine projection from the visual cortex in the cat. II. The projection from areas 18 and 19. Brain Res 39:319–335
16. Brodal P (1972) The corticopontine projection in the cat. The projection from the auditory cortex. Arch Ital Biol 110:119–144
17. Brodal P (1978) Principles of organization of the monkey corticopontine projection. Brain Res 148:214–218
18. Brodal P (1978) The corticopontine projection in the rhesus monkey. Origin and principles of organization. Brain 101:251–283
19. Brodal P (1979) The pontocerebellar projection in the rhesus monkey: An experimental study with retrograde axonal transport of horseradish peroxidase. Neuroscience 4:193–208
20. Brodal P, Walberg F (1977) The pontine projection to the cerebellar anterior lobe. An experimental study in the cat with retrograde transport of horseradish peroxidase. Exp Brain Res 29:233–248
21. Brown AG, Rose PK, Snow PJ (1977) The morphology of spinocervical tract neurons revealed by intracellular injection of horseradish peroxidase. J Physiol 270:747–764
22. Burne RA, Eriksson MA, Saint-Cyr JA, Woodward, DJ (1978) The organization of the pontine projection to lateral cerebellar areas in the rat: Dual zones in the pons. Brain Res 139:340–347
23. Burne RA, Mihailoff GA, Woodward DJ (1978) Visual corticopontine input to the paraflocculus: a combined autoradiographic and horseradish peroxidase study. Brain Res 143:139–146
24. Chiba M (1980) Patterns of organization of the corticopontine projection in the cat with particular reference to the pontocerebellar projection. J Hirnforsch 21:89–99
25. Cooper MH, Beal JA (1978) The neurons and the synaptic endings in the primate basilar pontine gray. J Comp Neurol 180:17–42
26. Cooper MH, Fox CA (1976) The basilar pontine gray in the adult monkey: A Golgi study. J Comp Neurol 168:145–174
27. Dhanarajan P, Rüegg DG, Wiesendanger M (1977) An anatomical investigation of the corticopontine projection in the primate (*Saimiri sciureus*). The projection from motor and somatosensory areas. Neuroscience 2:913–922
28. Dow RS (1942) Cerebellar action potentials in response to stimulation of the cerebral cortex in monkeys and the cat. J Neurophysiol 5:121–136
29. Eisenman LM (1980) Pontocerebellar projections to the paraflocculus in the rat. Brain Res 188:550–554
30. Eisenman LM, Noback CR (1980) The pontocerebellar projection in the rat: Differential projections to sublobules of the uvula. Exp Brain Res 38:11–17
31. Fink RP, Heimer L (1967) Two methods for selective silver impregnation of degenerating axons and their synaptic endings in the central nervous system. Brain Res 4:369–374
32. Gibson A, Baker J, Mower G, Glicksten M (1978) Corticopontine cells in area 18 of the cat. J Neurophysiol 41:484–495
33. Harvey RJ, Porter R, Rawson JA (1977) The natural discharges of Purkinje cells in paravermal regions of lobules V and VI of the monkey's cerebellum. J Physiol (Lond) 271:515–536
34. Hoddevik GH (1975) The pontocerebellar projection onto the paramedian lobule in the cat: An experimental study with the use of horseradish peroxidase as a tracer. Brain Res 95:291–307

35. Hoddevik GH (1977) The pontine projection to the flocculo-nodular lobe and the paraflocculus studied by means of retrograde axonal transport of horseradish peroxidase in the rabbit. Exp Brain Res 30:511–526
36. Hoddevik GH, Walberg F (1979) The pontine projection onto longitudinal zones of the paramedian lobule in the cat. Exp Brain Res 34:233–240
37. Hoddevik GH, Brodal A, Kawamura K, Hashikawa T (1977) The pontine projection to the cerebellar vermal visual area studied by means of the retrograde axonal transport of horseradish peroxidase. Brain Res 123: 209–227
38. Holländer H, Brodal P, Walberg F (1969) Electromicroscopic observations on the structure of the pontine nuclei and the mode of termination of the corticopontine fibres. An experimental study in the cat. Exp Brain Res 7:95–110
39. Jankowska E, Padel Y, Tanaka R (1975) Projections of pyramidal tract cells to α-motoneurones innervating hind-limb muscles in the monkey. J Physiol 249:637–667
40. Jansen J Jr (1957) Afferent impulses to the cerebellar hemispheres from the cerebral cortex and certain subcortical nuclei. Acta Physiol Scand [Suppl 143] 41:1–99
41. Jones EG, Wise SP (1977) Size, laminar and columnar distribution of efferent cells in the sensory-motor cortex of monkeys. J Comp Neurol 175:391–438
42. Kawamura K, Chiba M (1979) Cortical neurons projecting to the pontine nuclei in the cat. An experimental study with the horseradish peroxidase technique. Exp Brain Res 35:269–285
43. Lafleur J, Lean J de, Poirier LJ (1974) Physiopathology of the cerebellum in the monkey-I. Origin of cerebellar afferent nervous fibers from the spinal cord and brain stem. J Neurol Sci 22:471–490
44. Larsell O, Jansen J (1972) The Comparative Anatomy and Histology of the Cerebellum. The Human Cerebellum. Cerebellar Connections and Cerebellar Cortex. University of Minnesota Press, Minneapolis
45. Lynch JC, Mountcastle VB, Talbot WH, Yin TCT (1977) Parietal lobe mechanisms for directed visual attention. J Neurophysiol 40:362–389
46. Mihailoff GA (1978) Principal neurons of the basilar pons as the source of a recurrent collateral system. Brain Res Bull 3:319–332
47. Mihailoff GA (1978) Anatomic evidence suggestive of dendrodendritic synapses in the opossum basilar pons. Brain Res Bull 3:333–340
48. Mihailoff GA, King JS (1975) The basilar pontine gray of the opossum: A correlated light and electron microscopic study. J Comp Neurol 159:521–552
49. Mihailoff GA, Burne RA, Woodward DJ (1978) Projections of the sensorimotor cortex to the basilar pontine nuclei in the rat: an autoradiographic study. Brain Res 145:347–354
50. Mizuno N, Mochizuki K, Matsushima CAR, Sasaki K (1973) Projections from the parietal cortex to the brain stem nuclei in the cat, with special reference to the parietal cerebro-cerebellar system. J Comp Neurol 147:511–522
51. Mountcastle VB, Lynch JC, Georgopoulos A, Sakata H, Acuna C (1975) Posterior parietal association cortex of the monkey: Command functions for operations within extrapersonal space. J Neurophysiol 38:871–908
52. Nyby O, Jansen J (1951) An experimental investigation of the corticopontine projection in *Macaca mulatta.* Skr Nor Vidensk Akad Oslo Mat Naturvidensk K1 1–47
53. Oka H, Sasaki K, Matsuda Y, Yasuda T, Mizuno N (1975) Responses of pontocerebellar neurones to stimulation of the parietal association and the frontal motor cortices. Brain Res 93:399–407
54. Ramón Y, Cajal S (1911) Histologie du système nerveux de l'Homme et des Vertébrés, vol II. Maloine, Paris Translated by L Azoulay
55. Rosina A, Provini L, Vitali A, Bentivoglio M, Kuypers HGJM (1979) Divergence within the pontine projection to the neocerebellum as revealed by retrograde fluorescent double labeling technique. Neurosci Lett [Suppl] 3:127
56. Rüegg DG, Séguin JJ, Wiesendanger M (1977) Effects of electric stimulation of somatosensory and motor areas of the cerebral cortex on neurones of the pontine nuclei in squirrel monkeys. Neuroscience 2:923–927

57. Rüegg DG, Wiesendanger M (1975) Corticofugal effects from sensorimotor area I and somatosensory area II on neurones of the pontine nuclei in the eat. J Physiol (Lond) 247:745–757
58. Sanides D, Fries W, Albus K (1978) The corticopontine projection from the visual cortex of the cat: An autoradiographic investigation. J Comp Neurol 179:77–88
59. Sasaki K, Oka H, Kawaguchi S, Jinnai K, Yasuda T (1977) Mossy and climbing fibre responses produced in the cerebellar cortex in monkeys. Exp Brain Res 29:419–428
60. Shambes GM, Gibson JM, Welker W (1978) Fractured somatotopy in granule cell tactile areas of rat cerebellar hemispheres revealed by micromapping. Brain Behav Evol 15:94–140
61. Snider RS, Eldred E (1952) Cerebro-cerebellar relations in the monkey. J Neurophysiol 15:27–40
62. Tomasch J (1968) The overall information capacity of the major afferent and efferent cerebellar cell and fiber systems. Confin Neurol 30:359–367
63. Wiesendanger M, Rüegg DG, Wiesendanger R (1979) The corticopontine system in primates: Anatomical and functional considerations. In: Massion J, Sasaki K (eds) Cerebrocerebellar interactions. Elsevier/North Holland Biomedical Press, Amsterdam Oxford New York, pp 45–65
64. Wiesendanger R, Wiesendanger M, Rüegg DG (1979) An anatomical investigation of the corticopontine projection in the primate (*Macaca fascicularis* and *Saimiri sciureus*) – II. The projection from frontal and parietal association areas. Neuroscience 4:747–765
65. Wiitanen JT (1969) Selective silver impregnation of degenerating axons and axon terminals in the central nervous system of the monkey. Brain Res 14:546–548
66. Wise SP, Jones EG (1977) Cells of origin and terminal distribution of descending projections of the rat somatic sensory cortex. J Comp Neurol 175:129–158

Discussion

Martin: With regard to species differences seen in the corticopontine targets, do you feel these circuits are comparable in different species? Is it possible that species differences in the location of pontine neurons receiving specific cortical afferents simply represent variations in the final position assumed by neurons migrating to the base of the pons?

Brodal: These species differences probably do not represent functional differences, but there are some physiological data from Sasaki and co-workers in the monkey, which suggest that the circuits may not be totally comparable.

Martin: In any case the position of pontine neurons may not be the best basis for making comparisons between species.

Altman: In the monkey, does the anterior cortex tend to project to the medial pons and the posterior to the lateral pons? If this is correct and we can go from the monkey to the rat, one can draw a parallel because the medial pontine neurons arise earlier than the lateral ones. There is also some evidence that the anterior cortex forms earlier than the posterior cortex. So you would have a first come, first served basis and the difference in the cat may have something to do with the location of the visual cortex.

Brodal: You are probably right, but there is one problem with the projection from the premotor cortex. In the monkey, it is located medially and in the cat it is lateral, which would not follow this pattern. The rat in fact might be more like the monkey than the cat with regard to this topography.

Gould: I think there are some species differences that cannot be accounted for by compensatory olivocerebellar circuits. In the cat, the projections from the superior colliculus and the visual cortex to the pontine nuclei do not seem to overlap at all. In the monkey I think there is considerable overlap. Would you agree with that?

Brodal: I cannot say definitely, but I would think there is no more overlap in the monkey than in the cat. I am not so sure that there is a precise overlap in the monkey, but this could be studied by double labeling experiments.

Snider: What does area 8 overlap with? In particular, does it overlap with area 17?

Brodal: No, they do not overlap in the pons, but both cell groups converge in the cerebellum, which supports your physiological experiments.

Snider: Is there any overlap between areas 3, 1, and 2 and areas 4 and 6.

Brodal: The general rule in the monkey is that there is little overlap except for the projections from the leg cortex.

Snider: I am also interested in the overlap between superior temporal gyrus and area 17.

Brodal: There is very little, but there again they may come together in the cerebellar projection.

Thach: Some of the older studies on the pontocerebellar projection using the Gudden method showed a more definite stereotyped pattern of the projection than the HRP method. Is that possibly due to the Gudden method requiring larger lesions to show an effect and those with HRP being smaller?

Brodal: Yes, the Gudden method shows the overall topography, but what is more interesting is the topography within this topography.

Thach: Granted, but do your results contradict the previous results or are they compatible?

Brodal: No, they are not contradictory, but of course, the family is involved.

Martin: The question of cerebellar feedback to the basilar pons and other precerebellar nuclei is intriguing to me. What is that projection picking out in the pons? As you know it is very restricted. What is specific about those pontine regions to which the cerebellum projects?

Brodal: It seems to be (in the cat) to those regions which receive afferents from the sensory-motor cortex and project to the anterior lobe. That has also intrigued me. Of course, the reticulotegmental nucleus receives a much stronger cerebellar projection. But, there is no good reciprocity between this nucleus and the cerebellum. It is not a simple circuit. But, I really cannot answer your question.

Martin: In the opossum, the cerebellum also projects mainly to that part of the basilar pons receiving input from somatic motor and sensory cortices. How do your data correlate with models of corticopontocerebellar function, such as that proposed by Allen and Tsukahara? There seems to be a relative lack of projection from parietal association areas.

Brodal: Well, I don't feel I can say much about that, but there is a strong input from area 5. I don't think prefrontal cortex rostral to area 6 can be included in this circuitry either.

The Olivocerebellar Projection in the Cat

J. Voogd

The topical relations of the inferior olive and the cerebellum have been the subject of several recent reviews (Brodal 1980, Brodal and Kawamura 1980, Walberg 1980). In this paper the topography of the olivocerebellar system will be considered. Superficially there is a certain similarity in the shape of the principal nucleus of the inferior olive and the dentate nucleus, "l'olive cérébelleux" of the French authors. However, early attempts to correlate the principal nucleus of the inferior olive with the cerebellar hemisphere (the "neocerebellum") and the accessory olives with the vermis and the flocculus (the "palaeocerebellum") met with only limited success. In human cases with chronic cerebellar lesions of the hemisphere the rostral pole and the medial portion of the principal nucleus usually were intact and in some cases cell loss was even found in parts of the accessory olives (Holmes and Stewart 1908, Brouwer 1913, 1915; Brouwer and Coenen 1919, 1921).

Experimental investigations with myelin degeneration techniques after lesions of the inferior olive in laboratory animals (Klimoff 1899, Lüthy 1932, Voogd 1964) never revealed the full extent of the olivocerebellar projection, probably because the caliber of these fibers is too small (1–5 µm, Szentágothai-Schimert 1941). Until the advance of the modern antegrade axonal degeneration and transport techniques, Brodal's (1940) account of the olivocerebellar localization in cat and rabbit remained the only complete experimental investigation available for almost 30 years. His work was based on the study of retrograde changes in the inferior olive, after lesions of the cerebellar cortex in newborn animals (the so-called modified Gudden method). Although these experiments allow for a detailed localization of the changes in the inferior olive, their interpretation is hampered by the large size and the irregular shape of the lesions. Brodal's interpretation favored a lobular organization of the olivocerebellar projection, each of the cerebellar lobules receiving fibers from a single, discrete part of the olive. The principal nucleus was found to be connected with the lob-

Fig. 1. Diagram of the olivocerebellar projection in the cat (Brodal, 1940). *D*, dorsal acessory olive; *d. cap.*, dorsal cap; *d. l.*, dorsal leaf of principal nucleus of the inferior olive; *dm. c. col.*, dorsomedial cell column of medial olive; *Lob. a., b., and c.*, lobules a, b, and c of Bolk; *M*, medial accessory olive; *m*, medial; *(nucl.)β*, group *β* of the medial accessory olive; *N. fast*, fastigial nucleus; *N. int*, nucleus interpositus; *N. lat*, lateral cerebellar nucleus; *v. l.*, ventral leaf of principal nucleus; *v. l. o.*, ventrolateral outgrowth of principal nucleus; *1, 2, 3, 4*, lobules 1–4 of the anterior lobe. Brodal et al. (1975) with permission from the Wistar Press

Experimental Brain Research, Suppl. 6

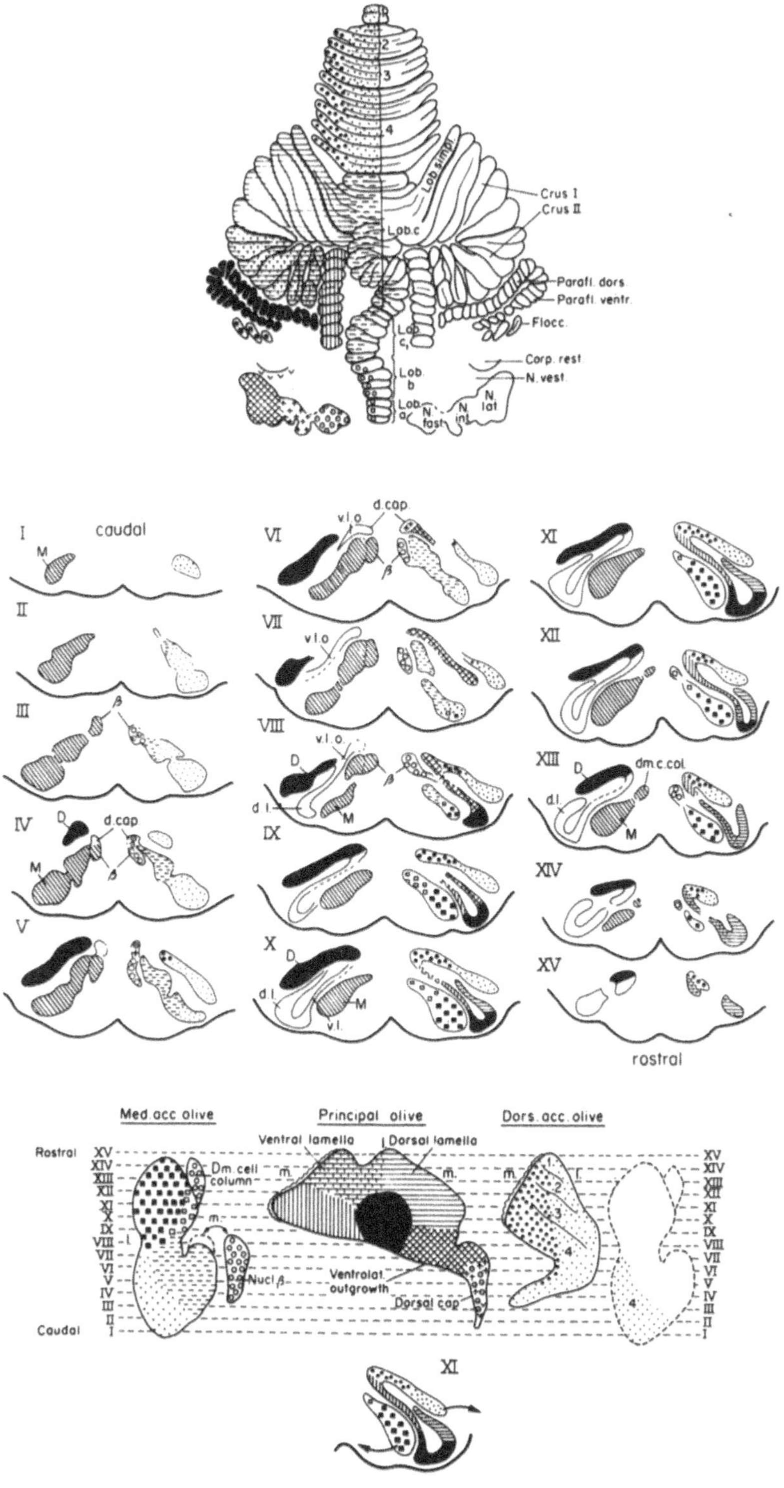
Lob. simpl.
Crus I
Crus II
Lob. c
Parafl. dors.
Parafl. ventr.
Flocc.
Lob. c1
Corp. rest.
N. vest.
Lob. b
Lob. a
N. fast.
N. int.
N. lat.
caudal
rostral
M
β
D
d.cap
v.l.o
d.l.
v.l.
dm.c.col.
Med. acc. olive
Principal olive
Dors. acc. olive
Ventral lamella
Dorsal lamella
Rostral
Caudal
Dm. cell column
Nucl. β
Ventrolat. outgrowth
Dorsal cap

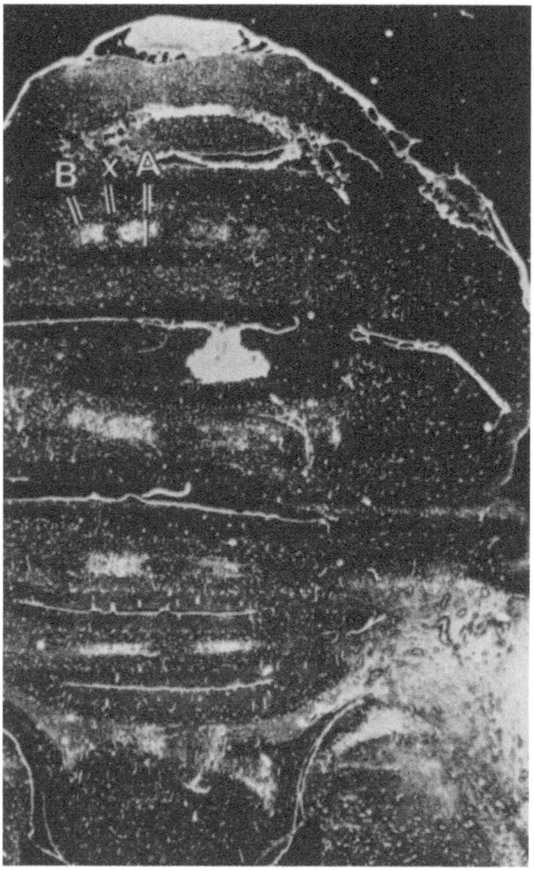

Fig. 2. Degenerated fibers in the *A* and *B* compartments of the vermis of the anterior lobe after a lesion of the caudal half of the inferior olive in the cat (H 7548, Groenewegen and Voogd 1977). In the dorsal folia of the lobe the *A* and *B* compartments are separated by a gap, corresponding to the presumed "*x*" compartment. Dark-field photograph of Nauta stained section

ules of the hemisphere (Fig. 1), the medial accessory olive with the entire vermis and the flocculus. For the dorsal accessory olive a projection to the anterior lobe was established, which extends beyond the vermis into an intermediate region between vermis and hemisphere, the so-called pars intermedia. In the cat the pars intermedia covers almost the whole of the hemisphere of the anterior lobe, but in the rabbit a third, most lateral zone is present in the anterior lobe, which receives olivocerebellar fibers from the rostral pole of the principal nucleus.

In the sixties we made some accidental observations in Nauta-stained cases with lesions of the reticular formation in the cat, which encroached upon the inferior olive. As reported in 1969, these experiments, with survival times of approximately 1 week, only showed the course of the degenerated olivocerebellar fibers in the white matter (Voogd 1969). It was not until 1974 that Desclin discovered the extremely rapid disappearance of the degenerated climbing fiber terminals from the molecular layer. Lesions of the caudal pole of the inferior olive, involving both the medial and dorsal accessory olives and the caudal extension of the principal nucleus (the so-called dorsal cap and the ventrolateral

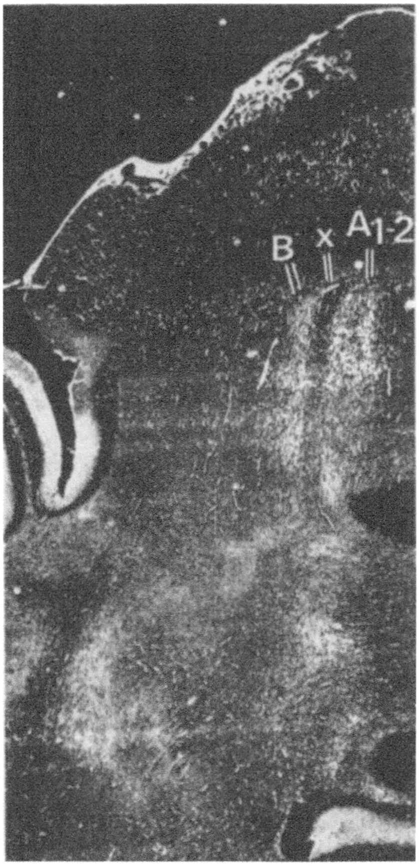

Fig. 3. Slightly more caudal section through the anterior lobe of the experiment depicted in Fig. 2. Note the presence of two bundles of degenerated fibers A_1 and A_2 in the A compartment. Compare with Figs. 3, 11, 12

outgrowth) gave rise to a bilateral degeneration in the white matter of the entire vermis, which was distributed in a medial and a lateral bundle (Figs. 2, 3). The medial bundle (A) showed a further subdivision into medial and lateral parts, the lateral bundle (B) was only present in the vermis of the anterior lobe and the simple lobule. After a lesion of the caudal pole of the dorsal accessory olive only the lateral bundle (B) was found to be degenerated. These observations were clearly at variance with Brodal (1940): different parts of the inferior olive apparently project to different longitudinal zones, which are continuous through successive lobules, often extending all over the length of the folial chains of the vermis or hemisphere. A single cerebellar lobule usually contains several of these zones, and the main feature of the olivocerebellar projection therefore proved to be its zonal, rather than its lobular, organization.

The longitudinal zonal type of cerebellar organization was not new to us. In earlier investigations in the cat with the Häggqvist modification of the Alzheimer-Mann stain (Alzheimer 1910, Häggqvist 1936, Voogd and Feirabend 1981) a similar organization had been proposed for the corticonuclear projection (Voogd 1964, 1967, 1969; Voogd and Bigaré 1980). In the cer-

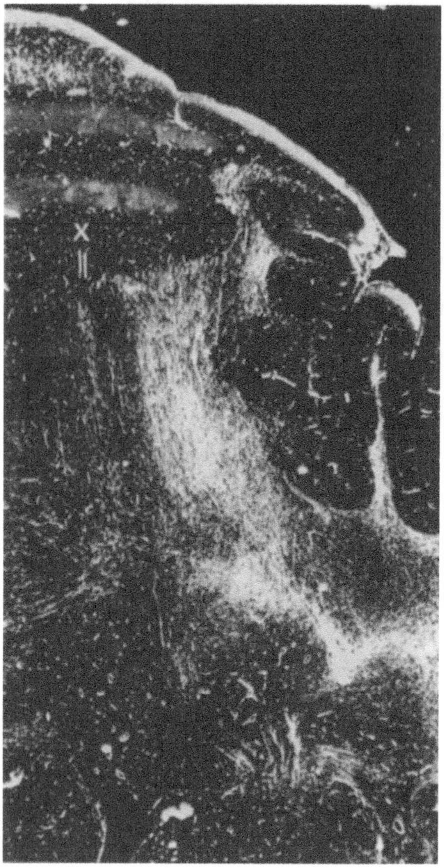

Fig. 4. Degenerated fibers in the white matter of the hemisphere of the anterior lobe after a lesion of the rostral half of the inferior olive in the cat (H 7579, Groenewegen and Voogd 1977). In the white matter of the vermis degenerated fibers are present only in the presumed "*x*" compartment

ebellar white matter the Purkinje cell fibers were found to be distributed in a number of parallel, parasagittal sheets, each originating from a (hypothetical) longitudinal zone of Purkinje cells, and terminating on a certain central cerebellar nucleus. The position in the vermis of the bundles of olivocerebellar fibers, moreover, proved to coincide with the position of two of the sheets of corticonuclear fibers. The medial "A" compartment of the vermal white matter contains the corticonuclear fibers from a medial zone to the fastigial nucleus and olivocerebellar fibers from the caudal part of the medial accessory olive, the lateral "B" compartment of the vermis includes the corticovestibular fibers to Deiters nucleus and the olivocerebellar fibers from the caudal tip of the dorsal accessory olive. These observations on the similarity in the organization of the corticonuclear and olivocerebellar projections, prompted a further search with more appropriate methods, such as antegrade axonal transport of tritiated amino acids, which came into use at that time (Cowan et al. 1972). The first demonstration of the termination of olivocerebellar fibers as climbing fibers in longitudinal strips in the molecular layer, after large injections of tritiated amino acids in the inferior olive, by Courville et al. (1974), therefore did not come as a surprise. Their observation of large, empty spaces in between the strips of labeled climbing fibers created a perennial problem which still concerns us and gave a fresh impulse to the search for other sources for the climbing fibers.

The origin of the olivocerebellar fibers to the vermis and the flocculus from caudal parts of the inferior olive is complemented by the origin of the fibers to the hemisphere from the rostral parts of the accessory olives and the principal nucleus (Fig. 4). As has been shown by Groenewegen (Groenewegen and Voogd 1976, 1977; Groenewegen 1978, Groenewegen et al. 1979) the projection of the rostral part of the inferior olive can be resolved into a number of zones, each corresponding to one of the corticonuclear projection zones as known from previous studies. Moreover olivocerebellar fibers were found to terminate on the central cerebellar nuclei, which receive the axons from Purkinje cells contacted by the climbing fiber terminals of the same olivocerebellar parent fibers (Fig. 5). However, the projection of the rostral part of the inferior olive is not

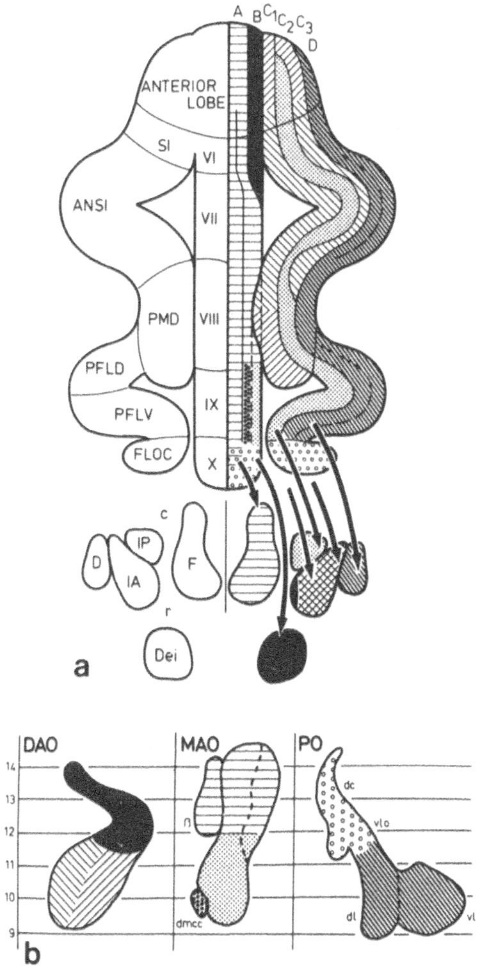

Fig. 5a, b. Diagram of the olivocerebellar projection in the cat. *ANS* or *ANSI*, ansiform lobule; *ANSU*, ansula, part of the Crus II of the ansiform lobule; *β* or *nβ*, cell group *β* of the medial accessory olive; *c*, caudal; *CR II*, Crus II of the ansiform lobule; *D*, dentate nucleus; *dc*, dorsal cap of the inferior olive; *DAO*, dorsal accessory olive; *Dei*, Deiters nucleus; *dl*, dorsal leaf PO; *dmcc*, dorsomedial cell column of the inferior olive; *F*, fastigial nucleus; *FLOC*, flocculus; *FPL*, fissura posterolateralis; *IA*, anterior interposed nucleus; *IP*, posterior interposed nucleus; *L*, lateral cerebellar nucleus; MAO, medial accessory olive; *PFL*, paraflocculus; *PFLD*, dorsal paraflocculus; *PFLV*, ventral paraflocculus; *PO*, principal nucleus of the inferior olive; *PMD* or *PMED*, paramedian lobule; *r*, rostral; *SI*, lobulus simplex; *vlo*, ventrolateral outgrowth of the principal nucleus of the olive; *Roman numerals* indicate the cerebellar lobules according to Larsell's nomenclature. Groenewegen et al. (1979) with permission from the Wistar Press

limited to the hemisphere. In addition to a projection to the C_2 zone, which extends all the way over the hemisphere, from the anterior lobe to the flocculus and to the posterior interposed nucleus, fibers from the rostral half of the medial accessory olive terminate in two zones in the lateral part of the caudal vermis (lobule IX, Fig. 6). The medial of these two zones originates from the dorsomedial cell column, a group of cells located dorsomedial to the rostral medial accessory olive, the lateral zone from the medial accessory olive proper. A similar situation exists in lobule VIII of the caudal vermis where fibers from the rostral half of the dorsal accessory olive (the C_1 zone) invade the lateral part of

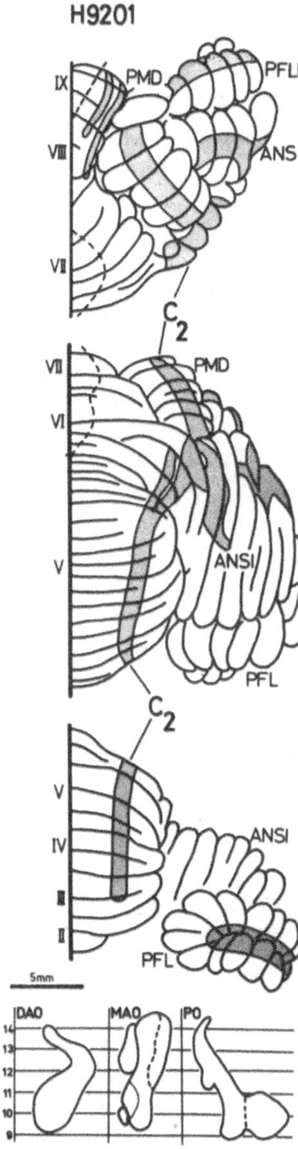

Fig. 6. The localization of labeled climbing fibers in the C_2 zone after an injection of tritiated leucine in the rostral part of the medial accessory olive in the cat. In the upper part of the figure graphic reconstructions of the caudal, dorsal, and rostral aspects of the cerebellum are depicted. *Shading* indicates the localization of the climbing fibers and of the effective injection site in the bottom diagram of the inferior olive at the bottom of the figure. Numbers to the left of this diagram refer to the stereotactic planes · P9–14. For abbreviations see Fig. 5. Groenewegen et al. (1979) with permission from the Wistar Press

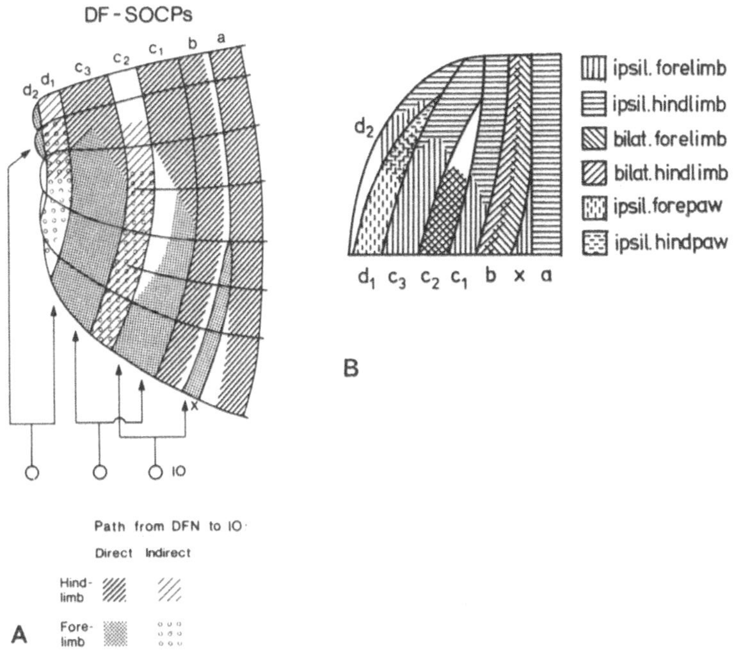

Fig. 7. **A** The termination of the dorsal spino-olivocerebellar path in lobules IV and V of the anterior lobe. Reproduced from Ekerot and Larson (1980a). **B** A diagram of the sagittal organization of the cerebellar anterior lobe as revealed by the projection patterns of the climbing fiber system. *DFN*, nuclei of the dorsal funiculus; *IO*, inferior olive. Oscarsson (1979) with permission from TINS

this lobule (Fig. 5). However, this projection is certainly less well documented than the projection from the medial accessory olive to lobule IX.

Another part of the vermis which receives olivocerebellar fibers from rostral parts of the inferior olive is located in between the A and the B zones in the anterior lobe vermis. It was not described as such in our earlier papers, but it is clearly indicated in our figures (Groenewegen and Voogd 1977, their Plates 2, 12, and 13), which are again reproduced in this paper (Figs. 2–4). In the case of a lesion of the caudal accessory olive the bundles of degenerated olivocerebellar fibers in the A and the B compartments cannot be separated in the ventral part of the anterior lobe, but become separated by a gap in the dorsal part of the lobe (Fig. 2). Caudally this gap widens (Fig. 3). In the case of a lesion of the rostral half of the inferior olive, degeneration in the anterior lobe is present both in the hemisphere and in the gap between the A and the B compartments in the dorsal part of the anterior lobe (Fig. 4). Our attention to this strip was drawn by the observations of Ekerot and Larson (1977, 1979 a, b) and Oscarsson (1979) of a so-called x zone in a corresponding position in some of their experiments (Fig. 7).

At this point the important contributions of electrophysiology to the concept of the longitudinal organization of the olivocerebellar projection should be mentioned. Oscarsson demonstrated spino-olivo-cerebellar paths which activate a number of parallel, longitudinal strips of climbing fibers (see Oscarsson 1969, 1973). The experiments of Armstrong et al. (1973a, b) showed the collateralization of climbing fibers in narrow, longitudinal zones (Fig. 8), and culminated in an accurate map of the olivocerebellar projection on the basis of antidromic activation of the inferior olive (Armstrong et al. 1974, Fig. 9). Initially these experiments were conducted independently of our anatomical approach. The strong similarity in the topography of Oscarsson's climbing fiber strips and the anatomical zones, made them adopt a modification of our nomenclature (Oscarsson and Sjölund 1977a, b).

This similarity should not hide the fact that the criteria used to define Oscarsson's climbing fiber strips and the anatomical zones are not identical. Oscarsson uses stimulation of certain ascending spinal tracts which are left standing after a subtotal cordotomy. The olivary relay in his spinal-olivo-cerebellar paths is not studied as such, and conclusions as to the exact site of origin of the climbing fibers in his pathways, therefore, are based on other evidence. His zones are thus characterized by the way they are activated from the periphery, the conduction velocity in these pathways, their topography, and the collateralization of the climbing fibers within and in between the zones. The latter two criteria are shared by our anatomical zones. The localization of the anatomical zones is primarily based upon their efferent, corticonuclear projection. Our conclusions on the localization in the olivocerebellar projection are largely

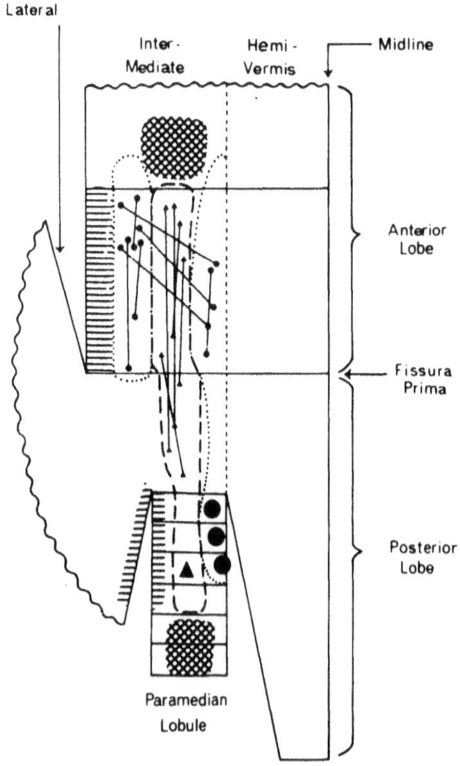

Fig. 8. Distribution of branches from climbing fibers which provided two branches accessible to stimulation. *Symbols* joined in pairs represent the stimulated branches of a single parent axon. *Small circles* represent branches of climbing fibers in C_1 and C_3 zones of fibers stimulated at the *large circle* in the C_1 zone in the paramedian lobule. *Triangles* represent climbing fibers in the C_2 zone. *Hatched areas* indicate other axon reflex climbing fiber connections. Armstrong et al. (1973b)

dependent on, or have been strongly influenced by, previous knowledge of the zonation in the corticonuclear projection.

This bias is not without danger, but in the case of the connections of the lateral B zone of the vermis of the anterior lobe our contention of the basic similarity in the topographical organization of the corticonuclear and olivocerebellar projections was completely confirmed by Andersson and Oscarsson (1977, 1978a, b). They found that the cells of Deiters nucleus, which we showed to receive

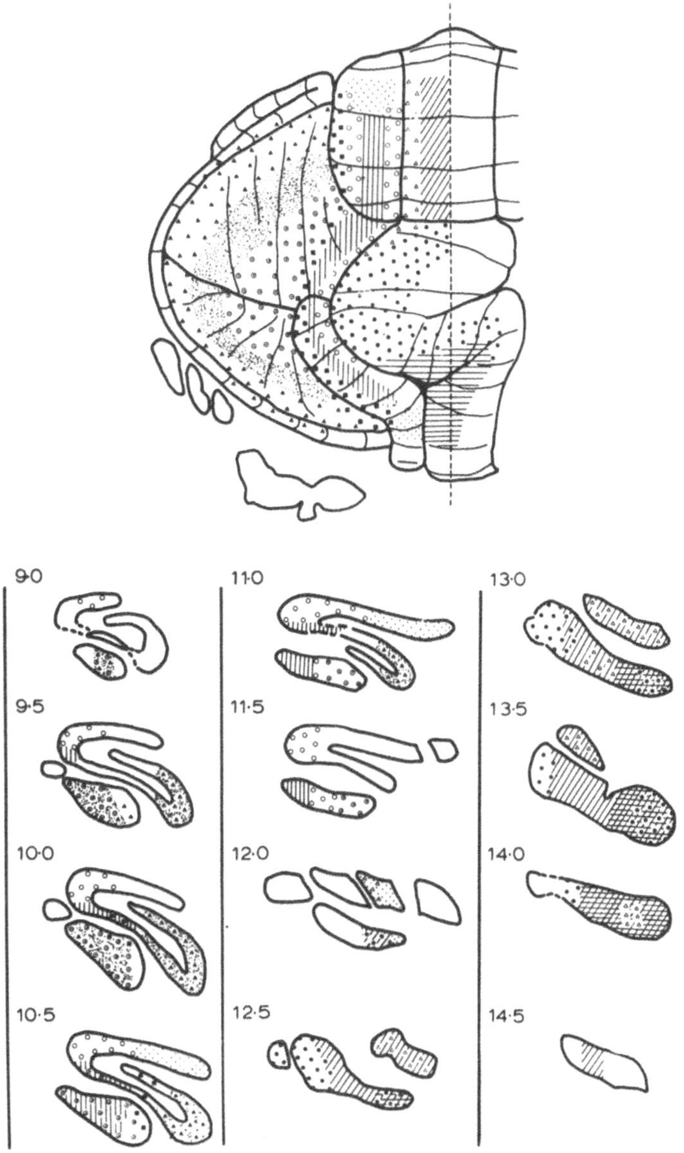

Fig. 9. Diagram of the topographical localization in the olivocerebellar projection in the cat, based on antidromic stimulation of the inferior olive. Armstrong et al. (1974) with permission from the Wistar Press

Purkinje cell fibers from the B zone and collaterals from the caudal pole of the dorsal accessory olive, are activated by collaterals of climbing fibers which terminate in the B-zone. In turn these climbing fibers gave rise to a Purkinje cell-mediated inhibition of the same cells of Deiters nucleus.

Collateralization of climbing fibers, although within the realm of the autoradiographic tracing technique, has not been extensively used by us, with one possible and notable exception. This exception concerns the projection of the rostral half of the dorsal accessory olive to two zones, C_1 and C_3. Their localization was known from myeloarchitectonic studies and concerns one of the main points of resemblance between Oscarsson's climbing fiber strips and the anatomical zones. In lobule II of the anterior lobe the C_1 and C_3 zones are continuous, but more dorsally they separate and the C_2 zone becomes intercalated between them. Both C_1 and C_3 are related to the anterior interposed nucleus, whereas C_2 is connected with the posterior interposed nucleus (Voogd 1969, Voogd and Bigaré 1980). Injection of tritiated leucine in the rostral part of the dorsal accessory olive usually results in simultaneous labeling in the C_1 and the C_3 zones (Groenewegen et al. 1979). This could be taken as evidence for transverse branching of olivocerebellar fibers, which provide climbing fibers to both zones. Transverse branching of climbing fibers was first described by Armstrong et al. (1973a, b, Fig. 8). Ekerot and Larson (to be published) analyzed the branching of climbing fibers destined for their c_1 and c_3 zones in more detail. According to them (Fig. 7), branches of the same climbing fiber always distribute to paired subzones: medial c_1+medial c_3; lateral c_3+d_2 and lateral c_1+x.

This type of distribution of the climbing fibers clearly differs from the concept advanced in our anatomical studies. Groups of cells, presumably located in the dorsal accessory olive, send climbing fibers to paired subzones, and these straddle other zones that receive a projection from different parts of the inferior olive. The borders between the pairs of subzones, which receive branches of single parent fibers, therefore do not coincide with the borders of the anatomical zones, but are located in the middle of them. In the ventral part of the anterior lobe the subzones c_1, c_3, and d_2 fuse. This fusion also can be seen in some of our experiments. In an experiment from Groenewegen (1978), H 9317 II (Fig. 10), with an injection in the rostral dorsal accessory olive, labeling in the hemisphere of lobule II reaches its lateral margin and labeling in an incipient d_2 zone is indicated[1]. The presence of paired subzones in the C_3 zone was also observed in our experiments (Groenewegen et al. 1979, Plate 12).

The irregularity in the branching of climbing fibers to the c_1 and the x zone poses a challenging problem. The irregularity lies in the fact that these fibers

1 The notation "d_2" for this zone may cause confusion, because this indication is derived from the anatomical D zones which were supposed to receive climbing fibers from the principal nucleus of the inferior olive and to project to the lateral cerebellar nucleus. Experiments in the cat, with HRP injected into the central nuclei, show that a zone in the extreme lateral part of lobules II and III, corresponding to the d_2 zone, projects to the anterior interposed nucleus. "D" zones projecting to the lateral cerebellar nucleus were not found to be present in the lobules II and III but to occupy the extreme lateral part of the more dorsal and caudal folia of the anterior lobe (Bigaré 1980, Voogd and Bigaré 1980)

skip the medial c_1 zone to terminate in its lateral part. In a reexamination of the Häggqvist material, a narrow compartment was found which originally was included with the A compartment (Figs. 11, 12). This area is located in between the A and the B compartments in the dorsal part of the anterior lobe. Its fibers are smaller than in the neighboring A and B compartments and it was therefore considered to belong to the "raphe", the area of small, presumably afferent fibers, separating A and B. However, upon closer inspection it is clear that this narrow compartment consists of a central bundle of slightly larger fibers, bordered by strips of thin fibers. If the central fibers are the fibers from Purkinje

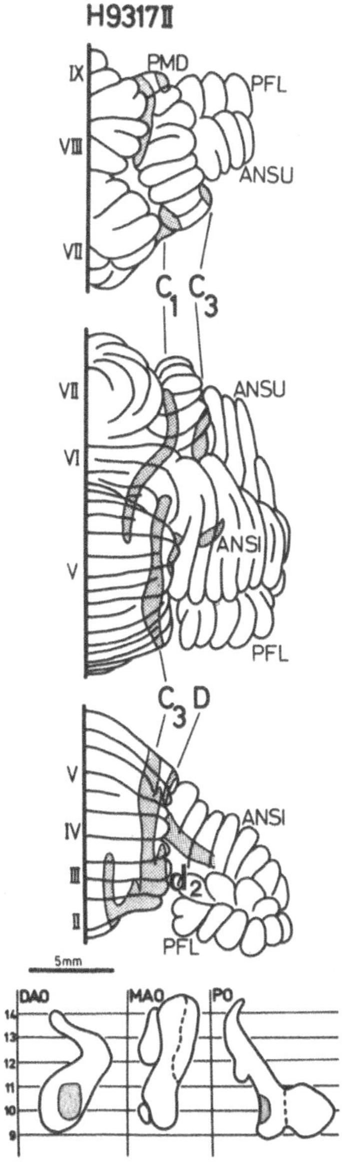

Fig. 10. The localization of labeled climbing fibers after an injection of tritiated leucine in the rostral part of the dorsal accessory olive. Compare with Fig. 6. Groenewegen (1978) with permission from the author. For abbreviations see Fig. 5

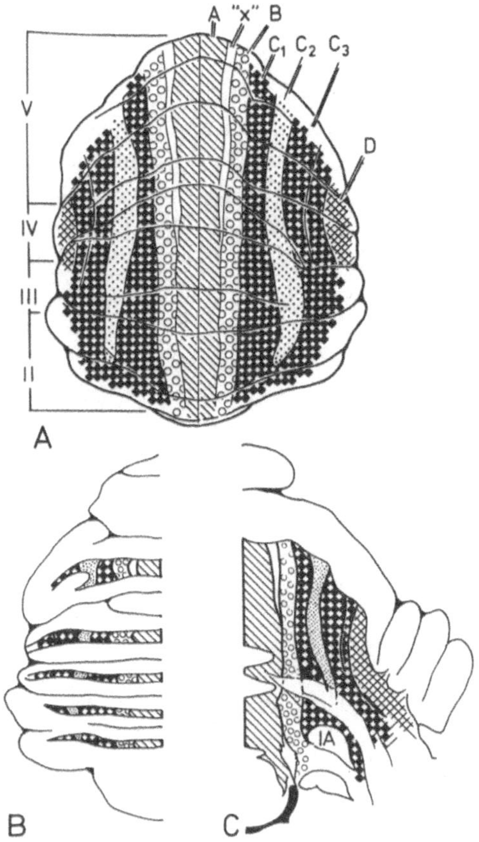

Fig. 11 A–C. Localization of the myeloarchitectonic compartments in the anterior lobe of the cat. **A** projection of the borders of the compartments on a rostral view of the anterior lobe; **B** rostrally located section through the anterior lobe; **C** caudally located section through the anterior lobe. For abbreviations see Fig. 5

cells of the x zone then they are certainly smaller than the Purkinje cell fibers of the A, B, and C_1 zones. Small calibre Purkinje cell fibers, as present in the presumed x compartment, are also found in the C_2 compartment. When this line of reasoning is followed, the irregularity in the branching of the climbing fibers to the x and the lateral c_1 zone could be explained by an origin of this set of climbing fibers from the medial accessory olive. In which case the lateral part of the c_1 zone of Ekerot and Larson (to be published) should be included in our C_2 zone and the irregularity in the branching of the fibers of the dorsal accessory olive to c_1, c_3, and d_2 would be restored.

As to the origin of the climbing fibers to the presumed x zone our material offers no conclusive evidence. As pointed out before, the rostral part of the medial accessory olive indeed projects to the C_2 zone, but whether fibers to the x zone originate from this nucleus or from the dorsal accessory olive cannot be decided. A termination in x and C_2 is present in case H 9318 with an injection sparing the rostral and caudal poles of the medial accessory olive, which also involves the dorsal accessory olive and the principal nucleus.

In recent publications on the olivocerebellar system more attention was devoted to the presence of a longitudinal pattern in its terminal field than to the mor-

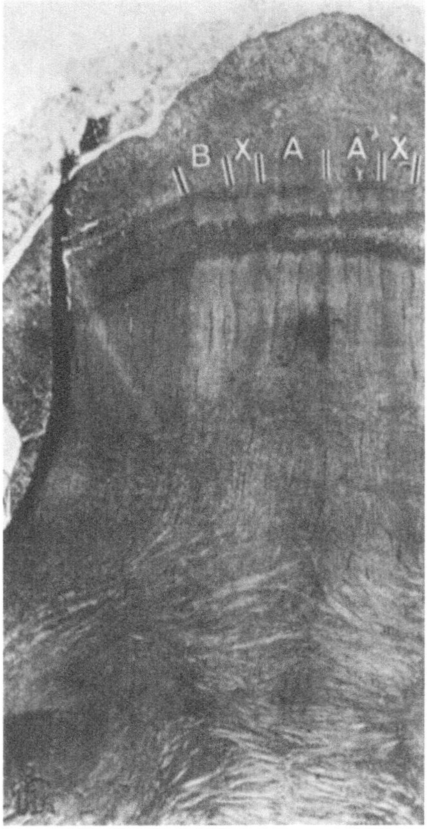

Fig. 12. Transverse Häggqvist stained section through the anterior lobe of the cat (H 9039)

phology of the olive. I will try to review the olivocerebellar projection from the point of view of the subdivision of the inferior olive and the interrelations of its composite parts. In most mammals the medial accessory olive (MAO) is a single, well-defined cell group. Its division into rostral and caudal parts, with their widely diverging projections to the A and C_2 zones, therefore came as a surprise (Groenewegen and Voogd 1976).

Topographic histochemistry of acetylcholinesterase (AChE) reveals more of the internal division of the MAO. According to Martin et al. (1975) for the opossum and Marani and Voogd (1977) for the cat, several rostrocaudally directed columns of high and low AChE activity are present in the caudal part of the MAO. In the opossum a medial column with a high AChE activity ("a") continues into the rostral part of the MAO, but in the cat (Fig. 13) the rostral part of this nucleus shows a low and uniform distribution of the enzyme. Cytoarchitectonic studies also suggested a mediolateral subdivision of the caudal MAO (Taber 1961, cat; Bowman and Sladek 1973, *Macaca*; Martin et al. 1975, opossum; Saigal et al., Olivocerebellar connections in sheep, unpublished work). In the cat two divisions (the "ventral" and "medial" parts) are recognized. In *Macaca*, the opossum, and sheep three divisions (a, b, and c) seem to

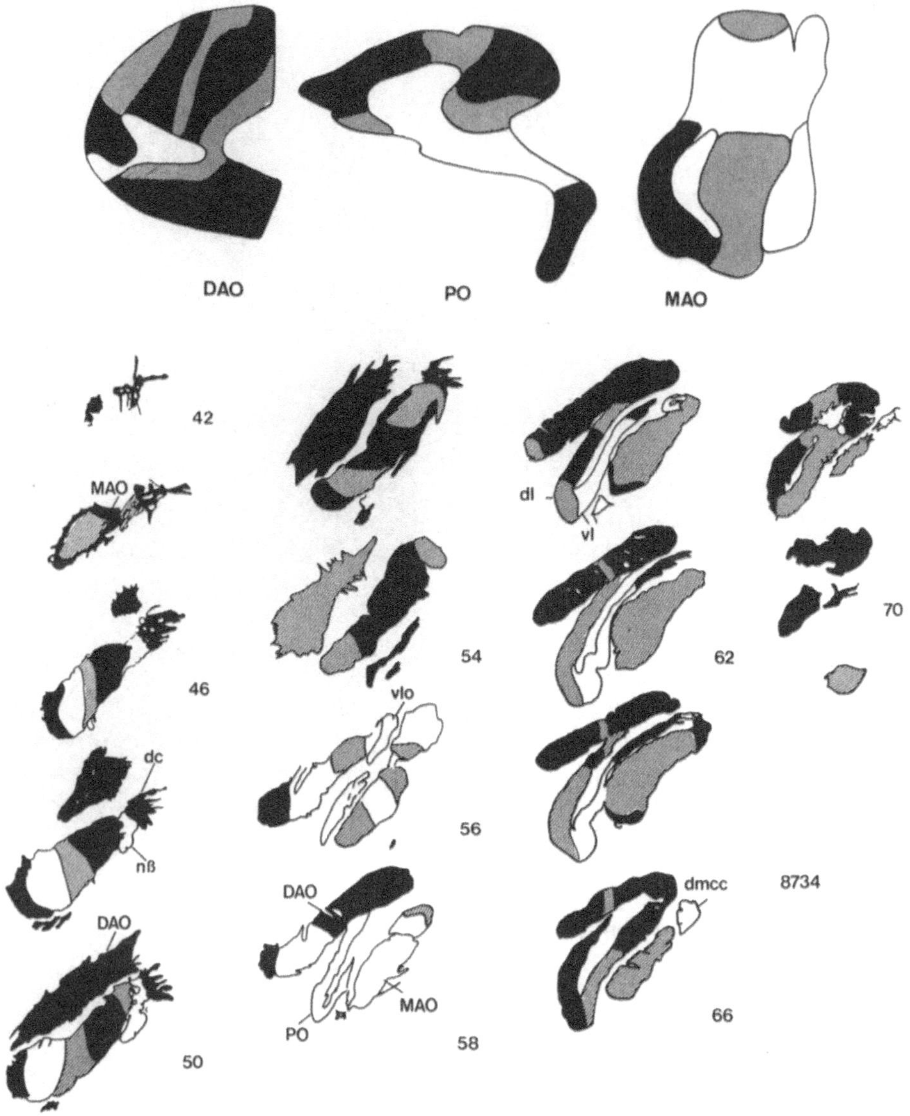

Fig. 13. Distribution of acetylcholinesterase in the inferior olive of the cat, indicated in a diagram of the olive constructed after Brodal (1940). High activity is indicated in *black*, medium activity is *shaded*. For abbreviations see Fig. 5. Marani et al. (1977) with permission from the Wistar Press

be present from medial to lateral. Division "c" in part, or as a whole, represents the "group β", which constitutes the third and most medial division in the cat. Dorsal to group β the principal nucleus makes its appearance in the shape of the "dorsal cap" which can be recognized in all species. No columnar division seems to be present in the rostral half of the MAO. Only the discrete "dorsomedial cell column" is present on its dorsomedial side. According to some authors it can be considered as the rostral prolongation of the group β (Brodal 1940).

Are all these subdivisions, or is the lack of subdivision, accounted for in the projection of the MAO to the cerebellum? Labeling in the caudal pole of the MAO following HRP injections in the vermis of the anterior lobe and the simple lobule (lobule VI), the pyramis (lobule VIII), and to some extent in lobule VII does not display a columnar distribution of the labeled cells (Hoddevik et al. 1976, Brodal and Walberg 1977). However, after injections of tritiated leucine or lesions of this part of the MAO two bundles of olivocerebellar fibers are present in the A compartment (Fig. 3) and two corresponding sets of labeled climbing fibers can be distinguished in the A zone (Groenewegen and Voogd 1977). These observations get support from the localization of labeled Purkinje cells and the cells of the contralateral inferior olive after injections of HRP in the fastigial nucleus of the cat (Bigaré 1980, Figs. 14, 15).

After an injection of HRP in the rostromedial fastigial nucleus (H 9869) labeled Purkinje cells are present in the medial vermis and in a medial column of cells in the caudal part of the MAO. After a rostrolateral injection (C 459) labeling is present more laterally in the vermis and the contralateral MAO. Similar observations were made in monkeys (Voogd et al., unpublished work). Injections of tritiated leucine in the "a" and "b" columns of the caudal MAO labeled two strips of climbing fibers (A_1 and A_2) in the entire vermis with the exception of lobules IX and X (Fig. 16). In another case with an injection which mainly involves the "b" column the labeling is limited to the A_1 zone.

Separate cell columns in the caudal pole of the MAO therefore project to separate A_1 and A_2 zones and to the corresponding parts of the fastigial nucleus. The next medial column is the group β, which was found to project to the uvula (lobule IX, Brodal 1940, 1976) and lobule VII (Hoddevik et al. 1976, Saigal et al., Olivocerebellar connections in sheep, unpublished work).

This projection to the caudal vermis and the caudal pole of the fastigial nucleus is visualized in C 402 11 (Figs. 14, 15) with an HRP injection of this part of the fastigial nucleus. In addition the dorsomedial cell column is labeled in this case. In terms of its projection to specific longitudinal zones (A_1, A_2, a separate A zone?) the position of the group β is not yet clear. The dorsomedial cell column was found to project to a separate zone in the lateral part of lobule IX (Groenewegen et al. 1979, Voogd and Bigaré 1980: the A_3 zone).

The most lateral zone in lobule IX and the entire C_2 zone in the hemisphere receive climbing fibers from the rostral half of the MAO. Groenewegen's material shows that paired subzones are present in some parts of the C_2 zone (see Fig. 4a from Groenewegen et al. 1979), but nothing is known about a separate origin of these subzones in the rostral MAO. Intermingling of A- and C_2-projecting cells at the border region of the rostral and caudal halves of the MAO

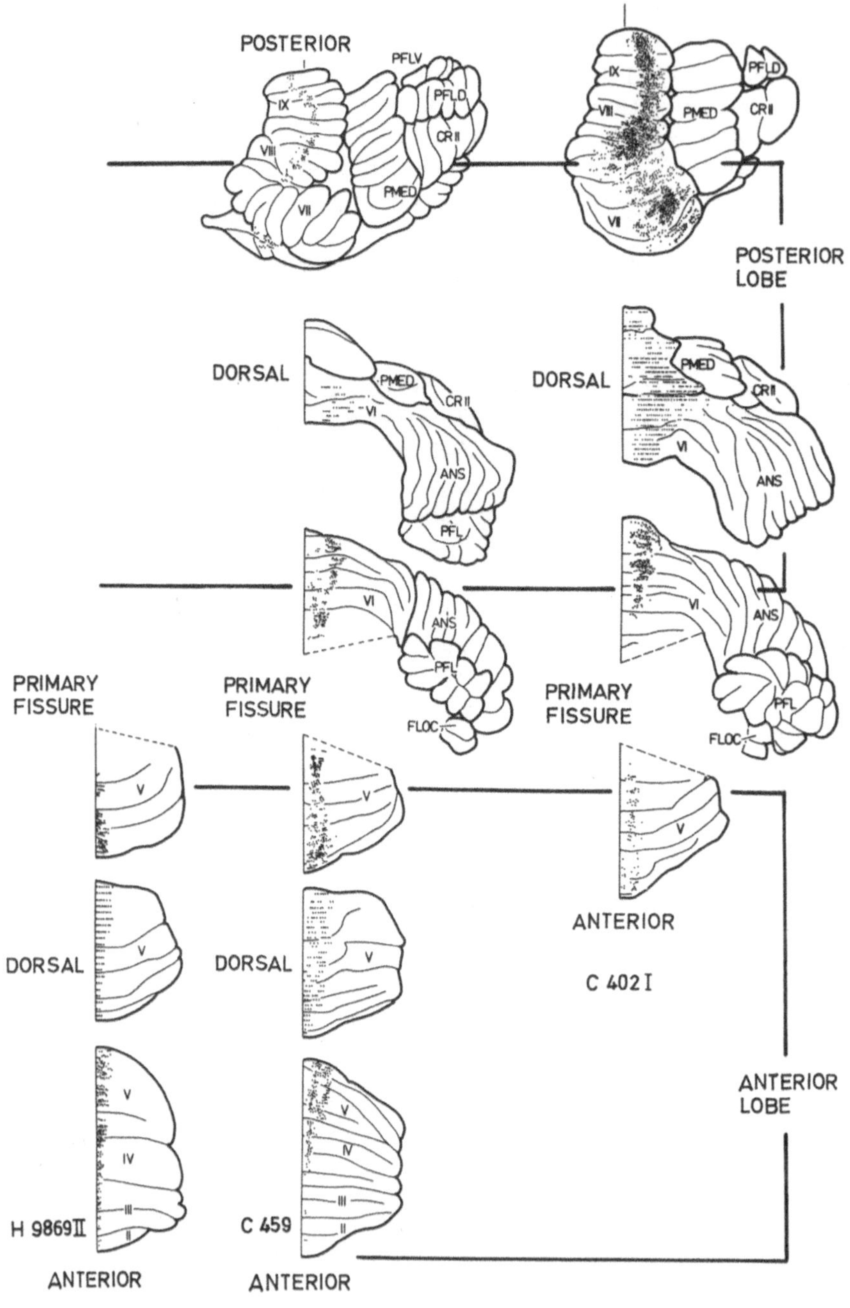

Fig. 14. The localization of labeled Purkinje cells after injections of HRP in the fastigial nucleus of the cat. Purkinje cells are indicated on graphic reconstructions of the cerebellar surface. At the *top* caudal and dorsal views of the posterior lobe are shown, followed by the rostral and caudal banks of the opened primary fissure, and a dorsal and a rostral view of the anterior lobe. For injection sites see Fig. 15. For abbreviations see Fig. 5. Bigaré (1980) with permission from the author

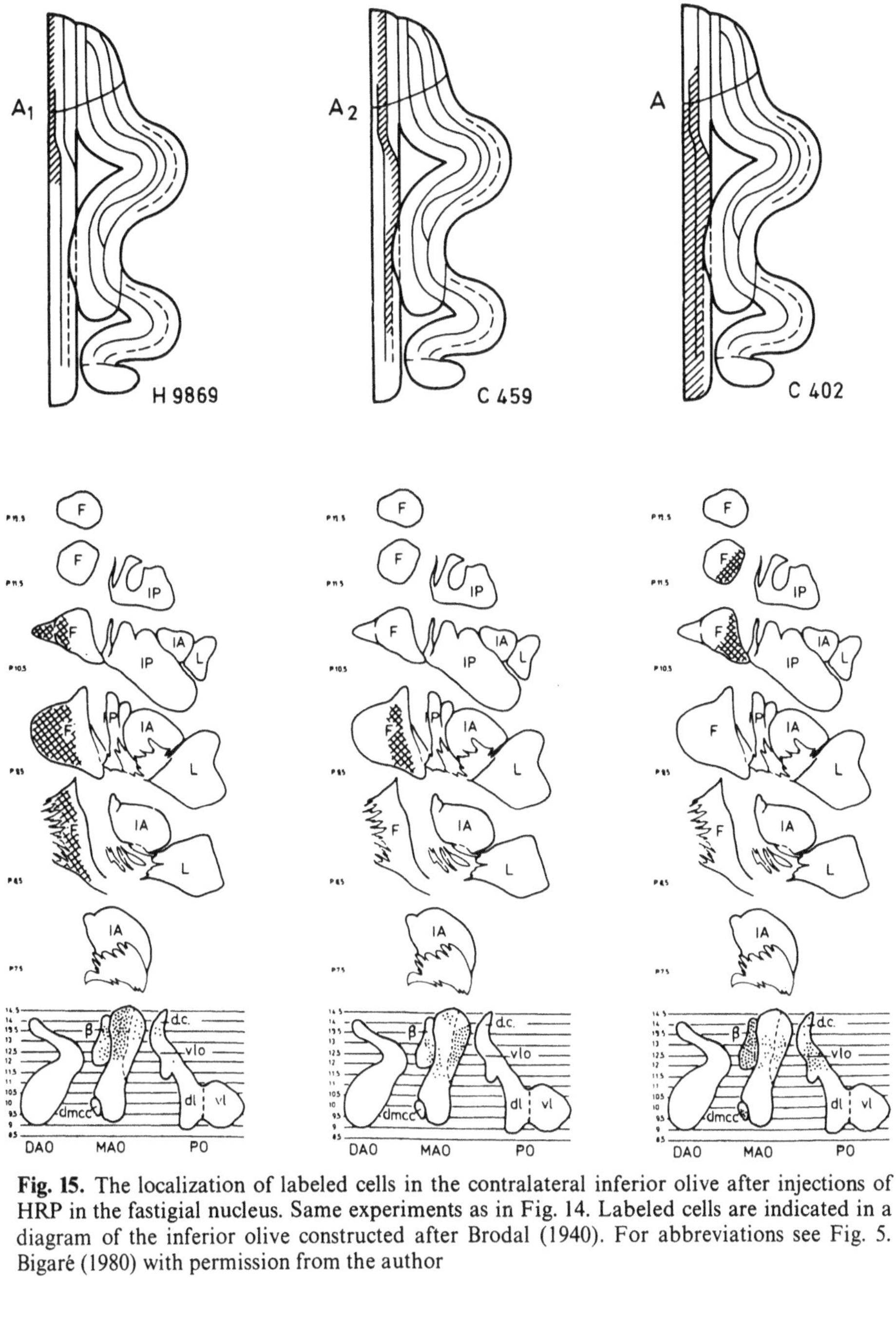

Fig. 15. The localization of labeled cells in the contralateral inferior olive after injections of HRP in the fastigial nucleus. Same experiments as in Fig. 14. Labeled cells are indicated in a diagram of the inferior olive constructed after Brodal (1940). For abbreviations see Fig. 5. Bigaré (1980) with permission from the author

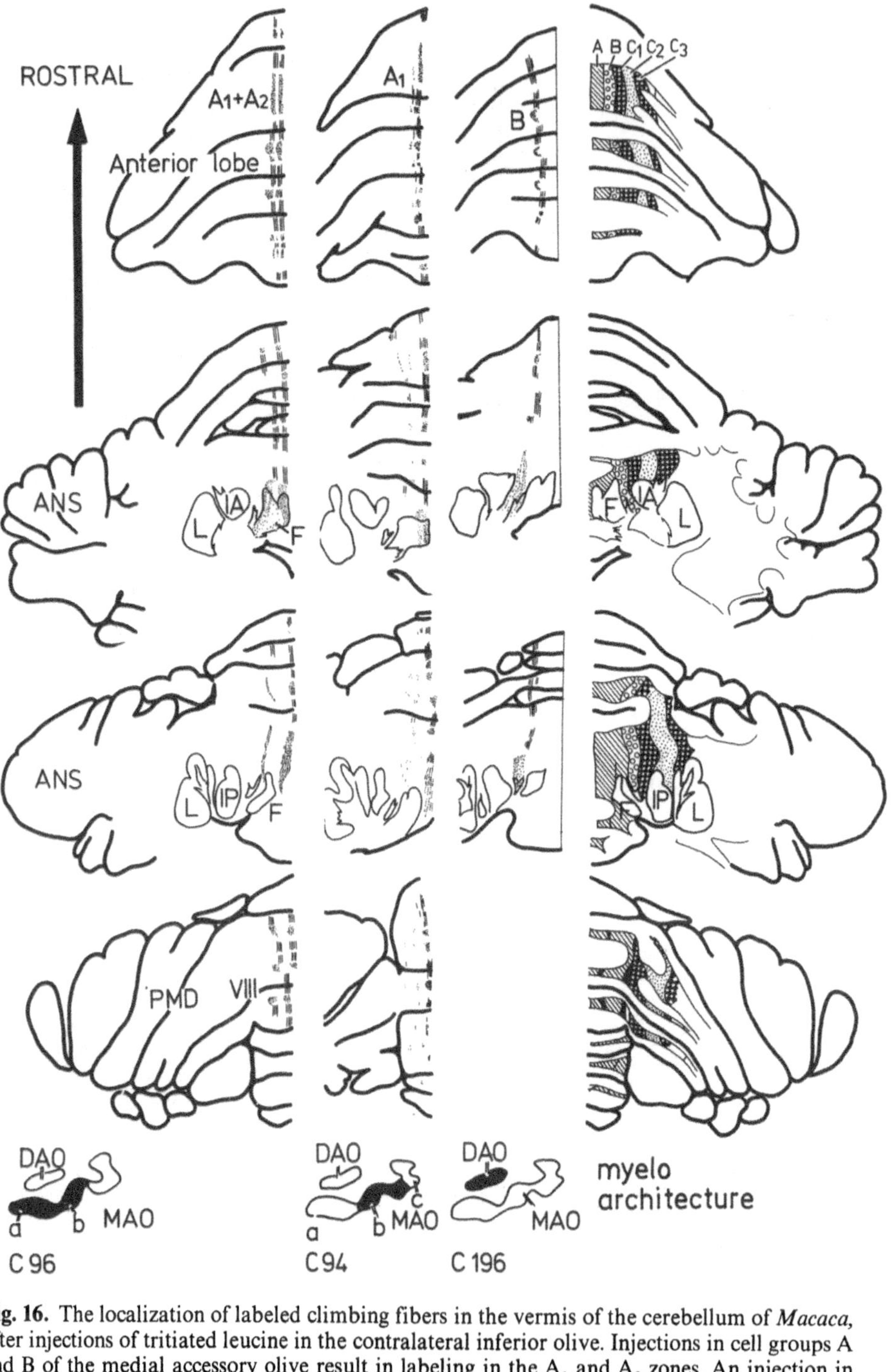

Fig. 16. The localization of labeled climbing fibers in the vermis of the cerebellum of *Macaca*, after injections of tritiated leucine in the contralateral inferior olive. Injections in cell groups A and B of the medial accessory olive result in labeling in the A_1 and A_2 zones. An injection in the dorsal accessory olive is followed by labeling in the B zone. To the *right* the borders of the myeloarchitectonic compartments in the white matter are indicated in drawings of corresponding Häggqvist stained sections. For abbreviations see Fig. 5

seems to be slight (compare Brodal et al. 1975, Brodal and Walberg 1977) and the existence of double projecting cells with axons to both zones has not yet been investigated. As pointed out before the occurrence of cells with branching axons in this region, which is still within the territory covered by the "dorsal spino-olivocerebellar climbing-fiber system" (Boesten and Voogd 1975, Groenewegen and Voogd 1976) would offer an alternative explanation for the origin of the branched climbing fibers terminating in the "x" and "c_1" zones (Ekerot and Larson, to be published).

The rostral MAO projects in a topological manner to different parts of the C_2 zone. Fibers to the segments of the zone located within the anterior lobe and the paramedian lobule originate caudal to the fibers to the ansiform lobule and the paraflocculus (Groenewegen et al. 1979, Walberg 1980). A contribution to the C_2 zone to the flocculus as described by Brodal (1940), Hoddevik and Brodal (1977) and Walberg et al. (1979) originally was denied by Groenewegen et al. (1979) but could be retrieved in the injections with tritiated leucine in the rostral tip of the MAO (Gerrits and Voogd, to be published). In these experiments labeling of climbing fibers can be traced from the ventral paraflocculus, through the posterolateral fissure, in a small mediocaudal portion of the flocculus (Fig. 17, H 8789).

The diverging projections of the dorsal accessory olive (DAO) to the B zone and the C_1 and C_3 zones are less well-documented than the projections from the MAO. The reasons for this are both technical and conceptual. The deep localization of the DAO makes it less accessible and only a few selective injections of this nucleus have been reported in investigations using the autoradiographic tracing technique. Moreover the zones supplied by the DAO are very close or even contiguous, and the use of retrograde tracer techniques therefore is fraught with difficulties. Where the anatomists succeeded in demonstrating the zones, physiologists complicated the issue by the demonstration of lateral branching of climbing fibers between these zones.

The laterally directed bend in the boomerang-shaped DAO seems to mark the transition of the caudal pole, projecting to the B zone and the large rostral portion from which the C_1 and C_3 zones originate. The B zone is unique because it only occurs in the anterior lobe and the simple lobule (Groenewegen and Voogd 1977). It lacks the dual representation in the anterior and posterior lobes and the branching climbing fibers which characterize the A, C, and D zones. The rostral border of the area in the DAO projecting to B is still enigmatic (Fig. 18). Armstrong et al. (1974) put it at the notch in the contour of the DAO. Brodal and Walberg (1977) found a projection of the entire DAO to the anterior lobe and did not distinguish between the B and the C_1 zone in their injections of the anterior lobe vermis. After HRP injections of the paramedian lobule no labeled cells were found in the caudal pole of the DAO (Brodal et al. 1975). The caudal limb of the DAO therefore should be the origin of the projection to the B zone, which is present in the anterior lobe, but absent in the posterior lobe. In the autoradiographic studies of Groenewegen and Voogd (1977) and Kawamura and Hashikawa (1979) this border was set more rostrally. When the available evidence is weighed I would be inclined to attach more importance to the methods using retrograde transport, or antidromic acti-

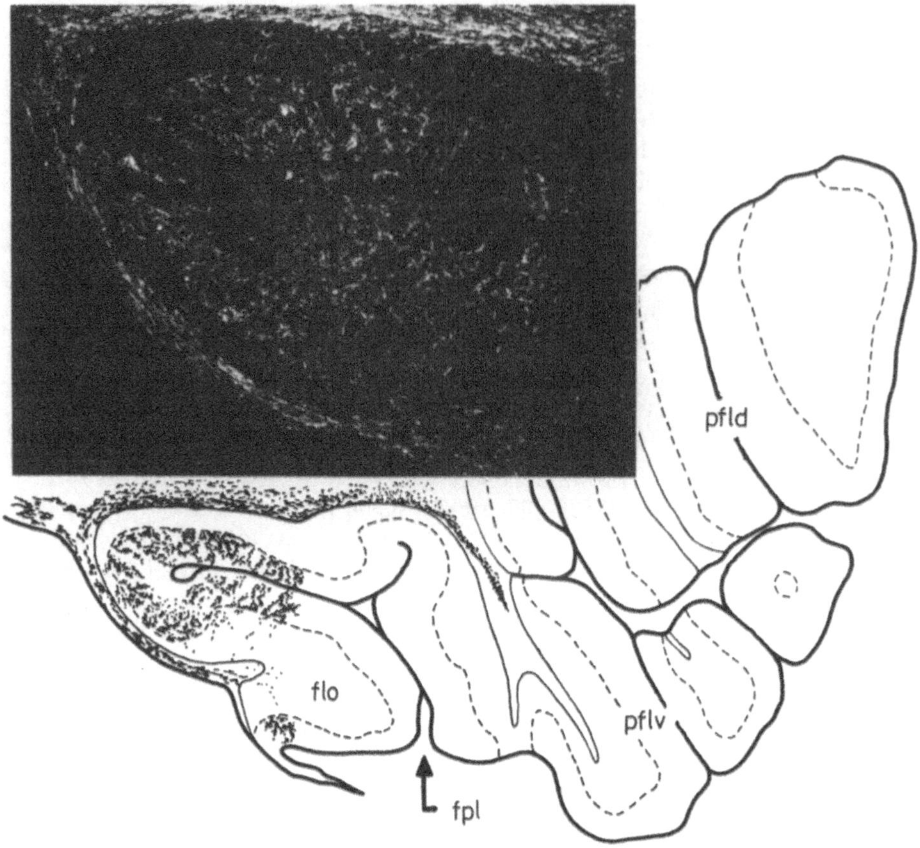

Fig. 17. The termination of the C_2 zone in the flocculus. Labeled climbing fibers are located in the ventral paraflocculus and the caudomedial part of the flocculus, after an injection of tritiated leucine in the rostral pole of the medial accessory olive. Experiment H. 8789. For abbreviations see Fig. 5

vation. Walberg and Brodal (1979) and Brodal and Kawamura (1980), however, included a more rostrolateral portion of the DAO in the projection area to the B zone and consequently found a representation of this zone in the ventromedial paramedian lobule, an area usually assigned to the C_1 zone (Oscarsson and Sjölund 1977a, b; Groenewegen et al. 1979). As a consequence of this line of reasoning Dietrichs and Walberg (1979) described the projection of the alleged B zone in the ventromedial paramedian lobule to the anterior interposed nucleus, the target of the C_1 zone in our investigations (Bigaré 1980, Voogd and Bigaré 1980).

Although the exact position of the border between the cells projecting to B and to C_1–C_3 has not been settled, there is no evidence for cells with branching axons between these zones. As yet the anatomical evidence is inconclusive on the exact origin in the rostral DAO of the sets of branching climbing fibers to combinations of the C_1, C_3, and d_2 zones in the anterior lobe and the paramedi-

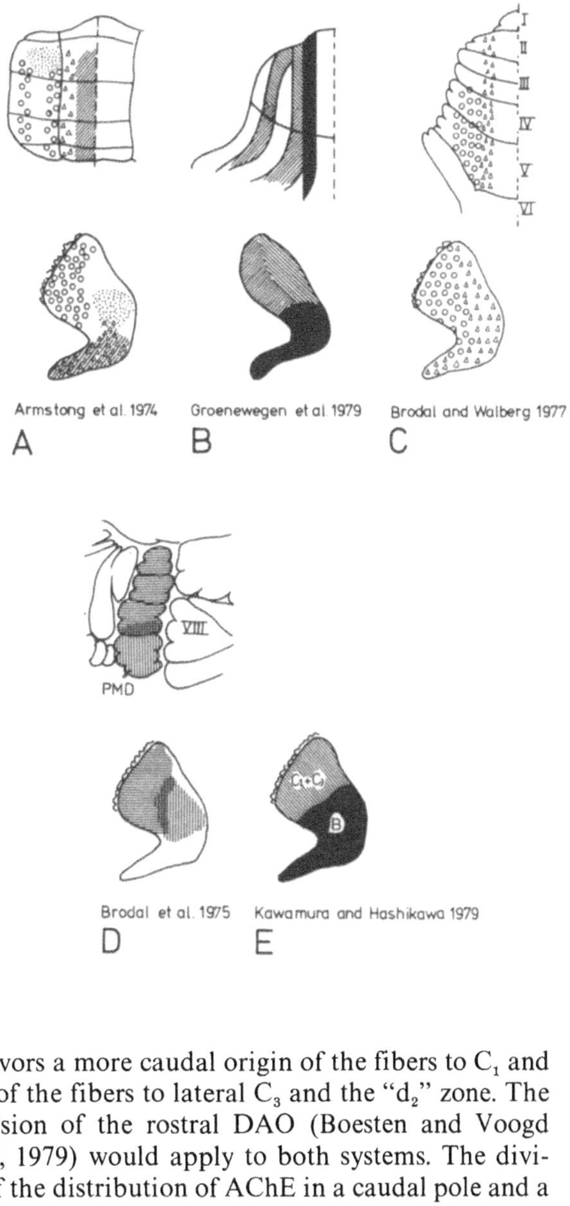

Fig. 18 A–E. The projection of the dorsal accessory olive. **A** according to Armstrong et al. (1974), after Brodal and Walberg (1977), compare with Fig. 9; **B** according to Groenewegen et al. (1979), compare with Fig. 5; **C** Projection to the anterior lobe according to Brodal and Walberg (1977); **D** Projection to the paramedian lobule according to Brodal et al. (1975); **E** according to Kawamura and Hashikawa (1979). For abbreviations see Fig. 5

an lobule. My interpretation favors a more caudal origin of the fibers to C_1 and medial C_3 and a rostral origin of the fibers to lateral C_3 and the "d_2" zone. The mediolateral somatotopic division of the rostral DAO (Boesten and Voogd 1975; Groenewegen et al. 1975, 1979) would apply to both systems. The division of the DAO on the basis of the distribution of AChE in a caudal pole and a rostromedial and a rostrolateral part (Fig. 13, Marani et al. 1977) therefore seems to be related to the output rather than to the input of the DAO.

The advance in knowledge about the principal nucleus of the inferior olive (PO) has been slow. Since Brodal (1940) the "dorsal cap" and the "ventrolateral outgrowth" have been considered as the caudal extension of the dorsal leaf of the PO. According to most authors (Alley et al. 1975, Hoddevik and Brodal 1977, Groenewegen and Voogd 1977, Walberg et al. 1979, Kawamura and Hashikawa 1979) the dorsal cap and ventrolateral outgrowth project to the nodule and the flocculus. The rest of the dorsal leaf of the PO is connected with the hemisphere only. In many mammals the ventral leaf of the PO is continuous with the dorsomedial cell column (Kooy 1916). In sheep a similar connection is present more caudally between the ventral leaf and the group β (Saigal et al., Olivocerebellar connections in sheep, unpublished work). After HRP injections into lobule IX of the caudal vermis, labeling is present in the group β, the dorsomedial cell column, and the adjoining part of the ventral leaf of the PO (Brodal 1976, Saigal et al., Olivocerebellar connections in sheep, unpublished work). The rest of the ventral leaf seems to project to the hemisphere only.

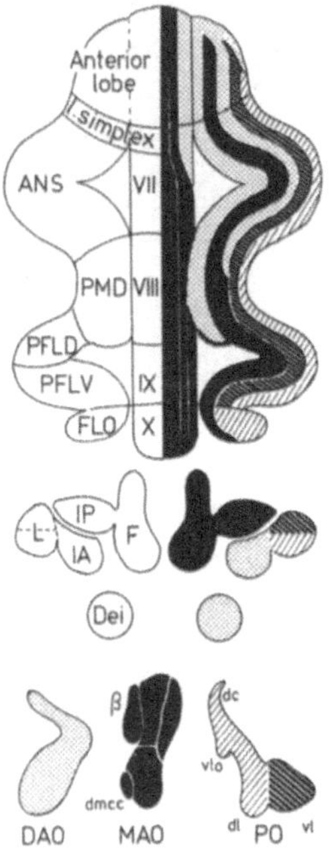

Fig. 19. The olivocerebellar projection in the cat. The projection from the medial and dorsal accessory olives and the dorsal and ventral leaf of the principal nucleus, as described in this paper, are indicated in different *shadings*. For a comparison and for the abbreviations consult Fig. 5

Both the dorsal and ventral leaf of the PO project to all main subdivisions of the hemisphere, with the possible exception of the anterior lobe for which only a contribution of the dorsal leaf has been evidenced (Brodal and Walberg 1977). On the basis of the corticonuclear projection of the D_1 and the D_2 zone to different parts of the lateral cerebellar nucleus (Voogd 1964, 1969; Voogd and Bigaré 1980, Bigaré 1980) and the topography of the reciprocal nucleo-olivary projection (Beitz 1976, Tolbert et al. 1975, Martin et al. 1976, Chan-Palay 1977), we (Groenewegen et al. 1979) considered it likely that the ventral leaf projects to the medial D_1 zone and the dorsal leaf to the lateral D_2 zone of the hemisphere. These expectations were borne out by observations of Rosina and Provini (to be published) after localized HRP injections in the simple and ansiform lobules of the cat, and are compatible with the report of Kotchabhakdi et al. (1978) on the projection of the inferior olive to these lobules. However, the reverse connection of the dorsal leaf to D_1 and of the ventral leaf to D_2 recently was described by Brodal and Walberg (1979) for the cat's paramedian lobule.

In summary we can conclude that the MAO and DAO project to different sets of interdigitating zones (Fig. 19). The MAO-dependent zones fuse in the caudal part of the cerebellum and project to the caudally and medially located posterior interposed and fastigial nuclei. The DAO-dependent zones fuse in the rostral part of the cerebellum (Oscarsson 1979) and do not reach so far caudally. They project to the rostrally located anterior interposed nucleus and the nucleus of Deiters. A similar rostrocaudal split is observed for the projection of the PO. The ventral leaf of the PO projects to vermal lobule IX and the D_1 zone and is related to the caudal parvocellular dentate. The dorsal leaf projects to vermal lobule X, the flocculus, and the D_2 zone and is related to the rostral magnocellular dentate. The significance of the coupling of dorsal and ventral leaf in the lateral bend of the PO is not understood.

Acknowledgments. The author wishes to express his gratitude to Frieda Bigaré, Nico Gerrits, Henk Groenewegen, Enrico Marani, and Jose Sedo for the use of their scientific material, to Prof. Dr. A. Karamanlidis and Dr. R. P. Saigal for the opportunity to collaborate on the olivocerebellar projection in the sheep and to Mrs. E.A.H. Bruyn and Mrs. M.J.C. Stokman for their secretarial assistance. Part of the research on which this paper was based was supported by FUNGO, subdivision of the Netherlands Organization for the Advancement of Pure Research Z.W.O.

References

1. Alley K, Baker R, Simpson JI (1975) Afferents to the vestibulocerebellum and the origin of the visual climbing fibers in the rabbit. Brain Res 98:582–589
2. Alzheimer A (1910) Beiträge zur Kenntnis der pathologischen Glia und ihrer Beziehungen zu den Abbauprodukten im Nervengewebe. In: Nissl F, Alzheimer A (eds) Histologische und histopathologische Arbeiten über die Großhirnrinde. G Fischer, Jena, 406–458
3. Andersson G, Oscarsson O (1977) The projection of Purkinje cell axons from sagittal microzones in the cerebellar cortex to single neurones in the lateral vestibular nucleus of the cat. Proc Int Union Physiol Sci (Paris) 13:23
4. Andersson G, Oscarsson O (1978a) Projections to lateral vestibular nucleus from cerebellar climbing fibre zones. Exp Brain Res 32:549–564
5. Andersson G, Oscarsson O (1978b) Climbing fiber microzones in cerebellar vermis and their projection to different groups of cells in the lateral vestibular nucleus. Exp Brain Res 32:565–579
6. Armstrong DM, Harvey RJ, Schild RF (1973a) Cerebello-cerebellar responses mediated via climbing fibers. Exp Brain Res 18:19–39
7. Armstrong DM, Harvey RJ, Schild RF (1973b) The spatial organization of climbing fibre branching in cat cerebellum. Exp Brain Res 18:40–58
8. Armstrong DM, Harvey RJ, Schild RF (1974) Topographical localization in the olivo-cerebellar projection: An electrophysiological study in the cat. J Comp Neurol 154:287–302
9. Beitz AJ (1976) The topographical organization of the olivo-dentate and dentato-olivary pathways in the cat. Brain Res 115:311–317
10. Bigaré F (1980) De efferente projectie van de cerebellaire schors van de kat. Thesis, University of Leiden
11. Boesten AJP, Voogd J (1975) Projections of the dorsal column nuclei and the spinal cord on the inferior olive in the cat. J Comp Neurol 161:215–238

12. Bowman JP, Sladek RJ (1961) Morphology of the inferior olivary complex of the rhesus monkey. J Comp Neurol 152:299–316
13. Brodal A (1940) Experimentelle Untersuchungen über die olivocerebellare Lokalisation. Z Gesamte Neurol Psychiatr 169:1–153
14. Brodal A (1976) The olivocerebellar projection in the cat studied with the method of retrograde axonal transport of horseradish peroxidase. IV. The projection to the uvula. J Comp Neurol 166:417–426
15. Brodal A (1980) Olivocerebellocortical projection in the cat as determined with the method of retrograde axonal transport of horseradish peroxidase. 2. Topographical pattern in relation to the longitudinal subdivision of the cerebellum. In: de Montigny C, Courville J (eds) Anatomy and physiology of the inferior olive. Raven Press, New York, pp 187–205
16. Brodal A, Kawamura K (1980) The olivocerebellar projection: A review. Adv Anat Embryol Cell Biol 64:1–140
17. Brodal A, Walberg F (1977) The olivocerebellar projection in the cat studied with the method of retrograde axonal transport of horseradish peroxidase. IV. The projection to the anterior lobe. J Comp Neurol 172:85–108
18. Brodal A, Walberg F, Hoddevik GH (1975) The olivocerebellar projection in the cat studied with the method of retrograde axonal transport of horseradish peroxidase. I. The projection to the paramedian lobule. J Comp Neurol 164:449–470
19. Brouwer B (1913) Über Hemiatrophia neocerebellaris. Arch F Psychiatr 51:539–577
20. Brouwer B (1915) Anatomische Untersuchung über das Kleinhirn des Menschen. Psychiatr Neurol Blad 19:104–129
21. Brouwer B, Coenen L (1919) Über die Olivia inferior. J Psychol Neurol 25:52–71
22. Brouwer B, Coenen L (1921) Untersuchungen über das Kleinhirn. Psychiatr Neurol Blad 25:201–220
23. Chan-Palay V (1977) Cerebellar dentate nucleus. Springer, Berlin Heidelberg New York
24. Courville J, Faraco-Cantin F, Diakiw N (1974) A functionally important feature of the distribution of the olivo-cerebellar climbing fibers. Can J Physiol Pharmacol 52:1212–1217
25. Cowan WM, Gottlieb DI, Hendrickson AE, Price JL, Woolsey TA (1972) The autoradiographic demonstration of axonal connections in the central nervous system. Brain Res 37:21–51
26. Desclin JC (1974) Histological evidence supporting the inferior olive as the major source of cerebellar climbing fibres in the rat. Brain Res 77:365–384
27. Dietrichs E, Walberg F (1979) The cerebellar corticonuclear and nucleocortical projections in the cat as studied with anterograde and retrograde transport of horseradish peroxidase. I. The paramedian lobule. Anat Embryol (Berl) 158:13–39
28. Ekerot C-F, Larson B (1977) Three sagittal zones in the cerebellar anterior lobe innervated by a common group of climbing fibres. Proc Int Union Physiol Sci (Paris) 13:208
29. Ekerot C-F, Larson B (1979a) The dorsal spino-olivocerebellar system in the cat. I. Functional organization and termination in the anterior lobe. Exp Brain Res 36:201–217
30. Ekerot C-F, Larson B (1979b) The dorsal spino-olivocerebellar system in the cat. II. Somatotopical organization. Exp Brain Res 36:219–232
31. Ekerot C-F, Larson B (1980) Termination in overlapping sagittal zones in cerebellar anterior lobe of mossy and climbing fiber paths activated from dorsal funiculus. Exp Brain Res 38:163–172
32. Ekerot C-F, Larson B (to be published) Climbing fiber branching in the cerebellar anterior lobe. Exp Brain Res
32a. Gerrits NM, Voogd J (to be published) The climbing fiber projection to the flocculus and adjacent paraflocculus in the cat. Neuroscience
33. Groenewegen HJ (1978) The olivocerebellar projection in the cat. Thesis, University of Leiden
34. Groenewegen HJ, Voogd J (1976) The longitudinal zonal arrangement of the olivocerebellar, climbing fiber projection in the cat. An autoradiographic and degeneration study. Exp Brain Res [Suppl] 1:65–71

35. Groenewegen HJ, Voogd J (1977) The parasagittal zonation within the olivocerebellar projection. I. Climbing fiber distribution in the vermis of cat cerebellum. J Comp Neurol 174:417–488
36. Groenewegen HJ, Boesten AJP, Voogd J (1975) The dorsal column nuclear projection to the nucleus ventralis posterior lateralis thalami and the inferior olive in the cat: an autoradiographic study. J Comp Neurol 162:505–518
37. Groenewegen HJ, Voogd J, Freedman SL (1979) The parasagittal zonation within the olivocerebellar projection. II. Climbing fiber distribution in the intermediate and hemispheric parts of cat cerebellum. J Comp Neurol 183:551–602
38. Häggqvist G (1936) Analyse der Faserverteilung in einem Rückenmarkquerschnitt (Th. 3). Z Mikrosk Anat Forsch 39:1–34
39. Hoddevik GH, Brodal A (1977) The olivocerebellar projection studied with the method of retrograde axonal transport of horseradish peroxidase. V. The projection to the flocculonodular lobe and the paraflocculus in the rabbit. J Comp Neurol 176:269–280
40. Hoddevik GH, Brodal A, Walberg F (1976) The olivocerebellar projection in the cat studied with the method of retrograde axonal transport of horseradish peroxidase. III. The projection to the vermal visual area. J Comp Neurol 169:155–170
41. Holmes G, Stewart TG (1908) On the connection of the inferior olives with the cerebellum in man. Brain 31:125–137
42. Kawamura K, Hashikawa T (1979) Olivocerebellar projection in the cat studied by means of anterograde axonal transport of labeled amino acids as tracers. Neuroscience 4:1615–1633
43. Klimoff J (1899) Über die Leitungsbahnen des Kleinhirns. Arch Anat Physiol, Anat Abth: 11–27
44. Kooy FH (1916) The inferior olive in vertebrates. Thesis, University of Groningen, Bohn, Haarlem
45. Kotchabhakdi N, Walberg F, Brodal A (1978) The olivocerebellar projection in the cat studied with the method of retrograde axonal transport of horseradish peroxidase. VII. The projection to lobulus simplex, Crus I and II. J Comp Neurol 182:293–314
46. Lüthy F (1932) Über anatomische Beziehungen der unteren Olive zum Kleinhirn. Zentralbl Neurochir 61:498
47. Marani E, Voogd J, Boekee A (1977) Acetylcholinesterase staining in subdivisions of the cat's inferior olive. J Comp Neurol 174:209–226
48. Martin GF, Dom R, King SJ, Robards M, Watson CRR (1975) The inferior olivary nucleus of the opossum (Didelphis marsupialis virginiana), its organization and connections. J Comp Neurol 160:507–534
49. Martin GF, Henkel CK, King SJ (1976) Cerebello-olivary fibers: their origin, course and distribution in the North American opossum. Exp Brain Res 24:219–236
50. Oscarsson O (1969) The sagittal organization of the cerebellar anterior lobe as revealed by the projection patterns of the climbing fiber system. In: Llinas R (ed) Neurobiology of cerebellar evolution and development. AMA-ERF Chicago, pp 525–537
51. Oscarsson O (1973) Functional organization of spinocerebellar paths. In: Iggo A (ed) Handbook of sensory physiology, vol. II. Somatosensory system. Springer, Berlin Heidelberg New York, pp 339–380
52. Oscarsson O (1979) Functional units of the cerebellum – sagittal zones and microzones. TINS 2:143–145
53. Oscarsson O, Sjölund B (1977a) The ventral spino-olivocerebellar system in the cat. I. Identification of five paths and their termination in the cerebellar anterior lobe. Exp Brain Res 28:469–486
54. Oscarsson O, Sjölund B (1977b) The ventral spino-olivocerebellar system in the cat. II. Termination zones in the cerebellar posterior lobe. Exp Brain Res 28:487–503
54a. Rosina A, Provini L (to be published) Olivary projection to the ansiform lobule: longitudinal and topographical organization. Neuroscience
55. Szentágothai-Schimert J (1941) Die Bedeutung des Faserkalibers und der Markscheidendicke im Zentralnervensystem. Z Anat 11:201–233
56. Taber E (1961) The cytoarchitecture of the brain stem of the cat. I. Brain stem nuclei of the cat. J Comp Neurol 116:27–69

57. Tolbert DL, Massopust LC, Murphy MG, Young PA (1976) The anatomical organization of the cerebello-olivary projection in the cat. J Comp Neurol 170:525–544
58. Voogd J (1964) The cerebellum of the cat. Thesis, University of Leiden. Van Gorcum, Assen
59. Voogd J (1967) Comparative aspects of the structure and fiber connections of the mammalian cerebellum. In: Fox CA, Snider RS (eds) The Cerebellum. Progress in Brain Research 25:94–135
60. Voogd J (1969) The importance of fiber connections in the comparative anatomy of the mammalian cerebellum. In: Llinas R (ed) Neurobiology of cerebellar evolution and development. AMA-ERF Chicago, pp 493–541
61. Voogd J, Bigaré F (1980) The topographical distribution of olivary and cortico-nuclear fibers in the cerebellum. A review. In: de Montigny C, Courville J (eds) Anatomy and physiology of the inferior olive. Raven Press, New York pp 207–234
62. Voogd J, Feirabend HKP (1981) Classical methods in neuroanatomy. In: Lahue R (ed) Methods in neurobiology, vol. 2. Plenum, New York London Washington Boston, pp 301–364
63. Walberg F (1980) Olivocerebellar projection in the cat as determined with the method of retrograde axonal transport of horseradish. I. Topographical pattern. In: de Montigny C, Courville J (eds) Anatomy and physiology of the inferior olive. Raven Press, New York, pp 169–186
64. Walberg F, Brodal A (1979) The longitudinal zonal pattern in the paramedian lobule of the cat's cerebellum. An analysis based on a correlation of recent HRP data with results of studies with other methods. J Comp Neurol 187:581–588
65. Walberg F, Kotchabhakdi N, Hoddevik GH (1979) The olivocerebellar projection to the flocculus and paraflocculus in the cat compared to those in the rabbit. A study using horseradish peroxidase as a tracer. Brain Res 161:389–394

Discussion

Gould: Could you characterize briefly the differences in the width of the zones in the cat and the monkey.

Voogd: The system in the cat and the monkey is exactly the same: A, B, C_1, C_2, C_3, D zones. However, the region which receives the projections from the principal olive in the monkey is greatly expanded.

Robertson: The width of the zones in the cat are thought to be 1 mm wide. How wide are they in the monkey? Our functional results suggest they are about 1½–3 mm.

Voogd: That may be.

Robertson: When we look at our functional compartments we see a large forearm area and right next to it a face area. There are obviously parallel fibers coursing between these two compartments. I was wondering what the functional role of these longitudinal compartments might be?

Voogd: That of course depends on the efferent projections. The only thing I can see is what connections are effected by these zones. In summary the zones have the following efferent connections:

A zone – Vestibular nuclei and bilateral reticular formation
B zone – Deiters nucleus
C_1, C_3 – Red nucleus
C_2 – Red nucleus, and nucleus of Darkschewitsch
D – Thalamic nuclei

You can enumerate these efferent connections which monitor a particular system, but it is not easy to make sense of it.
Balazs: There is a remarkable difference in the longitudinal zones of these two species. Where would the rat fit in?
Voogd: It is much like the cat, perhaps A and B are slightly larger with the other zones similar to the cat.
Palay: In the autoradiograms, I noticed very few grains in the molecular layer after injections in the inferior olive.
Voogd: All my pictures are at low magnification. It is usually very clear, but the labeling in the white matter is much heavier.
Sotelo: What is the survival time after injections?
Voogd: One week.
Sotelo: If you have these bands in the white matter perhaps they spread like a fan in the molecular layer and then the gaps are filled between the bands of labeled fibers. This of course relates to the question of all the climbing fibers coming from the inferior olive. I believe they do, even if you have the bands.
Voogd: No, it is not fanlike. The relation between the white matter and the molecular layer is that the climbing fibers are located more laterally in the white matter. The gaps between the labeled bands can be understood in terms of the long narrow columns of cells in the olive which give rise to the climbing fibers. Only a small part of this narrow column is labeled by an injection of leucine so you get a stripe of label. It is impossible to label all the cells in the same way so it is not surprising that you see these bands of label. Incomplete injections result in these gaps.
Sotelo: We have succeeded in labeling the whole vermis in a 5-day-old rat. Of course the olive is much smaller.
Simpson: Do you think it is possible that a Purkinje cell could project to two distinctly different target sites: I think you published a paper that said some cells in the A zone send their axons to the medial vestibular nucleus.
Voogd: Purkinje cells in the lateral part of the A2 zone go to fastigial nucleus and are then distributed to the vestibular nuclei. I do not know of other examples, but I expect from the flocculus you could get projections to the dentate and to the vestibular nuclei.

Spino-Olivocerebellar Circuits in the North American Opossum with Notes on Their Development *

G. F. Martin, G. A. Bishop, J. L. Culberson, J. S. King, C. Laxson, M. Linauts, and M. Panneton

Introduction

Kooy [22] viewed the inferior olivary nucleus of the marsupial opossum as a poorly developed forerunner of the same nucleus in eutherian mammals and it was not until connectional data became available that it was possible to discern subdivisions comparable to those described for other species [28, 45]. Because the North American opossum is a generalized mammal, the connections of its olive are of comparative interest and provide information concerning circuits which probably exist in all mammals. In addition, it is possible to study the early development of olivary connections in the opossum because its young are born 12–13 days after conception [16, 34] and are thus available for experimental manipulation.

The connections of the opossum olive have been described previously [24, 25, 28, 32] and the reader is referred to those reports for a more comprehensive account. In this report, we shall concentrate on those areas which receive direct and indirect projections from the spinal cord. It is our intent to describe the olivary targets of such axons and to emphasize that these areas also receive projections from other regions of the neural axis. In turn, we shall describe the cerebellar projections of olivary nuclei receiving spinal innervation so as to provide an overview of spino-olivocerebellar circuits. Preliminary data on the development of these connections will also be described.

Methods

The olivary targets of spinal axons were studied using degeneration methods. Lesions of the spinal cord were made at several levels and after 7–14 days the Fink-Heimer technique [12] was employed to impregnate degenerating axons within the olive. Technical details relative to these cases have been described elsewhere [28]. In subsequent experiments, horseradish peroxidase (HRP) was injected iontophoretically into the olive so as to label neurons projecting to it. Material from those cases was reacted for the presence of HRP with O-dianisidine as a chromagen [10]. In companion experiments ^{3}H-leucine was placed into each of the areas suggested by the HRP method to innervate the olive. The ^{3}H-marker was injected by means of a pressure system and after 9–11 days the

* This investigation was supported by U.S.P.H.S. Grants NS-07410 and NS-08798

Experimental Brain Research, Suppl. 6

perfused brains were cut and processed by the modification of the autoradiographic method described previously [24]. The autoradiographic material was used to determine if any of the areas labeled by the HRP method projected to regions of the olive receiving spinal input.

The organization of olivocerebellar connections was studied by means of the HRP method. Pressure or iontophoretic injections of the enzyme were made into different parts of the cerebellar cortex, and after 24 hours the perfused brains were removed and cut on a freezing microtome. Sections through the cerebellum and inferior olive were reacted for the presence of HRP with diaminobenzidine. The preparation of tissue from those experiments has also been described previously [25].

Observations on the development of afferent connections with the inferior olive were made on the brains of pouch-young opossums subjected to either thoracic cord transection, metencephalic hemisection, or cortical ablation. Details of the surgical procedures are described elsewhere [33]. After short survival times degenerating neurites were impregnated by the Fink-Schneider method [23]. Additional cases were used to determine if olivary axons had grown into the cerebellum by the time spinal neurites reached their definitive targets in the olive. In those experiments a paste of HRP was placed on the exposed cerebella of animals operated at the appropriate age. After 6–24 hours, they were sacrificed and perfused, and the removed brains were processed for HRP histochemistry with diaminobenzidine. Pouch-young opossums were obtained from females either pregnant when captured in the wild or bred at The Ohio State University. Litters found in the pouch that were not there on the previous day were considered to be 1 day old (embryonic day 12±). Because the date of birth was not known for animals born in the wild, snout-rump (S-R) lengths were obtained and their ages estimated from the growth curves of Cutts et al. [9].

Results

The Organization of Spino-Olivary Connections

Figure 1 illustrates the results obtained from a case subjected to a lesion of the spinal cord at C-5 and impregnated for degenerating axons by the Fink-Heimer method. The degeneration is plotted on the side of the lesion. In caudal sections (Fig. 1A–C) axonal debris is found within the medial and dorsal accessory nuclei. In the medial accessory complex it is limited to subnucleus a and the lateral part of subnucleus b. Beginning at about the level indicated by line E in Fig. 2, degenerating axons fill the dorsal accessory nucleus (Fig. 1C, D), but avoid the medial accessory complex. At progressively more rostral levels (Fig. 1E–G), degenerating axons are present within most of the dorsal accessory nucleus. In sections comparable to those shown in H and I of Fig. 4, however, they avoid its ventromedial extreme (the area indicated by the arrow in Fig. 1G; see also Figs. 5, 6).

Transection of the sacral cord elicits no degeneration within the olive, but axonal debris is found in all of the areas described above after lumbar, thoracic, and

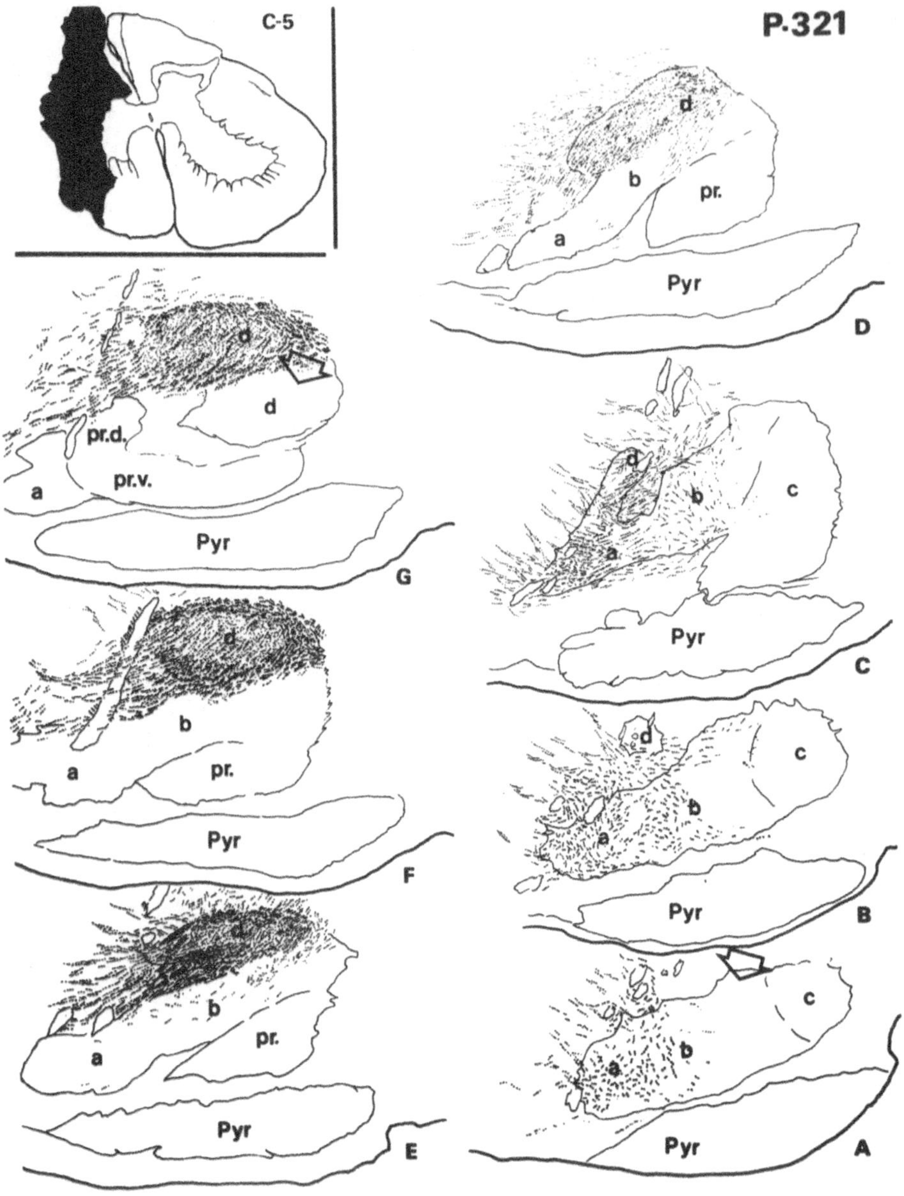

Fig. 1A–G. Plot of axonal degeneration in the olive (caudal **A** through rostral **G**) on the side of a lesion of the fifth cervical cord segment (*upper left*). The pyramidal tract (*Pyr*) and appropriate subdivisions of the olive are labeled. The *arrows* point to the specific regions refered to in the text. Martin et al. [28][1]

---

1 Abbreviations used in Figs. 1–19: *a*, subnucleus a of medial accessory complex; *Al*, nucleus alaris; *b*, subnucleus b of medial accessory complex; *bp*, brachium pontis; *c*, subnucleus c of medial accessory complex; *CcD*, nucleus cochlearis dorsalis; *CF*, campi Forelli; *CI*, colliculus inferior; *Cn*, culmen; *cp*, commissura posterior; *cr*, corpus restiformis; *CrI*, crus I; *CrII*, crus II; *CS*, colliculus superior; *Cu*, nucleus cuneatus medialis; *CuL*, nucleus cuneatus

cervical lesions. Comparison of the amount of axonal degeneration present in the olive of different cases gives the impression that caudal thoracic and rostral lumbar segments are particularly heavy contributors to spino-olivary connections. Lesions of the first or second cervical segment produce evidence for additional connections, however. Caudally, degenerating axons are still numerous in subnuclei a and b of the medial accessory nucleus, but they extend medially to the boundary between subnuclei b and c. In addition, a few degenerating axons are found in that part of the dorsal accessory nucleus indicated by the arrow in Fig. 1G. It did not appear that caudal levels of the dorsal column nuclei were involved in the lesions of C-1 and C-2.

Projections from Various Areas of the Neural Axis Which are Distributed to Nuclei of the Olive Receiving Spinal Input

Horseradish peroxidase injections of the inferior olive label spinal neurons, which are particularly abundant at caudal thoracic and lumbar levels. Unfortunately, such injections often spread to areas adjacent to the olive which also contain spinal axons. For that reason the material is not definitive concerning the cells giving rise to spino-olivary connections. The brainstem labeling was useful, however, because in subsequent autoradiographic experiments we were able to show that the areas labeled in the HRP cases did, indeed, innervate the olive. For example, olivary injections of HRP labeled neurons in the dorsal column nuclei contralaterally (curved arrows in Fig. 7A, B). When ^{3}H-leucine injections include those nuclei, labeled axons can be traced to areas of the olive receiving innervation from the spinal cord. The injection shown in Fig. 8 is centered within the nucleus cuneatus. In caudal sections (e.g., Fig. 8A) labeled axons are found contralaterally within subnucleus b of the medial ac-

---

1 Continued: lateralis; *d*, dorsal accessory nucleus; *Dcl*, declive; *Dent*, nucleus dentatus (lateralis); *DK*, nucleus Darkschewitsch; *Fac*, nucleus n. facialis; *Fast*, nucleus fastigius; *g*, genu n. facialis; *GLD*, nucleus corporis geniculati lateralis dorsalis; *GMc*, nucleus corporis geniculati medialis: pars centralis; *Hg*, nucleus n. hypoglossi; *IFLM*, nucleus interstitialis fasciculi longitudinalis medialis; *InP-a*, nucleus interpositus: pars emboliformis (nucleus interpositus anterior); *InPg*, nucleus interpositus: pars globosa (nucleus interpositus posterior); *IP*, interpeduncular nucleus; *K*, cap of Kooy; *LES*, lesion; *Lr*, nucleus linearis; *mth*, fasciculus mammillothalamicus; *OI*, nucleus olivaris inferior; *OS*, nucleus olivaris superior; *ped*, pedunculus cerebri; *PFl*, paraflocculus; *PMi*, lobus paramedianus inferior; *PMs*, lobus paramedianus superior; *pr.d.*, dorsal lamella of principal nucleus; *pr.v.*, ventral lamella of principal nucleus; *Pyc*, pyramis; *Pyr*, tractus pyramidalis; *RaO*, nucleus obscurus raphae; *RD*, nucleus reticularis medullae oblongatae dorsalis; *RGc*, nucleus reticularis gigantocellularis; *RGcv*, nucleus reticularis gigantocellularis pars ventralis; *RN*, nucleus ruber; *RP*, nucleus reticularis pontis; *RPc*, nucleus reticularis paravocellularis; *SPF*, nucleus subparafascicularis; *Sx*, lobus simplex; *TgI*, nucleus interstitialis tegmenti; *TgP*, nucleus profunda tegmenti; *TrMo*, nucleus motorius n. trigemini; *TrSc*, nucleus tractus spinalis n. trigemini: pars caudalis; *TrSi*, nucleus tractus spinalis n. trigemini: pars interpolaris; *TrSo*, nucleus tractus spinalis n. trigemini: pars oralis; *TrSv*, nucleus sensorius n. trigemini ventralis; *TSl*, nucleus tractus solitarii: pars lateralis; *Uv*, uvula; *VstI*, nucleus vestibularis inferior; *VstL*, nucleus vestibularis lateralis; *VstM*, nucleus vestibularis medialis; *xVB*, nucleus ventralis thalami basalis; *ZI*, zona incerta

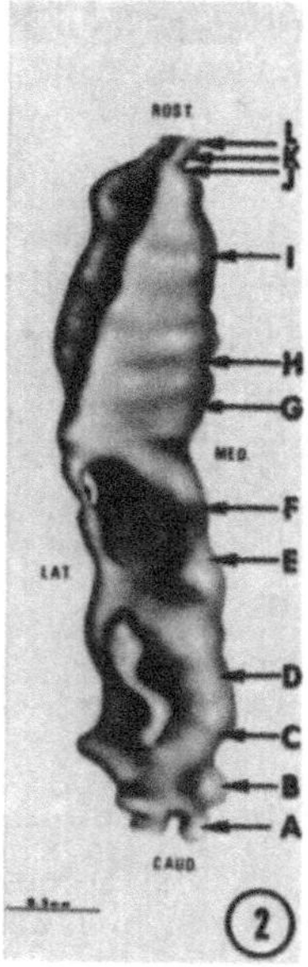

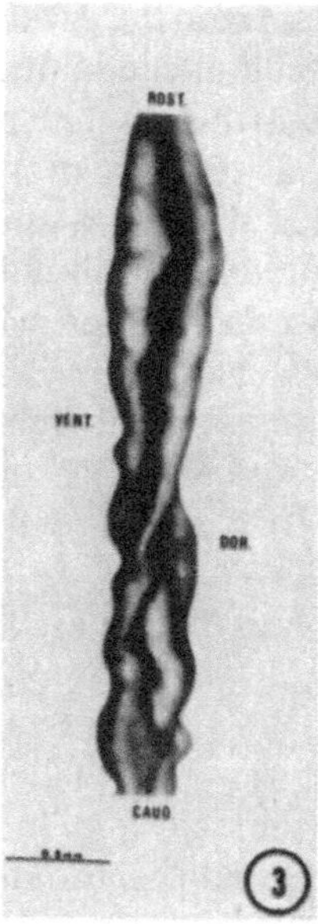

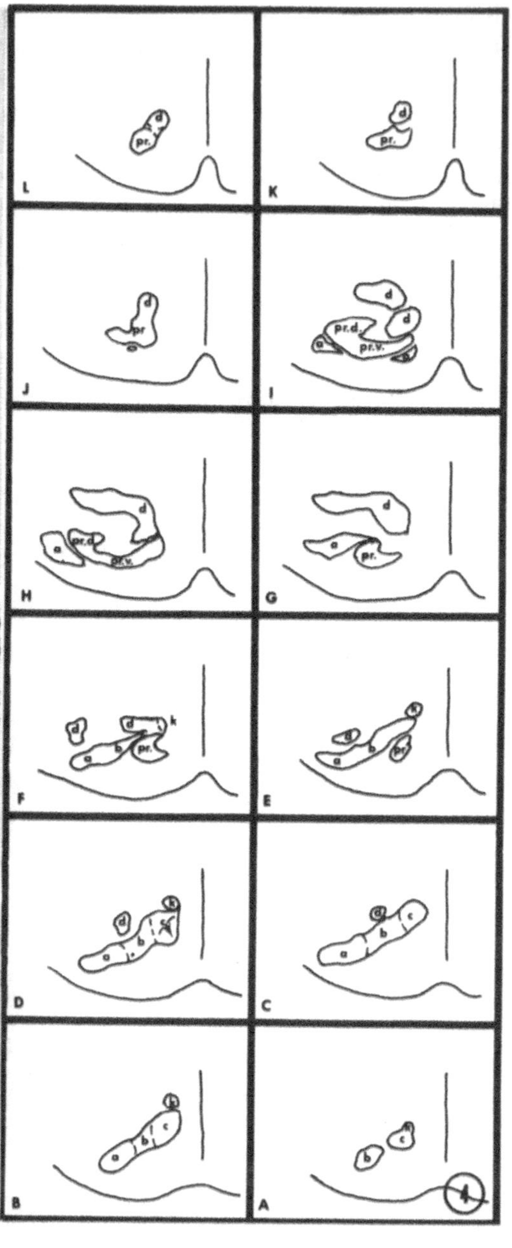

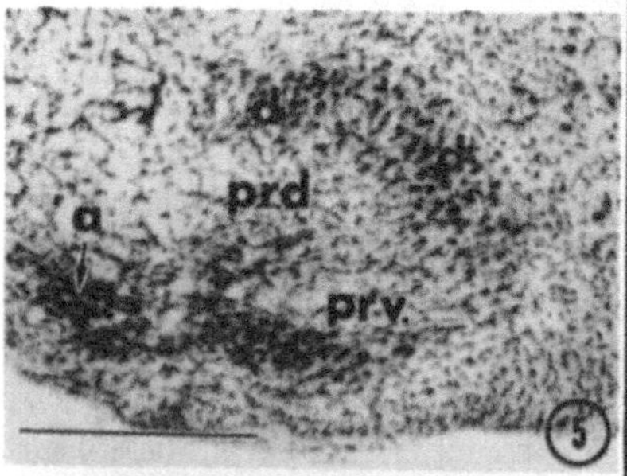

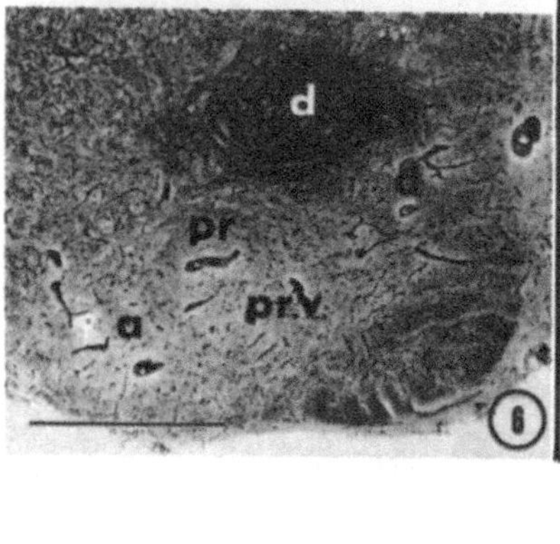

Fig. 2. Dorsal view of a wax reconstruction of the opossum olive. The *letters* indicate the level of sections from which the drawings in Fig. 4 were made. Martin et al. [28]

Fig. 3. Lateral view of the same reconstruction shown in Fig. 2. Martin et al. [28]

Fig. 4. Drawings of Nissl-stained sections through the opossum olive (caudal, **A,** through rostral, **L**) cut at the levels indicated in Fig. 2. Martin et al. [28]

cessory complex. Minimal label is found within subnucleus a, but none is present within subnucleus c. In more rostral sections, labeling is still present within subnucleus b contralaterally (Fig. 8B, C), but it eventually shifts to that part of the dorsal accessory nucleus avoided by *most* spinal axons (e.g., arrow, Fig. 8E). A small, but consistent amount of labeling is present in comparable areas ipsilateral to the injection. Olivary projections from the nucleus gracilis also reach

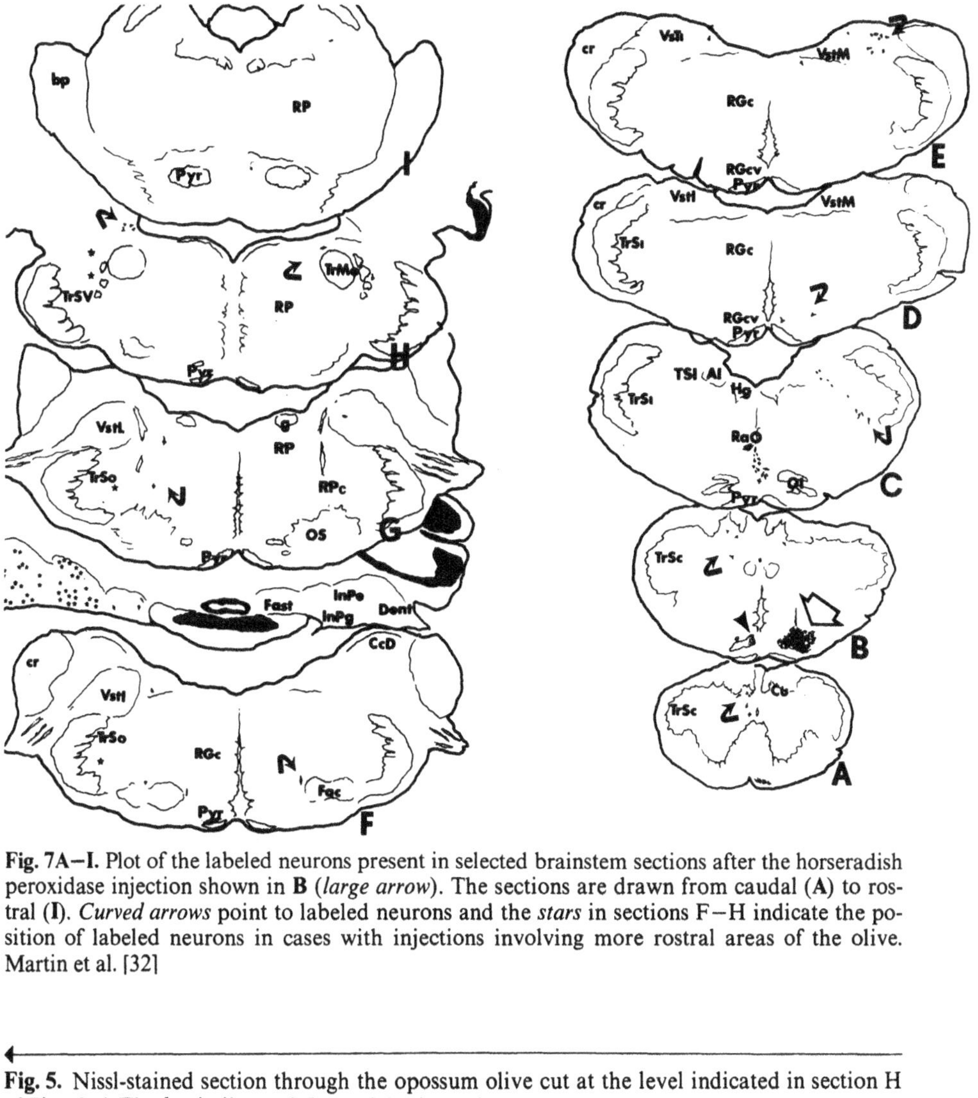

Fig. 7A–I. Plot of the labeled neurons present in selected brainstem sections after the horseradish peroxidase injection shown in **B** (*large arrow*). The sections are drawn from caudal (**A**) to rostral (**I**). *Curved arrows* point to labeled neurons and the *stars* in sections F–H indicate the position of labeled neurons in cases with injections involving more rostral areas of the olive. Martin et al. [32]

Fig. 5. Nissl-stained section through the opossum olive cut at the level indicated in section H of Figs. 2, 4. The *bar* indicates 0.5 mm. Martin et al. [28]

Fig. 6. Fink-Heimer impregnation of degenerating axons in the olive subsequent to a lesion of the cervical enlargement. The section was cut at the same level as that in Fig. 5 and degenerating axons are impregnated in lateral parts of the dorsal accessory nucleus. The *bar* indicates 0.5 mm. Martin et al. [28]

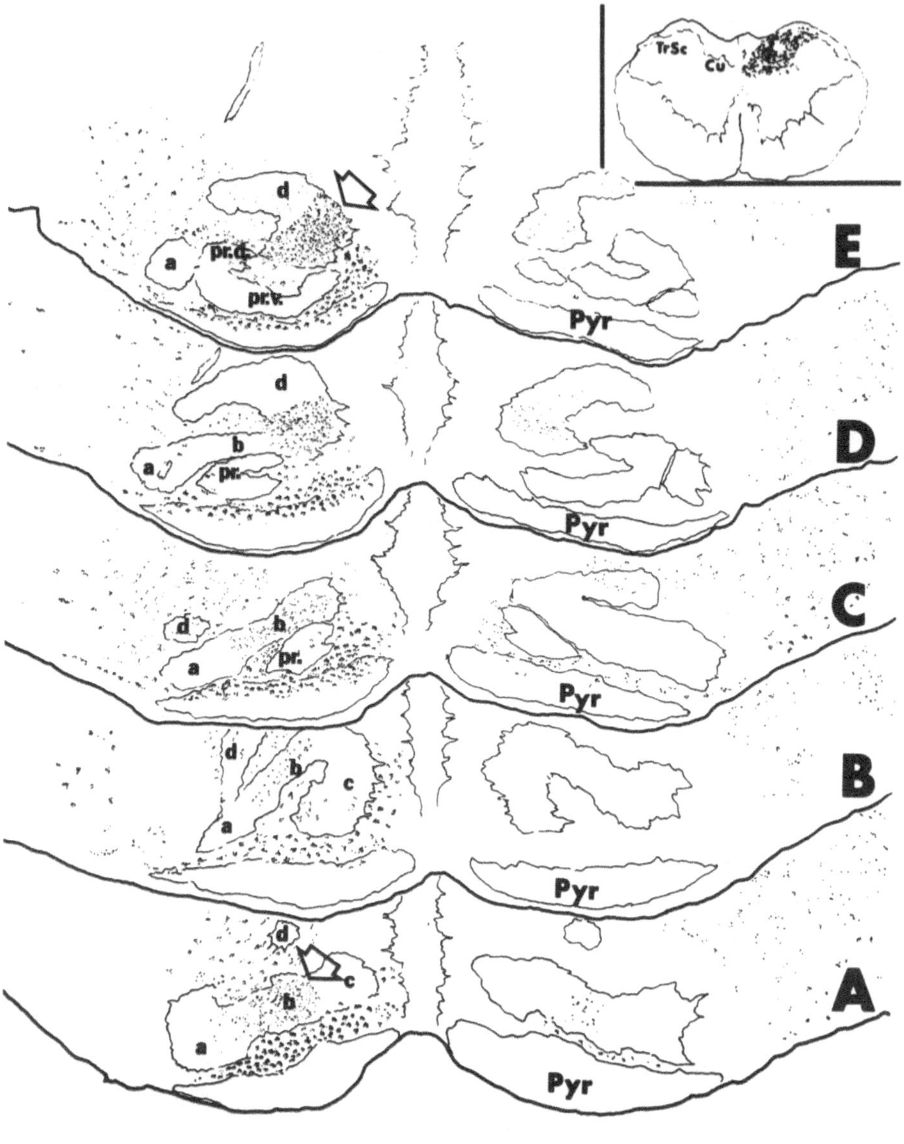

Fig. 8A–E. Plot of the olivary labeling produced by an injection of ^{3}H-leucine into the nucleus cuneatus and caudal spinal trigeminal nucleus (*upper right*). All sections, including those with the injection, are drawn as they appear through darkfield optics. Section **A** is the most caudal, whereas **E** is the most rostral. Major labeling in both sections is indicated by *arrows*. Martin et al. [32]

subnuclei a and b of the medial accessory nucleus; but they occupy only those parts of the dorsal accessory nucleus supplied by the majority of spinal axons [28].

Horseradish peroxidase injections of the olive label neurons within the ipsilateral nucleus of the tractus solitarius and medial to subnucleus interpolaris of

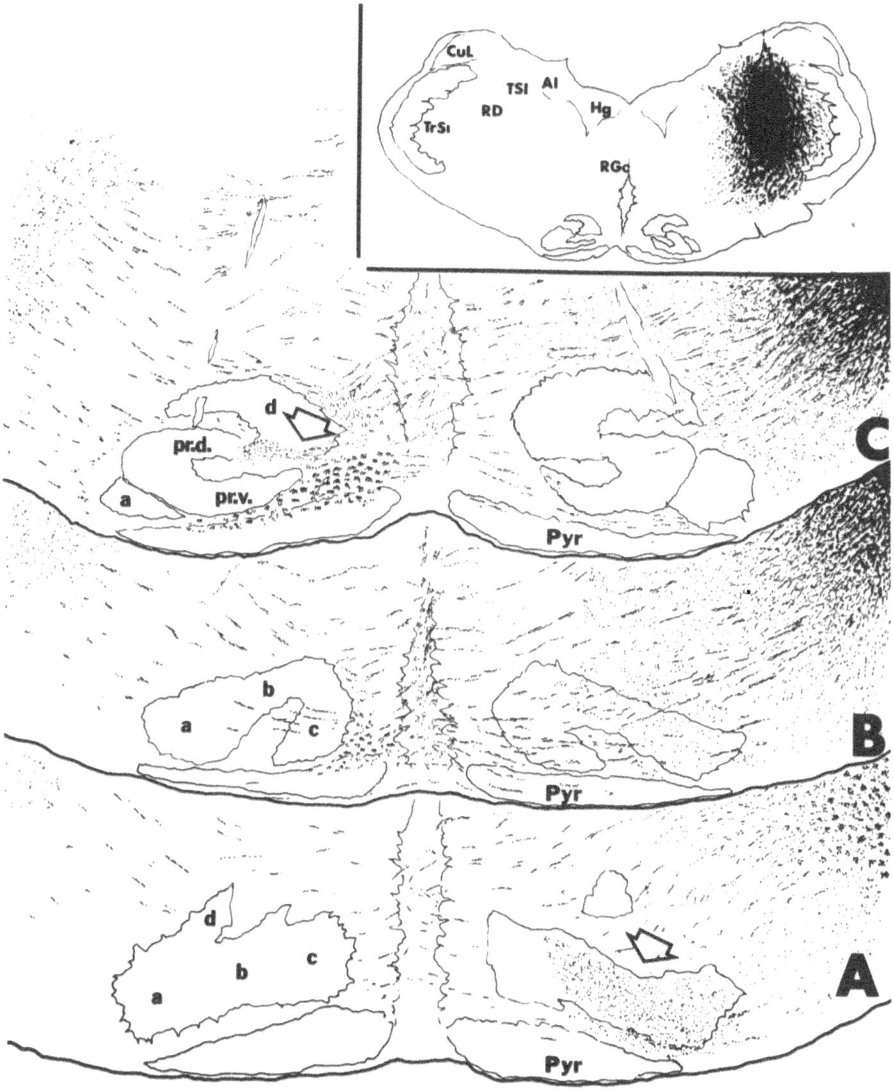

Fig. 9A–C. Plot of the olivary labeling produced by the injection of ^{3}H-leucine drawn at the *upper right*. All sections, including that through the injection site, are drawn as they appear through darkfield optics. Section **A** is the most caudal. Significant labeling is indicated by *arrows*. Martin et al. [32]

the spinal trigeminal complex (terminology of Oswaldo-Cruz and Rocha-Miranda [41]). The latter neurons are indicated by the curved arrow in Fig. 7C. When comparable areas are included in injections of ^{3}H-leucine (e.g., Fig. 9) labeled axons can be found, ipsilaterally, within caudal parts of subnuclei a and b of the medial accessory olive (arrow, Fig. 9A). The labeling indicated by the

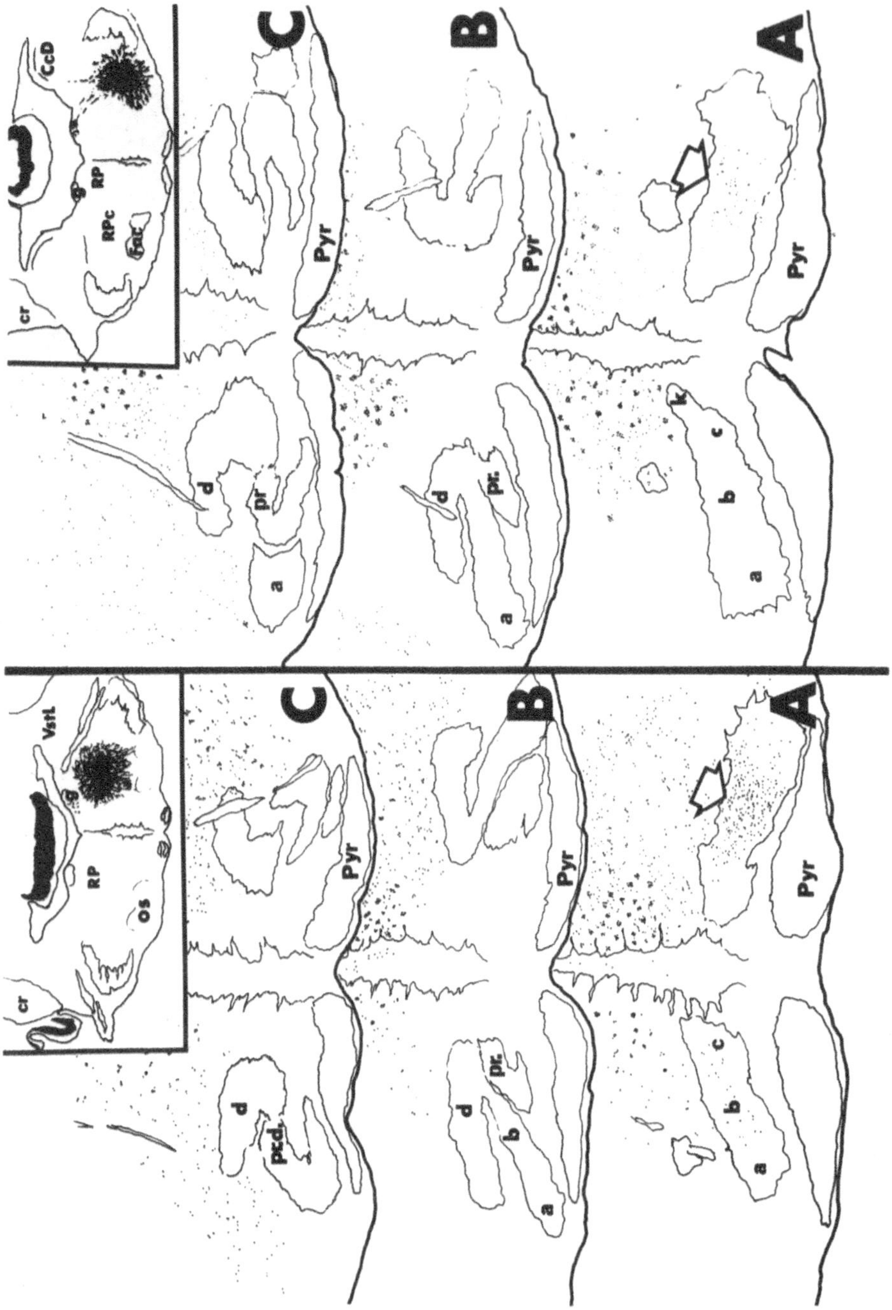

Fig. 10A–C. Plots of olivary labeling produced by reticular injections of ^{3}H-leucine. The injection sites (*upper right* for each case) and the olivary labeling are drawn as they appear through darkfield optics. In both cases, section **A** is the most caudal and olivary labeling is indicated by *arrows*. Martin et al. [32]

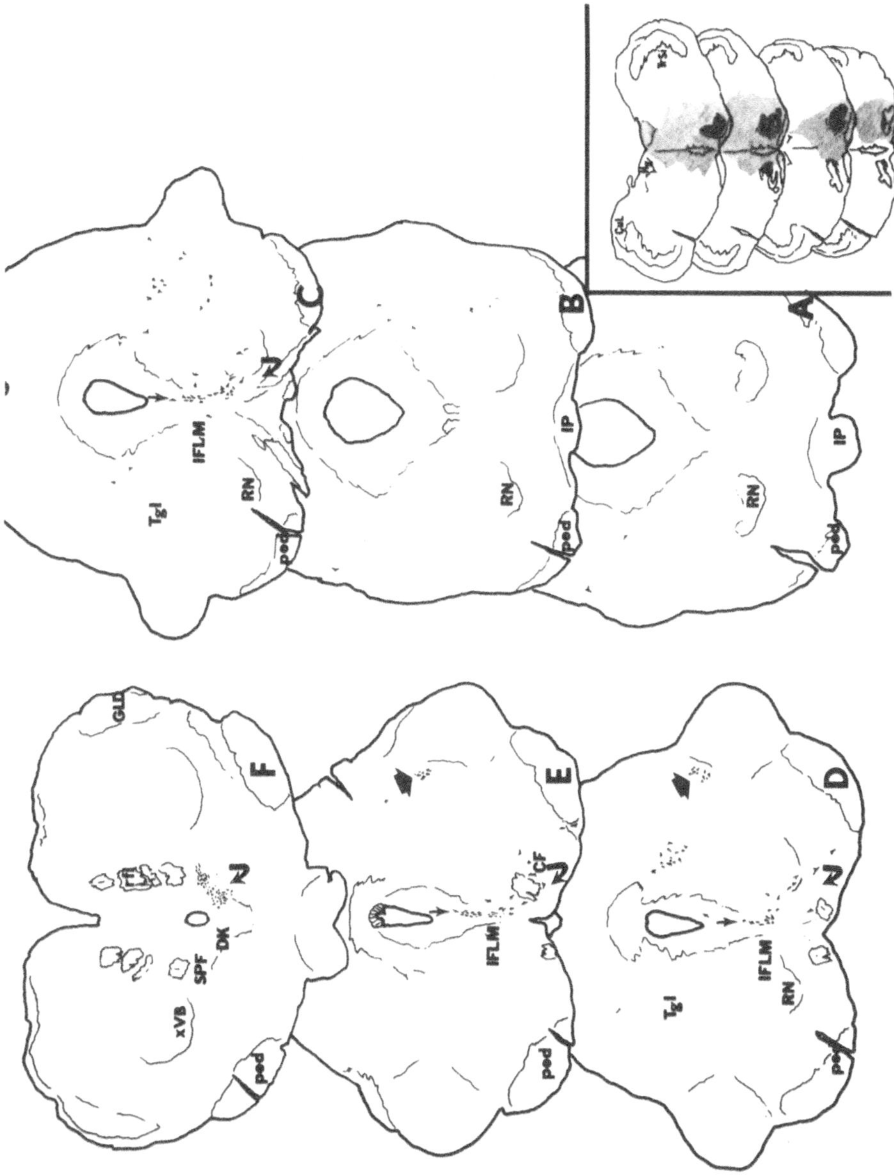

Fig. 11 A–F. Plot of the neuronal labeling present in the caudal thalamus and midbrain after the injection of HRP drawn in the *insert*. The sections are drawn from caudal (**A**) through rostral (**F**) and labeled neurons are indicated by *arrows*. Martin et al. [32]

arrow in Fig. 9C may be due to involvement of spinal trigeminal neurons because a similar distribution of silver grains is seen in autoradiograms from cases with injection of ^{3}H-leucine into more rostral areas of the spinal trigeminal complex.

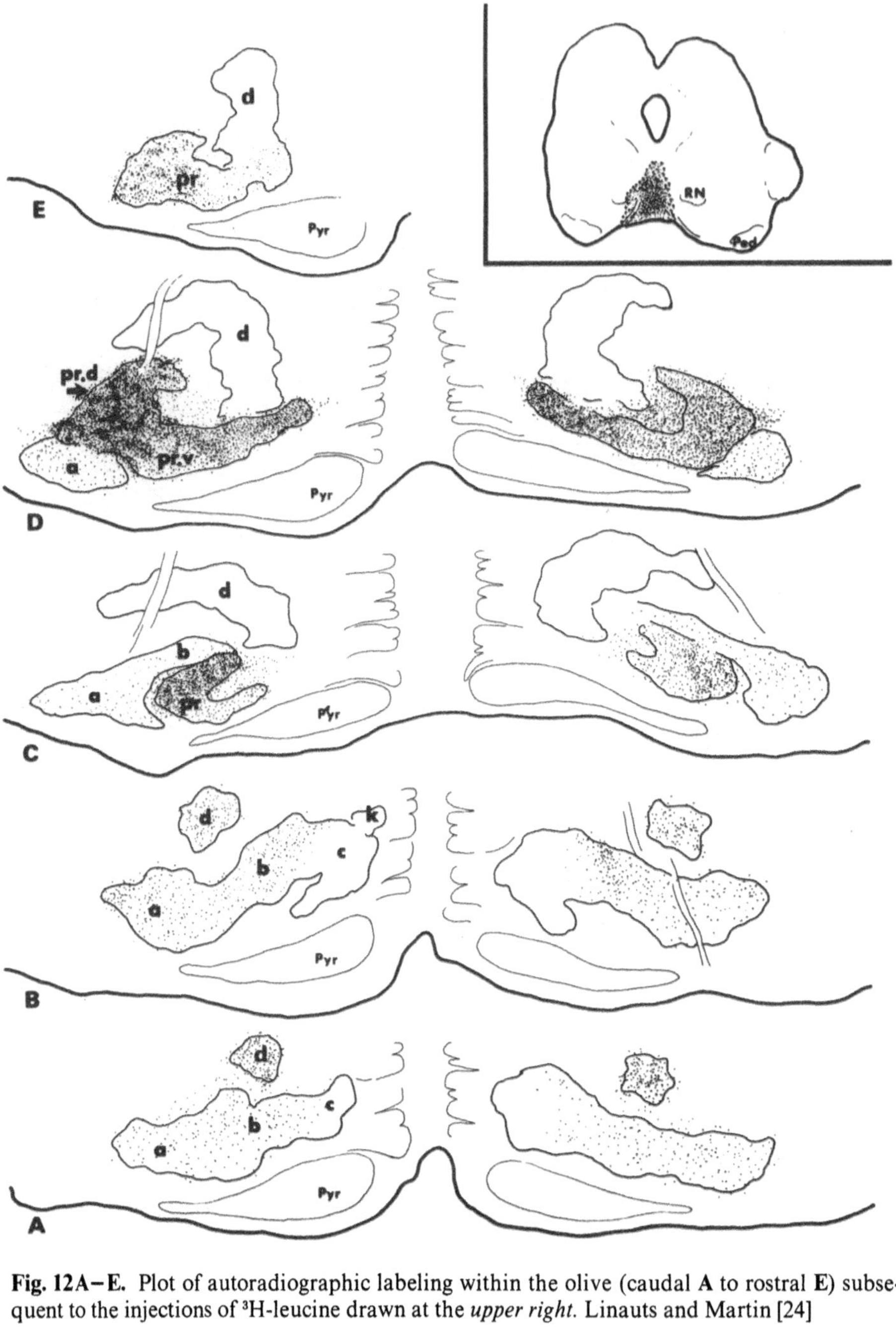

Fig. 12A–E. Plot of autoradiographic labeling within the olive (caudal **A** to rostral **E**) subsequent to the injections of ^{3}H-leucine drawn at the *upper right.* Linauts and Martin [24]

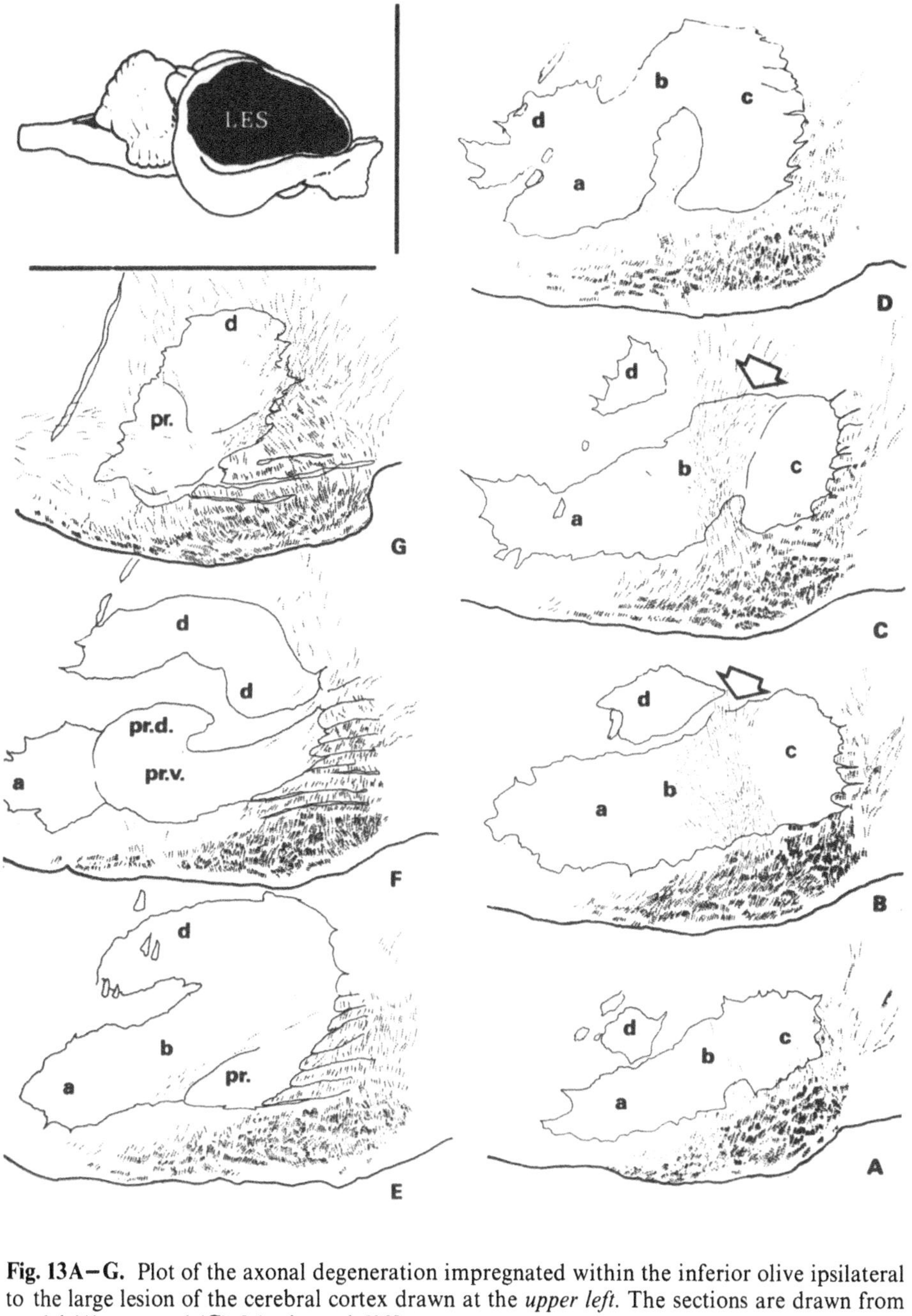

Fig. 13A–G. Plot of the axonal degeneration impregnated within the inferior olive ipsilateral to the large lesion of the cerebral cortex drawn at the *upper left*. The sections are drawn from caudal (**A**) to rostral (**G**). Martin et al. [28]

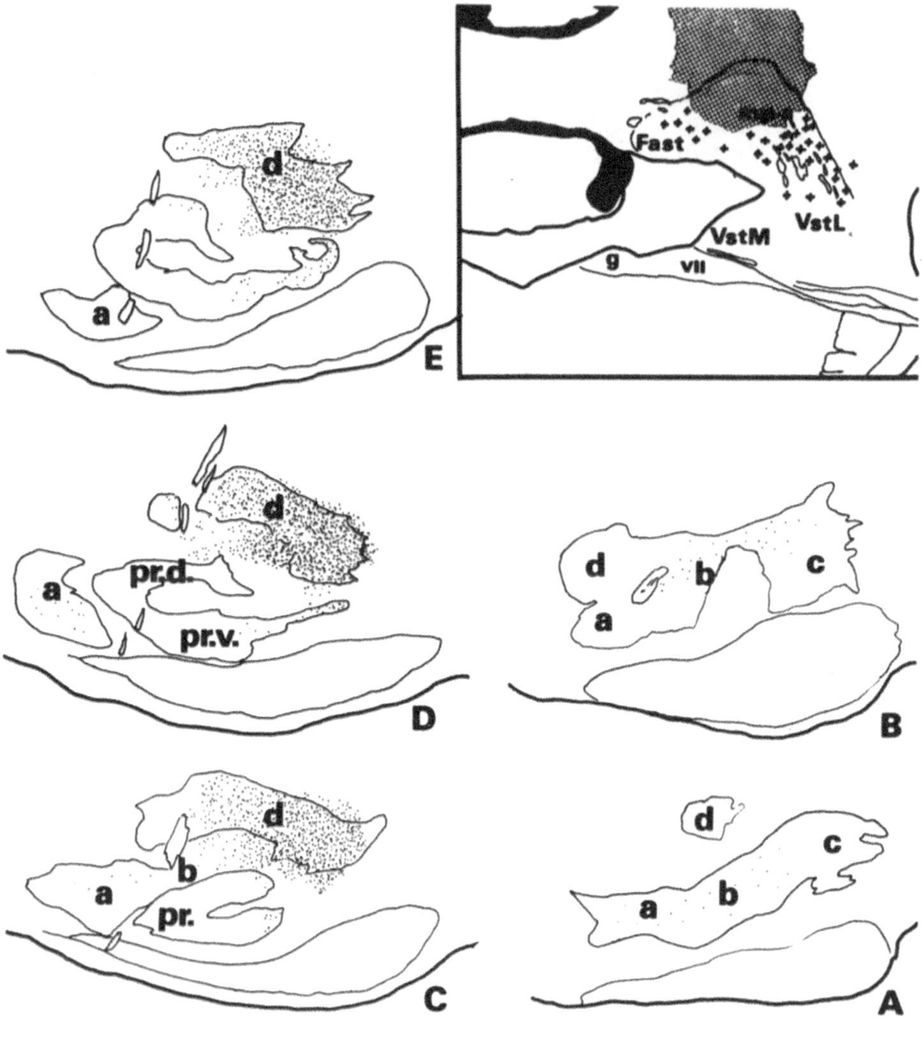

Fig. 14A–E. Plot of the autoradiographic labeling in selected section of the olive produced by the placement of ^{3}H-leucine drawn at the *upper right*. The bulk of the injection site is *stippled*, but lightly labeled neurons are indicated by *crosses*. The sections are drawn from caudal (**A**) through rostral (**E**). Martin et al. [29]

Olivary injections of HRP also label neurons in the nuclei obscurus and pallidus of the medullary raphe (Fig. 7C). Our ^{3}H-leucine injections which include those areas also spill over into the adjacent olive, but there is evidence for a projection to at least subnucleus b of the medial accessory nucleus. Evidence for such a connection is also provided by injections of ^{3}H-serotonin into the olive. Autoradiograms from such cases reveal labeled axons and terminals (electron microscopy) in subnucleus b (King, Hop, and Burry, unpublished work).

Reticular neurons were labeled subsequent to injections of HRP into the olive and the autoradiographic technique shows that reticulo-olivary connections exist [31]. Some of the autoradiographic cases provide evidence that reticular neurons of the medulla project to caudal (spinal) parts of the medial and dorsal accessory nuclei as well as to rostrolateral parts of the dorsal accessory nucleus (see Martin et al. [31]). It is difficult to interpret such cases, however, because of the proximity of the injection site to the olive. In contrast, brains with injections of ^{3}H-leucine into caudal areas of the nucleus reticularis pontis (terminology of Oswaldo-Cruz and Rocha-Miranda [41]) provide definitive results. Such injections produce labeling which precisely outlines subnucleus b of the medial accessory olive (arrows in P-404 and P-582, Fig. 10A).

Large deposits of HRP which are centered in the inferior olive label neurons in multiple areas of the midbrain (Fig. 11). We have previously described the olivary projections from each of these areas [24] but one is of particular significance for this account. In Fig. 11C–E, the small, straight arrows point to labeled neurons which are lined up in a dorsal to ventral direction medial to the interstitial nucleus of Cajal and within the periaqueductal gray. It is of interest that neurons are labeled in comparable areas, including the nucleus of Darkschewitsch, even after relatively small injections of HRP into caudal parts of the accessory nuclei. The significance of such labeling can be appreciated from Fig. 12. When ^{3}H-leucine is placed so as to include neurons comparable to those referred to above, evidence is found for projections to subnuclei a and b of the medial accessory nucleus, caudally, as well as to the caudal part of the dorsal accessory nucleus (Fig. 12A, B). Other cases [24] show that the labeling of the principal nucleus (Fig. 12C–E) was produced by spread of the marker to the interstitial nucleus of Cajal and the medial red nucleus.

It is worth noting that ^{3}H-leucine injections of tegmental areas comparable to those labeled in Fig. 11 C, D (tgl) provide evidence for projections to the ventromedial part of the dorsal accessory nucleus rostrally (e.g., Fig. 9, ref. [24]). Some of these axons may reach areas supplied by rostral cervical and cuneate projections, but most of them outline the trigeminal area.

It might seem reasonable that the motor cortex would project heavily to areas of the olive innervated by spinal axons. This may not be the case, however. Figure 13 is a plot of the axonal degeneration produced within the pyramid and olive by decortication on the ipsilateral side. Although degenerating axons reach the medial extreme of subnucleus b (arrows, Fig. 13 B, C), most parts of subnucleus b and all of subnucleus a are free of axonal debris. Degenerating axons pass through rostral areas of the dorsal accessory nucleus (Fig. 13G), but there is little evidence for terminal fields. Comparable conclusions have been reached by examining autoradiographic material from cases subjected to injections of ^{3}H-leucine into the motor-sensory cortex.

Deposits of HRP into the olive label neurons in the deep cerebellar nuclei of the contralateral side (Fig. 7F) and Fig. 14 shows the autoradiographic results obtained by placement of ^{3}H-leucine into the nucleus interpositus anterior. As illustrated in Fig. 14C–E, labeling is heavy within those rostral parts of the dorsal accessory nucleus receiving spinal and dorsal column innervation. The exact location of the labeling varies from case to case depending upon the lo-

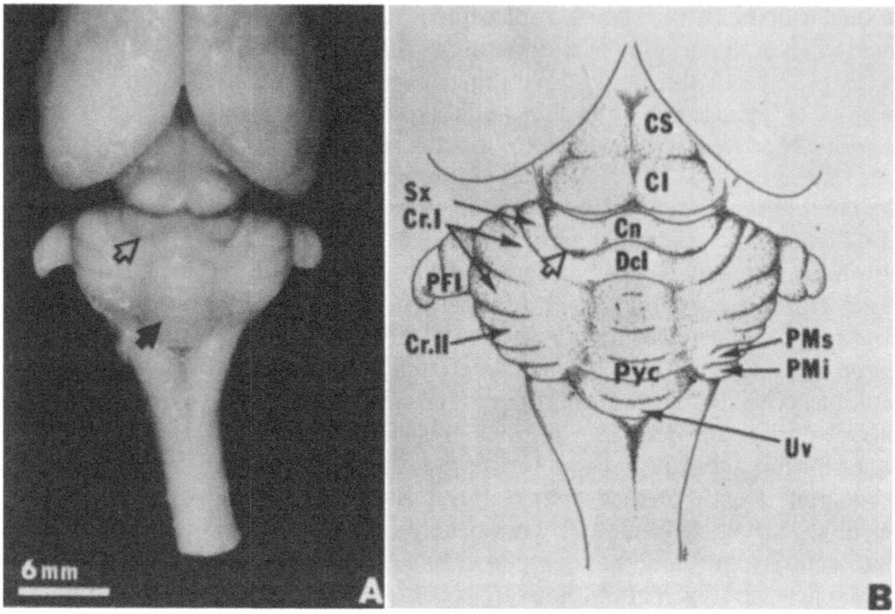

Fig. 15. Dorsal view of the opposum brain (**A**) on which the primary and secondary fissures of the cerebellum are indicated by *arrows*. The drawing on the right (**B**) identifies various folia as well as the inferior and superior colliculi. Martin et al. [25, 32]

cation of the injection site. There is evidence that rostral parts of the nucleus interpositus anterior project most laterally in the dorsal accessory nucleus. Injections of ^{3}H-leucine into the nucleus interpositus posterior label rostral and intermediate levels of the medial accessory nucleus, but not the caudal areas innervated by spinal axons. The latter areas receive a small projection from the nucleus fastigius. The lateral nucleus of the cerebellum projects strongly to the principal nucleus of the olive, but does not innervate olivary areas receiving spinal input.

Projections to the Cerebellar Cortex from Olivary Nuclei Receiving Spinal Projections

Figure 15 shows a dorsal view of the opossum cerebellum and indicates the nomenclature employed herein. Observations from 29 adult opossums with injections of HRP into different folia of the cerebellum show that those portions of the olive receiving spinal input project to the anterior lobe, the pyramis, and the paramedian lobule. Such areas also receive spinal input through mossy fiber channels [17, 30].

The results obtained by an injection of HRP into the anterior lobe (culmen) just lateral to the midline are illustrated in Fig. 16. On the side contralateral to the injection, olivary labeling is extensive in subnucleus a of the medial accessory complex (Fig. 16B, C) and a few neurons are labeled in lateral parts of sub-

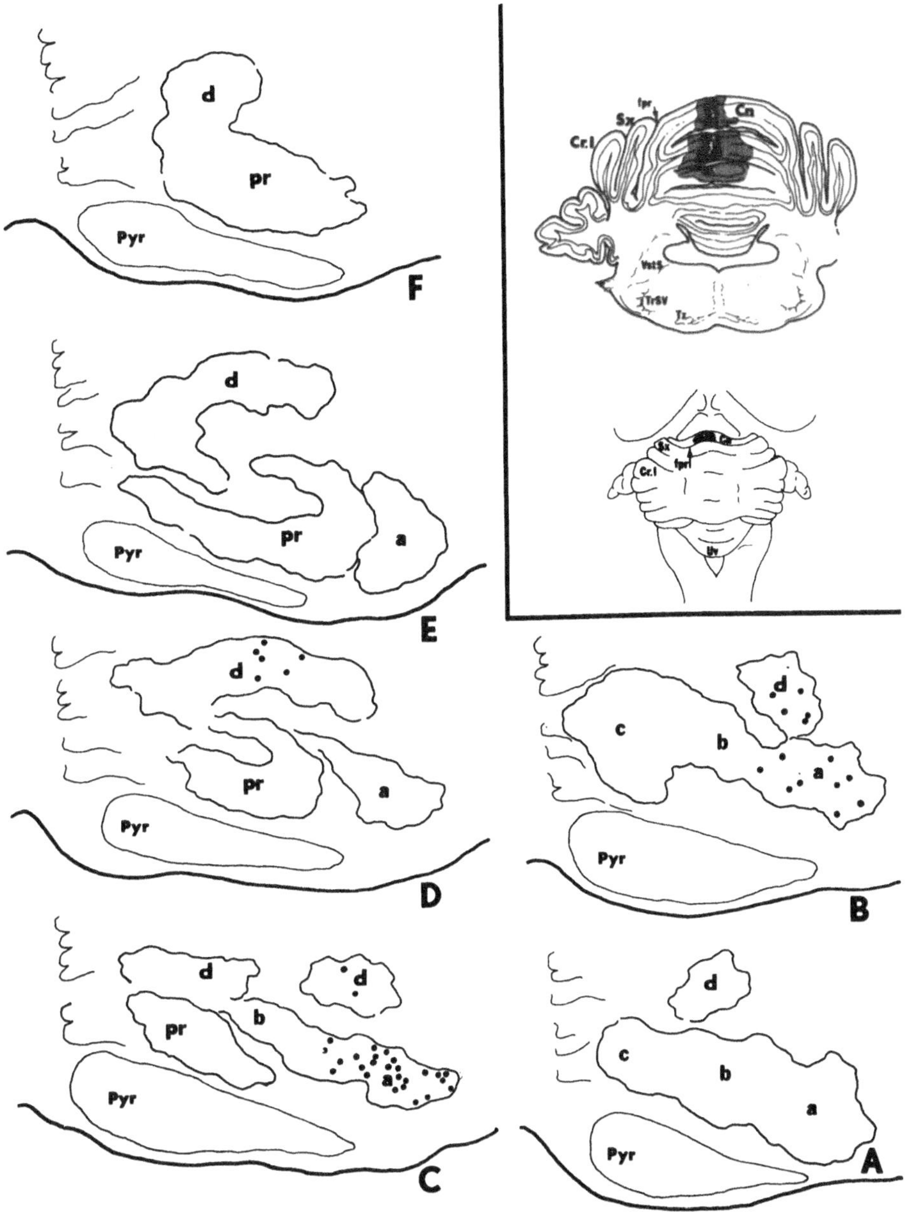

Fig. 16A–F. Plot of the olivary labeling produced by the HRP injection of the cerebellum drawn at the *upper right*. Labeled neurons are indicated by *dots* on drawings of sections through the contralateral olive from caudal (**A**) through rostral (**F**). Linauts and Martin [25]

nucleus b as well as in intermediate areas of the dorsal accessory nucleus (Fig. 16B–D). The most caudal portions of the medial and dorsal accessory nuclei do not contain reactive neurons in this case. In another brain, however, the lingula and preculmen were included in a paramidline injection, labeling

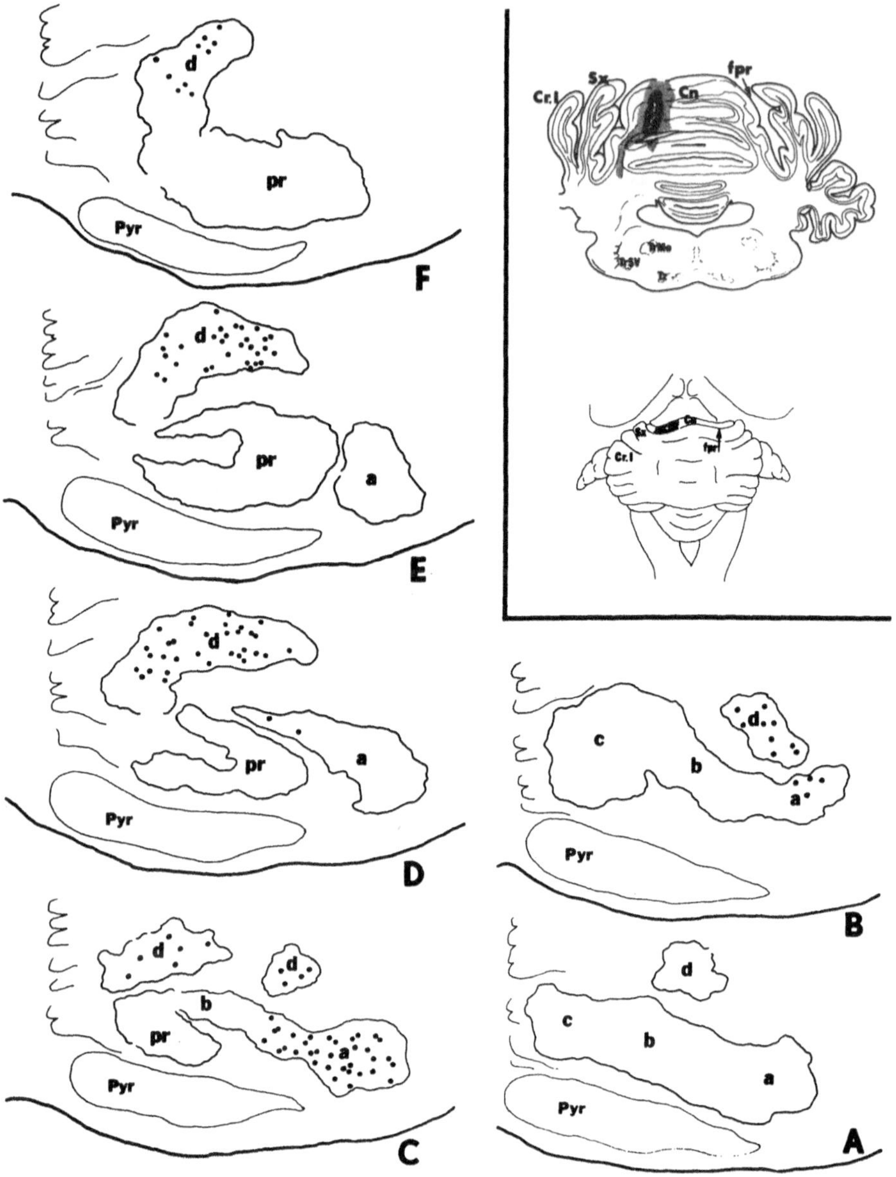

Fig. 17A–F. Plot of the olivary labeling produced by the HRP injection of the cerebellum shown at the *upper right*. Labeled neurons are indicated by *dots* on drawings of sections through the contralateral olive from caudal (**A**) through rostral (**F**). Linauts and Martin [25]

neurons in those parts of subnuclei a and b which are unlabeled in Fig. 16A as well as in all spinal targets of the dorsal accessory nucleus. Reactive neurons are found in comparable areas of subnuclei a and b subsequent to HRP injections of the pyramis. In contrast to the case shown in Fig. 16 where the greatest labeling is present in spinal areas of the medial accessory nucleus, Fig. 17 illustrates

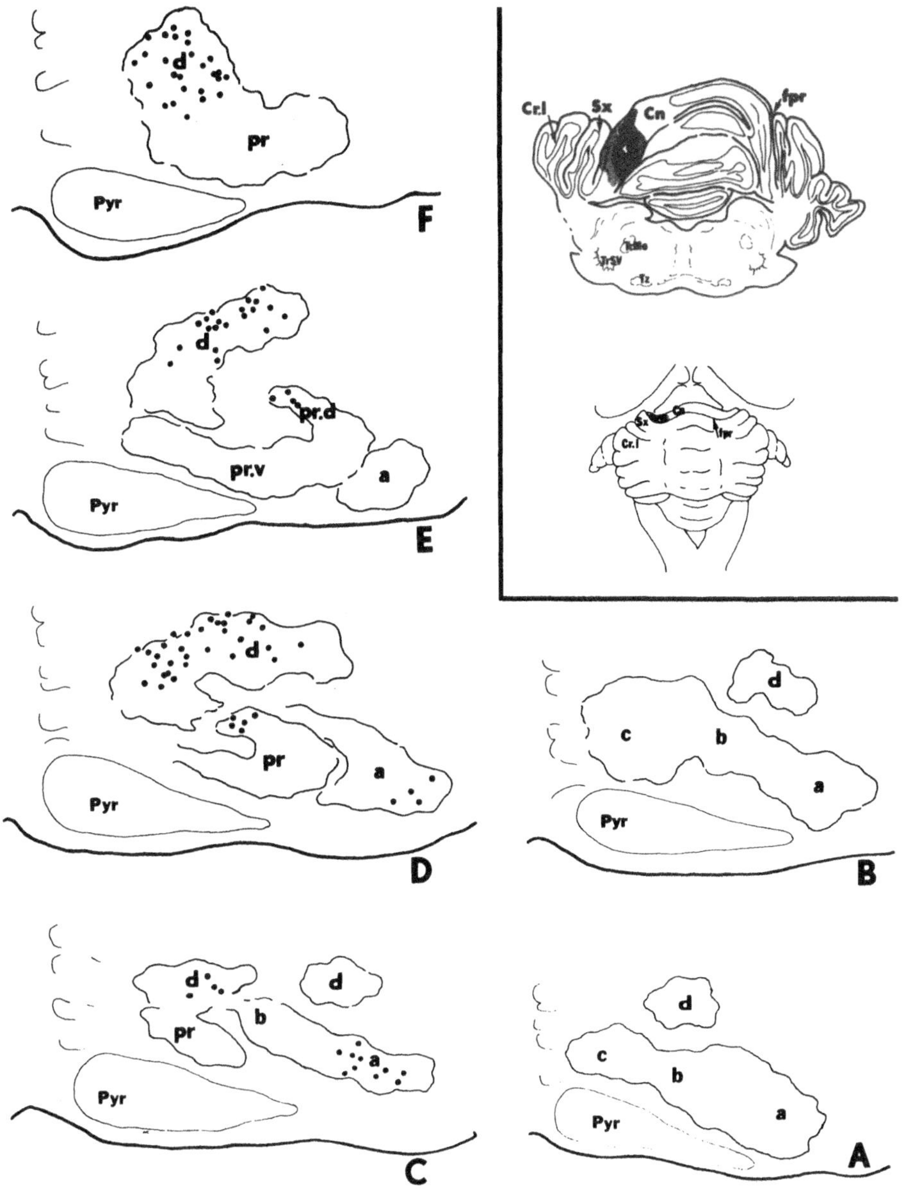

Fig. 18 A–F. Plot of the olivary labeling produced by the HRP injection of the cerebellum shown at the *upper right*. Labeled neurons are indicated by *dots* on drawings of sections from caudal (**A**) through rostral (**F**). Linauts and Martin [25]

the results of an experiment where the labeling is most extensive in the dorsal accessory nucleus. Comparison of the injections in the two brains shows that the one producing the greatest labeling of the dorsal accessory nucleus is the most lateral. It should be noted from Fig. 17B–F that the dorsal accessory labeling is in areas innervated by spinal (Fig. 1) and cuneate axons (Fig. 8), but spares the

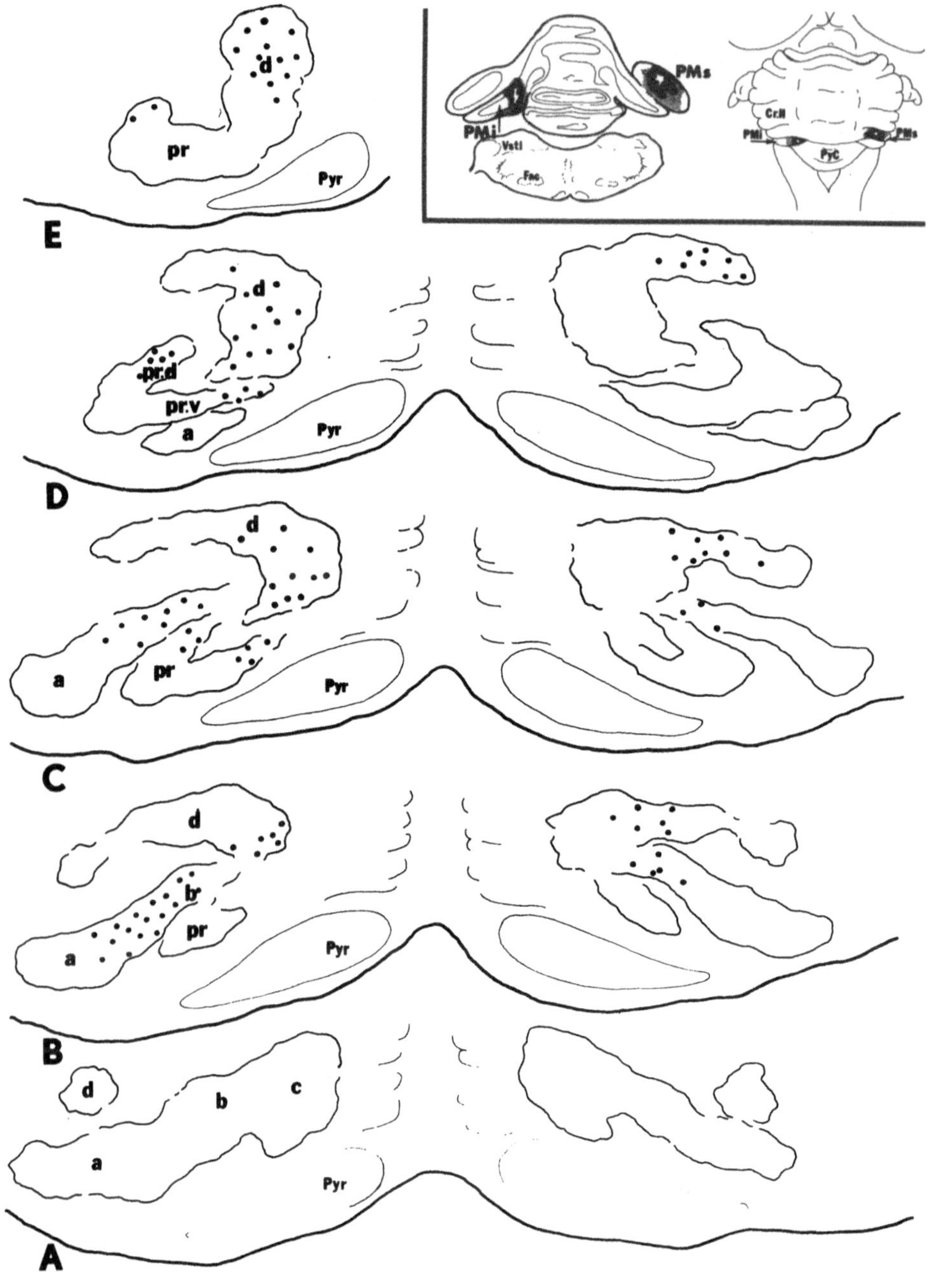

Fig. 19 A–E. Plot of the olivary neurons labeled by the injections of the cerebellum drawn at the *upper right.* Labeled neurons are indicated by *dots* on sections drawn from caudal (**A**) through rostral (**E**) levels. Linauts and Martin [25]

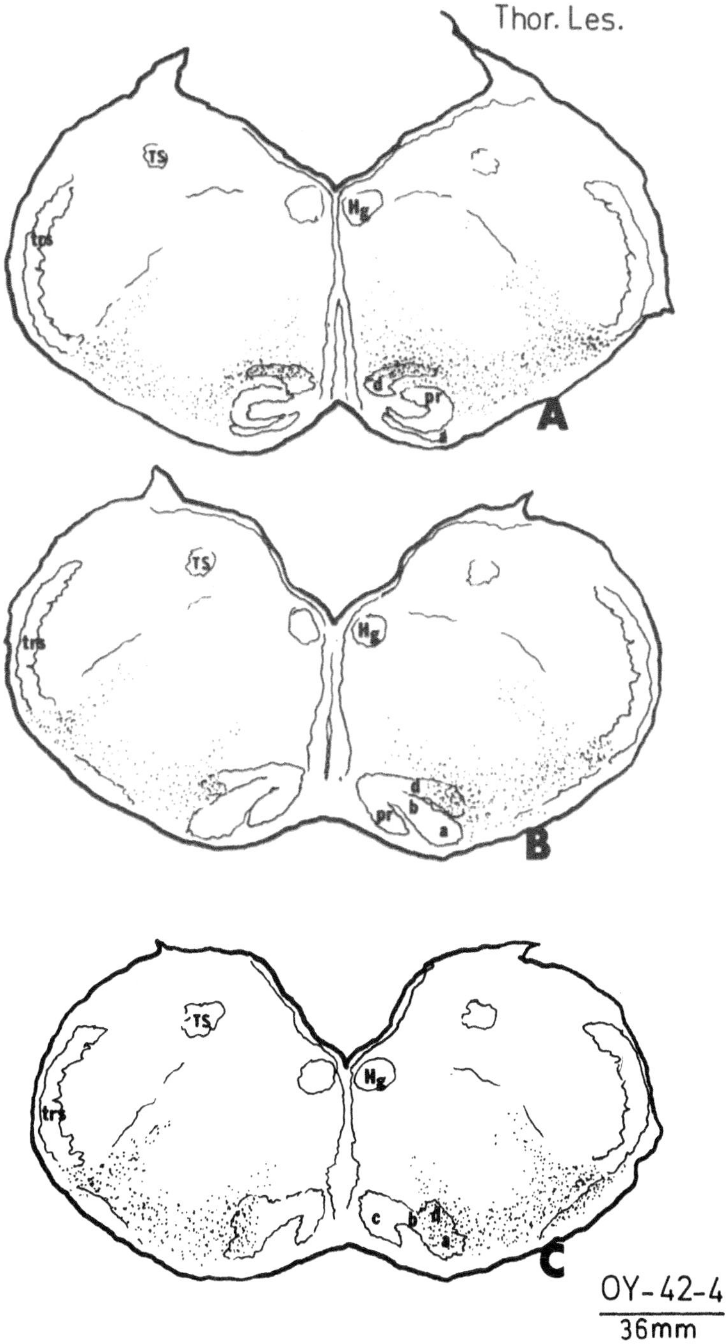

Fig. 20 A–C. Plot of the degeneration argyrophilia produced in selected myelencephalic sections by the Fink-Schneider technique after thoracic cord transection in a 36-mm opossum. The sections are drawn from rostral (**A**) to caudal (**C**). Martin et al. [33]

region receiving trigeminal input (Fig. 9). The latter region contains labeled neurons after injections of the lobus simplex, crus I, and crus II, as well as after rostral paramedian lobe injections (left side of Fig. 19C, D).

Injections of the anterior lobe lateral to that shown in Fig. 17 also label the dorsal accessory nucleus. In addition, reactive cells are found within the dorsal lamella of the principal olive (Fig. 18D, E). Note that in both Figs. 17D and 18D a few labeled neurons are found at those intermediate levels of the medial accessory nucleus which receive neither spinal (Fig. 1E, F) nor dorsal column (Fig. 8D) inputs.

In Fig. 19 the results of two paramedian lobule injections can be seen in the same brain. Different parts of the dorsal accessory nucleus are labeled on the two sides. The injection of the inferior folia of the paramedian lobule labeled neurons in that part of the dorsal accessory nucleus receiving the major input from the spinal cord and from the nucleus gracilis (e.g., Fig. 19D, right side), whereas the injection of the superior folia labeled neurons in the cuneate and trigeminal targets of the dorsal accessory nucleus (Fig. 19C, D, left side). Note that both lamellae of the principal olive were labeled by the more lateral injection (left side of Fig. 19D) as well as nonspinal parts of the medial accessory nucleus (left side of Fig. 19B, C). Caudal portions of the medial and dorsal accessory nuclei were unlabeled after paramedian lobule injections.

The Development of Spino-olivocerebellar Circuits

The inferior olive can be identified in the ventromedial myelencephalon of the opossum 3–5 days after birth (15.0 mm, S-R length). Although there is evidence that a few spinal neurites reach the edge of the olive 7 days after birth (19 days after conception), they do not grow into all of their adult targets until later. Figure 20 is a plot of the degeneration argyrophilia produced by the Fink-Schneider technique 12 h after transecting the thoracic cord of a 36-mm (S-R length) opossum. This specimen had been in the pouch for approximately 12 days (24 days after conception). Degenerating axons are present within subnuclei a and b of the medial accessory complex caudally (Fig. 20C), and within those parts of the dorsal accessory nucleus which receive spinal innervation in the adult animal (Fig. 20A, B). Electron microscopic observations reveal that the olivary neuropil is very immature at this stage and that spinal neurites are small and unmyelinated [27].

Several cases are available with metencephalic hemisections at ages comparable to that of the animal illustrated in Fig. 20. The strategy was to injure all of the axons from mesencephalic levels which had grown past the lesion site and then to impregnate them by the Fink-Schneider method. The processed material contained degeneration argyrophilia in all of the olivary nuclei known to receive midbrain projections in the adult animal – including subnuclei a and b of the medial accessory complex, caudally, and ventromedial portions of the dorsal accessory nucleus, rostrally. Metencephalic hemisections also damage the developing cerebellum and the impregnated material suggests that cerebellar axons reached most, if not all, of their olivary targets. In contrast, axons

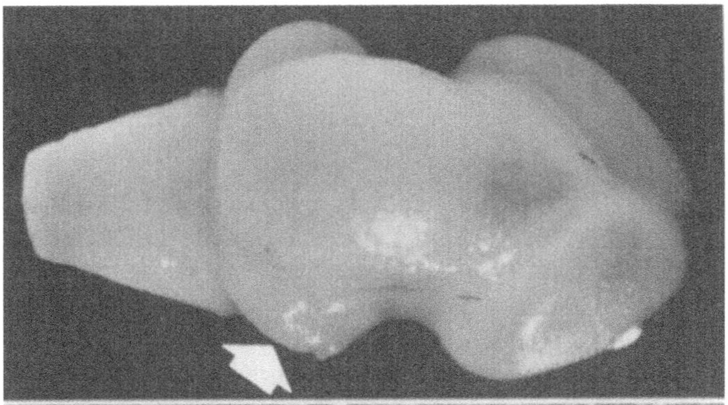

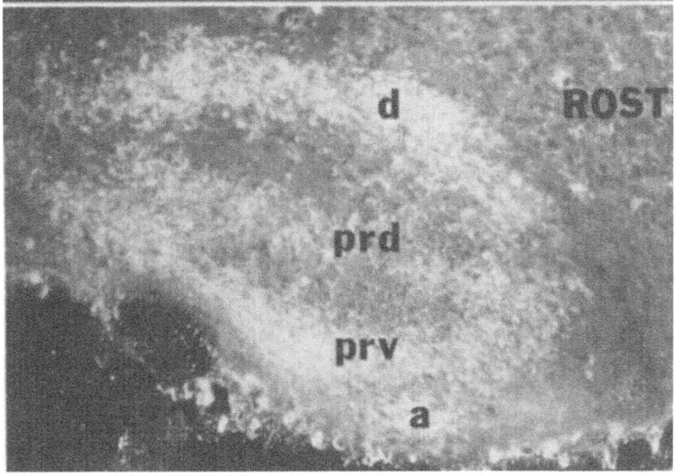

Fig. 21. (*Above*) Dorsal view of the brain from a 38-mm S-R length opossum showing the small cerebellum (*arrow*). Spino-olivocerebellar circuits are present in immature form by this stage. The brain measures 9 mm from its rostral tip to the caudal end of the medulla

Fig. 22. (*Below*) Darkfield photomicrograph of a sagittal section through the olive contralateral to an HRP placement into the cerebellum of a 36-mm S-R length opossum. Labeled neurons fill all subdivisions of the olive. The olive measures 1 mm from rostral (*ROST*) to caudal

from the cerebral cortex do not reach the olive until considerably later. The first evidence for cortico-olivary connections is present in animals measuring 45–55 mm which have been in the pouch for 25–30 days. At that stage cortical lesions elicit short-latency degeneration in the portion of the medial accessory complex receiving cortical projections in the adult animal (see Fig. 13).

Since spino-olivary axons reach their adult targets by at least 36 mm, S-R length (about 16 days in the pouch), we attempted to determine if olivary axons had grown into the cerebellum by the same age. A dorsal view of the brain from a 38-mm opossum is shown in Fig. 21. In one successful case a paste of HRP was placed on the cerebellum of a 37-mm (S-R length) animal and the reacted sections revealed that neurons were labeled throughout the contralateral olive (Fig. 22). Of particular interest is the fact that labeled neurons were present in those areas of the olive receiving spinal input.

Discussion

The caudal part of the medial accessory olive is a target of spinal projections in the opossum [18, 28]. Spinal axons innervate subnuclei a and b and those arising from rostral levels of the cervical cord reach the most medial part of subnucleus b. Generally comparable results have been reported for placental mammals [3, 5, 6, 19, 35, 36, 43]. Subnucleus b also receives spinal information through projections from the nuclei gracilis and cuneatus in the opossum (also see ref. [28]). Similar connections have been described for the cat [3, 4, 5].

In the opossum, spinal zones of the medial accessory olive are characterized by the presence of a number of overlapping connections. Projections from the spinal cord, the nucleus gracilis, the nucleus cuneatus, the nucleus of the tractus solitarius and subjacent areas, certain areas of the spinal trigeminal complex, the raphe nuclei of the medulla, specific areas of the reticular formation, and ventromedial regions of the rostral midbrain converge on subnucleus b. Some of these connections have also been described for placental mammals [4, 26, 42]. In addition, cortical axons may reach that part of subnucleus b supplied by axons from rostral cervical levels. It is of interest, however, that spinal (caudal) portions of subnuclei a and b receive relatively little feedback from the cerebellum. Although a light projection from the nucleus fastigius has been reported for the opossum [29] and cat [3], its existence has been questioned in the cat and rat [2, 7, 8, 44].

The parts of the medial accessory olive receiving spinal input innervate a vermal zone just lateral to the midline of the anterior lobe and pyramis. A projection from the comparable part of the olive to a similar zone, zone A, has been described in the cat [14]. The location of zone A in the opposum has been estimated by Haines et al. (this volume) on the basis of its projection to the nucleus fastigius.

In the opossum, caudal and rostrolateral parts of the dorsal accessory nucleus receive a major projection from the spinal cord as well as input from the nucleus gracilis [18, 28]. Comparable connections have been described for the cat [3, 5]. The caudal part of the dorsal accessory nucleus is also innervated by axons which arise within the ventromedial midbrain [24, 28] and, perhaps, from reticular neurons of the medulla [31]. The rostrolateral part of the dorsal accessory nucleus may also receive projections from closely related reticular or raphe neurons [31]. In addition, most of the dorsal accessory nucleus is heavily innervated by the cerebellum. This projection is highly organized and arises primarily within the nucleus interpositus anterior [2, 7, 11, 13, 29, 44].

The parts of the dorsal accessory nucleus referred to above project laterally within the anterior lobe as well as to inferior folia of the paramedian lobule. Taken as a whole, the areas of the anterior lobe receiving such connections may be homologous to zone B as well as zones C1 and C3 as those terms are used in the cat [14, 15]. It should be noted that in the cat, zone B is supplied by axons from the caudal half of the dorsal accessory nucleus and that it does not extend into the paramedian lobule [14]. Such may also be the case in the opossum since the caudal end of the dorsal accessory nucleus is not labeled by paramedian lobule injections.

The part of the dorsal accessory nucleus receiving cuneate and rostral cervical projections may also be innervated by the midbrain tegmentum (see also [24]). The area of the dorsal accessory nucleus in question receives a heavy projection from the nucleus interpositus anterior and supplies axons to lateral parts of the anterior lobe as well as to superior folia of the paramedian lobule. In the cat, the comparable part of the dorsal accessory nucleus projects to zones C1 and C3 [14]. The work by Haines et al. (this volume) suggests that zones C1, C2, and C3 are very small and close together in the opossum. It is worth noting that our most lateral injections of HRP into the anterior lobe, as well as those in the paramedian lobule, labeled the principal olive, providing evidence for representation of zone D (see this volume, Chap. 14).

It can be concluded from our data that those divisions of the opossum cerebellum receiving spinal information through mossy fiber channels [17, 30] also receive climbing fibers from areas of the olive supplied by spinal axons. In addition, it appears that the spinal information reaching the cerebellum through the olive can be modified by activity in several areas of the neural axis. In the opossum, this is particularly true of those signals reaching the marsupial homologue of zone A through subnucleus b of the medial accessory olive. In the cat [37–39], zone A can be activated by ipsilateral hindlimb stimulation through both the ventral funiculus spino-olivocerebellar pathway (VF-SOCP) and the dorsal funicular spino-olivocerebellar pathway (DF-SOCP). If true for the opossum, these data would correlate with the fact that subnucleus b receives connections from caudal levels of the spinal cord as well as from the nucleus gracilis. Because part of subnucleus b is also innervated by the nucleus cuneatus and rostral levels of the cervical cord, one might expect that at least a portion of zone A would receive information from the forelimb through the DF-SOCP. In the cat [14], zone A has its major effect through the nucleus fastigius and, in the opossum at least, the nucleus fastigius projects lightly to the part of the medial accessory olive which innervates zone A.

Climbing fiber activity reaching the marsupial counterpart of zone B may be modified by midbrain and local reticular neurons and, in part, by the nucleus interpositus anterior. Interpositus axons may not reach the caudal extreme of the dorsal accessory nucleus. In the cat zone B can be activated by bilateral stimulation of the hindlimbs through both the VF-SOCP and the DF-SOCP (see ref. [40] for discussion). In the cat (see discussion in ref. [14]) and possibly in the opossum, spinal and gracile axons converge on the part of the dorsal accessory nucleus innervating zone B. According to Groenewegen et al. [15], zone B projects to the lateral vestibular nucleus (see also ref. [1]). However, in our material there is no suggestion that the lateral vestibular nucleus innervates the inferior olive.

The parts of the opossum olive innervating areas comparable to zones C1 and C3 in the cat appear to be topographically organized. The rostrolateral part of the dorsal accessory nucleus receives spinal, gracile and, possibly, reticular input as well as projections from specific parts of the nucleus interpositus anterior. It is tempting to speculate that it is this area of the olive which projects to hindlimb regions of zones C1 and C3. In contrast, ventromedial parts of the dorsal accessory nucleus receive cuneate and rostral cervical projections, light projections from the midbrain tegmentum and strong projections from certain areas of the nucleus interpositus anterior. It may be this area which innervates the forelimb portions of zones C1 and C3. The reader is referred to Oscarsson and Sjölund [40] as well as Groenewegen et al. [15] for discussions of these circuits as they have been defined in the cat. Zones C1 and C3 apparently project to the nucleus interpositus anterior [15] which, in turn, innervates those areas of the olive supplying climbing fibers to zones C1 and C3.

Our experiments in the pouch-young opossum reveal that direct spino-olivocerebellar circuits develop very early. Because of its unique embryology the opossum may provide an opportunity to correlate the initial appearance and subsequent maturation of these systems with the development of spinally activated climbing fiber responses.

In summary, spinal areas of the olive are not exclusively spinal. Processing of spinal information through climbing fiber channels may be modified by activity in several areas of the brain. It is of interest that spinal axons do not contribute to the synaptic glomeruli within the olive [20, 21]. These data must be considered in models of spino-olivocerebellar function.

Acknowledgments. The authors wish to recognize the technical skills and dedication of Mary Ann Jarrell. The photographic help of Mr. Karl Rubin and the typing of the manuscript by Ms. Malinda Amspaugh are also appreciated.

References

1. Andersson O, Oscarsson O (1978) Climbing fiber microzones in cerebellar vermis and their projections to different groups of cells in the lateral vestibular nucleus. Exp Brain Res 32:565–579
2. Beitz AJ (1976) The topographical organization of the olivo-dentate and dentato-olivary pathways in the cat. Brain Res 115:311–317
3. Berkley KJ, Worden IG (1978) Projections to the inferior olive of the cat. I. Comparisons of input from the dorsal column nuclei, the lateral cervical nucleus, the spino-olivary pathways, the cerebral cortex and the cerebellum. J Comp Neurol 180:237–252
4. Berkley KJ, Hand PJ (1978) Projections to the inferior olive of the cat. II. Comparison of input from the gracile, cuneate and the spinal trigeminal nuclei. J Comp Neurol 180:253–264
5. Boesten AJP, Voogd J (1975) Projections of the dorsal column nuclei and the spinal cord on the inferior olive in the cat. J Comp Neurol 161:215–238
6. Breazile JE, Kitchell RL (1968) Ventrolateral spinal cord afferents to the brain stem in the domestic pig. J Comp Neurol 133:363–372
7. Brown JT, Chan-Palay V, Palay SL (1977) A study of afferent input to the inferior olivary complex in the rat by retrograde axonal transport of horseradish peroxidase. J Comp Neurol 176:1–22
8. Chan-Palay V (1977) Cerebellar dentate nucleus. Organization, cytology and transmitters. Springer, Berlin Heidelberg New York
9. Cutts JH, Krause WJ, Leeson CR (1978) General observations on the growth and development of the pouch young opossum. Biol Neonate 33:264–272

10. De Olmos JS (1977) An improved method for the study of central nervous connections. Exp Brain Res 29:541–551
11. Dom R, King JS, Martin GF (1973) Evidence for two direct cerebello-olivary connections. Brain Res 57:498–501
12. Fink RP, Heimer L (1967) Two methods for selective silver impregnation of degenerating axons and their synaptic endings in the central nervous system. Brain Res 4:369–374
13. Graybiel AM, Nauta HJW, Lasek RJ, Nauta WJH (1973) A cerebello-olivary pathway in the cat: an experimental study using autoradiographic tracing techniques. Brain Res 58:205–211
14. Groenewegen HJ, Voogd J (1977) The parasagittal zonation within the olivo-cerebellar projection. I. Climbing fiber distribution in the vermis of cat cerebellum. J Comp Neurol 174:417–488
15. Groenewegen HJ, Voogd J, Friedman SL (1979) The parasagittal zonation within the olivocerebellar organization. I. Climbing fiber distribution in the intermediate and hemispheric parts of the cat cerebellum. J Comp Neurol 183:551–602
16. Hartman CG (1952) Possums. University of Texas Press, Austin
17. Hazlett J, Martin GF, Dom R (1971) Spino-cerebellar fibers of the opossum, *Didelphis marsupialis virginiana.* Brain Res 33:257–271
18. Hazlett JS, Dom R, Martin GF (1972) Spino-bulbar, spino-thalamic and medial lemniscal connections in the American opossum. J Comp Neurol 146:95–118
19. Jane JA, Schroeder DM (1971) A comparison of dorsal column nuclei and spinal afferents in the European hedgehog (*Erinaceus europeaus*). Exp Neurol 30:1–17
20. King JS (1976) Synaptic clusters (glomeruli) in the inferior olivary nucleus. J Comp Neurol 165:387–400
21. King JS, Martin GF, Bowman MH (1975) The direct spinal area of the inferior olivary nucleus: an electron microscopic study. Exp Brain Res 22:13–24
22. Kooy FH (1917) The inferior olive in vertebrates. Folia Neurobiol 10:205–369
23. Leonard CM (1973) A method for assessing stages of neuronal maturation. Brain Res 53:412–416
24. Linauts M, Martin GF (1978a) An autoradiographic study of midbrain-diencephalic projections to the inferior olivary nucleus in the opossum (*Didelphis virginiana*). J Comp Neurol 179:325–354
25. Linauts M, Martin GF (1978b) The organization of olivo-cerebellar projections in the opossum, *Didelphis virginiana*, as revealed by the retrograde transport of horseradish peroxidase. J Comp Neurol 179:355–382
26. Loewy AD, Burton H (1978) Nuclei of the solitary tract: efferent projections to the lower brain stem and spinal cord of the cat. J Comp Neurol 181:421–450
27. Maley BE, King JS (1980) Early development of the inferior olivary complex in pouch young opossums. I. An electron microscopic study. J Comp Neurol 194:741–760
28. Martin GF, Dom R, King JS, Robards M, Watson CRR (1975) The inferior olivary nucleus of the opossum (*Didelphis marsupialis virginiana*), its organization and connections. J Comp Neurol 160:507–534
29. Martin GF, Henkel CK, King JS (1976) Cerebello-olivary fibers: their origin, course and distribution in the North American opossum. Exp Brain Res 24:219–236
30. Martin GF, Andrezik JA, Crutcher K, Linauts M, Panneton M (1977a) The lateral reticular nucleus of the opossum (*Didelphis virginiana*). J Comp Neurol 174: 151–186
31. Martin GF, Beattie MS, Hughes HC, Linauts M, Panneton M (1977b). The organization of reticulo-olivo-cerebellar circuits in the North American opossum. Brain Res 137:253–266
32. Martin GF, Culberson J, Laxson C, Linauts M, Panneton M, Tschismadia I (1980a) Afferent connections of the inferior olivary nucleus with preliminary notes on their development. Studies using the North American opossum. In: Courville J, DeMontigny C, Lamarre Y (eds) The inferior olivary nucleus – anatomy and physiology. Raven Press, New York, pp 35–72
33. Martin GF, Culberson JL, Tschismadia I (1980b) The development of major projections to the inferior olivary nucleus. Experimental studies using the North American opossum. Anat and Embryol (Berl) 160:187–202

34. McCrady E (1938) The embryology of the opossum. Amer Anat Memoirs, 16. The Wistar Institute of Anatomy and Biology, Philadelphia
35. Mehler WR (1969) Some neurological species differences – *a posteriori*. Ann NY Acad Sci 167:424–468
36. Mizuno N (1966) An experimental study of the spino-olivary fibres in the rabbit and the cat. J Comp Neurol 127:267–292
37. Oscarsson O (1969) Termination and functional organization of the dorsal spino-olivo-cerebellar path. J Physiol (Lond) 200:129–149
38. Oscarsson O (1976) Spatial distribution of climbing and mossy fibre inputs into the cerebellar cortex. Exp Brain Res [Suppl] pp: 36–42
39. Oscarsson O, Sjölund B (1974) Identification of five spino-olivo-cerebellar paths ascending through the ventral funiculus of the cord. Brain Res 69:331–335
40. Oscarsson O, Sjölund B (1977) The ventral spino-olivocerebellar system in the cat. I. Identification of five paths and their termination in the cerebellar anterior lobe. Exp Brain Res 28:469–486
41. Oswaldo-Cruz E, Rocha-Miranda CE (1968) The brain of the opossum (*Didelphis virginiana*). Instituto de Biofisica, Universidade Federal do Rio de Janeiro, Rio de Janeiro
42. Ricardo J, Koh ET (1978) Anatomical evidence of direct projections from the nucleus of the solitary tract to the hypothalamus, amygdala, and other forebrain structures in the rat. Brain Res 153:1–26
43. Schroeder DM, Jane JA (1971) Projections of dorsal column nuclei and spinal cord to brain-stem and thalamus in the tree shrew, *Tupai glis*. J Comp Neurol 142:309–350
44. Tolbert DL, Massopust LC, Murphy MG, Young PA (1976) The anatomical organization of the cerebello-olivary projection in the cat. J Comp Neurol 170:525–544
45. Watson CRR, Herron P (1977) The inferior olivary complex of marsupials. J Comp Neurol 176:527–538

Discussion

Robertson: The climbing-fiber response in zone B of the medial accessory olive is probably not solely the result of afferents from the hindlimb terminating there. There are collaterals or terminals from other areas and a bilateral termination.

Martin: I don't doubt that.

Brodal: In one of your illustrations with a cortical lesion you showed a projection to the olive. In the cat and monkey this seems to be a weak projection.

Martin: Don't let me mislead you by that illustration. You go through a lot of sections of the olive before you find the area receiving cortical innervation. It is indeed a weak projection.

Voogd: The cells that you showed between the interstitial nucleus of Cajal and the central gray, are they different from Darkschewitsch?

Martin: Neurons are labeled in the nucleus Darkschewitsch after olivary injections of HRP, but the ones you refer to are not within the confines of that nucleus.

General Discussion: Radial Connectivity in the Cerebellar Cortex: A Novel View Regarding the Functional Organization of the Molecular Layer

R. Llinás

One of the delights of a meeting such as the one we have here is that it serves as a forum to present new views to colleagues who are knowledgeable and interested and who comprise the central core of the field in question. Obviously the cerebellum has been one of the loci in which the relationship between structure and function has been best documented. It is one of the few areas in the central nervous system where an account has been given of the interaction between the different neuronal elements which constitute it. It is true, nevertheless, that some nagging problems remain.

I would like to address myself to one such problem and to suggest a possible solution. The proposed solution is of significance, if correct, because it represents a major departure from our conception of the functional organization of the molecular layer.

The problem at hand is the following. The parallel fibers extend over a rather wide area of the cerebellar cortex covering many millimeters [8] – in some cases (for instance, in the frog) the whole cerebellum. Furthermore, modern analyses of the problem, for instance, that of Mugnaini and collaborators [2, 5], indicate that the parallel fibers have a lateral spread which may be as long as 6 mm. Physiologically the parallel fibers exercise an excitatory action on Purkinje cells throughout their length [3]. Thus, it would be expected that activation of a localized region of the granule cell layer by mossy fibers would generate a Purkinje cell activity along the whole length of the activated set of parallel fibers. The problem arises when one compares such anatomical results with the physiological results reported by Oscarsson [6] and by Welker and collaborators [9] who demonstrated that activation of peripheral nerves or sensory stimuli will generate activity in rather restricted areas of the cerebellar cortex. Oscarsson's experiments indicate that the spatial distribution of electrical activity of Purkinje cells matches beautifully the spatial distribution, into rostrocaudal bands, for the mossy fiber afferent system as described by Voogd [10]. An even more detailed description of the spatial distribution of mossy fibers in the granular layer has been determined by Welker and collaborators [11] by means of detailed electrical recording from the granule cells and Purkinje cells. These authors have shown that the very specific mossy fiber inputs activated by trigeminal stimulation in the rat and cat produce very well localized activity in the granular layer. More important, however, such granule cell activity is translated into *the exclusive activation of the Purkinje cells lying immediately above the area of activated granule cells.* Indeed, Welker and colleagues [1] demonstrate that such Purkinje cell activity does not exceed spatially the area of distri-

Experimental Brain Research, Suppl. 6

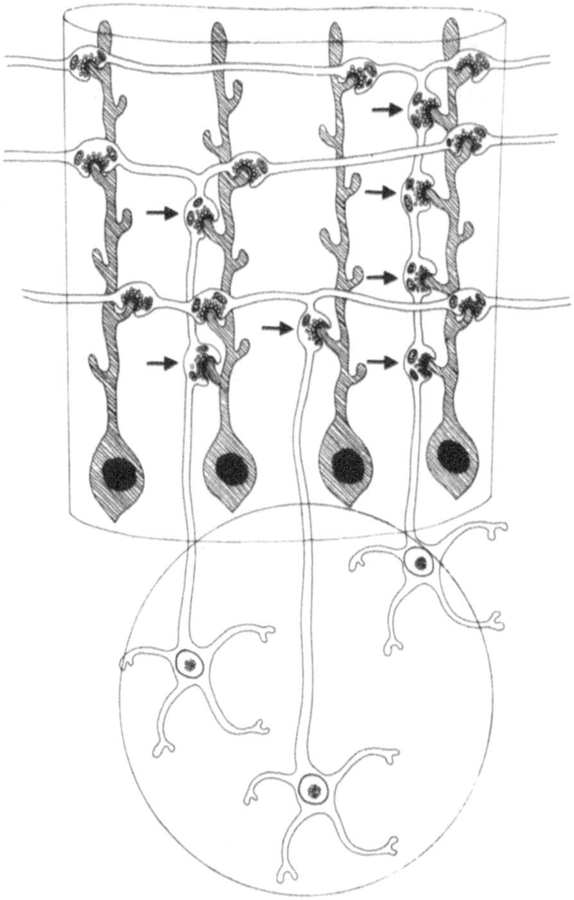

Fig. 1. Radial organization of the synaptic junctions between the ascending portion of the granule cell axons and the dendrites of Purkinje cells. The granule cells (in the *circle*) generate ascending axons which penetrate the molecular layer of the cortex (*cylinder*). Along their path, these axons generate synaptic contacts (*arrows*) with Purkinje cell (*shaded*) dendritic spines as well as with the dendrites of the inhibitory interneurons of both granular and molecular layers. Because an ascending axon will contact a given Purkinje cell repeatedly, this descending portion will have a more powerful synaptic action on the Purkinje cells located immediately above their cells of origin; thus the radial organization of molecular layer input

bution of granule cell activity; that is to say, spatially the *maximal degree of Purkinje cell activity is related to the distribution of granule cell activity and not to distribution of their parallel fibers.*

In thinking about this problem, the possibility came to mind that the spatial distribution of activity of Purkinje cells following mossy fiber activation could be due to the fact that the *granule cell axons make synaptic contact with Purkinje cells as they reach the molecular layer prior to their bifurcation.* Thus a given set of ascending granule cell axons will generate a statistically larger number of contacts with Purkinje cells lying immediately above than with Purkinje cells lying either to the left or right of the bifurcation point of their axons. Such view is illustrated in Fig. 1. If this were the case, the basic organization of the molecular layer would be such that the ascending axons of the granule cells would serve as the main, mossy-fiber mediated, input to the Purkinje cells and to the molecular and granule layer interneurons, while the horizontal axons of the granule cells would serve a more modulatory function.

The present hypothesis does not de-emphasize the importance of the parallel fibers. It simply calls attention to the fact that the *granule cell axons may have two distinct functions*, one relating to their ascending portion, which gives it a *radial organization* and the *spatial specificity* observed experimentally, and a more modulatory role relating to their parallel fiber portion. This is basically similar to the scheme proposed some years ago regarding horizontal and vertical integration of Purkinje cells [4], only vertical integration has a solid morphological basis rather than being the spatial distribution of parallel-fiber activity.

Having had this thought, I remembered seeing in Enrico Mugnaini's paper [5] some beautiful examples of ascending parallel fiber synapses on Purkinje cell dendrites. These findings were also reported by Palay and Chan-Palay [7]. Since then, Dr. Mugnaini has confirmed his finding that ascending axons of parallel fibers will contact given Purkinje cells may times.

Note Added in Proof. While at the time of the symposium, only preliminary physiological data were obtained, recent experiments in collaboration with Dr. M. Sugimori indicate that, in guinea pig cerebellar slices, local stimulation of the granular layer lying immediately under the Purkinje cell produces graded synaptic depolarization and firing of these large cells. Such synaptic potentials are clearly distinguishable from the climbing fiber input and may be reversed by passing current through the recording electrode. Because such depolarization is apparent only when the granule cells located immediately under the Purkinje cell are activated, and because the slices are as thin as 50 μm giving basically no lateral spread to the parallel fibers, the data clearly indicate that the ascending axons of the parallel fibers must have a strong excitatory action on the Purkinje cells.

References

1. Bower JM, Woolston DC, Gibson JM (1980) Congruence of spatial patterns of receptive field projections to Purkinje cell and granule cell layers in the cerebellar hemispheres of the rat. Soc Neurosci Abst 6:511
2. Brand S, Dahl A-L, Mugnaini E (1976) The length of parallel fibers in the cat cerebellar cortex. An experimental light and electron microscopic study. Exp Brain Res 26:39–58
3. Eccles JC, Llinás R, Sasaki K (1966) Parallel fibre stimulation and responses induced thereby in the Purkinje cells of the cerebellum. Exp Brain Res 1:17–39
4. Llinás R (1970) Neuronal operations in cerebellar transactions. In: Schmitt FO (ed) The Neurosciences: Second Study Program. Rockefeller Univ Press, New York, pp 409–426
5. Mugnaini E (1972) The histology and cytology of the cerebellar cortex. In: Larsell O, Jansen J (eds) The Comparative Anatomy and Histology of the Cerebellum: The Human Cerebellum, Cerebellar Connections and Cerebellar Cortex. Univ Minnesota Press, Minneapolis, pp 201–262

6. Oscarsson O (1979) Functional units of the cerebellum – Sagittal zones and microzones. Trends in Neuroscience 2:143–145
7. Palay SL, Chan-Palay V (1974) Cerebellar Cortex: Cytology and Organization. Springer, Berlin Heidelberg New York
8. Ramón y Cajal S (1911) Histologie du système nerveux de l'homme et des vertébrés. Maloine, Paris
9. Shambes GM, Gibson JM, Welker W (1978) Fractured somatotopy in granule cell tactile areas of rat cerebellar hemispheres revealed by micromapping. Brain Behav Evol 15:94–140
10. Voogd J (1969) The importance of fiber connections in the comparative anatomy of the mammalian cerebellum. In: Llinás R (ed) Neurobiology of Cerebellar Evolution and Development. American Medican Assn, Chicago, pp 493–514
11. Woolston DC, Kassel JJ, Gibson JM, Welker WI (1979) Branching of trigeminal mossy fiber axons and the precision of body surface representation in the cerebellum. Soc Neurosci Abst 5:108

Discussion

Voogd: I think Dr. Llinás has made an interesting suggestion. I have no great objection.

Llinás: It is relevant also as far as the quantification of the cortex is concerned because it has been done on the basis of synapses produced by parallel fibers on Purkinje cells rather than the ascending part of the granule cell axons.

Palay: When you make horizontal sections you see that the ascending granule cell axons are assembled in clumps which are repeated again and again. You could say that they have a vertical orientation. There are grave difficulties though because the synapses within these clumps are on the same kinds of thorns or spines that the parallel parts contact. It conceivably might be that instead of making only one contact, the same axon may make several contacts on the same Purkinje cell. But the number of varicosities is really not so great as Dr. Mugnaini's Golgi impregnation suggests. I wonder if Dr. Mugnaini might also worry about that particular Golgi impregnation.

Mugnaini: Actually this problem must be looked at more closely. We have previously pointed out that not only do these ascending axons contact Purkinje cells, but they also climb along Golgi cell dendrites and one single fiber may make a series of synapses on the same Golgi cell. So, I think we have to look into this a little more precisely in order to be able to answer your question. Was that picture an exception? The answer is no!

Palay: No, that wasn't my question. When you make electron micrographs you may see many preterminal formations, but the number per axon is rather small, probably five or six per axon, and they could synapse on a variety of cell types, not only on Purkinje cells. However, I suspect that most of them are with the thorns of Purkinje cells. But, the question about the Golgi impregnation was related to the apparent droplet formation in the axon; they do not all necessarily represent synaptic varicosities.

Mugnaini: The varicosities are there and they are about 5 μm apart.

Sotelo: This is the moniliform state of an axon which is an artifact of the impregnation. In the rat I have looked at many ascending parts of the parallel fier and they are varicose but never to the extent you have shown in your material.

Mugnaini: I have been worrying a lot myself about the moniliform state. The stellate cell dendrites are particularly susceptible to this. Actually it is difficult to make a rapid Golgi preparation without this problem. However, as far as the parallel fibers are concerned they are not subject to this same kind of artifact. I have looked with the electron microscope and I have been unable to find an example in which the parallel fibers become moniliform.

Altman: Dr. Llinás, as a physiologist why don't you think of a physiological solution. Under physiological conditions parallel fibers cannot activate all the Purkinje cells under the parallel fiber beam because most of the Purkinje cells are under inhibition.

Llinás: But then one has to suggest that inhibition gets to the Purkinje cell prior to the parallel-fiber input. This generates a latency problem. The first input that the Purkinje cell will see is parallel-fiber excitation, which is monosynaptic. The disynaptic inhibition must, of necessity, occur later.

Altman: I don't understand your answer because when you stimulate the cortical surface you are only activating the parallel fibers. You are not activating through the granule cell system the inhibitory elements of the Purkinje cells, basket cells, stellate cells. But if you come from the granule cell layer maybe you cannot activate all Purkinje cells because your mossy fiber activation also results in inhibition.

Llinás: No, the problem is the following: Mossy fibers come to a particular region of granule cells. This clear spatial relationship is seen from Voogd's and Oscarrson's findings in the vermis and those in the hemisphere by Welker and his collaborators. One has a well-localized, mossy-fiber input to the granule layer, as demonstrated by recordings from the granular layer. Under these conditions the Purkinje cells which are firing are only those immediately above. This does not make sense if the total extent of the parallel fibers is active and if the parallel fiber portion of the granule cell axons is the main activator of Purkinje cells, under normal conditions.

Krnjevic: Surely to get activation of a given Purkinje cell you must get synchronous convergence of a sufficient number of afferent fibers (EPSPs) on that particular cell. So what you need is a particular arrangement of synapses and the right latencies. You could get a parallel arrangement of this kind.

Llinás: Precisely, what you want is an axon hitting a Purkinje cell several times rather than one axon/one Purkinje cell.

Krnjevic: But that's not the only way of doing it. A number of parallel fibers could converge and get EPSPs simultaneously on certain Purkinje cells. You would get excitation of those cells and not of any others.

Llinás: That cannot explain the precise spatial organization of Purkinje cell activity.

Ito: I have a similar question to answer Dr. Altman's point. Perhaps I may ask also about the possibility of Purkinje cell collaterals. They could inhibit neighboring Purkinje cells so that only a single class of Purkinje cells can fire.

Llinás: You know as well as everyone else that collateral inhibition of Purkinje cells is not very powerful on other Purkinje cells.

Thach: I should think your own evidence along with Sasaki and Eccles might have supported such an arrangement if it were in fact the case. As you stimulate with your local stimulus a beam of parallel fibers, with your recording electrode on "out" you are going to get to a point governed by the length of the parallel fiber, about half-way, where you can antidromically activate granule cells and thus the Purkinje cells down that vertical axon. Past that you would see a sudden falloff in Purkinje excitation since you are far enough down the parallel fiber that there would be no vertical activation.
Llinás: Yes, except you realize that given any artifically activated beam of parallel fibers, the ascending granule cell axons will be spatially separated from one another and thus their action would be basically lost. Now, the activation of mossy fibers generates a well-organized column of granule cell ascending axons, having a potency somewhere in between a climbing fiber and parallel fibers. Rather than the 200 or so synapses per Purkinje cell that a climbing fiber provides, there may be five or ten per ascending axon. Given the number of such ascending axons in an area, this should be a rather potent input.
Mugnaini: The number of granule cells/mm is pretty important because those numbers allow you to calculate the exact number of ascending parallel fiber axons. You have approximately 1000 cells per mm^3 so the number of axons would be 1000.
Palay: But in each one of those ascending columns there must be hundreds of ascending axons in a cluster.
Mugnaini: Yes, they come in clusters of a few up to 12.
Thach: Why don't you activate that column just as effectively antidromically with a parallel-fiber shock say up to 1.5 mm lateral?
Llinás: Local surface stimulation of parallel fibers cannot produce the same distribution of ascending axonal activity as mossy-fiber activation of the granular layer. Surface stimulation will activate all fibers in a given plane (20 μm or so deep) but not all fibers in an ascending column. Ascending fibers belonging to given columns will terminate at different depths and their parallel portions will have different lengths.
Martin: I think it is a very provocative hypothesis.

Investigations of the Olivocerebellar and Spino-Olivary Pathways

D. M. Armstrong, N. C. Campbell, S. A. Edgley, R. F. Schild, and J. R. Trott

Introduction

The inferior olivary nucleus projects almost exclusively to the cerebellum and as a source of cerebellar input it is sufficiently important that the functional integrity of the cerebellum seems absolutely dependent on the presence of an intact olivocerebellar projection. However, despite much research the precise nature of the olivary contribution to the cerebellar regulation of movements remains largely obscure. This state of affairs is particularly galling because olivocerebellar axons evoke highly characteristic "complex spike" events (CS) in the Purkinje (P) cells and additionally because the olive receives abundant inputs from the spinal cord – a circumstance that might suggest it should be relatively easy to correlate olivary discharges with specific peripheral events.

The purpose of this contribution is to discuss a few aspects of the connections and activity of the olivary nucleus which seem likely to be significant for attempts to understand the functional role of the olivocerebellar system in relation to movement control. Three main questions will be addressed and in each case a brief review of previous work will be followed by an account of recent or current studies by the authors. The questions posed are: (a) What is the distribution of olivocerebellar fibres within the cerebellar cortex and in what manner do they terminate? (b) What are the sources in the spinal cord of afferents to the olive and in what regions of the olive do they terminate? (c) What correlations, if any, exist between the occurrence of olive cell discharges and peripheral events during walking?

Termination of the Olivocerebellar fibres

In the past 2 decades there has been protracted argument regarding the question of whether all olivocerebellar fibres terminate as climbing fibres (CFs) and the related, and no less intriguing, question of whether all CFs arise from the inferior olive. The second query is of particular importance for the interpretation of physiological experiments in which climbing-fibre activity is sampled by means of microelectrode recordings from the P cells which they innervate. The evidence was reviewed by Armstrong in 1974 [4] and again in 1978 [5], and it was concluded that the electrophysiological evidence overwhelmingly supported an affirmative answer to the first question. It also seemed to indicate that certainly the vast majority of CFs arise from the inferior olive. To the arguments advanced in 1974 and 1978 it can be added that whilst recordings from olive cells have invariably revealed discharge patterns entirely appropriate for neurons supposed to initiate CS in P cells, in no case have recordings from any other group of brain stem neurons revealed discharges with the required characteristics.

However, given the nature of both questions posed above it is likely that anatomical rather than electrophysiological experiments will provide the definitive answers and it was noted that neuroanatomists were cautious in their views. In part at least this arose from the relative difficulty of demonstrating degeneration of CF terminals in the cerebellar molecular layer after lesions placed in any likely source of these afferents. In this situation the results of orthograde axonal transport studies become of especial interest and in 1978 it was noted that such experiments by Voogd and his colleagues [33, 35] and by Courville and Faraco-Cantin [23] were interpreted as indicating that the olivocerebellar projection was entirely crossed, that it provided terminations in the molecular layer throughout the cerebellar cortical sheet, and that the fibres terminated exclusively as CFs. In one other tracer study, by Murphy, O'Leary, and Cornblath [49], labelled terminals believed to be CFs were found in the molecular layer after large injections of tracer into the pons. However, it is possible in this case that the labelling was due to uptake and transport by cells (e.g., in locus coeruleus) providing the aminergic afferents which terminate in both molecular and granular layers [e.g. 22].

In summary, therefore, it appeared that most evidence, both electrophysiological and anatomical, indicated that the inferior olive provides CFs to all parts of the cerebellar cortex and that the olive is by far the most important and perhaps the only source.

However, more recently, an important orthograde transport study of the olivocerebellar projection in the rat has been reported by Chan-Palay, Palay, Brown and Van Itallie [21]. The tracer used was ^{35}S-methionine injected into the ventral brain stem to produce injection sites encompassing the whole of one olive. Terminal labelling was found in all cerebellar lobules and although the bulk of it was contralateral lighter labelling was present ipsilaterally. However, the most striking finding was that on both sides of the cerebellum the label was distributed into narrow sagittal bands of molecular layer alternating with slightly narrower unlabelled bands. Moreover when injections were made into both olives, the sagittal banding persisted, indicating that the crossed and uncrossed projections reach the same strips of cortex. These findings were taken to indicate that the very substantial numbers of CFs which presumably exist within the unlabelled bands must derive from some (unknown) source outside the inferior olive. Since then, another tracer study (in the cat) has given similar findings [38]. Clearly these results reopen the argument regarding CF origins and we have therefore felt it worthwhile to undertake another study in the rat but using tritiated leucine, a more conventional tracer than ^{35}S-methionine.

Methods

Male albino rats weighing 275–375 g were used and a retropharyngeal approach to the olive was made in the barbiturate-anaesthetised animal. Removal of the basioccipital bone and the underlying dura gave a clear view of the pyramids and hypoglossal rootlets and these were used as landmarks. Pressure injections of tracer solution were made into the left olive via a glass micropipette (50–60 µm tip diameter). In the rostrocaudal dimension the nucleus spans 2.5–2.8 mm and in the first experiments it proved impossible by a single injection to produce an injection site which included the whole nucleus. In the cases reported here four to five injections were therefore made at distances of 0.3–1.5 mm from the midline and spaced over a rostrocaudal distance of approximately 2.5 mm. Each injection comprised 0.2 µl of an aqueous solution of L-[4,5-^{3}H]leucine (Radiochemicals Centre, Amersham), previously concentrated by evaporation under nitrogen to yield a radioactive concentration of 60–70 µCi/µl.

The animals were allowed to survive 2–4 days and then anaesthetised and perfuse-fixed with Holt-Hicks solutions. Brain stem and cerebellum were post-fixed for 7 days, embedded in gelatin and serially frozen-sectioned at 25 µm in the coronal plane. Sections were defatted and dipped in Kodak NTB 2 or Ilford G5 emulsion and exposed for 3 weeks at 4 °C. They were lightly stained with cresyl violet after development (Kodak D19 or D19b developer, respectively) and examined under bright- and dark-field illumination using a Zeiss Ultraphot III microscope.

Four animals were pretreated at least 3 days prior to tracer injection with the drug regime of Llinàs et al. [44] which employs 3-acetyl pyridine and harmaline to destroy the inferior olive pharmacologically and niacinamide to protect other areas of the central nervous system.

Results

Olive cells were judged to have taken up (and transported) the tracer if the concentration of silver grains over the soma was higher than over the surrounding neuropil. On this basis the composite injection site encompassed most of one inferior olive in four normal animals selected from a series of more than 20 in most of which the nucleus was only partially filled.

Figure 1 A is a low-power photomicrograph showing part of an injection site: it shows a section 2 mm from the caudal pole of the olive and therefore includes the principal and both accessory olives. Figure 1 B shows another site at higher magnification to demonstrate the characteristically dense accumulations of silver grains which overlay the somata of the olivary neurons. In all cases, serial sections spanning the rostrocaudal extent of the olive were scrutinized to identify any region which had escaped labelling (vide Figs. 3, 4, which document the olivary involvement in two different cases). In each animal some small portions of the nucleus were unlabelled, sometimes because the injection site was too restricted and sometimes because around one or more pipette tracks a small "is-

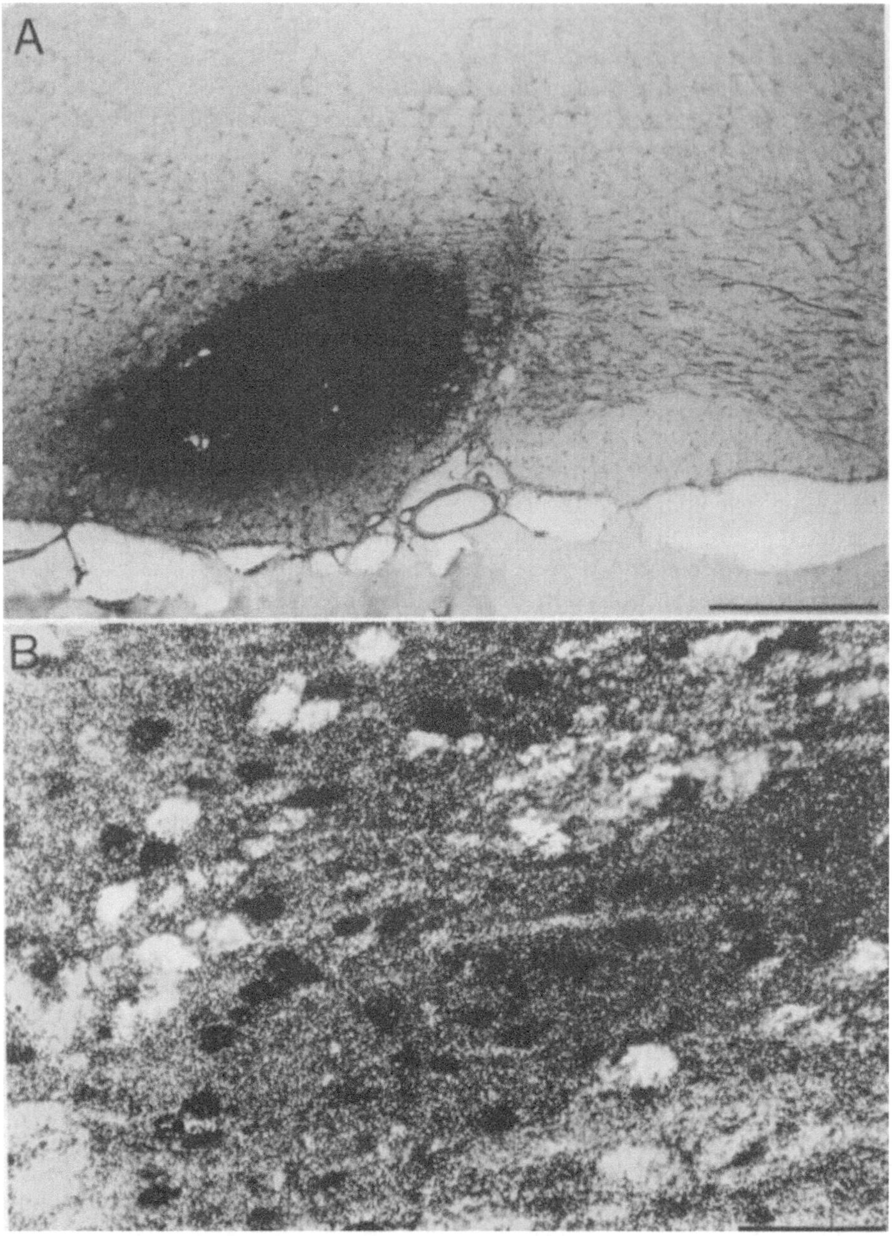

Fig. 1A, B. Injection site produced in the inferior olive by injection of ^{3}H-leucine. **A** Transverse section through the ventral medulla showing injected olive to *left*. Section 2 mm rostral to caudal pole of nucleus. Same case as Fig. 3. *Bar* is 0.5 mm. **B** Higher-power micrograph showing typical appearance of labelled olivary neurons in another case. *Bar* is 50 μm

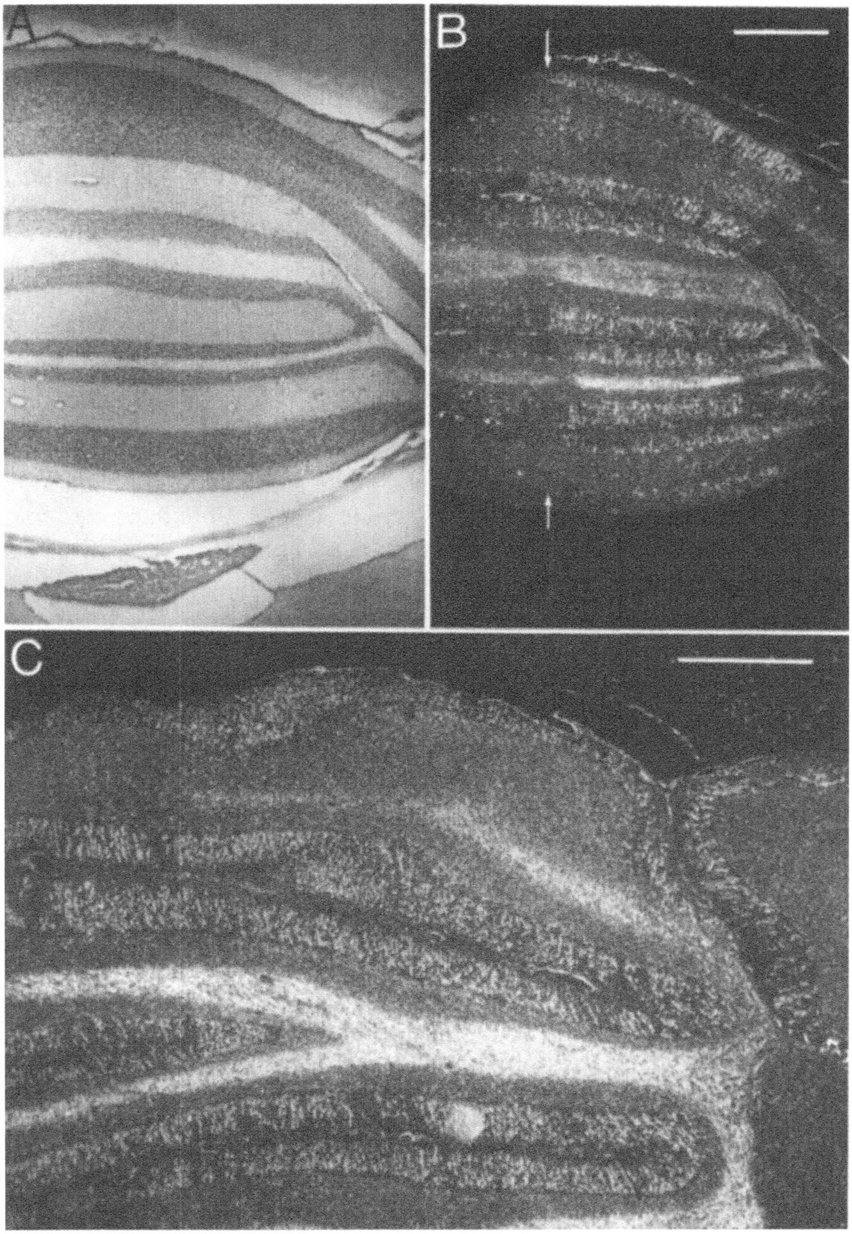

Fig. 2A–C. Axonal transport to molecular layer of cerebellar cortex after olivary injection of ^{3}H-leucine. **A, B,** Bright- and dark-field micrographs, respectively, of same vermal region. Coronal section. Cerebellar midline shown by *arrows*. Note heavy labelling in molecular layer contralateral to injected olive. Same case as Fig. 3. *Calibration* is 0.5 mm. **C** Dark-field micrograph of coronal section through cerebellar hemisphere in another case. *Calibration* is 0.5 mm

land" of cells failed to take up tracer, presumably because of damage by the injection. In all cases there was some spread of tracer into the pyramid and into the reticular formation dorsal and/or dorsolateral to the olive.

In each case heavy labelling was widely distributed in the molecular layer on the contralateral side of the cerebellum but ceased abruptly at or near the anatomical midline. In some cases of the larger series labelling was present on both sides of the cerebellum but in these the injection site invariably included the most medial portion of the contralateral olive. Our results are therefore consistent with the proposition that the CF projection from the rat olive is entirely crossed.

The type of molecular layer labelling observed in all cases is exemplified by Fig. 2. Figure 2A shows a bright-field photomicrograph of a coronal section in which the cerebellar midline is indicated by arrows; the whole width of the hemivermis contralateral to the injection (right of the arrows) is included together with the medial part of the ipsilateral hemivermis. Figure 2B is a dark-field micrograph of the same region and shows conspicuous labelling through most of the molecular layer on the contralateral side. Note that in each of the four folia the intensity of labelling decreases abruptly at or near the cerebellar midline. High-power examination and grain counting showed that ipsilateral labelling was not significantly different from background level off the section. By contrast, on the contralateral side the labelling is more or less continuous (apart from a few tiny gaps which are not systematically distributed) over lengths which extend mediolaterally for as much as 0.9–1.5 mm. Within these labelled areas the silver grains are distributed in closely spaced but discrete lines which extend from the P cell layer towards the pial surface. In coronal sections the planar dendritic trees of the cells and the accompanying CF arborizations are mainly intercepted edge on so that such a distribution is compatible with its having resulted from axonal transport in the CFs. Two other observations were in accord with this view. Firstly, in areas where the curvature of the folia brought the plane of the P cell dendrites into the plane of section the grains were arranged to produce beautiful tree-like formations. Secondly, labelling was confined to the deeper three-quarters of the molecular layer, in agreement with the known morphology of the CF branches which contact the main dendrites of the P cells.

Figure 3 shows the injection site for the case of Fig. 2A, B together with a diagrammatic reconstruction of the cerebellar molecular layer arrived at by examination of the serial coronal sections. Regions with heavy labelling of the molecular layer are stippled and in these areas the labelling was fairly uniform in intensity. The unstippled regions are those in which molecular labelling was absent. However, it is important to note that these include some areas in which there was patchy or sporadic labelling either of individual CFs or of small groups. The unstippled regions therefore represent an attempt to indicate the *maximum* extent of the "unlabelled" molecular layer. In this case the vermis was labelled throughout virtually its whole extent and if it is assumed that the olivocerebellar localisation in the rat is broadly similar to that in the cat this can be attributed to the fact that tracer uptake occurred throughout the whole of both accessory olives in their caudal halves. In the lobulus simplex, crura,

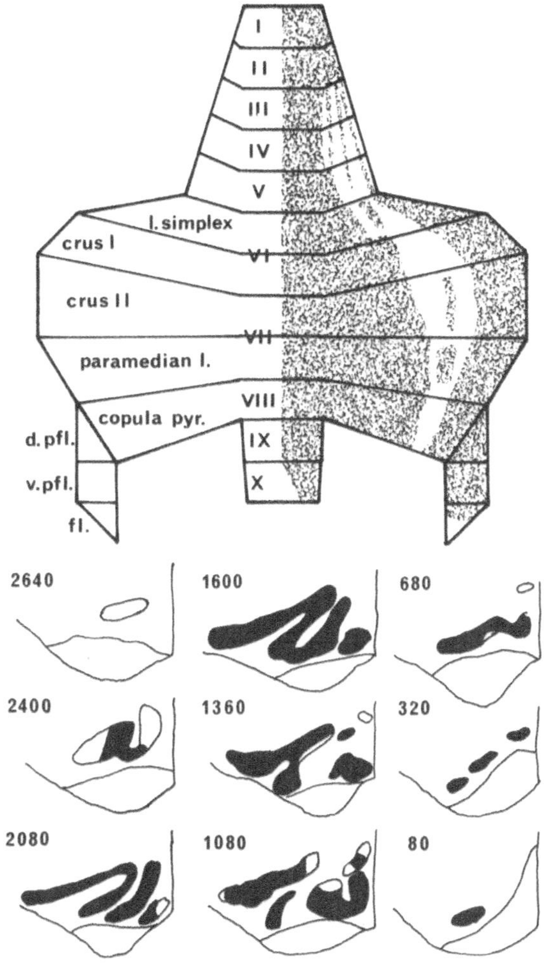

Fig. 3. Injection site and extent of axonal transport to cerebellar molecular layer in one animal. *Stippling* in cerebellar diagram shows area of molecular layer with labelling similar to that in Fig. 2B, C. *Unstippled areas* were unlabelled or lightly labelled (see text). *Roman numerals* identify lobules according to Larsell [41]. *d. pfl.* and *v. pfl.*, respectively dorsal and ventral paraflocculus; *fl.*, flocculus. Injection site in series of transverse sections spanning the olive. Distance of each from caudal pole of nucleus shown in μm. *Midline* to *right*; pyramid indicated. Olive neurons throughout the filled areas had taken up ^{3}H-leucine (see text)

paramedian lobule and copula pyramidis labelling was extensive but incomplete and on the same basis the gaps here can be accounted for by the failure of the injection site to include the rostral tip of the olive and by the presence in the middle of the nucleus of some cells which did not take up tracer, presumably because of damage (see above). Only in the intermediate (i.e. paravermal) portion of the anterior lobe (part of which is visible near the left edge of Fig. 2A) is there any real alternation of labelled with unlabelled strips of the kind consistently found by Chan-Palay et al. [21].

However, in other cases the findings for this region were quite different as may be seen from Fig. 4 which presents a case in which the injection site excluded only part of the rostral dorsal accessory olive and a few cells in other regions. The molecular layer was labelled throughout the anterior lobe except for a small region near the midline in lobules II and III. In the posterior lobe vermis an "unlabelled" (in fact lightly labelled) strip extended throughout lobules V to

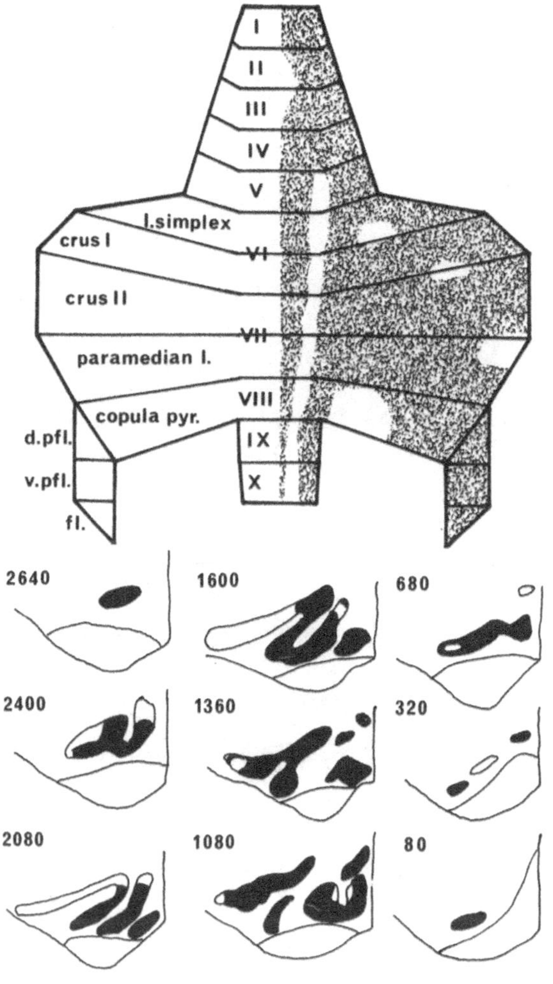

Fig. 4. Injection site and axonal transport to molecular layer in another case. Conventions as Fig. 3

X. In the hemisphere some patches were "unlabelled" but these were not arranged in longitudinal strips and except in the copula pyramidis all were lightly labelled.

Findings for the hemisphere in another case very similar to that of Fig. 4 are illustrated in Fig. 2C, which is a dark-field micrograph showing a large part of the (contralateral) hemisphere as seen in a coronal section. Except for a few small and scattered gaps the molecular layer in all three visible folia is labelled throughout its mediolateral extent and it is perhaps worth emphasising that this field measures 3.4 mm from side to side.

In all four cases there was spread of injectate beyond the confines of the inferior olive at some rostrocaudal level and although this spread was never extensive it might be argued that some of the molecular layer labelling should be ascribed to the existence in the reticular formation of hypothetical cells providing CFs or otherwise terminating in the molecular layer. To control for this possibility ^{3}H-

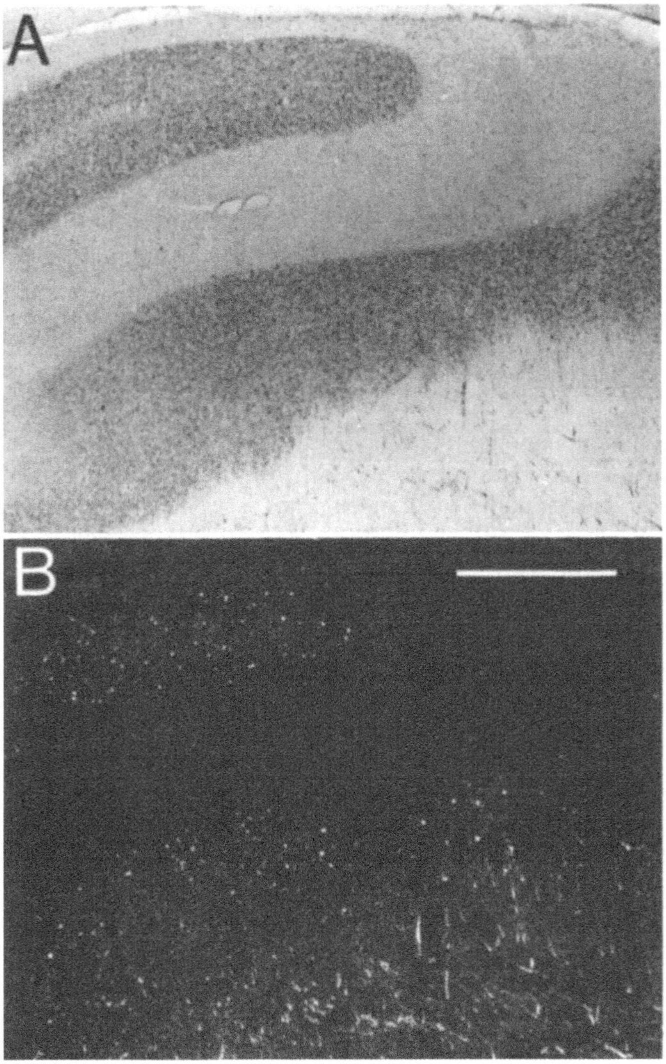

Fig. 5A, B. Axonal transport to cerebellum following ^{3}H-leucine injection into olivary region 4 days after pharmacological destruction of olivary neurons. **A, B** Bright- and dark-field micrographs, respectively, of same cerebellar area. Labelled fibres in white matter and grain clumps in areas of granular layer are visible in both **A** and **B**. **B** shows absence of label in molecular layer. *Calibration* 0.5 mm

leucine injections were made in four animals after pharmacological pretreatment to destroy the inferior olives (see Methods). These animals were grossly ataxic and the histology showed that both olivary nuclei were absent. In the injected nucleus many labelled cells were present but they were small and quite unlike the characteristically plump, rounded cells of the normal olive. The corresponding cells in the contralateral olivary region were judged to be glial cells and no more than 10–20 normal olive cells were present. The injection sites in

these control animals were very similar in location to those in normal animals but owing to marked shrinkage of the olives there was more extensive encroachment into the reticular formation.
In these cases no labelling above background level was found in any part of the molecular layer. However, there was extensive labelling in the cerebellar white matter and in the granular layer. These findings are illustrated by the micrographs of Fig. 5, where lines of grains can be seen overlying fibres in the white matter, and numbers of grain clumps can be seen in the granular layer. This labelling presumably overlies mossy fibres and their terminal rosettes. Labelled rosettes were also encountered in normal animals but were substantially fewer.

Discussion

Our findings support the view that in the rat as in the cat the olivocerebellar axons terminate (probably exclusively) as climbing rather than mossy fibres. Thus, labelling in the molecular layer was widespread after tracer injections into the intact olive but entirely absent after similar injections made after histologically verified destruction of the olivary neurons. Although some mossy-fibre terminals were labelled in the normal animals such labelling survived destruction of the olives. Moreover, the number of labelled rosettes was correlated with the extent to which the injection site extended beyond the confines of the olive, being greater in the control animals in which shrinkage of the olives resulted in labelling of more brain stem reticular neurons.
Our results also indicate, seemingly unequivocally, that the climbing-fibre projection in the rat is entirely crossed: when the injection site was confined to one olive, molecular layer labelling was confined to the contralateral half of the cerebellum, ceasing very abruptly at the midline. This finding is in complete accord with the results of several studies in the cat [20, 23, 33, 35, 38], but it is clearly at odds with the findings of Chan-Palay et al. [21] in the rat. We have no explanation for this discrepancy. We do not believe that any uncrossed labelling has been overlooked because on the crossed side it was sufficiently intense to outline individual CFs throughout their arborization in the molecular layer.
A second major difference between our findings and those of Chan-Palay et al., relates to the distribution of molecular layer labelling in relation to the cerebellar cortical sheet. We have found no evidence for a pattern of regularly alternating strips of labelled and unlabelled cortex repeatedly demonstrable in different animals. Our usual finding from coronal sections was that the molecular layer was labelled throughout lengths of folium well in excess of 1 mm. In many cases the folia were labelled along their whole length. This was not due to any extracellular diffusion of tracer which might have escaped from the CFs because the grains were so distributed as to indicate that radioactivity was confined within the terminal arborizations.
Strip-like zones free of label (or lightly labelled) were sometimes found, but they could always be accounted for on the basis of incomplete injection of the olive. Their position varied between the four animals (and also in the larger series of partial "fills"), and the larger the injection site the smaller were the

areas of unlabelled cortex. Assuming that the topographical organization of the olivocerebellar projection is broadly similar in the rat and cat the location of the unlabelled zones correlated quite well with the location of any unlabelled olivary neurons.

The extensive labelling in our animals is not readily ascribable to tracer spread to any hypothetical extra-olivary source of CFs (such as reticular neurons near the olive) because it was absent when the olive had been destroyed. In pretreated animals there was no histological evidence of damage to the reticular formation and there was increased labelling of mossy-fibre rosettes, indicating that axonal transport in surviving cerebellar afferents was unimpaired. This combination of findings is best explained by supposing that the reticulocerebellar fibres terminate as mossy fibres and that the increase in the number labelled results from the wider spread of injectate which occurred in the absence of olive cells.

Since our findings indicate that the inferior olives provide CFs to all parts of the cerebellar cortex they clearly differ in important respects from those of Chan-Palay et al. Explanations must be sought and two possibilities suggest themselves. On the one hand it is conceivable that the intense radioactivity of the ^{35}S-methionine they used may have produced an apparent injection site significantly larger than the volume of tissue within which tracer was taken up and transported. In this connexion it may be noted that in our hands several injections of ^{3}H-leucine were required – and even then filling of the olive was never quite complete. A second, and perhaps more interesting possibility, is that the olivary neurons differ biochemically so that around half of the cells incorporate and transport methionine whilst the remainder fail to do so. If the two types were in groups suitably juxtaposed it is possible that a pattern of labelled alternating with unlabelled bands of terminals might be produced in the cerebellum. Experiments using ^{3}H-methionine are currently being undertaken to discriminate between these two possibilities.

The Spino-olivary Projections in the Cat

In a recent series of papers Oscarsson and Sjölund [53, 54, 55] have reported a detailed investigation of the functional organization of those spino-olivocerebellar paths which ascend in the ventral funiculus of the cat spinal cord (VF-SOCPs). Five such paths were identified which, unlike other SOCPs, are mediated via spinal neurons projecting directly to the inferior olive. They terminated in different regions of the vermal and paravermal (i.e. intermediate) cerebellar cortex (see Fig. 6A) and were termed the C_1, C_3, A, B_1, and B_2 paths according to the location of their termination zones relative to Voogd's [34, 35] longitudinal subdivision of the cortex.

The different VF-SOCPs differ considerably in their electrophysiological properties which suggests that their respective spino-olivary relay neurons may be located in different regions of the spinal grey matter. This possibility prompted two of us to undertake a study [7, 8] in which horseradish peroxidase (HRP) was injected into the inferior olive and the distribution of retrogradely

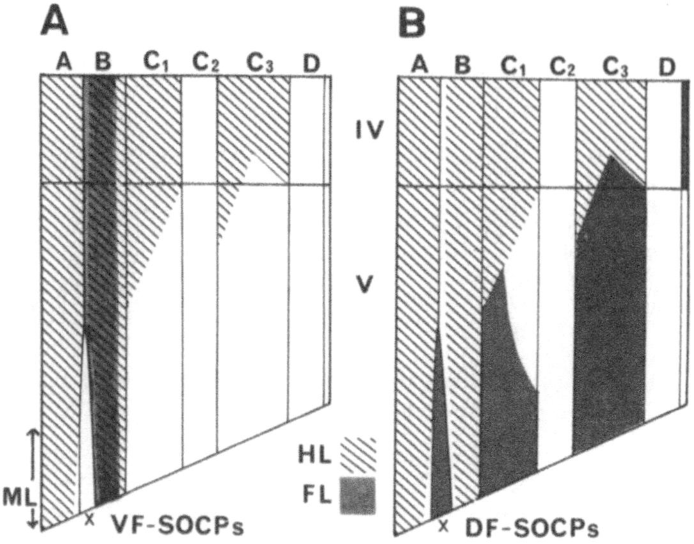

Fig. 6 A, B. Termination zones in cerebellar anterior lobe for electrophysiologically identified spino-olivocerebellar paths to lobules IV and V. Diagrammatic. *ML*, midline; *HL*, hindlimb; *FL*, forelimb. **A** *VF-SOCPs* terminating in A, B, C_1, and C_3 zones of Voogd as determined by Oscarsson and Sjölund [53]. X and C_2 zones not supplied. **B** *DF-SOCPs* to same region as determined by Oscarsson [51] and by Ekerot and Larson [27]. Indirect pathways omitted

labelled spinal neurons was determined. The results are summarized in Figs. 7, 8, which respectively show the labelled neurons in the lumbosacral (LS) and cervicothoracic (CT) enlargements. Lumbosacral neurons greatly outnumbered those in the CT enlargement, an observation which accords with the electrophysiological finding of four hindlimb VF-SOCPs (A, B_2, C_1, and C_3) as compared with a single forelimb path (B_1). Ninety-five percent of LS cells were contralateral to the injected olive which suggests that the vast majority of LS spino-olivary fibres are crossed, a conclusion reached independently by Oscarsson and Sjölund [55]. Most fibres arising at the CT level were also crossed but a significant minority (24%) of labelled cells was ipsilateral to the injection site.

In the full report of this work the distribution of labelled cells in the individual cases was so far as possible correlated with the intra-olivary location of the injection site and on this basis, and taking into account the electrophysiological properties of the VF-SOCPs, it was suggested that the retrogradely labelled cells in the LS dorsal horn (see Fig. 7) were likely to be the spinal relays for the C_1 and C_3 VF-SOCPs (which overlap heavily in the olive owing to the existence of olive cells providing axonal branches to both zones). It was also suggested that the cells in the intermediate grey matter at CT and LS levels (see Figs. 7, 8) functioned as relays respectively for the B_1 (forelimb) and B_2 (hindlimb) VF-SOCPs. Finally, the highly circumscribed group of cells in the ventromedial LS grey matter (see Fig. 7) was postulated as relay for the (hindlimb) A VF-SOCP, though it seemed possible that some functional overlap existed (in the sense that some intermediate cells might also act as A path relays).

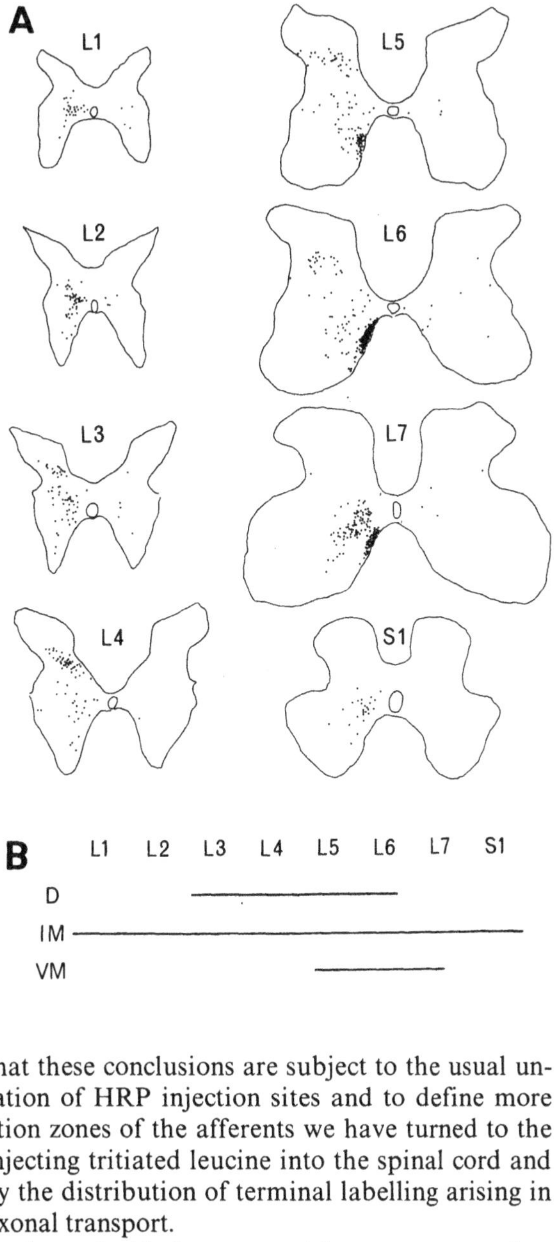

Fig. 7 A, B. Location in lumbosacral cord of all spino-olivary neurons retrogradely labelled after HRP injections into inferior olive. **A** Transverse cord sections, each from the middle of the segment indicated. *Left* is contralateral to injected olive for all sections. Cells from 12 animals pooled. **B** Rostrocaudal extent of the three cell populations evident in **A** relative to cord segmentation. *D*, cells in dorsal horn; *IM*, cells in intermediate grey matter; *VM*, cells at medial border of ventral horn

However, it was emphasised that these conclusions are subject to the usual uncertainty which attends evaluation of HRP injection sites and to define more accurately the olivary termination zones of the afferents we have turned to the complementary approach of injecting tritiated leucine into the spinal cord and using autoradiography to study the distribution of terminal labelling arising in the olive through orthograde axonal transport.

For purely technical reasons we have decided to proceed in two stages and to concentrate initially on defining the olivary areas receiving terminations from source cells throughout the cross section of the grey matter in the segments belonging to the two spinal enlargements; as a second stage, we intend to attempt differential labelling of the different cell groups as defined by the HRP study. The present report is confined to results of the first stage investigation. The experiments have confirmed previous data (see below) concerning the spino-olivary projections and have also provided fresh information, particularly re-

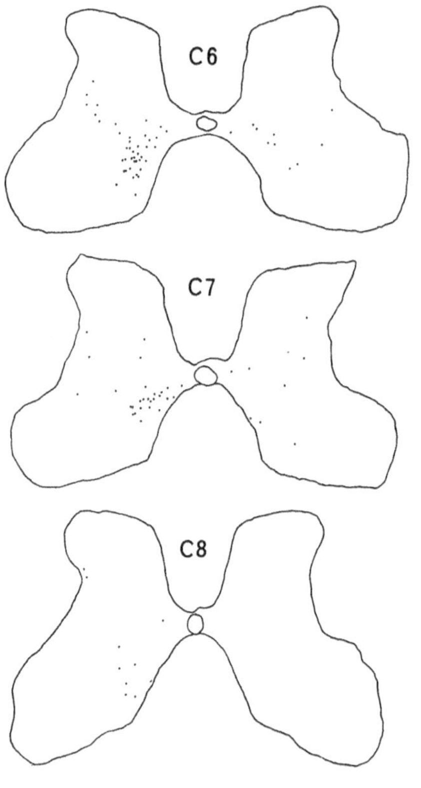

Fig. 8. Location of retrogradely labelled spino-olivary neurons in three segments of the cervicothoracic enlargement. *C-6, C-7,* ten experiments pooled; *C-8,* three experiments only

garding projections from the CT enlargement. The results also permit some deductions regarding fine-grain localization in the olivocerebellar pathway: they suggest as a working hypothesis that in those portions of the accessory olives receiving direct spino-olivary afferents (i.e. those supplying CFs to Voogd's A, B, C_1, and C_3 zones) the olivary neurons may be arranged in approximately rostrocaudal substrips or columns each of which supplies CFs to a longitudinal microzone within the appropriate Voogd zone.

For the present purpose the orthograde transport technique has the outstanding advantage that it readily permits separate tracing of terminals provided by spino-olivary cells at different segmental levels. In this respect it is markedly superior to techniques in which terminal degeneration is mapped after interruption of the spino-olivary axons at different levels of the spinal cord. Lesions at upper cervical levels inevitably interrupt axons arriving from both enlargements so that projection fields for the CT enlargement can be identified only by subtracting away the degeneration which results from lesions below the enlargement.

Despite this difficulty several detailed degeneration studies have been carried out, beginning with the now classical investigation by Brodal et al. [19]. This demonstrated terminations in the caudal halves of both accessory olives. Subsequent investigations notably by Mizuno [48] and Boesten and Voogd [15] have confirmed this finding, differing only in showing degeneration throughout the dorsal accessory olive with the exception of its rostromedial part. Neither Brodal et al. nor Mizuno found any evidence for differential localization of terminals from the two enlargements but Boesten and Voogd found that in the medial accessory olive degeneration after cervical tractotomy extended further rostrally and medially than after a thoracic lesion.

Methods

Results have been obtained from 16 adult cats of both sexes. Each was anaesthetised with pentobarbitone sodium and with aseptic precautions the arch of one LS or CT vertebrata was exposed. A burr hole was made in the dorsal lamina, and a slit in the underlying dura. A small area of pia was removed just medial to the dorsal root entry zone and a micromanipulator was used to introduce a glass pipette (tip diameter ca. 70 µm) vertically into the cord to a depth between 2.5 and 4 mm. The pipette was filled with an aqueous solution of ^{3}H-leucine (see first Section/Methods). A pressure injection comprising 1.0–1.5 µl of solution was made over a 10-min. period and the pipette was left in situ for 5–10 min. before withdrawal. The wound was closed in layers. In eight cases the injected segment lay between C4 and T2 and in eight between L1 and S1.

After a survival period of 3–6 days the animal was reanaesthetised and perfuse-fixed. The entire spinal cord was exposed and segments were identified by counting roots. In some cases the injection centred on the junction of two segments, in others it was confined to a single segment. The injected segment(s) and a brain-stem block including the whole inferior olive were frozen-sectioned (the latter in the stereotaxic transverse plane) and autoradiographs were prepared as described in the first Section (Methods). The results have been displayed on diagrammatic transverse sections through the olive and, to facilitate comparison with Boesten and Voogd [15] and Brodal et al. [19], also on reconstructed horizontal projections of the accessory olives.

Results

In all but one case the injection resulted in labelling of neurons throughout wide areas of the spinal grey matter on the side on which the pipette entered. In some cases there was spread across the midline into the medial part of the contralateral grey especially at the level of the central canal. Two large injection sites, respectively in the cervical and the lumbar enlargement, are shown at low magnification in Fig. 9 A, B.

Terminal labelling was found within the olivary complex in all but one case. It was invariably restricted to the accessory olives and was markedly heavier after LS than CT injections, in accord with our HRP study [7, 8]. Because LS differed systematically from CT cases in the distribution as well as the intensity of terminal labelling, it is convenient to present the results separately.

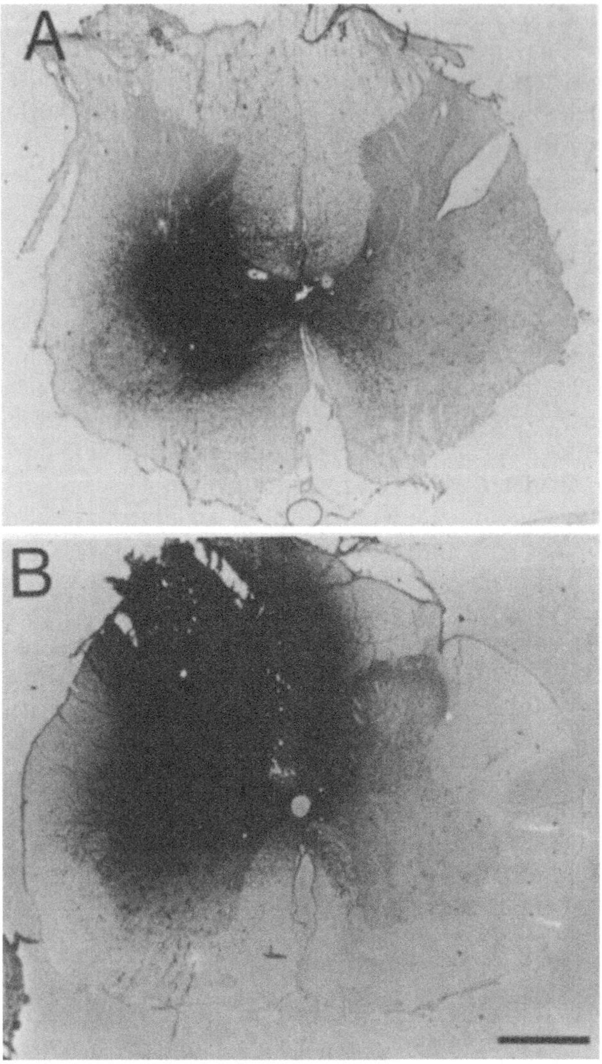

Fig. 9 A, B. Autoradiographs of spinal cord after large injections of ^{3}H-leucine. **A, B** show injection sites at L-5 and C-7/8, respectively. In both cases cellular uptake of tracer occurred throughout most of ipsilateral and also in medial part of contralateral grey matter. *Calibration* 1 mm

Lumbosacral Projections. Injections were placed in L-3 (two cases), L-5 (two cases), L-6, L-7, and L-7/S-1. In one further case injections were made into two adjacent segments producing a large injection site involving L-6 together with adjoining parts of L-5 and L-7. Terminal labelling was present in one or both olives in seven of these eight cases. Absence of labelling in the negative case is explicable because the injection site (at L-5) was confined to the lateral part of the ventral horn (cf. Fig. 7).

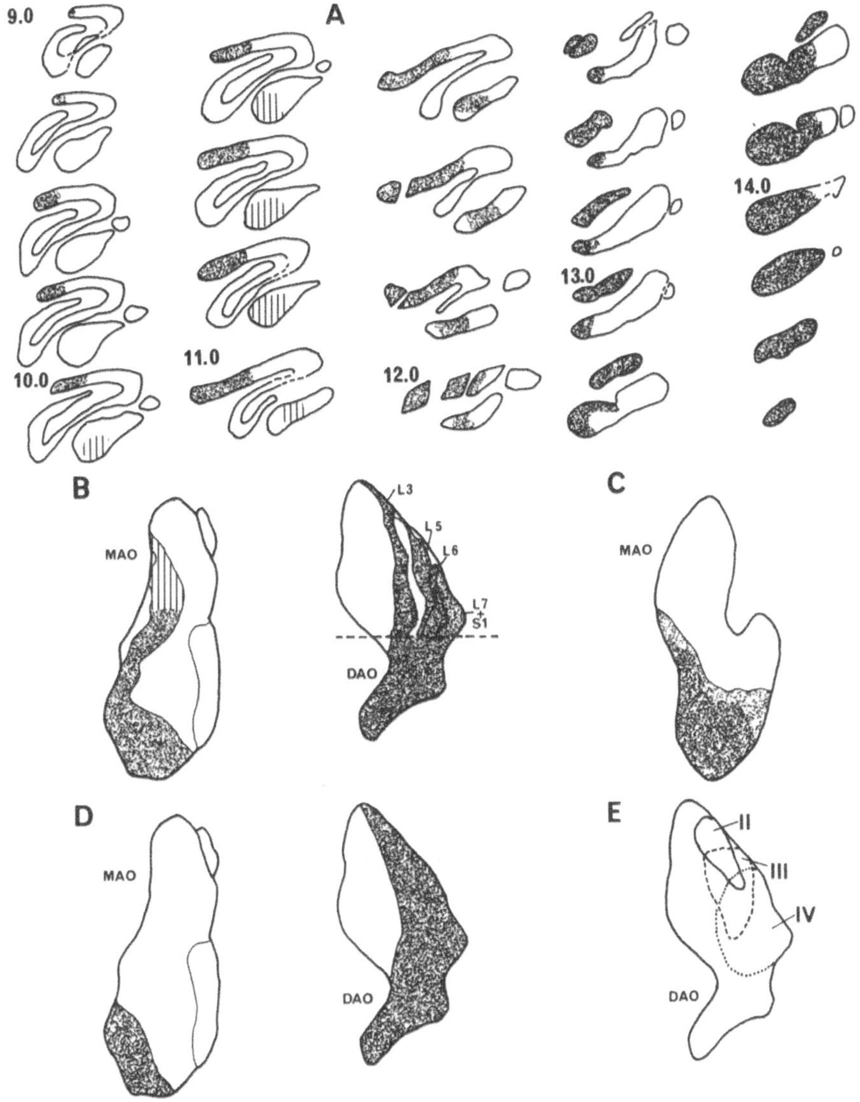

Fig. 10 A–E. Termination zones for spino-olivary fibres originating in the lumbosacral enlargement. **A** *Stippling* shows terminal labelling as found a in stereotaxic transverse sections through olive after ^{3}H-leucine injections into cord. For *hatching*, see text. Results from seven cases pooled. Projections entirely crossed with respect to spino-olivary cell bodies. Stereotaxic AP coordinates shown at 1-mm intervals; sections equally spaced. **B** Data from **A** transferred to horizontal reconstructions of the accessory olives. *MAO*, medial accessory olive. *DAO*, dorsal accessory olive. Rostral at *top*. In *MAO* medial border of subnucleus is to *right* and in *DAO* medial border is to *left* in this and all other horizontal reconstructions. *Lines* in rostral *DAO* enclose areas labelled after injection of the individual *LS* cord segments identified by *numerals*. *Horizontal dashed line* divides rostral from caudal *DAO*. **C** Lumbosacral projection to *MAO* as determined by Brodal et al. [19]. Redrawn. **D** Lumbosacral projections to *MAO* and *DAO* according to Boesten and Voogd [15]. Redrawn. **E** Distribution in rostral *DAO* of neurons retrogradely labelled after HRP injections into different lobules of anterior lobe as indicated by *Roman numerals*. Brodal and Walberg [18]

In five of the seven effective cases the injection site was confined to the ipsilateral hemi-cord and label was present only in the contralateral olive. In the other two cases there was involvement of the contralateral spinal grey, and in both there were some labelled terminals in the ipsilateral olive. In one case both contralateral spread and ipsilateral olivary labelling were minimal; in the other the injection involved both sides of the cord and the intensity of terminal labelling was almost as great ipsilaterally as contralaterally. Collectively these results indicate that the LS spino-olivary axons are entirely crossed relative to their parent cells. This result agrees well both with the results of our HRP study [7, 8] and with the studies of VF-SOCPs by Oscarsson and Sjölund [55].

When cases with injection sites in the same or neighbouring segments were compared the pattern of olivary labelling was very consistent. Thus, the large injection site involving three segments was accompanied by labelling which extended to all those olivary regions labelled after the single injections into L-5, L-6, and L-7. In addition, in the case with a bilateral injection site (at L-5), the spatial distribution of label was identical on the two sides. Finally, the distribution in the L-7 and L-7/S-1 cases was also virtually identical. We are confident therefore that our cases provide a reliable picture regarding the organization of the LS spino-olivary projections.

When all seven cases are pooled onto a single set of transverse sections through the olivary complex, the result in Fig. 10A is obtained. The only feature not so far duplicated is the presence of very light terminal labelling (shown by hatching) in the rostrolateral medial accessory olive (MAO). Although confirmation will be sought in other animals it should be noted that this result was obtained from the bilateral injection at L-5 (vide supra) and similar labelling was present in both MAOs.

To facilitate comparison with the results from degeneration experiments horizontal reconstructions of the accessory olives are presented in Fig. 10B. Comparison with Fig. 10C demonstrates that the present results entirely confirm the positive results obtained in MAO by Brodal et al. [19] and with Fig. 10D shows that in addition they confirm the wider distribution in the dorsal accessory olive (DAO) as reported by Boesten and Voogd [15].

Where our results depart somewhat from previous findings is in relation to any topographical organization within the LS spino-olivary projections, a feature which degeneration techniques are not well adapted to reveal (see above). In the rostral half of DAO (i.e. above the dashed line in Fig. 10B) a well-marked topographical localisation exists which is hidden within the pooled results of Fig. 10A. Each injection into one segment invariably led to terminal labelling within only a restricted region of the area shown in Fig. 10A and as the segmental level changed there was a corresponding shift in the location of this region. The restricted nature of the labelling in individual cases and the change in position with change in segmental level are both well shown by comparison of Fig. 11B and D which are dark-field photomicrographs showing rostral DAO after injections respectively into L-3 and L-6 (the same fields are shown brightfield at lower magnification in A and C respectively). In these and the other cases labelling in the rostrolateral DAO was restricted to a narrow, strip-like region which was approximately 350 μm wide but up to 2.5 mm in rostrocaudal

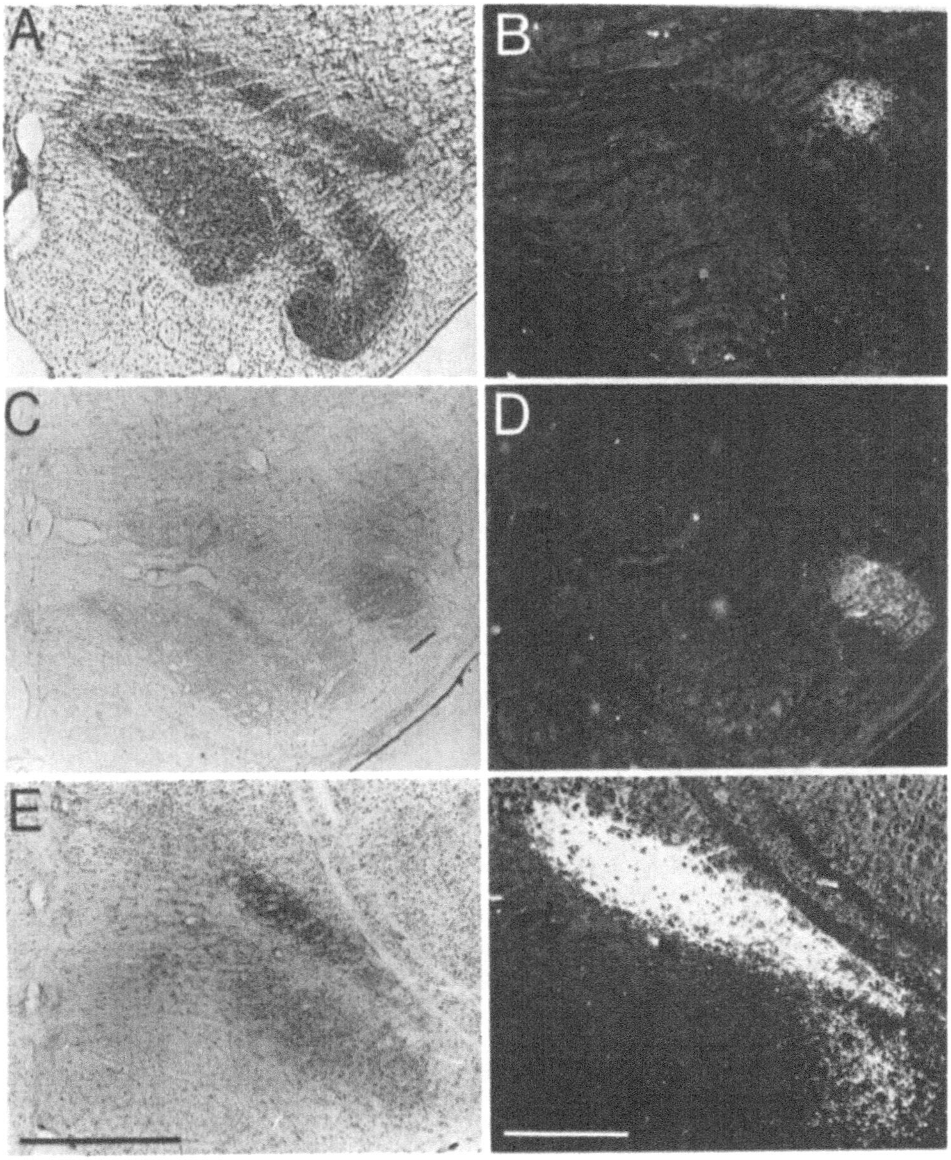

Fig. 11A–F. Terminal labelling in the accessory olives following ^{3}H-leucine injections into the lumbosacral cord. **A, B** Bright- and dark-field micrographs, respectively, of neighbouring sections showing label in rostral DAO after L-3 injection. Stereotaxic plane AP 9.75. Note magnification higher in **B**. **C, D** As **A** and **B** but injection at L-6; stereotaxic plane AP 11.0. **E, F** As **A** and **B** but showing label in caudal halves of MAO and DAO. Injection at L-6; level of section AP 12.75. Note labelling very heavy throughout DAO and moderate in lateral MAO. One mm *calibration* in E applies to **A, C, D, E;** 0.5 mm *calibration* in **F** applies to **B, F**

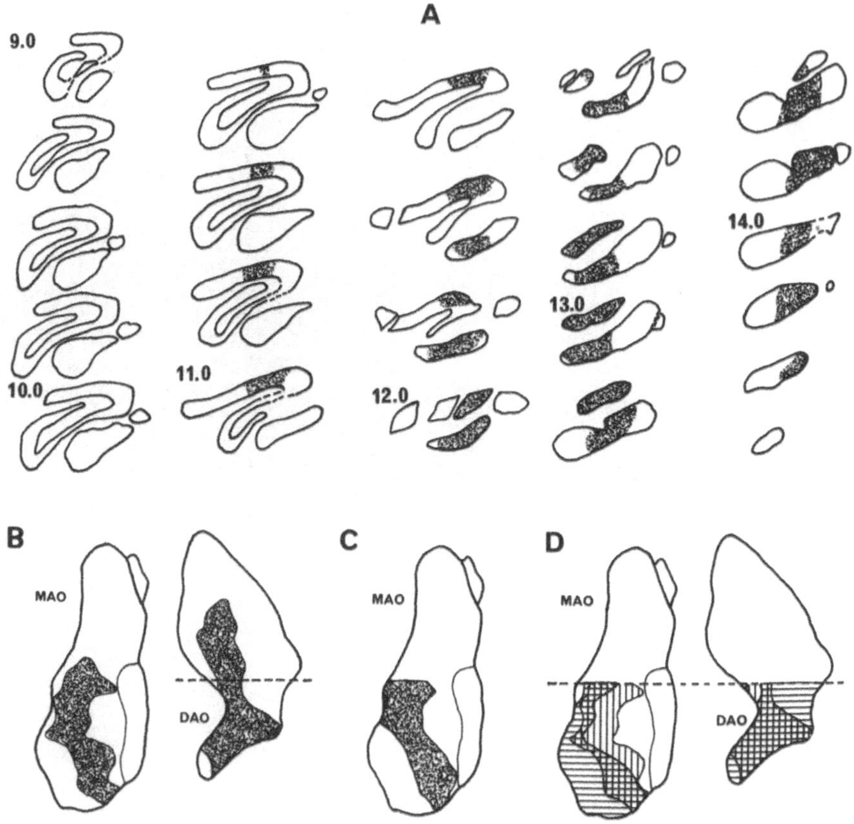

Fig. 12A–D. Termination zones for spino-olivary fibres originating in the cervicothoracic enlargement. **A** Terminal labelling as seen in transverse sections. Eight cases pooled. Projection to rostral *DAO* entirely crossed. Projections to caudal halves of *MAO* and *DAO* predominantly crossed. Ipsilateral labelling was within same areas. Conventions as in Fig. 10A. **B** Data of **A** transferred to horizontal plane. Conventions as Fig. 10B. **C** Cervicothoracic projection onto *MAO* demonstrated by Boesten and Voogd [15]. Note that a meagre ipsilateral projection was also found, in agreement with present study. These authors found that the distribution of terminal degeneration in *DAO* following hemicordotomy at C-3 was "found in the same areas (of *DAO*)" as after thoracic hemicordotomy (see Fig. 10D). **D** Superimposition of Figs. 10B and 12B to show extent of overlap between cervicothoracic (*vertical hatching*) and lumbosacral projections (*horizontal hatching*) to caudal *MAO* and *DAO* (below *horizontal dashed line*)

extent. Injections into successively more rostral LS segments labelled strips which were located progressively more medially and which in addition extended further toward the rostral pole of the olive. The approximate bounds of the strips found are shown in Fig. 10B.

In the caudal halves of both accessory olives localisation was much less marked. Thus in MAO labelling was present in all five cases in which injections were placed at or below L-5 (see Fig. 11E, F), and the distribution was virtually identical in each case (if the hatched region is excluded). Of the two more rostral injections (both L-3), one showed no termination in caudal MAO and the

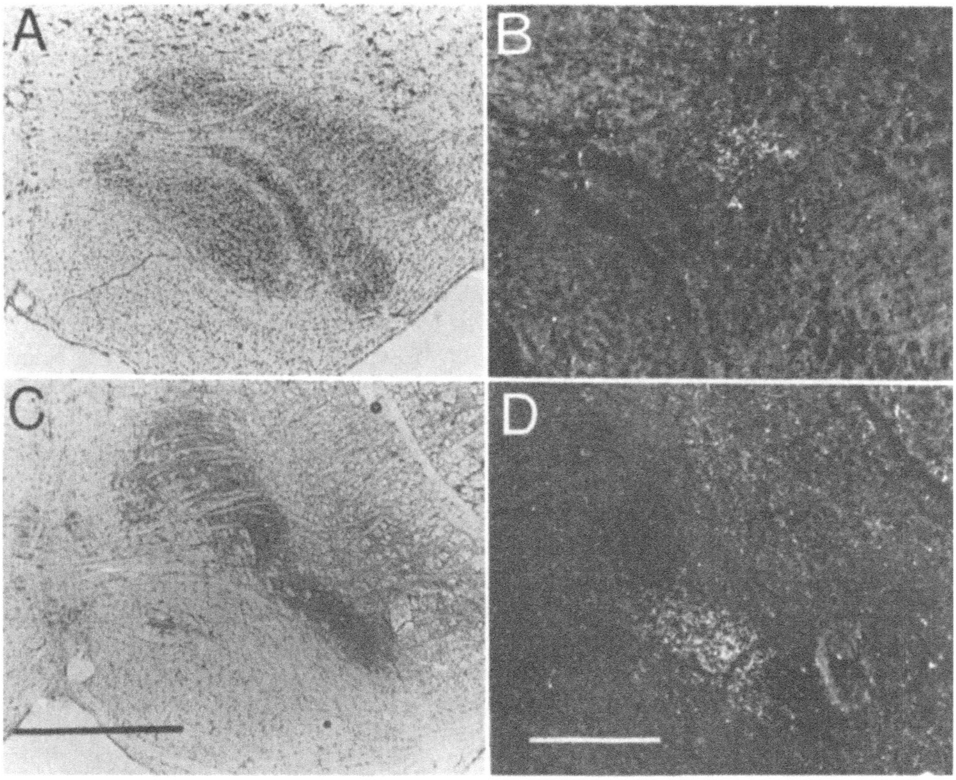

Fig. 13 A–D. Terminal labelling in accessory olives after injections into cervicothoracic enlargement. **A, B** Bright- and dark-field micrographs, respectively, of same section showing sparse and spatially restricted labelling in rostral DAO after injection at T-1/2. Plane of section AP 10.75. Note higher magnification in **B. C** and **D**, as **A** and **B** but termination in MAO at level AP 12.25 after injection at C-5/6. Note label is in lateral half of MAO but does not extend to lateral edge. One mm *calibration* in **C** applies **A** also; 0.5 mm *calibration* in **D** applies **B** also

other showed terminal labelling confined to the extreme lateral rim of the subnucleus.

In caudal DAO, terminations were present throughout the area below the broken line in Fig. 10 B after the injections at L-5 and L-6 (see Fig. 11 E, F) and in the case involving L-5 to L-7. After injections below this level (i.e. at L-7 and L-7/S-1) labelling was confined to the lateral half of the subnucleus. This same lateral area was also lightly labelled after both L-3 injections.

Cervico-thoracic Projections. All the injections were found to centre on the junction between two segments. They were at C-4/5, C-5/6, C-7/8 (two cases), C-8/T-1 (two cases), and T-1/2; in an additional case several injections were made producing an injection site which involved C-6, C-7, C-8, and T-1. In all cases terminal labelling was present in one or both olives although it was never as intense or widespread as after any of the LS injections.

In four cases (C-4/5, C-7/8, C-8/T1, and the case involving several segments) the injection site was restricted to the ipsilateral cord and in three of these (the first three) there was sparse terminal labelling in the ipsilateral olive. This finding indicates, in agreement with our HRP findings, that the CT differs from the LS enlargement in providing some uncrossed olivary afferents. However, they are few relative to the crossed fibres.

The result of pooling the findings made in all eight cases is shown in Fig. 12A, B. Also shown (Fig. 12C) is the projection which could be deduced by Boesten and Voogd [15] and although in MAO there is a measure of agreement between the two results it is immediately clear that large differences also exist. Some of these are explicable on the basis that the olivary regions involved in our study are also in receipt of LS input. However, this argument cannot be applied to the termination zone in rostral DAO. Termination here was always very light and also circumscribed as may be seen from Fig. 13A, B. Nevertheless, it was present (and identical in distribution) in six of the eight cases, in fact all those with injection below C-5/6. After unilateral injection (three cases) it was never present ipsilaterally. It would appear therefore that this light projection is entirely crossed and originates from the lower segments of the CT enlargement.

By contrast, the heavier projections to the caudal halves of the accessory olives (see Fig. 13C, D for termination in MAO) arose from all CT levels and were bilateral, though predominantly crossed. Ipsilateral labelling was always confined to areas corresponding to those labelled contralaterally.

Discussion

It is clear that the orthograde axonal transport technique is well suited for the study of the spino-olivary projections; it has shown terminations in all regions in which they were found in degeneration studies (see Figs. 10, 12), whilst in addition revealing some new termination areas for afferents from the CT enlargement.

Of particular interest is the demonstration that both LS and CT enlargements provide a crossed projection to the rostral DAO. According to Armstrong et al. [11], Groenewegen et al. [35], and Kawamura and Hashikawa [38] this region projects to Voogd's C_1 and C_3 cerebellar zones in the intermediate cortex with its medial portion projecting to what may be called "forelimb-related" areas such as lobule V of the anterior lobe and its lateral portion to "hindlimb" areas such as lobule IV (a different view is taken by Brodal and Walberg [18] as discussed later). Our LS projection which terminates in the lateral portion is a confirmation of findings by Mizuno [48] and by Boesten and Voogd [15] and presumably provides the anatomical substrate for the C_1 and C_3 VF-SOCPs conveying input from the hindlimbs (see Fig. 6A and ref. [53]). It may be noted in passing that gracilo-olivary fibres terminate in the same region [13, 14, 15, 34] and subserve a short-latency hindlimb dorsal funiculus path (DF-SOCP) which also has its cerebellar termination zone in hindlimb areas of the C_1 and C_3 zones (see Fig. 6B and ref. [27]).

Our CT projection to rostral DAO terminates in the medial portion where spino-olivary terminations have not previously been reported. The same area is however known to receive cuneo-olivary fibres [14, 34] which mediate a DF-SOCP terminating in forelimb areas of the C_1 and C_3 zones [27]. This suggests that the projection should provide the substrate for a forelimb VF-SOCP terminating in one or both of the C_1 and C_3 zones. However, reference to the detailed map of VF-SOCP termination zones in the anterior lobe (Fig. 6A) shows that no such path has yet been demonstrated to terminate in the predicted position (i.e. the "forelimb" portion of the C_1 and C_3 zones). One possible explanation resides in the very sparse nature of the new projection: it may constitute an input which is insufficiently powerful to discharge olive cells unless they are concurrently facilitated by cuneo-olivary or by descending inputs. This is not unlikely because the susceptibility of individual SOCPs to descending control is well known and differs considerably for different paths [e.g. 3, 27, 58].

Returning to the LS projection to rostral DAO, it is of considerable interest that successively more rostral segments projected in a precise and orderly manner to successively more rostral and medial strips or columns of olive cells. Both for the DF-SOCP terminating in Voogd's C_3 zone [28] and for the VF-SOCP to the B zone [2], climbing fibres (and therefore olive cells) with similar peripheral receptive fields have been shown to contact Purkinje cells located in narrow longitudinal substrips or "microzones" within the larger Voogd zone. If such a microzonal arrangement is characteristic also of the VF-SOCPs to the C_1/C_3 zones (as seems likely from ref. [57]) then our findings may indicate that each cortical microzone receives its climbing fibres from a narrow, longitudinally oriented column of olive cells within the larger population supplying the whole Voogd zone.

An additional clue as to the functional significance of the topographical localisation in the LS projection to the lateral part of rostral DAO is perhaps provided by data of Brodal and Walberg [18] regarding the olivocerebellar projection which originates from this area. Following HRP injections into individual lobules of the anterior lobe the distribution of retrogradely labelled olive cells was such as to indicate that cells projecting to lobules II, III, and IV form concentrations which overlap but are centred successively further caudally (see Fig. 10E). It was in fact concluded that rostral DAO projects to the *vermis* of the anterior lobe but other workers are agreed (see above) that the projection is to the "intermediate" area (i.e. to the "hindlimb" area of Voogd's C_1 and C_3 zones). A vermal projection would not in any case be consistent with the presence of gracilo-olivary terminals in this part of the olive and with the location of the corresponding DF-SOCP responses in the C_1 and C_3 zones (see above). Scrutiny of Brodal and Walberg's case reports shows that the findings are not in fact inconsistent with projections to the C_1 and C_3 zones particularly in view of their comment that purely vermal injection sites are difficult to achieve owing to diffusion of HRP along the cerebellar folia. If this reinterpretation (that rostrolateral DAO projects to the C_1 and C_3 zones) is accepted then it appears that in this olivary area the rostrocaudal ordering of the projection to lobules II and IV will lead to an intersection between the lumbar afferent and the olivocerebellar localisation such as to ensure that spino-olivary input from an individual cord segment will be distributed to the C_1 and C_3 zones in more than one lobule in the rostral part of the anterior lobe (compare Fig. 10B, E). In other words, a tendency will exist for the creation of longitudinal microzones within the Voogd zone, a conclusion reached by a different route above. A similar "longitudinally distributive" function can also be ascribed to the branching of olivocerebellar axons, which often results in one olive cell providing climbing fibres to two or more of the lobular compartments within a single Voogd zone [e.g. 9, 10, 29, 54].

Finally, as regards this region of the olive, it may be noted that if the deductions from our HRP experiments are correct and the hindlimb C_1 and C_3 VF-SOCPs are indeed mediated via neurons in the LS dorsal horn then the existence of CT input to the rostral DAO may imply a corresponding population of spino-olivary neurons in the dorsal horn within the CT enlargement. Reference to Fig. 8 shows that only a handful of appropriately located neurons were found in segments C6, C7, and C8 but their paucity is not surprising since the HRP injection sites only minimally involved the medial part of rostral DAO.

Regarding the projections to the caudal half of MAO, it is generally agreed [11, 17, 18, 33, 37, 38] that this region projects to Voogd's zone A and the LS afferents to this region presumably, therefore, mediate the hindlimb VF-SOCP shown electrophysiologically to terminate in this zone [53]. However, like Boesten and Voogd [15], we have found evidence also for a (mainly crossed) CT projection and it is puzzling, therefore, that electrophysiological investigations have not revealed a forelimb VF-SOCP terminating in the A zone (see Fig. 6A). At present it can only be suggested, as for the CT projection to rostral DAO, that traffic confined only to this pathway does not lead to olive discharges. This ad hoc explanation is, however, unattractive in view of the relatively substantial nature of the projection.

The extent to which there is convergence between the CT and LS projections to caudal MAO is of some interest, and Fig. 12D shows the extent of overlap as deduced by superimposing Figs. 10B and 12B. One result of the partial overlap is to create within the subnucleus three strips or columns of termination which are approximately rostrocaudally orientated (in fact slightly skewed). Proceeding from the lateral edge we encounter successively a zone receiving only LS afferents, a zone of CT/LS overlap, and a zone receiving only CT input. To these may be added a fourth, medially located zone in which no spino-olivary terminations were found. Here again, therefore, there is evidence for organization of the spino-olivary input on a columnar basis and it may be noted that as mapped by Groenewegen et al. [34] the terminals provided to caudal MAO by the gracile nucleus also distribute within a "columnar" territory (which overlaps heavily with that occupied by our CT projection). These gracilo-olivary fibres presumably subserve the A zone DF-SOCP demonstrated electrophysiologically [27, 51]. If future electrophysiological studies succeed in demonstrating a microzonal arrangement within the A zone VF-SOCP then our findings will probably support extension to the caudal MAO of the concept that individual microzones receive their climbing-fibre innervation from approximately rostrocaudal columnar subgroups of olive cells.

Some independent information regarding fine-grain localisation in the olivocerebellar projection from caudal MAO is in fact available from the studies of Brodal and Walberg [18] and Hoddevik et al. [37]. After injections of HRP into the different lobules of the anterior lobe vermis no systematic differences were noted in the distribution of retrogradely labelled olive cells, but it is satisfying to note that the overall distribution accords well with the area shown here to receive spino-shirary projections. The only discrepancy relates to the lateral edge of caudal MAO which contained no labelled cells although on the basis of the present results they would be expected. However, after injections into lobule VIII in the posterior lobe, labelled cells were found (indeed confined) in just this region [37], and we may note that lobule VIII is innervated by branches of the same olivary neurons which project to the A zone in the anterior lobe; moreover it receives VF-SOCP input from the hindlimbs in excellent accord with the present results [54].

In the caudal part of DAO the present study has demonstrated rather extensive overlap between the LS projection previously known from degeneration studies and a fairly substantial CT input not previously recognised. There appears to be no substantial region which exclusively receives CT afferents although in the lateral part of the subnucleus there is a significant area receiving only LS afferents. The caudal half of DAO projects to Voogd's zone B [11, 33, 38] and once again it is instructive to correlate the present findings with electrophysiological results regarding the VF-SOCPs. Within zone B, Andersson and Oscarsson [2] have established the existence of five longitudinally arranged CF microzones which differ in their patterns of peripheral input. The most medial receives only forelimb input, but with progressive lateral movement in the cortex successive microzones are met in which the balance between forelimb and hindlimb inputs is progressively shifted until the most lateral receives input exclusively from the hindlimb. If the CFs to this microzone derive from the region of DAO receiving only LS spino-olivary fibres we have again an indication that a longitudinal substrip within one of Voogd's zones may be innervated from a discrete subpopulation of neurons within DAO.

In conclusion, it is clear from our results that the different spino-olivary projections differ in the degree of their topographical localization, which is most marked in the LS projection to rostrolateral DAO. Nevertheless, there are signs of a columnar type topography in all the projections. When our findings are correlated with electrophysiological studies of the SOCPs it seems likely that the functional microzones recently detected in the cerebellar cortex are each CF-innervated from an approximately rostrocaudal subpopulation of olive cells within the olivary subnucleus supplying the Voogd zone. The microzones reportedly overlap [2] and no doubt the olivary columns show corresponding overlap. Admittedly, this schema has been deduced indirectly from evidence which is sometimes only suggestive. However, although it must remain tentative, it may provide a valuable working hypothesis, not least because it will be difficult using current anatomical techniques, to study the olivocerebellar projection directly at the level of spatial resolution required to demonstrate the origin of the microzones.

Finally, the postulated schema is by no means incompatible with a degree of differential localisation of the olive cells projecting to different cerebellar lobules, as indicated by recent HRP studies [18, 37, 40]. Given the widespread branching shown by olivary axons and provided that olivary areas supplying different lobules are suitably juxtaposed it is perfectly possible for the two localisations to interact so as, in general, to create longitudinal microzones which extend across a varying number of cerebellar lobules.

Activity of Inferior Olivary Neurons During Locomotion in the Cat

As emphasised above, substantial numbers of cells in the accessory olives receive abundant direct and indirect inputs from the spinal cord; besides the multiple VF-SOCPs and DF-SOCPs already mentioned, LF-SOCPs have also been defined electrophysiologically [42, 43]. Furthermore, although Oscarsson [52] has emphasised that some of these paths may forward information regarding events in spinal motor centres, there is nevertheless abundant evidence both in anaesthetised and in resting, intact animals that CS are readily evoked in many P cells by exteroceptive stimuli [see, for example, 6, 25, 26, 36, 39, 56]. In particular, the CFs supplying many P cells in the anterior lobe are exquisitely sensitive to inputs from phasic cutaneous mechanoreceptors and may readily be discharged at short and consistent latency by manœuvres such as tapping the skin, particularly that of the feet. On the basis of this evidence one of the authors suggested in 1974 [4] that some CFs and their parent olive cells might serve as "event detectors" signalling to the cerebellar cortex the precise timing of peripheral events which synchronously excite cutaneous mechanoreceptors in large numbers, i.e. events such as foot placement during locomotion or the acquisition of a target surface during exploratory voluntary movements. A similar suggestion has since been made by Rushmer et al. [56] who pointed out that since phasic cutaneous mechanoreceptors respond both to the onset and offset of skin indentation [45], it is likely that the CFs would discharge at both the make and the break of contact between the skin and an external surface.

If olivary neurons do indeed fulfil such a postulated exteroceptive role it should be possible in behaving animals to detect temporal correlations between olive-cell discharges (or CS in P cells) and the occurrence of peripheral events such as foot fall and lift during locomotion or the grasp and release of solid objects during manipulative tasks (though the existence of such correlations could not in itself *prove* that the CS were generated by peripheral input).

In cats, only two investigations have so far been made which might provide evidence for such correlations. Thus McElligot [47] has recorded from P cells in animals trained to step across a row of elevated pegs. However, the results have been reported only in brief with the main emphasis on methodology. One other attempt has been reported by Boylls [16] who succeeded in recording directly from olivary neurons projecting to Voogd's A zone in the decerebrate walking cat preparation. Only a few single neurons were recorded, which is not surprising in view of the difficulties of the preparation, but evidence was found for some tendency of the cells to discharge at preferred times during the step cycle.

In monkeys, CS have been recorded by several workers using animals executing stereotyped voluntary movements of the forelimbs, and these studies [32, 36, 60,

61] have failed to establish any close correlations between CS and specific peripheral events, even for olive cells which were demonstrably sensitive to cutaneous stimulation imposed on the passive animal [36]. Such failures have lent favour to an alternative and stimulating type of hypothesis which assigns to the olivocerebellar system a role in processes of motor learning that may require plastic modification of the electrophysiological properties of the cerebellar cortical circuitry [1, 31, 46].

Nevertheless, it remains true that CS in the cerebellar areas related to the limbs have been studied almost exclusively in monkeys and in relation to only a limited range of movement tasks. This consideration has prompted us to undertake a study of P-cell discharges during the locomotion of chronically prepared cats trained to walk on a moving belt. CS have been recorded from some P cells in the anterior lobe and determinations made of their time of occurrence relative to the stepping activity of the limbs.

Methods

Young adult cats were trained to relax during the procedures for mapping somatosensory receptive fields and also to walk steadily on a belt moving at speeds between 0.3 and 0.7 m/s. At such speeds the animals adopted an alternative (pacing) type of gait and in all cases they walked confidently with head and tail erect. Training was achieved solely through encouragement, and no aversive techniques were used. Each animal was subsequently operated on with general anaesthesia and aseptic technique. A small post-tentorial craniotomy was made which permitted access to the paravermal (intermediate) part of cerebellar lobule V and a capped titanium cylinder was affixed to the skull by means of dental acrylic cement. The dura remained intact and was protected by an overseal of medical grade silastomer. A socket was attached to the skull which permitted attachment during recording sessions of a solid state preamplifier. In addition electromyographic (EMG) electrodes were implanted into both triceps brachii (TB) muscles and in some cases cufftype stimulating electrodes were applied to the ipsilateral superficial radial nerve in the forearm. The leads from all peripheral electrodes were taken subcutaneously to a small connector mounted on the skull. Further details are given in ref. [12].

During recording sessions the cylinder cap was replaced by a small autoclavable micromanipulator used to advance glass-insulated tungsten microelectrodes through the silastomer and meninges into the cerebellum. The animals appeared oblivious to this procedure and no attempt was made to restrict movements of the head. The cylinder was angled forwards by 30° relative to stereotaxic vertical so that the electrodes passed through several cortical layers in lobule V before reaching the nucleus interpositus.

When stable single units were isolated, recordings were obtained during locomotion at different speeds and at rest, and in some cases the peripheral receptive field was mapped. Electroneurograms, EMGs, and an index of belt speed were tape-recorded and subsequently analysed with the aid of a PDP 11-34 computer to produce inter-CS interval histograms, raster displays, and event histograms.

Results

Extracellular recordings have been obtained from large numbers of P cells and neurons of the nucleus interpositus anterior. The latter were identified from their antidromic responses to stimulation in the midbrain near the red nucleus and the former on the basis of depth, pattern of tonic discharge, and the presence of both simple and complex spikes [cf. 6, 12]. Any units showing amplitude modulation of the action potentials or other signs of unstable recording conditions were rejected but it should be noted that one advantage of monitoring olive-cell discharge indirectly by recording the CS of their target P cells is that any slight relative movements between brain and microelectrode cannot produce spurious changes in the discharge of the cell of interest (i.e. the olivary neuron).

It has proved reasonably straightforward to obtain stable records from P cells but rather more difficult to obtain recordings in which CS can reliably be discriminated from the tonic simple spike (SS) activity. The difficulty arises because in many units the CS have consisted of an initial full-sized spike followed by severely attenuated secondary spikes [cf. 6]. However, we have been aided in the attempt to isolate CS by the fact that in a proportion of cases we recorded CS in the absence of SS. We believe that such records do not represent the activity of a specialised class of P cells in which tonic SS are absent, but rather that they were obtained from the main dendrites of normal P cells; very slight electrode advance often carried the tip into the layer of P cell bodies and resulted in the appearance of SS apparently in the same unit. Other workers have previously recorded CS in isolation in both unanaesthetised and anaesthetised preparations [e.g. 30, 39, 59, 61], and those recorded by Thach [59] are very similar in form to the present responses. On some occasions SS first appeared when walking began, either because of increased mossy-fibre input or perhaps because the brain moved slightly relative to the electrode (on such occasions CS amplitude did not change).

Figure 14A and B are records obtained during locomotion from two units typical of those discharging CS only. In each case the continuous record is accompanied by a fast swept record to the left which superimposes several successive CS. The traces above each continuous unit record are EMG signals recorded from the ipsilateral TB muscle which shows one burst of activity during each step cycle in the forelimb. Figure 14C shows a mixture of CS (marked by arrows) and SS recorded from a third unit; we have chosen to illustrate a unit in which SS occurred relatively infrequently as a short burst of impulses once per step cycle. However, in most units the rate of SS discharge was much higher, although usually showing frequency modulations phase-locked to the step cycle [cf. 50].

To date, in three cats we have recorded discriminable CS from 15 P cells during steady locomotion and efforts to increase the sample are in progress. All units were in tracks shown histologically to pass through several layers of cortex in lobulus V just rostral to the fissura prima. Mediolaterally the tracks ranged from just lateral to the paravermal vein to 1.5 mm further laterally and the large majority, therefore, passed through the C_1 and C_2 zones in the "intermedi-

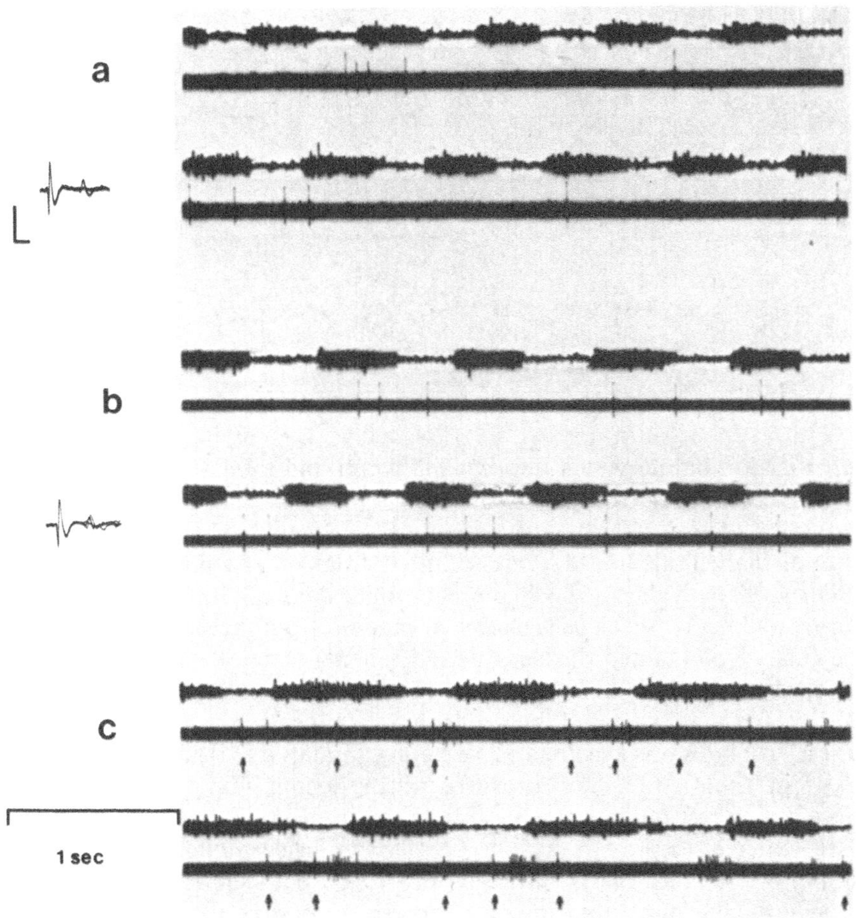

Fig. 14a–c. Complex spikes recorded in lobule V of cerebellar anterior lobe whilst the cat walked steadily on a moving belt. **a, b, c** show different units. *Top* trace in each is EMG from triceps brachii of forelimb ipsilateral to the unit. In each case *lower* record follows directly from *upper*. Complex spikes in **c** are identified by *arrows*. 1-s *time bar* applies to all three records. Frames on *left* in **a** and **b** show superimposed traces of the CS on much faster time scale. Bandwidth 1–10 kHz. In both cases the initial spike is followed only by one variable wavelet (cf. ref. 59). Other CS included several stunted spikes (cf. ref. 10). *Calibration bars* for superimposed traces: *times bar* is 1 ms and applies to **b** also. *Vertical bar* ist 1 mV for **a,** 2 mV for **b,** negative *upwards*. Speed of walking for **a, b, c** 0.3 ms^{-1}

ate" part of the anterior lobe. Receptive field mapping was carried out whenever possible and though the majority of units recorded during locomotion were lost before this procedure could be completed, mapping was then carried out for other P cells lying nearby. Collectively such mappings indicated that the units recorded during locomotion lay in cerebellar cortical areas receiving both mossy- and climbing-fibre inputs from the forelimb. Complex spike events were most readily evoked by light taps to the distal part of the ipsilateral forelimb, particularly to the foot. In some cases weak shocks were applied to the

Table 1. CS during locomotion

Unit	Belt speed (ms^{-1})	Mean step duration (s)	Number of steps	Number of CS	CS/step	Max. inter-CS interval (s)	Mean CS rate (s^{-1})
1	0.5	0.83	141	167	1.2	2.6	1.4
2	0.6	0.68	172	268	1.6	1.4	2.2
3	0.55	0.72	135	153	1.1	2.7	1.5
4	0.3	0.78	60	74	1.2	2.1	1.4
5	0.3	1.04	82	115	1.4	1.7	1.4
6	0.3	1.00	108	202	1.9	2.1	1.9
7	0.3	0.78	71	111	1.6	1.8	2.0

superficial radial nerve via the implanted cuff and the latencies of CS evoked by this route ranged from 12–20 ms.

Inspection of Fig. 14A, B, C shows immediately that in all three records CS were discharged at the slow rates familiar from other studies. This is further emphasised by Table 1 which presents some data relating to CS discharged during walking by seven cells chosen at random from the sample. For each cell the data were obtained during a period ranging from 50 to 120 s, throughout which the animal walked steadily at the belt speed indicated. The discharge rates, which were typical of the whole sample, ranged from 1.4 to 2.2/s. A similar range of rates was encountered in resting animals [cf. 6] and in fact for cells 6 and 7 in Table 1 the rates measured during locomotion were identical with those during rest periods comparable in duration. As Table 1 shows, the rates were sufficient to provide for one CS per step cycle though only in one case (cell 6) was the rate nearly sufficient for two CS per step. However, as Table 1 also shows, the maximum interval between successive CS was in every case longer than the step cycle, so that not all steps were accompanied by CS. This can indeed be seen directly in the records of Fig. 14 where for each unit at least one step is unaccompanied by a CS (whilst in others two or more may occur). This point is further documented by inter-CS interval histograms which showed that a considerable proportion of the steps making up a walking bout were necessarily without CS. Examples of such histograms are shown for two units in Figs. 15A, 16A.

The finding that CS do not occur in association with each step does not of course exclude that these events may occur preferentially at one or more fixed times during the step cycle. Two forms of computer-generated display have been used to investigate this possibility by "averaging" the CS during many successive step cycles, a procedure necessitated by the low overall rate at which CS appeared. In one display the times elapsing during each of many successive steps were aligned vertically to produce rasters in which each dot represents a CS. The other display took the form of a postevent histogram in which activity during successive steps was summed to provide an indication of the probability of occurrence of CS at different times during the step cycle. For both displays the start of the step cycle was taken as the time at which electrical activity be-

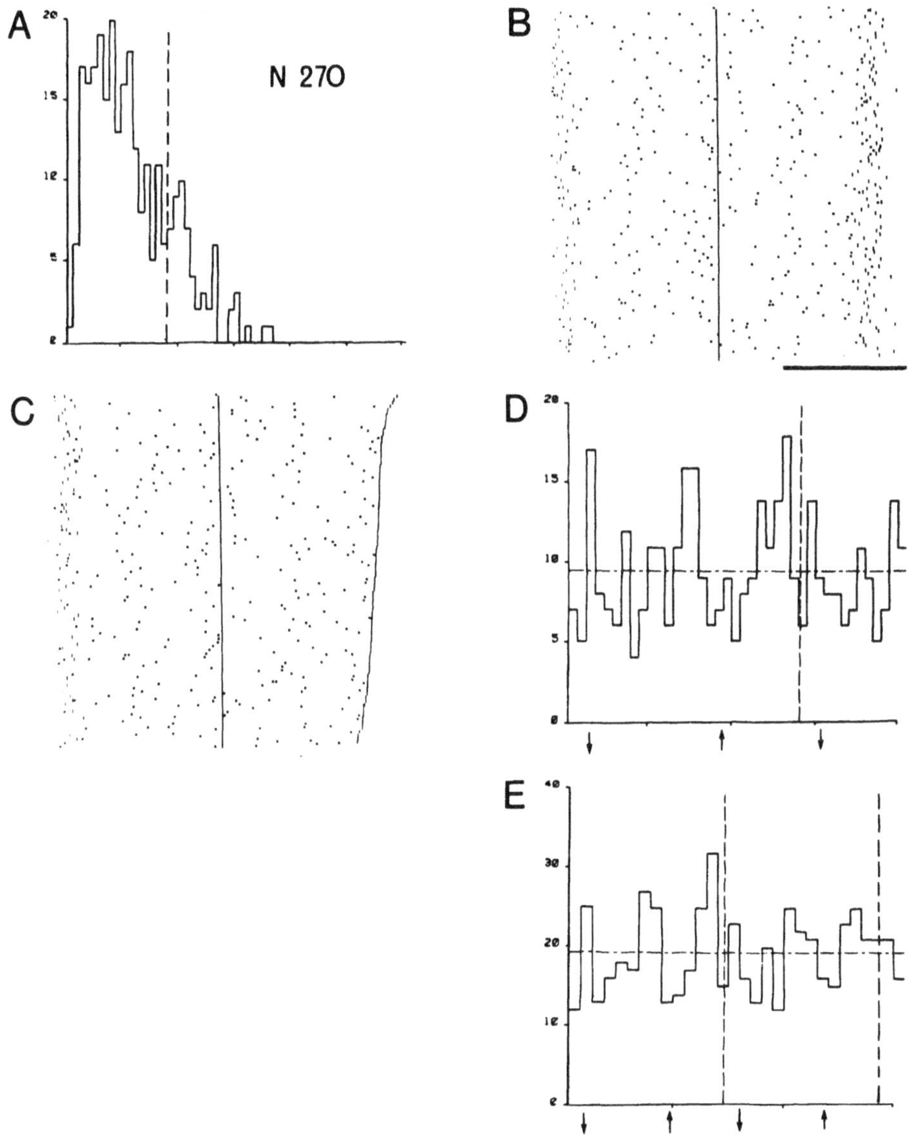

Fig. 15 A–E. Computer-generated raster and histogram displays of CS activity recorded from a single P cell during locomotion. **A** Frequency histogram of intervals between successive CS. *Vertical scale* is number of intervals. Forty ms binwidth. *N*, number of intervals. *Vertical broken line* is mean duration of step cycle during period of data collection (680 ms). Speed of locomotion 0.6 ms^{-1}. **B** Raster display of CS discharged during locomotion. *Vertical centre line* marks time of onset of EMG in TB. Each line of raster spans two paces, onset of first of these and end of second are shown by *short vertical lines* (for further explanation see text). *Time bar* 500 ms. Ninety-nine lines displayed. **C** Same data as **B** but rasterlines rank-ordered according to duration of pace to *right* of *centre line*. **D** Histogram showing number of CS discharged at different times in the step cycle. Formed by overlap summation of segments of unit record each beginning at the onset of the successive bursts of EMG in TB. Horizontal axis spans 1 s equivalent to ca. 1.3 step cycles. Each *vertical broken line* indicates end of one step/beginning of next; 173 steps and 270 CS. Mean duration of step 680 ms. Binwidth 25 ms. *Vertical scale* is number of CS per bin. *Downward arrows* indicate approximate time of ground contact for ipsilateral forefoot. *Upward arrows*, approximate time of foot lift. **E** As D but horizontal axis spans 1.5 s equivalent to ca. 2 step cycles. Binwidth 50 ms

gan in the TB muscle of the forelimb ipsilateral to the cerebellar microelectrode. Other studies in our laboratory have elucidated the temporal relationships during steady stepping between foot fall and lift and the cycles of electrical activity in most major muscles of the cat forelimb [24]. Over the range of belt speeds and step durations employed in the present study (respectively 0.3–0.7 ms^{-1} and 1.0–0.65 s), foot fall is delayed relative to the onset of TB activity by a time equal to approximately 8% of the whole step cycle, whilst foot lift occurs 5% after the end of activity in the same muscle.

Examples of both kinds of display are shown for one unit (not one of those in Fig. 14) in Fig. 15B–E. In the raster display of Fig. 15B the central vertical line represents the time of onset of TB activity. Each line in the raster therefore represents two complete steps, the beginning of the first and the end of the second being indicated by a short vertical line. There is naturally some small variation in the duration of successive steps and Fig. 15C shows a slightly modified form of raster in which the same steps as in Fig. 15B have been rank-ordered vertically according to duration. Inspection of the rasters shows that this unit did not display any obvious tendency for CS to occur precisely phase-locked to any particular moment in the step cycle, although on a somewhat broader time scale it is evident that CS were more likely to occur in some periods than others. The impression is gained that as compared with other periods, CS occurred more often around the middle of the step and again at around the end of one step and the onset of the next.

This visual impression is confirmed by the postevent histogram of Fig. 15D formed from a large number of steps (173) including those in the raster. The horizontal axis spans a time period of 1 s equivalent to ca. 1.3 step cycles (vertical broken line marks the average duration of a step). Effectively the continuous record of unit activity has been broken into time segments of equal length each beginning at the onset of TB activity and many successive segments have been superimposed. The mean probability of occurrence of a CS in any one 25-ms bin is shown by the horizontal broken line and it is clear that during the step cycle there are considerable variations about the mean. Although considerable bin-to-bin fluctuation is present it is evident that CS occurred at all times during the step cycle and that the probability for a CS is relatively high in the third bin of the first step, in the middle of the step cycle and at around the transition from one step cycle to the next. These "peaks" are also seen when the data are displayed using 50 ms binwidths as shown in Fig. 15E, which additionally displays data from a second step cycle, the horizontal axis spanning a time period of 1.5 s. Both the step cycles display a peak in the middle and at around the transition from one step to the next (because of the natural variation in the duration of successive steps it is not surprising that the amplitude of the peaks diminishes as time beyond zero increases). The overall distribution of the peaks did not change when smaller binwidths were employed.

Although it is clear that in this unit the probability for a CS did vary systematically during the step cycle it is nevertheless important to note that the probability "peaks" in this and other units were mostly rather broad. Since the steps were rather regular this suggests that if the CS are triggered by some particular event in the step cycle then their temporal coupling to that event must neces-

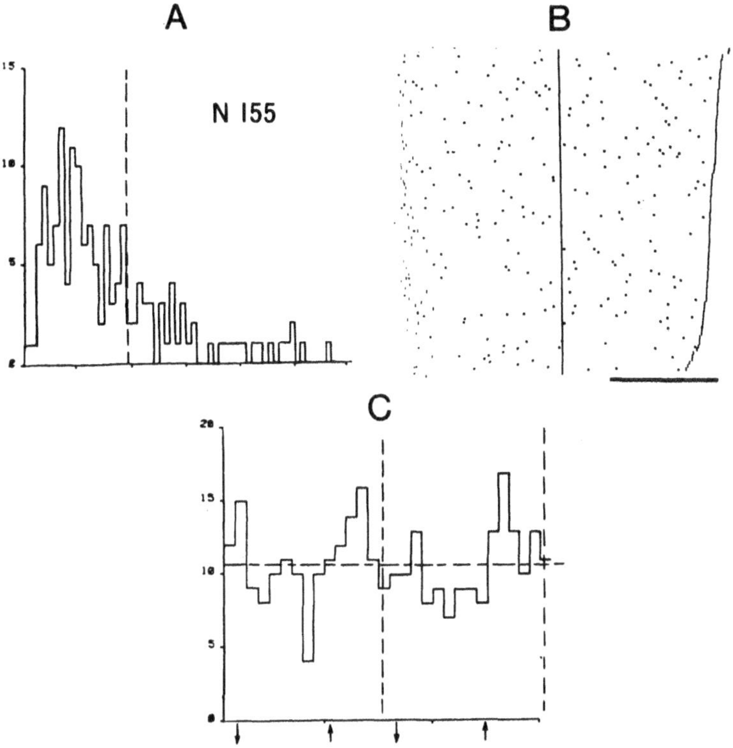

Fig. 16 A–C. Computer-generated raster and histogram displays of CS activity recorded from a second P cell during locomotion. **A** Frequency histogram of intervals between successive CS. *Vertical scale* is number of intervals. Binwidth 40 ms. *N,* number of intervals. *Vertical broken line* is mean duration of step cycle during period of data collection (720 ms). Speed of locomotion 0.55 ms^{-1}. **B** Rank-ordered raster display of CS discharged during locomotion. *Vertical centre line* marks time of onset of EMG in TB. Each line of raster spans two paces, onset of first of these and end of second are shown by *short vertical lines. Time bar* 500 ms; 99 lines displayed. **C** Histogram showing number of CS discharged at different times in the step cycle. Same format as Fig. 15E; 136 steps and 155 CS. Mean duration of step 720 ms. *Downward arrows* indicate approximate time of ground contact for ipsilateral forefoot. *Upward arrows,* approximate time of foot lift

sarily be loose. Furthermore, it should be noted that even for that bin in Fig. 15E which contains most CS, they amount to only 32 occurring in this 50 ms time segment of the step during no less than 173 successive steps. Moreover among the 13 bins making up the step cycle the maximum variation in probability amounted only to a factor of three (i.e. it varied from 32 to 11 CS per 50-ms bin).

Displays similar to those of Fig. 15C, E are shown for another unit in Fig. 16B, C. Here the raster provides no convincing evidence for phase-locking between CS and step cycle, though the histogram perhaps reveals a brief increase in probability near the start of the step cycle and a more noticeable increase towards the end. This pattern is repeated in both paces spanned by the 1.5-s time axis.

Some units showed no consistent relationship between CS probability and the step cycle even when over 100 steps were averaged, but for those units which did show cyclical fluctuations (the majority) the findings in the two cells illustrated are typical in respect of the amplitude of the fluctuations. It is clear, therefore, that although there was often some phase-locking between CS and parts of the step cycle it was never very striking.
Regarding the times at which probability was highest, some peaks occurred at around the time of foot fall for the ipsilateral forefoot (i.e. 60–80 ms after TB onset; downward arrows beneath the histograms). Such peaks are evident in Figs. 15D, E, 16C. Peaks also occurred at the time of foot lift (indicated by upward arrows) and an example is seen in Fig. 16C. However, other peaks occurred at times unrelated to these events (e.g. Fig. 15D, E), even in units in which CS were readily evoked in the resting animal by taps to the ipsilateral forefoot but not by tactile stimuli applied elsewhere on the body surface. In the whole sample of units, each displayed 1, 2 or 3 peaks and some of these were approximately coincident with either fall or lift of the ipsilateral forefoot. However, as the broadness of many peaks showed, the synchronization with these events was not precise.

Discussion

It must be emphasised at the onset that the sample of units so far studied is very small so that no far-reaching conclusions can be drawn. However, even these results have been difficult to obtain and we hope that presentation is justified by the intrinsic interest of any such recordings obtained in freely moving animals. At any rate the results are consistent across the sample in showing that during steady locomotion at walking speeds the olive cells discharged at the same slow rates characteristic of resting animals. In this respect our findings are similar to those made in monkeys carrying out discrete and stereotyped forelimb movements [i.e. 36, 60, 61]. They also resemble those made by Boylls [16] for a small number of olive cells within the caudal part of the medial accessory olive in decerebrate cats walking on a moving belt. Like Boylls, we find that substantial numbers of paces can occur in which there is no discharge by the olive cell under study.
When averaging techniques were used to investigate the possibility that CS occur at preferred times during the step cycle only modest cyclical changes in discharge probability were found with "peaks" once or twice per step cycle and some units gave no evidence of preferred timing. These findings were made amongst the population of cells making up the C_1 and C_2 zones in lobule V and presumably, therefore, they reflect the discharge pattern of olive cells located in rostral DAO and rostral MAO which respectively project to the C_1 and C_2 zones. They closely resemble the findings of Boylls who found (in olive cells projecting to the A zone in lobule V), that amongst a sample of five olivary neurons, three discharged without apparent relation to the events of the step cycle while two showed two preferred discharge periods (described as "broad probability bumps") per step cycle. On the whole, like Boylls, we find "that the

discharges [of 'stepping-related' olive cells] retain only a loose latency relationship with their triggering events in the step cycle whatever these might be".
Our working hypothesis suggested that those olive cells receiving abundant spinal inputs may subserve exteroceptive functions during active movement as well as at rest. However, although large populations of phasic mechanoreceptors in the distal parts of the limbs must be excited at foot fall and lift, the resulting afferent volley did not give rise in any P cell to a high probability of CS discharge. At best any one cell discharged at an appropriate time in perhaps one out of five steps, and moreover such discharges made up only a small proportion of the total CS during a sequence of steps. Our findings therefore do little to substantiate the working hypothesis and in that narrow sense they are disappointing. However, in a wider context they are nevertheless of considerable interest. They were made amongst a population of P cells in which CS are reliably evoked at short latency by tactile stimulation of the forefoot when the animal is at rest and they therefore resemble the results of Harvey et al. [36], who found in monkeys that although CS were readily evoked by taps to the limb in the passive animal, jerks imposed during voluntary movements were remarkably ineffective. Several findings in anaesthetised or decerebrate animals indicate that powerful descending controls are available to regulate the SOCPs either at the olivary or the pre-olivary levels [e.g. 27, 53, 58]. Our results and those of Harvey et al. seem to indicate that during both locomotor and manipulative behaviours such controls operate to reduce the traffic in SOCPs which in the absence of active movement are open for transmission.

Summary and Conclusions

Results are presented from three separate investigations of the olivocerebellar system. The first, an anatomical study, indicates that in the rat as in the cat the olivocerebellar projection is entirely crossed and that it supplies climbing fibres to the whole extent of the cerebellar cortex. There is thus no necessity to postulate the existence of alternative large scale sources of these afferents.
The second study has revealed more completely than hitherto the extent of the spino-olivary projections in the cat. Afferents from the cervicothoracic enlargement terminate in much wider areas of the accessory olives than previously realised, though these projections remain numerically less important than those of the lumbar cord. Some degree of ("columnar") topographical organization was present in all the spino-olivary input to the rostral dorsal accessory olive, where afferents originating in different lumbar segments projected to different narrow columns of olivary neurons. When the findings are correlated with electrophysiological studies of the spino-olivocerebellar paths they provide indirect evidence to support the concept that narrow and approximately rostrocaudal columns of olive cells project to longitudinal microzones within the larger zones of the cerebellar cortex defined by Voogd.
The third, electrophysiological study has provided data regarding the discharge patterns during locomotion of a small population of olive cells projecting to the intermediate part of lobule V. These neurons receive abundant peripheral in-

puts (via several SOCPs and mainly from the forelimb). However, during steady walking they discharge at low rates and show only modest cyclical changes in discharge probability which are not strongly time-locked to any aspect of the sequence of activities making up the step cycle. These results are taken to indicate that during locomotion the relevant SOCPs are subject to substantial central inhibition.

Acknowledgements. Supported by the Medical Research Council of Great Britain. We wish to thank Mrs. L. Gregory for her expert histological assistance, Mr. C. Makepeace for photography and Mrs. A Lear for typing the manuscript.

References

1. Albus JS (1971) A theory of cerebellar function. Math Biosci 10:25–61
2. Andersson G, Oscarsson O (1978) Climbing fiber microzones in cerebellar vermis and their projection to different groups of cells in the lateral vestibular nucleus. Exp Brain Res 32:565–579
3. Andersson G, Sjölund B (1978) The ventral spino-olivocerebellar system in the cat. IV. Spinal transmission after administration of clonidine and L-dopa. Exp Brain Res 33:227–240
4. Armstrong DM (1974) Functional significance of connections of the inferior olive. Physiol Rev 54:358–417
5. Armstrong DM (1978) The mammalian cerebellum and its contribution to movement control. In: Porter R (ed) Internat Rev Physiol, 17. Neurophysiology III. University Park Press, Baltimore, p 239
6. Armstrong DM, Rawson JA (1979) Activity patterns of cerebellar cortical neurones and climbing fibre afferents in the awake cat. J Physiol 289:425–448
7. Armstrong DM, Schild RF (1979) Spino-olivary neurones in the lumbo-sacral cord of the cat demonstrated by retrograde transport of horseradish peroxidase. Brain Res 168:176–179
8. Armstrong DM, Schild RF (1980) Location in the spinal cord of neurones projecting directly to the inferior olive in the cat. In: Courville J et al. (eds) The inferior olive. Anatomy and Physiology. Raven Press, New York, pp 125–144
9. Armstrong DM, Harvey RJ, Schild RF (1973a) Branching of inferior olivary axons to terminate in different folia, lobules or lobes of the cerebellum. Brain Res 54:365–371
10. Armstrong DM, Harvey RJ, Schild RF (1973b) The spatial organization of climbing fibre branching in the cat cerebellum. Exp Brain Res 18:40–58
11. Armstrong DM, Harvey RJ, Schild RF (1974) Topographical localization in the olivo-cerebellar projection: an electrophysiological study in the cat. J Comp Neurol 154:287–302
12. Armstrong DM, Rawson JA (1979) Responses of neurones in nucleus interpositus of the cerebellum to cutaneous nerve volleys in the awake cat. J Physiol 289:403–423
13. Berkley KJ (1975) Different targets of different neurons in nucleus gracilis of the cat. J Comp Neurol 163:285–304
14. Berkley KJ, Hand PJ (1978) Projections to the inferior olive of the cat. II. Comparisons of input from the gracile, cuneate and the spinal trigeminal nuclei. J Comp Neurol 180:253–264
15. Boesten AJP, Voogd J (1975) Projections of the dorsal column nuclei and the spinal cord on the inferior olive in the cat. J Comp Neurol 161:215–238
16. Boylls CC (1980) Contributions to locomotor coordination of an olivo-cerebellar projection to the vermis in the cat: experimental results and theoretical proposals. In: Courville J et al. (eds) The inferior olive. Anatomy and Physiology. Raven Press, New York, pp 321–348
17. Brodal A (1940) Experimentelle Untersuchungen über die olivocerebellare Lokalisation. Z Gesamte Neurol Psychiat 169:1–153

18. Brodal A, Walberg F (1977) The olivocerebellar projection in the cat studied with the method of retrograde axonal transport of horseradish peroxidase. IV. The projection to the anterior lobe. J Comp Neurol 172:85–108
19. Brodal A, Walberg F, Blackstad T (1950) Termination of spinal afferents to inferior olive in cats. J Neurophysiol 13:431–454
20. Brodal A, Walberg F, Hoddevik GH (1975) The olivocerebellar projection in the cat studied with the method of retrograde axonal transport of horseradish peroxidase. J Comp Neurol 164:449–470
21. Chan-Palay V, Palay SL, Brown JT, Van Itallie C (1978) Sagittal organization of olivocerebellar and reticulocerebellar projections: autoradiographic studies with ^{35}S-methionine. Exp Brain Res 30:561–576
22. Chu N-S, Bloom FE (1974) The catecholamine-containing neurons in the cat dorsolateral pontine tegmentum: distribution of the cell bodies and some axonal projections. Brain Res 66:1–21
23. Courville J, Faraco-Cantin F (1978) On the origin of the climbing fibers of the cerebellum. An experimental study in the cat with an autoradiographic tracing method. Neuroscience 3:797–809
24. Drew TB, Armstrong DM (1980) Motor cortex discharges during locomotion in the cat. In: Abstr XXVIII Congr Physiol Sci, Budapest, vol 14:387, Abstr 1267
25. Eccles JC, Sabah NH, Schmidt RF, Táboříková H (1972a) Cutaneous mechanoreceptors influencing impulse discharges in cerebellar cortex. III. In: Purkyně cells by climbing fiber input. Exp Brain Res 15:484–497
26. Eccles JC, Sabah NH, Schmidt RF, Táboříková H (1972b) Integration by Purkinje cells of mossy and climbing fiber inputs from cutaneous mechanoreceptors. Exp Brain Res 15:498–520
27. Ekerot C-F, Larson B (1979a) The dorsal spino-olivocerebellar system in the cat. I. Functional organization and termination in the anterior lobe. Exp Brain Res 36:201–217
28. Ekerot C-F, Larson B (1979b) The dorsal spino-olivocerebellar system in the cat. II. Somatotopical organization. Exp Brain Res 36:219–232
29. Faber DS, Murphy JT (1969) Axonal branching in the climbing fiber pathway to the cerebellum. Brain Res 15:262–267
30. Fujita Y (1968) Activity of dendrites of single Purkinje cells and its relationship to so-called inactivation response in rabbit cerebellum. Z Neurophysiol 31:131–141
31. Gilbert PFC (1974) A theory of memory that explains the function and structure of the cerebellum. Brain Res 70:1–18
32. Gilbert PFC, Thach WT (1977) Purkinje cell activity during motor learning. Brain Res 128:309–328
33. Groenewegen HJ, Boesten AJP, Voogd J (1975) The dorsal column nuclear projections to the nucleus ventralis posterior lateralis thalami and the inferior olive in the cat: an autoradiographic study. J Comp Neurol 162:505–518
34. Groenewegen HJ, Voogd J (1977) The parasagittal zonation within the olivocerebellar projection. I. Climbing fiber distribution in the vermis of cat cerebellum. J Comp Neurol 174:417–488
35. Groenewegen HJ, Voogd J, Freedman SL (1979) The parasagittal zonation within the olivocerebellar projection. II. Climbing fiber distribution in the intermediate and hemispheric parts of the cat cerebellum. J Comp Neurol 183:551–602
36. Harvey RJ, Porter R, Rawson JA (1977) The natural discharges of Purkinje cells in paravermal regions of lobules V and VI of the monkey's cerebellum. J Physiol (Lond) 271:515–536
37. Hoddevik GH, Brodal A, Walberg F (1976) The olivocerebellar projection in the cat studied with the method of retrograde axonal transport of horseradish peroxidase. II. The projection to the vermal visual area. J Comp Neurol 169:155–170
38. Kawamura K, Hashikawa T (1979) Olivocerebellar projections in the cat studied by means of anterograde axonal transport of labelled amino acids as tracers. Neuroscience 4:1615–1633
39. Kolb FP, Rubia FJ (1980) Information about peripheral events conveyed to the cerebellum via the climbing fiber system in the decerebrate cat. Exp Brain Res 38:363–373

40. Kotchabhakdi N, Walberg F, Brodal A (1978) The olivocerebellar projection in the cat studied with the method of retrograde axonal transport of horseradish peroxidase. VII. The projection to lobulus simplex, crus I and II. J Comp Neurol 182:293–314
41. Larsell O (1952) The morphogenesis and adult pattern of the lobules and fissures of the cerebellum of the white rat. J Comp Neurol 97:281–356
42. Larson B, Miller S, Oscarsson O (1969a) Termination and functional organization of the dorsolateral spino-olivocerebellar path. J Physiol (Lond) 203:611–640
43. Larson B, Miller S, Oscarsson O (1969b) A spinocerebellar climbing fibre path activated by the flexor reflex afferents from all four limbs. J Physiol (Lond) 203:641–649
44. Llinás R, Walton K, Hillman DE, Sotelo C (1975) Inferior olive: its role in motor learning. Science 190:1230–1231
45. Loeb GE, Bak MJ, Duysens J (1977) Long-term unit recording from somatosensory neurons in the spinal ganglia of the freely walking cat. Science 197:1192–1194
46. Marr D (1969) A theory of cerebellar cortex. J Physiol (Lond) 202:437–470
47. McElligot JG (1976) Cerebellar neuronal firing patterns in intact and unrestrained cat during walking. In: Herman RM, Grillner S, Stein PSG, Stuart DG (eds) Neural control of locomotion. Plenum, New York, p 781
48. Mizuno N (1966) An experimental study of the spino-olivary fibers in the rabbit and the cat. J Comp Neurol 127:267–292
49. Murphy MG, O'Leary JL, Cornblath B (1973) Axoplasmic flow in cerebellar mossy and climbing fibers. Arch Neurol 28:118–123
50. Orlovsky GN (1972) Work of the Purkinje cells during locomotion. Biophysics 17: 935–941
51. Oscarsson O (1969) Termination and functional organization of the dorsal spino-olivocerebellar path. J Physiol 200:129–149
52. Oscarsson O (1973) Functional organization of spinocerebellar paths. In: Iggo A (ed) Handbook of Sensory Physiology, II. Somatosensory System. Springer, Berlin Heidelberg New York, p 339
53. Oscarsson O, Sjölund B (1977a) The ventral spino-olivocerebellar system in the cat. I. Identification of five paths and their termination in the cerebellar anterior lobe. Exp Brain Res 28:469–486
54. Oscarsson O, Sjölund B (1977b) The ventral spino-olivocerebellar system in the cat. II. Termination zones in the cerebellar posterior lobe. Exp Brain Res 28:487–503
55. Oscarsson O, Sjölund B (1977c) The ventral spino-olivocerebellar system in the cat. III. Functional characteristics of the five paths. Exp Brain Res 28:505–520
56. Rushmer DS, Roberts WJ, Augter G (1976) Climbing fibre responses of cerebellar Purkinje cells to passive movement of the cat forepaw. Brain Res 106:1–20
57. Rushmer DS, Woollacott MH, Robertson LT, Laxer KD (1980) Somatotopic organization of climbing fiber projections from low threshold cutaneous afferents to pars intermedia of cerebellar cortex in the cat. Brain Res 181:17–30
58. Sjölund B (1978) The ventral spino-olivocerebellar system in the cat. V. Supraspinal control of spinal transmission. Exp Brain Res 33:509–522
59. Thach WT (1967) Somatosensory receptive fields of single units in cat cerebellar cortex. J Neurophysiol 30:675–696
60. Thach WT (1968) Discharge of Purkinje cells and cerebellar nuclear neurons during rapidly alternating arm movements in the monkey. J Neurophysiol 31:785–797
61. Thach WT (1970) Discharge of cerebellar neurons related to two maintained postures and two prompt movements. II. Purkinje cell output and input. J Neurophysiol 33:537–547

Structural Organization of the Fastigial Nucleus

A. J. Beitz

Introduction

The fastigial or medial cerebellar nucleus is phylogenetically the oldest of the four cerebellar nuclei and has been shown to influence functionally eye movements [3], posture and equilibrium [13], and autonomic activity [25]. The involvement of the fastigial nucleus in this broad spectrum of functional activity is probably mediated by its unique efferent projections to the thalamus, brain stem, and spinal cord [10]. Although this nucleus appears to be homologous in the rat, cat, monkey, and man with regard to both its connections and its functional activity [10, 13, 23, 25], the basic morphological subdivisions comprised the fastigial nucleus of these four species are apparently different. This difference is highlighted by a differential location of the small- and large-cell populations in the rodent, feline, and primate medial cerebellar nucleus. This variability in nuclear subdivisions as well as the lack of correlation between the reported morphological divisions of the nucleus and the known functional divisions of the nucleus raise important questions concerning fastigial organization. The first question raised regarding the organization of this nucleus is whether morphological subdivisions are present which can be correlated with the known functional divisions of the nucleus? Secondly, can these subdivisions be recognized in the rat, cat, and primate fastigial nuclei? Finally, does a common morphological plan exist which underlies the organization of this nucleus in the above mentioned species?

This chapter constructs a morphological blueprint of the fastigial nucleus, describes the existing intrinsic structure of this nucleus in rat, cat, monkey, and man and compares and contrasts it with more recent, detailed information from our laboratory concerning the basic organization of this nucleus in the rat. A detailed analysis of the morphological organization of the rodent medial nucleus in conjunction with a study of the cellular organization underlying its efferent projections has lead us to propose a rostral and caudal morphological subdivision of the nucleus, as described below. Evidence is also presented which suggests that a longitudinal zonal arrangement may exist in the fastigial nucleus. The rostrocaudal subdivisions and the three longitudinal zones may form the basic architectural plan which underlies the organization of this nucleus.

Experimental Brain Research, Suppl. 6

Morphological Subdivisions of the Fastigial Nucleus

In the rat, Goodman [17] first described a subdivision of the medial cerebellar nucleus which they designated the dorsolateral protuberance (DLP). It is characterized by a predominance of large neurons and thus is distinguished from the remainder of the nucleus which contains a mixture of small, medium, and large cells. Korneliussen [22] further subdivided the medial nucleus into a dorsolateral protuberance; a middle subdivision and a caudomedial subdivision based on the distribution of both myelinated fibers and small, medium, and large neurons (Fig. 1). These three basic subdivisions described by Korneliussen, were subsequently confirmed by Beitz and Chan-Palay [6].
In contrast to the above subdivisions recognized in the rodent medial cerebellar nucleus, the feline medial nucleus was originally shown by Snider [33] to consist of a large-celled medial division and a small-celled lateral division. This bipartitioning of the nucleus by Snider was subsequently refuted by Jansen and Jansen [21], who indicated that large cells predominated in the rostral half of the medial nucleus while small cells were a major contingent of its caudal portion. This suggestion of rostrocaudal differences in the nucleus was strengthen-

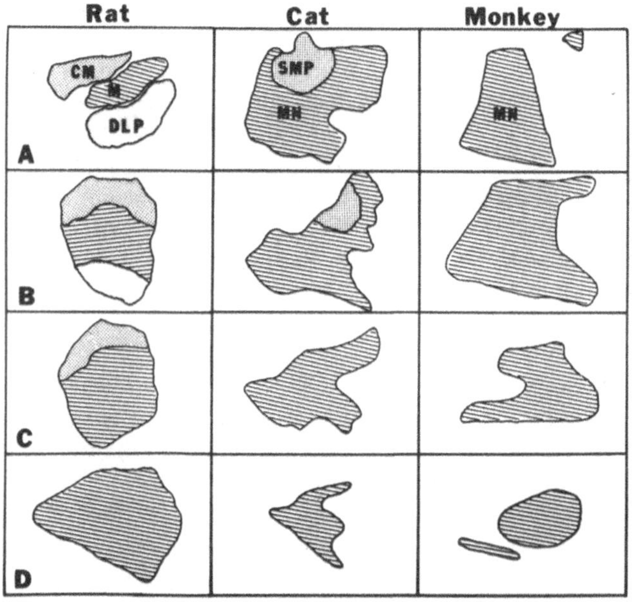

Fig. 1. Drawings of four horizontal sections (**A, B, C, D**) through the medial cerebellar nucleus (*MN*) of the rat, cat, and monkey illustrating the location of nuclear subdivisions in each species. The three nuclear subdivisions of the rodent medial nucleus, the caudomedial subdivision (*CM*), the middle subdivision (*M*), and the dorsolateral protuberance (*DLP*) are illustrated on the *left*. A single subdivision of the feline medial nucleus, the subnucleus medialis parvicellularis (*SMP*) of Flood and Jansen, is represented in the *center* of the drawing, while the medial nucleus of the monkey, which contains no discernable subdivisions, is shown at the *right*. The most ventral horizontal section in each case is represented in **A** and the dorsal portion of the nucleus is shown in **D**

ed by the work of Voogd [35], which demonstrated a difference in rostral and caudal portions of the medial nucleus in Haggquist-stained material. This rostrocaudal division of the nucleus in the cat may well be comparable to the anteroposterior subdivisions recently recognized in the rat [6, 7], as described below. Finally, Flood and Jansen [15] identified a small-celled group in the ventral part of the middle third of the nucleus which they called the *subnucleus medialis parvicellularis.* Presumably it corresponds to the small-celled lateral division of the fastigial nucleus of Snider.

In the monkey, the medial nucleus is second in size of the cerebellar nuclei. Courville and Cooper [12] described a group of small cells located in the most ventral part of this nucleus, but they did not feel that this cell group should be considered as a separate subdivision. In light of the findings of Courville and Cooper, it is interesting to note that an analysis of cell size in the medial nucleus of the rat has indicated that the rodent nucleus also contains a predominance of small cells in its most ventral portion which do not form a distinct nuclear subdivision [6].

The human fastigial nucleus was differentiated by Ziehen [36] into a medially situated nucleus fastigii and a lateral nucleus lacunosus. The two are closely related but are structurally different. The medial nucleus fastigii is compact and consists of small, closely arranged cells. The nucleus lacunosus has a more reticular appearance consisting of large, lightly staining cells that are irregularly arranged and among which pass fascicles of fibers. Based on its location and its complement of large cells, the nucleus lacunosus may correspond to the large-celled dorsolateral protuberance of the rat.

It is clear from examining the literature that the majority of schemes for subdividing the fastigial nucleus are based on the distribution of small and large neurons within the nucleus. Thus, a small-celled subdivision is described in the rat, cat, monkey, and human as indicated above. However, differences in the location of the small-celled segment in the rodent, feline, and primate fastigial nuclei raise some question of the true homology of this subdivision among these mammals. In contrast to these morphological subdivisions which are based on differences in cell size, both physiological and hodological studies have provided evidence for a bipartitioning of the medial nucleus into rostral and caudal portions [4, 10, 21, 27, 28]. Thus Moruzzi and Pompeiano [28] reported differences in postural asymmetry following caudal lesions and then rostral lesions of the medial cerebellar nucleus in decerebrate cats. The syndrome resulting from lesions of the rostral part of the nucleus was designated an ipsilateral fastigial atonia while caudal medial nuclear lesions gave rise to crossed fastigial atonia.

Miura and Reis [27] found that a reproducible pressor response could be induced from a small area localized to the rostral portion of the feline medial nucleus. Moreover, horizontal canal inputs are localized predominantly in the caudal portion of the nucleus [16]. The only morphological evidence for a rostrocaudal subdivision of the medial nucleus, however, is found in the work of Voogd [35] and the studies of Jansen and Jansen [21] as indicated above. One of the aims of the recent investigations in our laboratory was to determine if morphological differences exist in those portions of the medial nucleus which have been previously demonstrated to differ with regard to both their physiology and connectivity. The results of our study of neuronal numbers, density, and orientation in the medial nucleus [6] indicate that differences in both cellular density and neuronal arrangement exist between the anterior and posterior parts of the nucleus. Thus, calculations of neuronal density through a series of frontal sections showed the highest cell density in the caudal part of the nucleus (3.41×10^7 cm^3), while rostral portions of the nucleus displayed a lower packing density (2.40×10^7 cm^3). The caudal part of the nucleus is further distinguished by a predominant caudolateral to rostromedial orientation of its neuronal population. The majority of cells in the rostral part of the medial nucleus, however, show either a diagonal orientation preference from caudomedial to rostrolateral or a longitudinal rostral to caudal arrangement. The rostral and caudal halves of the medial cerebellar nucleus are thus two morphologically distinct regions. These two structurally different divisions of the medial nucleus are comparable to the areas of the nucleus that have been demonstrated in the literature to be functionally separable.

In order to determine if both the rostral and caudal subdivisions, identified in our Nissl preparations, and the three nuclear subdivisions proposed by Korneliussen [22] were related to the efferent connections of the rodent medial nucleus, iontophoretic injections of horseradish peroxidase (HRP) were made into various brain stem sites known to receive direct fastigial output (Beitz, 1981, Longitudinal zonation and morphological subdivisions within the medical cerebellar of the rat, unpublished work). The retrograde transport method was selected for this study instead of the autoradiographic technique for two major reasons. First of all, it is extremely difficult to confine injections of tritiated amino acids to only one of the subdivisions of the rodent medial cerebellar nucleus. Secondly, the number of retrogradely labeled cells in each subdivision of the medial nucleus could be easily quantitated following HRP injections into brain stem nuclei. Thus, the relative contribution of each subdivision to a particular efferent projection could be analyzed.

The results of this study substantiated the presence of rostral and caudal subdivisions in the rodent medial nucleus but failed to demonstrate a differential contribution from the DLP, middle subdivision, and caudomedial subdivision to specific brain stem targets. Thus, all three of these nuclear subdivisions contained labeled cells in each of our HRP cases (except one case involving an injection into the nucleus ventralis posterolateralis (VPL nucleus) of the thalamus in which only the caudomedial and middle subdivisions contained labeled cells). These findings indicate that the three subdivisions originally described by Korneliussen in the rat medial nucleus do not appear to subserve the topographical organization of the efferent projections of this nucleus. In contrast to these three subdivisions, the rostral and caudal subdivisions are clearly related to specific efferent projections (Table 1). The caudal division provides the sole source of fastigial fibers to the nucleus pontis oralis, the nucleus of the posterior commissure, and the VPL nucleus of the thalamus. The rostral division of the medial nucleus, on the other hand, provides the major source of fastigial projections to the lateral reticular nucleus and the gigantocellular reticular nucleus. The evidence from both our morphological and hodological studies in con-

Table 1. A summary of the distribution of HRP-labeled neurons in the three longitudinal zones and the rostral and caudal subdivisions of the medial cerebellar nucleus from ten representative cases. The case number and HRP injection site is indicated on the left and the total number of labeled cells observed in each longitudinal zone and each subdivision is listed in the appropriate columns for each case

HRP injection site	Contra zone A	Contra zone B	Contra zone C	Contra rostral subdivision	Contra caudal subdivision	Ipsil. zone A	Ipsil. zone B	Ipsil. zone C
1) R-90 N. parasolitarius	9	0	4	12	1	0	0	0
2) R-92 N. pontis oralis and caudalis	70	3	28	6	95	0	13	0
3) R-93 Medial and inferior vestibular n. caudal LVN	9	31	6	27	19	11	2	16
4) R-95 Paramedian reticular n.	10	0	4	1	13	0	2	0
5) R-103 N. posterior commissure	9	6	1	0	15	0	0	0
6) R-105 Lateral reticular n.	5	0	4	7	2	0	0	0
7) R-107 VPL	0	0	11	0	11	0	0	0
8) R-108 LVN, SVN	28	70	36	77	57	4	6	7
9) R-115 N. gigantocellularis	29	0	84	89	24	0	1	0
10) R-117 Pontis oralis	10	1	8	0	19	0	0	0

junction with the physiological evidence available in the literature would suggest that a bipartitioning of the fastigial nucleus into rostral and caudal portions may well form the basis of its morphological and functional organization.

Cellular Organization of the Fastigial Nucleus

Cell Size

The cells of the fastigial nucleus were first classified as either large or small by Ramón y Cajal [32]. This observation was subsequently confirmed in several mammalian species [9] including the rat [6], cat [33], monkey [20], and man [8, 19]. Jansen and Brodal [20] in the rabbit and Jansen and Jansen [21] in the cat, however, added cells of an intermediate size. According to the latter authors small, medium, and large cells are found throughout the nucleus but the large cells occur predominantly in the rostral half and in the tail end of the nucleus. More recently three cell types were also recognized in the rat [17, 22] and in the monkey [12]. A discrepancy clearly exists in the literature regarding the number of neuronal populations that exist in the fastigial nucleus. In an attempt to clarify this problem a recent extensive study of the cell populations which comprise the nucleus revealed the presence of two subpopulations of cells: a set of large cells which have neuronal areas greater than 180 µm, and a set of small cells with areas less than 180 µm [6]. These findings substantiated the original description provided by Ramón y Cajal and in addition provided quantitative evidence that small cells outnumber the large cells (small cell/large cell ratio = 1:0.76) within the rodent medial nucleus and that they are especially prominent in the caudomedial subdivision where the small cells comprise 75% of the total cell population.

Cell Shape and Cell Types

Most studies agree that the large cells are polygonal, multipolar, and stain deeply with thionin because of their coarse Nissl bodies, while the small cells are round or fusiform, contain a large nucleus, and are paler because of their much finer Nissl substance [12, 15, 14, 35]. In the rat fastigial nucleus, moreover, seven cell types have been identified in Nissl preparations based on cell

Fig. 2. 1a–7a Photomicrographs from Nissl preparations illustrating the seven cell types which comprise the medial cerebellar nucleus. **1b–7b** Camera lucida drawings of the seven cell types as seen in Golgi Kopsch preparations. **1c–7c** the seven neuronal varieties are shown containing HRP reaction product in their soma and proximal dendrites. These cells were labeled following iontophoretic injections of HRP into brain stem sites as described in the text. The cell types illustrated in **1–7** are: **1a–c**, neurons of the nuclear boundary; **2a–c**, large multipolar neurons; **3a–c**, fan-shaped neurons; **4a–c**, bouquet neurons; **5a–c**, large fusiform neurons; **6a–c**, small multipolar neurons; and **7a–c**, small bipolar neurons

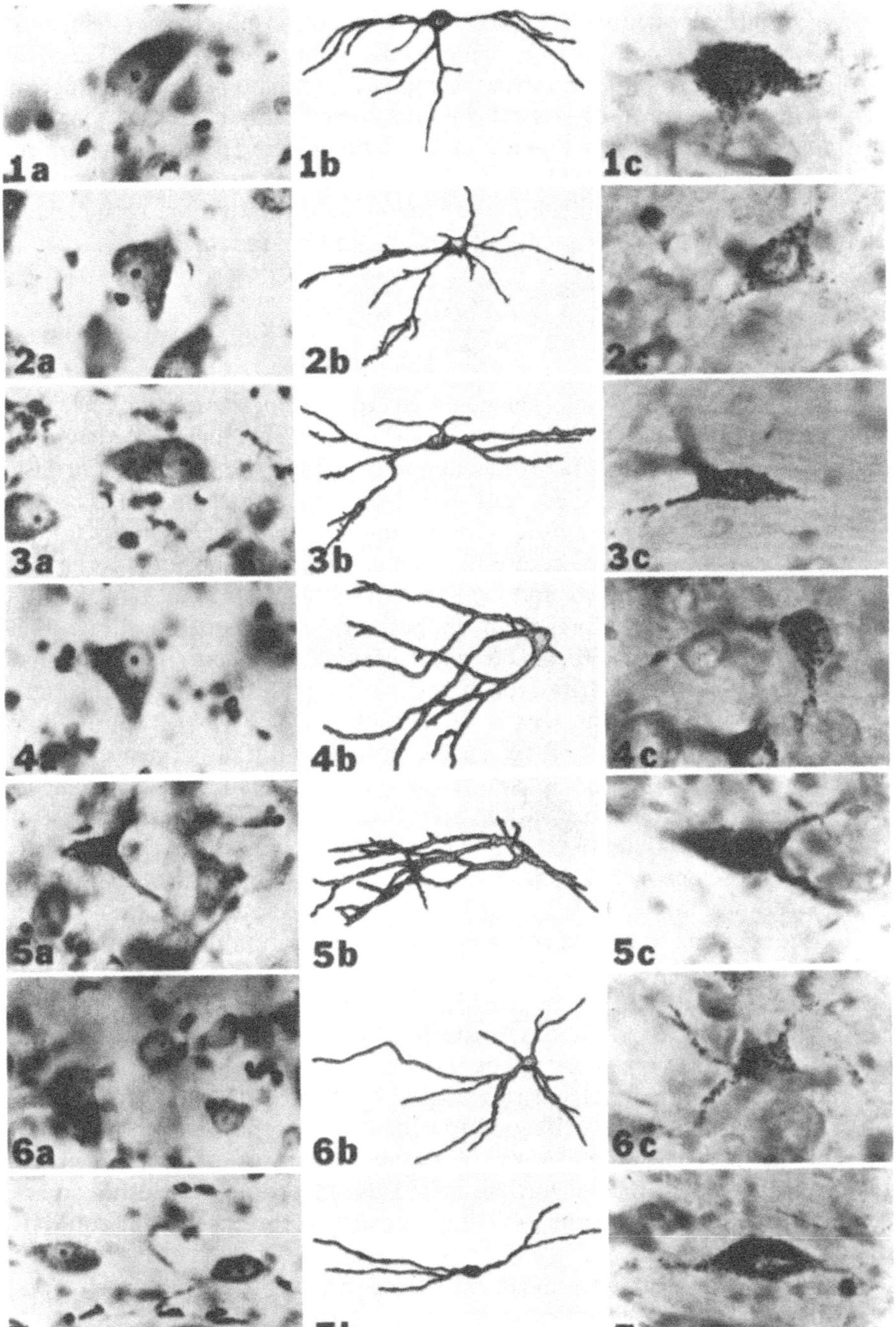
1a
1b
1c
2a
2b
2c
3a
3b
3c
4a
4b
4c
5a
5b
5c
6a
6b
6c
7a
7b
7c

size, shape, location, and staining characteristics [6] (Fig. 2). Large fusiform and large multipolar neurons, characterized by their peripheral complement of clumped Nissl substance, form the major constituents of the rodent DLP. The middle subdivision, on the other hand, contains three cell types: large triangular neurons, fusiform neurons, and small spindle-shaped cells. These cell types differ from those of the DLP both with regard to their location and their intrinsic Nissl pattern. The final two cell types, the large fusiform neurons and the small multipolar neurons, predominate in the caudomedial subdivision. As indicated below these seven cell types are also identifiable in Golgi preparations.

Neuronal Organization

The first detailed description of the neuronal structure of the medial nucleus in Golgi preparations was given by Ramón y Cajal [32] in which three neuronal categories were designated: (a) triangular cells, (b) stellate cells, and (c) fusiform cells. The dendrites of these cells were described as thick, long, and radiating from the cell body. Very little information was added to Ramón y Cajal's description of neuronal architecture in the medial nucleus until the recent account provided by Matsushita and Iwahori [26] in the rat and cat. Utilizing the Golgi-Kopsch and rapid Golgi methods these investigators demonstrated that the perikarya of the large (30–40 μm) and medium (20–30 μm) neurons generate at least six to eight dendrites, the majority of which exhibit a radial pattern and measure 350–400 μm in length. The small neurons (12.5–20 μm) which gather in the ventral portion of the nucleus also exhibit a radial dendritic pattern but the dendrites are shorter and fewer in number than those of the medium and large cells. These observations are generally in agreement with those of Sotelo and Angaut [34] in the cat and O'Leary et al. [29] in the rabbit. In addition these authors concur that there is extensive overlap of dendritic fields of individual neurons in the fastigial nucleus. Considerable disagreement exists, however, among the above investigators as to the location of dendritic spines along the dendrites. Matsushita and Iwahori [26] indicate that the spines are more numerous in distal than in proximal portions of the dendrites. This finding is in direct contrast to the observations of Sotelo and Angaut [34] who described the spines as very numerous on the somata and proximal portions of the dendrites. On the other hand, O'Leary et al. [29] described spines as being variably detected on dendrites belonging to cells of all shapes and sizes and occasionally upon their somata as well. A recent analysis of Golgi-impregnated neurons in the rodent medial nucleus found the majority of dendritic spines along the distal dendritic segment [7], thus supporting the observations of Matsushita and Iwahori.

As indicated above, Ramón y Cajal initially described three general cell types (triangular, stellate, and fusiform neurons) in the medial cerebellar nucleus. A review of the pertinent literature, however, reveals that apart from small and large multipolar neurons, specific neuronal cell types were not described in subsequent studies in the rat [26], the cat [26], or the rabbit [29]. In an attempt to delineate the neuronal organization of the rodent medial nucleus in Golgi preparations we have recently confirmed the presence of three general cell classes as described by Ramón y Cajal [7]. In addition, it was found that each of the three varieties could be subdivided into two or more subclasses. Thus, two types of triangular neurons were identified in the rodent medial nucleus and they were designated the bouquet neuron and the fan-shaped neuron (Fig. 2). The large multipolar neuron and the small multipolar neuron comprise two subgroups of Ramón y Cajal's stellate cell type, while the large fusiform neuron, the neuron of the nuclear boundary, and the small bipolar neuron are subgroups of Ramón y Cajal's fusiform cell type. Ramón y Cajal also described the dendrites of these cells as thick, long, and radiating from the cell body. The dendrites of the large multipolar neurons, the fan-shaped neurons and the large fusiform neurons all exhibit these features.

Thus, a total of seven cell types have been identified in Golgi preparations of the medial cerebellar nucleus based on cell size, shape, location, and dendritic pattern [7]. Two cell types predominate in the DLP: the neuron of the nuclear boundary and the large multipolar neuron. These two subclasses of cells are also easily recognized in Nissl preparations and maintain a caudolateral to rostromedial orientation across the nucleus. The bouquet neuron, the fan-shaped neuron, and the small bipolar neuron are most abundant in the middle subdivision and appear to correspond to the large triangular, the fusiform, and the small spindle-shaped cells observed in Nissl stained material. Finally, the large fusiform neuron and the small multipolar neuron characterize the caudomedial subdivision and can be correlated with the large fusiform cells and the small rounded cells, respectively, observed in Nissl preparations.

With the exception of the large fusiform neurons, which are only present in the caudal portion of the nucleus, the rostral and caudal halves of the medial nucleus contain the same cell types. A careful examination of these two regions, however, has revealed that they differ with regard to the organization of the neurons present [7]. This difference is highlighted by the fan-shaped neurons which maintain a caudolateral to rostromedial orientation in the posterior part of the nucleus and a caudomedial to rostrolateral orientation anteriorly. Other cell varieties also differ in these two nuclear regions. The small multipolar neurons, for instance, have ellipsoidal dendritic territories in the caudal half of the nucleus while rostrally these cells display spherical dendritic fields. These findings support the concept of a bipartitioning of the medial cerebellar nucleus into rostral and caudal subdivisions.

Axonal Organization

Regarding the site of axonal origin from cells in the fastigial nucleus, the axons of the neurons of the nuclear boundary, the large fusiform neurons, and the small bipolar neurons were observed to arise either from the perikaryon or from the thicker stem of a dendrite [7]. The axon of the bouquet neuron and the large and small multipolar neuron typically arises from the cell body, while the preferential site of origin of the axon hillock of the fan-shaped neuron is from one of the primary dendrites. The direction taken by the axons is different depending on the level of the fastigial nucleus in a rostrocaudal extent [26]. Generally the axons are seen to course ventrally for a short distance, turn rostrally or caudally and then course in a ventrolateral or ventromedial direction before leaving the nucleus. In the caudal portion of the medial nucleus the axons take a ventrolateral course and join fibers running from the cerebellar cortex to the vestibular nuclei. Rostrally, however, axons of fastigial neurons travel ventromedially giving rise to fibers of the hook bundle. These findings lend further support to a rostrocaudal bipartitioning of the fastigial nucleus. The large projection neurons have been observed to give off fine recurrent collaterals of various lengths that terminate within the nucleus [26, 29, 32]. Matsushita and Iwahori [26] also described the axonal pathways of small cells, indicating that these axons generate collaterals or ramify into very fine branchlets which terminate in the vicinity of the cell body. However, these investigators could not determine with certainty whether the main axon terminated within the nucleus or excited as a projection axon. These findings are in accord with that of O'Leary et al. [29] who in addition described the short axon cells as having endogenous termini.

In order to determine if the small cells described above can serve as projection neurons and to ascertain if each of the seven cell types, which we have identified in the medial nucleus, send their axons out of the cerebellum, iontophoretic injections of HRP were made into brain stem sites known to receive fastigial efferent projections (see Beitz, above). The results of our study indicated that all seven cell types may serve as projection neurons distributing their axons to various brain stem nuclei. Iontophoretic injections involving the vestibular nuclei, for instance, resulted primarily in labeling of fan-shaped neurons, small bipolar neurons, and large multipolar neurons. Small multipolar neurons and small bipolar neurons were predominantly labeled following injections into the nucleus of the posterior commissure, while large multipolar neurons and neurons of the nuclear boundary appear to be the major cell type projecting to the nucleus reticularis gigantocellularis. Each cell type is shown containing HRP granular reaction product in its soma and proximal dendrites in Fig. 2.

Longitudinal Zones Within the Fastigial Nucleus

Evidence has accumulated in the past two decades from morphological, physiological, and pharmacological studies which suggest that the entire cerebellum may be organized on a plan involving narrow sagittal zones [2, 11, 18, 24, 30, 31, 34]. The majority of studies to date have focused their attention on the longitudinal zonation of the cerebellar cortex. Groenewegen and Voogd [18] and Chan-Palay et al. [11], however, in their comprehensive investigations of the olivocerebellar projections provided evidence that the collaterals of olivocerebellar fibers have a zonal representation in the medial cerebellar nucleus as well. Further evidence to support a scheme of sagittal zonation within the nucleus comes from the work of Armstrong and Schild [1], which demonstrates that the medial aspect of the rodent cerebellar vermis projects to the medial aspect of the medial cerebellar nucleus while the lateral vermis projects to the lateral pole of the nucleus. The results of their study would suggest at least two zones within the nucleus, a medial and a lateral zone. This correlates well with physiological investigations which have shown functional differences between the medial and lateral aspects of the fastigial nucleus [16, 25].

More recently we have tentatively identified four longitudinal zones within the medial nucleus [6, 7], based on a detailed analysis of Nissl and Golgi preparations (Fig. 3 a). Zones A and C contain elliptical cells and are located on the medial and lateral aspect of the nucleus, respectively. Neurons of the nuclear boundary and fan-shaped neurons predominate in zone A, while small bipolar neurons, as well as fan-shaped neurons and neurons of the nuclear boundary, comprise zone C. An intermediate zone B is distinguished within the nucleus by a predominance of round cells in Nissl preparations. In Golgi-impregnated material this zone is characterized by the presence of bouquet neurons and small and large multipolar neurons. The fourth longitudinal region, zone D, contains a mixture of round and elliptical cells and is somewhat indistinct, occupying most of the caudomedial subdivision.

In order to determine if these longitudinal zones were related to the efferent output of the medial nucleus, iontophoretic injections of HRP were made into brain stem regions known to receive efferent projections from the fastigial nucleus [see Beitz, above]. Horizontal sections through the medial nucleus were analyzed for the distribution of retrogradely labeled cells to determine if labeling occurred in a zonal arrangement. The results of this analysis would suggest that the medial cerebellar nucleus consists of three major longitudinal regions (Fig. 3 b) which correspond to zones A, B, and C described above rather than the four zones tentatively identified in Nissl preparations. These three zones extend into the caudomedial subdivision dividing it into three portions. Thus, no evidence was found using this method to support the existence of zone

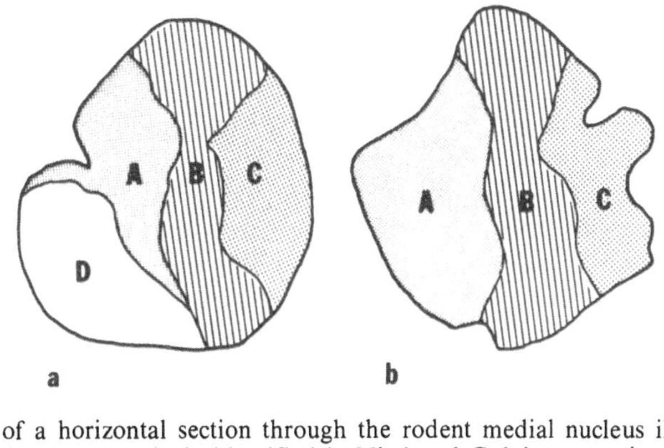

Fig. 3. **a** Schematic drawing of a horizontal section through the rodent medial nucleus illustrating the four longitudinal zones tentatively identified in Nissl and Golgi preparations, based on the distribution of round versus elliptical neurons. Zones *A* and *C* contain elongated cells, while Zone *B* is comprised of a majority of round neurons. Zone *D* is confined to the caudal part of the nucleus and contains a mixture of round and elongated cells. **b** A schematic drawing depicting the three longitudinal zones identified in our retrograde transport experiments. Zones *A, B,* and *C* are comparable to their counterparts identified in Nissl preparations. These three zones extend caudally into the region tentatively identified as Zone *D* in Nissl preparations so that this area actually forms the caudal portion of Zones *A, B,* and *C*

D, tentatively identified in the caudal portion of the nucleus. A quantitative analysis of the number of cells labeled in each zone following injections of HRP into various brain stem nuclei is shown in Table 1. These findings suggest a differential projection from each zone to specific brain stem sites. Zone B, for instance, was found to supply a majority of fibers to the contralateral vestibular nuclei while zone C appears to furnish the predominant input to the ipsilateral vestibular complex. Zone A, on the other hand, is the predominant source of fibers to the nucleus of the posterior commissure and the nucleus pontis oralis and caudalis. Although labeling was confined to a single longitudinal zone in only one of the HRP cases analyzed to date, the observation that one zone in each experiment did contain a majority of labeled cells, as well as the observation that cells containing HRP reaction product usually appeared to form narrow rostrocaudal bands across the nucleus, would support a scheme of sagittal zonation within the medial cerebellar nucleus.

Summary

An analysis of the structural organization of the medial cerebellar nucleus in the rat has been presented and compared with the known architectural arrangement of this nucleus in the cat, monkey, and man. It is difficult to homologize the three traditional nuclear subdivisions which comprise the rodent medial nucleus with the known subdivisions described in the feline and primate fastigial nucleus. In addition, the previous morphological schemes for subdividing the medial nucleus cannot be correlated with the rostrocaudal functional divisions of the nucleus, as indicated above. Hodological studies in our laboratory (see Beitz, above) have also provided evidence which suggest that the three subdivisions of this nucleus in the rat are not topographically related to the efferent output of the fastigial. The DLP, middle and caudomedial subdivisions thus do not appear to form the structural basis around which the fastigial nucleus is organized.

We have recently proposed rostral and caudal subdivisions of the rodent medial nucleus as described in the text. These two morphological subdivisions are evident in Golgi impregnations through the medial nucleus and their existence receives further support from studies utilizing the retrograde transport method which demonstrate specific labeling in one division or the other. This rostrocaudal bipartitioning of the rodent medial nucleus may compare to the anteroposterior regions recognized by Voogd [35] in the cat. This rostrocaudal division correlates well with the known hodological and functional organization of the nucleus and we propose that it may serve as the fundamental morphological foundation upon which fastigial function is built.

Superimposed on this basic morphological scheme is a series of three longitudinally oriented zones. Zone A is the most medially placed, consists primarily of fan-shaped neurons and neurons of the nuclear boundary and contains the greatest number of labeled cells following HRP injections into the nucleus of the posterior commissure, the nucleus pontis oralis and caudalis, or the paramedian reticular nucleus. The intermediate zone, zone B, contains numerous small and large multipolar neurons and is heavily labeled after HRP injections into the contralateral vestibular complex. Zone C is the most laterally situated band and contains a predominance of small bipolar neurons and fan-shaped neurons. It appears to provide a major contribution of fibers to the VPL of the thalamus and to the ipsilateral vestibular complex. This longitudinal zonation within the fastigial nucleus may underlie the functional differences demonstrated between the medial and lateral aspects of the nucleus by Martner [25] and Furuya et al. [16] and form an integral part of the scheme of sagittal organization of the cerebellum proposed by Oscarsson [31].

A careful analysis of both Nissl and Golgi preparations has thus provided evidence for both a bipartitioning of the medial cerebellar nucleus into rostral and caudal subdivisions and a longitudinal division of the nucleus into a series of sagittally oriented zones [6, 7]. A more recent analysis of the distribution of labeled cells within the nucleus, following iontophoretic injections of HRP into brain stem and thalamic nuclei known to receive fastigial projections, supports the presence of these two divisions and three longitudinal zones (see Beitz, above). The utilization of both traditional morphological techniques and the recently developed axonal transport techniques have thus provided new insights into the organization of this cerebellar nucleus. We propose that the rostrocaudal subdivisions and the longitudinal zones may form the basic architectural plan which underlies the organization of the fastigial nucleus.

References

1. Armstrong DM, Schild RF (1978) An investigation of the cerebellar corticonuclear projections in the rat using a autoradiographic tracing method. I. Projections in the vermis. Brain Res 141:1–19
2. Armstrong DM, Harvey RJ, Schild RF (1974) Topographical localization in the olivocerebellar projection: an electrophysiological study in the cat. J Comp Neurol 154:287–302
3. Azzena GB, Giretti ML (1967) Responses of the oculomotor units to deep cerebellar stimulation. Brain Res 6:523–534
4. Batton RR, Jayaraman A, Ruggiero D, Carpenter MB (1977) Fastigial efferent projections in the monkey: an autoradiographic study. J Comp Neurol 174:281–306
5. Deleted in production
6. Beitz AJ, Chan-Palay V (1979a) The medial cerebellar nucleus in the rat: Nuclear volume, cell number, density and orientation. Neuroscience 4:31–45
7. Beitz AJ, Chan-Palay V (1979b) A Golgi analysis of neuronal organization in the medial cerebellar nucleus of the rat. Neuroscience 4:47–63
8. Brun R (1927) Das Kleinhirn: Anatomie, Physiologie und Entwicklungsgeschichte. Abh Neurol Psychiatr Schweiz Arch Neurol Psychiatr 7:1–77
9. Brunner H (1919) Die zentralen Kleinhirnkerne bei den Säugetieren. Arb Neurol Inst Univ Wien 22:200–277
10. Carpenter MB, Batton RR (1982) Connections of the fastigial nucleus in the cat and monkey. In: Palay SL, Chan-Palay V (eds) The cerebellum – new vistas. Springer, Berlin Heidelberg New York, pp 250–295
11. Chan-Palay V, Palay SL, Brown JT, Van Itallie C (1977) Sagittal organization of olivocerebellar and reticulocerebellar projections: autoradiographic studies with ^{35}S-Methionine. Exp Brain Res 30:561–576
12. Courville J, Cooper CW (1970) The cerebellar nuclei of *Macaca mulatta:* a morphological study. J Comp Neurol 140:241–254

13. Dow RS, Moruzzi G (1958) The physiology and pathology of the cerebellum. University of Minnesota Press, Minneapolis
14. Eager RP (1968) Some fine structural features of the neural elements composing cerebellar nuclei in the cat. J Comp Neurol 132:233–262
15. Flood S, Jansen J (1961) On the cerebellar nuclei in the cat. Acta Anat (Basel) 46:52–72
16. Furuya N, Kawano K, Shimazu H (1975) Functional organization of vestibulofastigial projection in the horizontal semicircular canal system in the cat. Exp Brain Res 24:75–87
17. Goodman DC, Hallett RE, Welch RB (1963) Patterns of localization in the cerebellar corticonuclear projections of the albino rat. J Comp Neurol 121:51–67
18. Groenewegen HJ, Voogd J (1977) The parasagittal zonation within the olivocerebellar projection. I. Climbing fiber distribution in the vermis of cat cerebellum. J Comp Neurol 174:417–488
19. Jakob A (1928) Das Kleinhirn. In: von Mollendorf (ed) Springer, Berlin (Handbuch der mikroskopischen Anatomie des Menschen, vol IV/1, pp 674–916)
20. Jansen J, Brodal A (1942) Experimental studies on the intrinsic fibers of the cerebellum. The cortico-nuclear projection in the rabbit and the monkey (Macacus rhesus). Skr Norske Vidensk, Akad I Mat Nat Kl 11 no. 3:1–50
21. Jansen J, Jansen J (1955) On the efferent fibers of the cerebellar nuclei in the cat. J Comp Neurol 102:607–632
22. Korneliussen HJ (1968) On the morphology and subdivision of the cerebellar nuclei of the rat. J Hirnforsch 10:109–122
23. Larsell O, Jansen J (1972) The comparative anatomy and histology of the cerebellum: the human cerebellum, cerebellar connections and cerebellar cortex. University of Minnesota Press, Minneapolis, p 65–87
24. Marani E, Voogd J (1977) An acetylcholinesterase band pattern in the molecular layer of the cat cerebellum. J Anat 124:335–345
25. Martner J (1975) Cerebellar influences on autonomic mechanisms: An experiment study in the cat with special reference to the fastigial nucleus. Acta Physiol Scand [Suppl] 425:1–42
26. Matsushita M, Iwahori N (1971) Structural organization of the fastigial nucleus – I. Dendrites and axonal pathways. Brain Res 25:597–610
27. Mirua M, Reis DJ (1969) Cerebellum: a pressor response elicited from the fastigial nucleus and its efferent pathway in brainstem. Brain Res 13:595–599
28. Moruzzi G, Pompeiano O (1956) Crossed fastigial influence on decerebrate rigidity. J Comp Neurol 106:371–392
29. O'Leary JL, Smith JM, Inukai J, Mejia HH (1972) Architectonics of the cerebellar nuclei in the rabbit. J Comp Neurol 144:399–428
30. Oscarsson C (1969) The sagittal organization of the cerebellar anterior lobe as revealed by the projection patterns of the climbing fiber system. In: Llinás R (ed) Neurobiology of cerebellar evolution and development. AMA-ERF, Chicago, p 525–532
31. Oscarsson O (1979) Functional units of the cerebellum – sagittal zones and microzones. TINS, p 143–145
32. Ramón y Cajal S (1911) Histologie du système nerveux de l'homme et des vertébrés, vol II. Maloine, Paris. Translated by L Azoulay
33. Snider RS (1940) Morphology of the cerebellar nuclei in rabbit and cat. J Comp Neurol 72:399–415
34. Sotelo C, Angaut P (1973) The fine structure of the cerebellar nuclei in the cat. I. Neurons and neuroglial cells. Exp Brain Res 16:410–430
35. Voogd J (1964) The cerebellum of the cat. Ph. D. thesis, Van Gorcum, Leiden
36. Ziehen T (1934) Mikroskopische Anatomie des Gehirns. In: van Bardelebens (ed) Handbuch der Anatomie des Menschen, vol 4/2. Fischer, Jena, pp 863–1546

Discussion

Carpenter: Do you regard those small bipolar neurons that reach the rostral and caudal poles of the nucleus as local circuit neurons?
Beitz: They may be involved in that function. Since small bipolar neurons were labeled following injections in various brain stem nuclei they may have collaterals within the nucleus as well as projections to areas outside the fastigial nucleus. We were unable to trace the axons of these particular cells in our Golgi preparations; therefore I cannot address that question at this time.
Eccles: Do you think all of these neurons are excitatory, with none inhibitory and none completely enclosed within the nucleus for their projections?
Beitz: If one were to do immunohistochemistry with glutamic acid decarboxylase (GAD) to see if small cells are labeled and therefore contain the neurotransmitter gamma aminobutyric acid (GABA), that would provide evidence that they may indeed be inhibitory. Without immunohistochemical and electrophysiological data I really can't address that question.
Llinás: Is there any morphology that you know of that would go together with GAD staining? Can we say that the inhibitory neurons or most of the inhibitory neurons fall into a particular category, or go to a particular place in the brain stem?
Mugnaini: We have done some preliminary experiments which may address this question. In these experiments (in collaboration with Dr. W. Oertel and coworkers at the NIH), we used a very sensitive antibody to GAD, which in the cerebellar cortex stains Golgi, stellate, and Purkinje neurons. The perikarya of these cells stain lightly, but their axons are heavily stained. When you examine the deep cerebellar nuclei there are at most a few cell bodies which seem to be very lightly stained. The picture is predominated by deeply stained Purkinje axon terminals. We have therefore injected colchicine into the lateral ventricles. The colchicine is transported through the ventricular system and remains available for quite a while, thereby blocking axoplasmic transport. When you look at the deep nuclei with GAD antibody stain, the lateral and interposed nuclei contain a large number of positive medium-sized and small neurons. These labeled neurons are not homogeneously distributed. Very few of them are found in areas of lateral nucleus described as containing mostly large cells. In the lateral nucleus most of these cells are located within the fan of fibers at the hilus. Many small reactive cells are also located in the region between the anterior and posterior interposed nuclei. However, very few neurons in the fastigial nucleus proper are stained by GAD antibody. In fact, in the fastigial nucleus the picture is pretty much the same with or without colchicine pretreatment. With ventricular injections you run the risk that the colchicine will not diffuse equally into all of the nuclei. Therefore I cannot make a strong statement about the findings in fastigial nucleus. We have done some experiments in which colchicine has been delivered to the deep nuclei directly with a micropipette, but this material has not been studied yet. One further note of caution; in all immunocytochemical studies of this sort, there is the complication that by blocking axoplasmic transport you are forcing the cell to pile up various cytoplasmic substances, not just the enzyme you are looking for. Therefore, you run

the risk of getting a higher concentration of whatever impurity the antiserum may stain. The preliminary findings I have presented must be interpreted with caution.

Voogd: I'd like to ask you something of a comparative nature. When you look in rats, the dorsolateral protuberance of the fastigial nucleus is very obvious, while in the cat it is almost impossible to find the equivalent nuclear region. I think Armstrong and Schild [2] have given convincing evidence, based on leucine injections into rat cerebellar cortex, that the medial part of posterior lobe hemisphere, say, ansiform lobule and medial parts of paramedian lobule, project to this dorsolateral protuberance. This means, in rat at least, that this dorsolateral protuberance, which faces the junctional region of vermis and hemisphere of posterior lobe, receives Purkinje cell axons from part of the hemisphere. We can confirm this in normal Haggquist-stained material. This is the first and *only* real evidence that the fastigial nucleus, specifically its dorsolateral protuberance, receives afferents from the hemisphere. As far as I know, and from our experience in the cat, when you inject HRP into fastigial nucleus, even in its lateral part, labeled Purkinje cells are always limited to the vermis. There appears to be something in the rat which is absent, very small, or differently located than in the cat. Could you comment on that?

Beitz: I agree with you. The first real evidence for a hemispheral projection to the dorsolateral protuberance was provided by Goodman et al. [3], based on lesions of the hemisphere. They showed degeneration confined to the dorsolateral protuberance. Looking at Armstrong and Schild's [2] paper, my feeling is that more than just the dorsolateral protuberance is labeled with hemispheral injections; the extent of the labeling probably corresponds to my zone C. In addition, following some of their vermal injections labeling occurred in my zone A [1]. So, I agree with you. There seems to be a cortical representation in the fastigial nucleus that I think is probably a longitudinally oriented pattern.

Voogd: May I also ask a question about the efferents of the dorsolateral protuberance? In one of your slides it appeared that the dorsolateral protuberance was the main source of the direct fastigiobulbar pathway in the rat. Is that correct?

Beitz: That's not entirely correct. There is a major component in the ipsilateral vestibular projection that arises from the dorsolateral protuberance, but these fibers also arise from what I would call zone A. The main point is that in all our brain stem injections there was never a *single* fastigial subdivision labeled. In many cases there was one subdivision more heavily labeled or containing a quantitatively greater number of cells than the others. For instance, with injections into the nucleus gigantocellularis, the dorsolateral protuberance was very heavily labeled, more so than any of the other subdivisions, but all other subdivisions also contained labeled cells. My feeling from the 20 or so experiments we've done to date is that the efferent organization transcends these three subdivisions and that it may be related to the rostrocaudal divisions of the nucleus rather than this longitudinal pattern.

Voogd: There also appears to be something special concerning the efferent projection of the fastigial nucleus in the rat. As far as I know, only in rodents has the ipsilateral descending branch of the superior cerebellar peduncle been de-

scribed. Is there a chance that *this* pathway could originate from the dorsolateral protuberance?
Beitz: It's possible, but without doing anterograde studies, I really can't answer that point.
Snider: I'm always disturbed by the term "paleocerebellum". Would you like to speculate on which is the oldest part of the nucleus fastigii?
Beitz: Most investigators consider the dorsolateral protuberance to be neofastigial and the remainder to be paleofastigial. In looking at the phylogeny of the nucleus I would consider the caudomedial subdivision and probably portions of the middle subdivision to be the oldest parts.

References

1. Armstrong DM, Schild RF (1978a) An investigation of the cerebellar corticonuclear projections in the rat using an autoradiographic tracing method. I. Projections from the vermis. Brain Res. 141:1–19
2. Armstrong DM, Schild RF (1978b) An investigation of the cerebellar corticonuclear projections in the rat using an autoradiographic tracing method. II. Projections from the hemisphere. Brain Res 141:235–249
3. Goodman DC, Hallett RE, Welch RB (1963) Patterns of localization in the cerebellar corticonuclear projections of the albino rat. J Comp Neurol 121:51–67

Connections of the Fastigial Nucleus in the Cat and Monkey *

M. B. Carpenter and R. R. Batton, III

Introduction

The fastigial nucleus is easily distinguished from all other deep cerebellar nuclei by its position, size, and unique neural connections. This nucleus receives a strictly ipsilateral, topographically organized input from all lobules of the cerebellar vermis, so that the vermal cortex is represented sequentially in the fastigial nucleus [39]. In addition, the fastigial nucleus receives crossed projections from the dorsomedial cell column and nucleus β of the contralateral medial accessory olivary nucleus [12, 15, 17], bilateral projections from the medial and inferior vestibular nuclei [24, 28, 31, 93], and bilateral projections from certain perihypoglossal nuclei [103]. Like the other deep cerebellar nuclei, the fastigial nucleus receives small inputs from the paramedian reticular nuclei [95].
The efferent projections of the fastigial nucleus also are unique in that: (a) they do not enter the superior cerebellar peduncle, but emerge as separate crossed and uncrossed bundles, (b) a large part of the efferent fibers cross within the cerebellum, (c) efferent fibers project to nuclei at all levels of the brain stem, and (d) fastigial projections to the vestibular nuclei and portions of the brain stem reticular formation are bilateral while those to the thalamus and spinal cord are crossed [4, 6, 10, 27, 54, 69, 101, 104, 106, 109, 111, 112]. Unlike other deep cerebellar nuclei the fastigial nucleus is traversed in various regions by corticovestibular fibers from the vermal cortex that project to portions of the lateral and inferior vestibular nuclei [7, 92, 107].
Although there have been many studies of the afferent and efferent connections of the fastigial nucleus based upon degeneration techniques, almost all lesions in this nucleus concomitantly interrupt fibers which traverse it. Thus, degeneration studies introduce variables which make interpretations of findings both difficult and unreliable. Recently developed axoplasmic transport techniques using tritiated amino acids and autoradiography, and the enzyme horseradish peroxidase provide an opportunity to determine more accurately the connections of the fastigial nucleus [40, 41, 76, 77]. These methods have been used in the present study.

* Supported by research grant NS-14802 from the National Institute of Neurological and Communicative Disorders and Stroke of the National Institutes of Health and grants 9I9C07005 and 9I9C07016 from the Department of Defense, Uniformed Services University of the Health Sciences

Experimental Brain Research, Suppl. 6

Cerebellar Nuclei

All deep cerebellar nuclei are thought to originate as condensations of cells which migrate outward from the germinal neuroepithelium of the fourth ventricle [70]. The four deep cerebellar nuclei start to differentiate simultaneously at early developmental stages and there is no evidence in the rat indicating that individual cerebellar nuclei differ with respect to ontogenetic origin or age. An autoradiographic study in the mouse describes cells arising in the primative ependymal layer of the fourth ventricle on the 11th day which migrate outward into the mantle layer [82]. These cells separate into two main groups: (a) a deep group that subsequently differentiate into the large neurons of the roof nuclei, and (b) a second group that migrates deep to the molecular layer and ultimately differentiates into Purkinje cells. Although precursors of Purkinje cells form early, they do not become distinctly large cells and are not arranged in a single layer until 10 days after birth.

Four distinct deep cerebellar nuclei are recognized in most mammals, although many authors have illustrated them as a capriciously indented continuous cell mass [51]. A morphological study in the monkey distinguishes also four cerebellar nuclei on the basis of fiber patterns, differences in cellular morphology, and in the distribution of cell sizes in individual nuclei [38]. The principal advance appears to be the distinction between the two components of the interposed nuclei (i.e., anterior and posterior) and the dentate nucleus. The strongest argument supporting the validity of four individual deep cerebellar nuclei is based on observations indicating that each nucleus has unique connections.

Fastigial Nucleus

The fastigial nucleus, the most medial of the deep cerebellar nuclei, lies in the roof of the fourth ventricle and is second in size to the dentate nucleus. The irregular contours of the nucleus give it a variety of shapes in different planes of section, but the main cell mass has an ellipsoidal configuration with the long axis oriented rostrocaudally. Cell strands emerging from the lateral border of the nucleus extend ventrolateral towards the vestibular nuclei. In the monkey, there are no recognized subdivisions in the nucleus but clusters of cells appear to form subgroups. Lateral parts of the nucleus are traversed by numerous corticovestibular fibers [107]. The fastigial nucleus is characterized by a population of densely packed cells of varying size. Cells in the dorsal two-thirds of the nucleus are large and medium-sized, while small and very small cells predominate in ventral regions. Large and medium-sized cells are polygonal, stain deeply with cresyl violet and contain coarse clumps of chromatin. Small cells are round or fusiform, rather pale and have fine, evenly distributed chromatin. The very smallest cells lie in the roof of the fourth ventricle and it is not clear whether they are neurons or glial cells. Cells in the fastigial nucleus of the monkey range in size from 10 to 65 μm with the greatest number of cells in the range between 17 and 35 μm [38].

Golgi studies of the rat fastigial nucleus indicate that both large and medium-

Fig. 1. Cat C-1450. Projection drawings of cerebellum and brain stem demonstrating the HRP injection site in the right fastigial nucleus (*crosshatched* area surrounding needle track in **A–C**) and retrograde transport of the enzyme to Purkinje cells in the ipsilateral cerebellar vermis and to cells in brain stem nuclei (*black dots*). **A–D** are in rostrocaudal sequence. A photomicrograph of the HRP injection site is shown in Fig. 3A[1]

sized cells have dendrites radiating in all directions that bear spines which are most numerous on distal branches [79]. There is extensive overlap of dendritic fields in the nucleus, but no evidence of Golgi type II cells. Axons of fastigial neurons project ventromedial and ventrolaterally; those passing ventrolateral appear to project to the vestibular nuclei, while those passing ventromedially cross to the opposite side and presumably enter the uncinate fasciculus. Approximately equal numbers of cells give rise to crossed and uncrossed axons, but axons crossing to the opposite side appear most numerous in rostral regions of the nucleus. No commissural fibers appear to interconnect the fastigial nuclei.

Fastigial Afferent Projections

Attempts to determine the origin and terminations of fastigial afferents by degeneration techniques have employed two methods: (a) the study of retrograde cell changes following cerebellar lesions, and (b) the study of anterograde degeneration following lesions in the cerebellar cortex, brain stem nuclei, and in the vestibular nerve and ganglion.

1 Abbreviations used in Figures: *AC*, anterior commissure; *ACN*, accessory cuneate nucleus; *AIN*, anterior interposed nucleus; *AP*, area postrema; *β*, nucleus beta of medial accessory olivary nucleus; *CG*, central gray; *CI*, inferior colliculus; *CL*, central lateral nucleus; *CM*, centromedian nucleus; *CN*, cuneate nucleus; *CS*, superior colliculus; *CST*, corticospinal tract; *D*, dentate nucleus; *DAO*, dorsal accessory olivary nucleus; *DM*, dorsomedial nucleus; *DN*, dentate nucleus; *DSCP*, decussation of superior cerebellar peduncle; *f*, cell group f (Brodal and Pompeiano, '57); *FN*, fastigial nucleus; *FS*, fastigiospinal tract; *GP*, globus pallidus; *HB*, habenular nucleus; *IC*, internal capsule; *ICP*, inferior cerebellar peduncle; *IVN*, inferior vestibular nucleus; *JRB*, juxtarestiform body; *LC*, locus ceruleus; *LG*, lateral geniculate body; *LP*, lateral posterior nucleus; *LRN*, lateral reticular nucleus; *LVN*, lateral vestibular nucleus; *MAO*, medial accessory olivary nucleus; *MCP*, middle cerebellar peduncle; *MG*, medial geniculate body; *ML*, medial lemniscus; *MLF*, medial longitudinal fasciculus; *MVN*, medial vestibular nucleus; *NC*, nucleus cuneatus; *NG*, nucleus gracilis; *NPC*, nuclei of the posterior commissure; *NPS*, nucleus parasolitarius; *NRG*, nucleus reticularis gigantocellularis; *OC*, optic chiasm; *OT*, optic tract; *PIN*, posterior interposed nucleus; *PF*, parafascicular nucleus; *PN*, nucleus prepositus; *PRN*, paramedian reticular nucleus; *Pul*, pulvinar; *PVN*, paraventricular nucleus; *RN*, red nucleus; *RIN*, reticulotegmental nucleus; *SCP*, superior cerebellar peduncle; *SF*, solitary fasciculus; *SI*, substantis innominata; *SN*, substantia nigra; *SO*, superior olivary nucleus; *STN*, subthalamic nucleus; *SVN*, superior vestibular nucleus; *UF*, uncinate fasciculus; *VCN*, ventral cochlear nucleus; *VLo*, ventral lateral nucleus, pars oralis; *VM*, ventromedial nucleus; *VPI*, ventral posterior inferior nucleus; *VPLc*, ventral posterolateral nucleus, pars caudalis; *VPLo*, ventral posterolateral nucleus, pars oralis; *VPM*, ventral posteromedial nucleus; *x*, cell group x; *III*, oculomotor nerve; *V*, trigeminal nerve or nucleus; *VI*, abducens nerve; *VII*, facial nerve or nucleus; *VIII*, vestibular nerve; *X*, vagus nerve; *XII*, hypoglossal nerve or nucleus

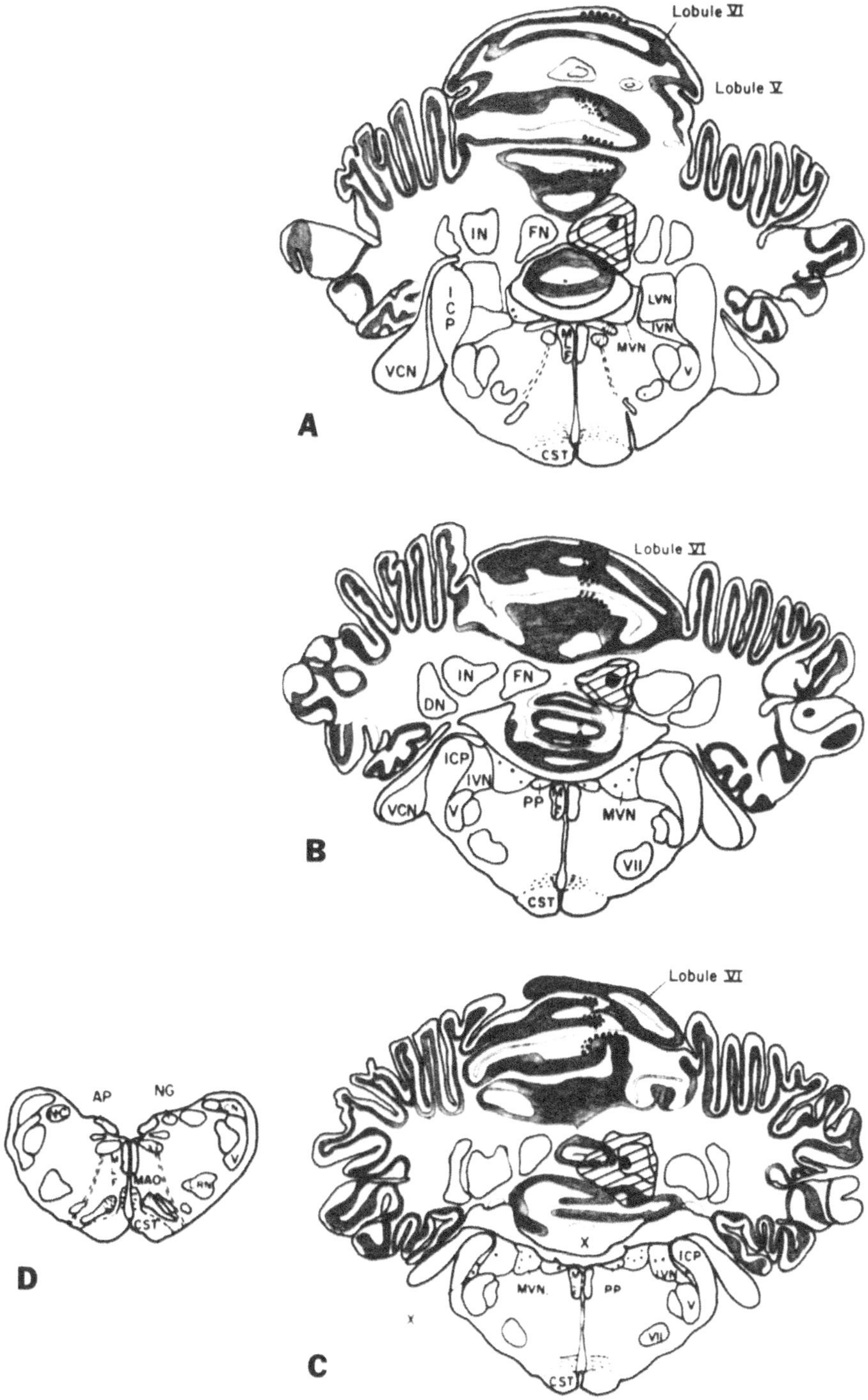
Lobule VI
Lobule V
IN
FN
I C P
LVN
IVN
MVN
VCN
V
CST
A
Lobule VI
IN
FN
DN
ICP
IVN
PP
VCN
V
MVN
VII
CST
B
Lobule VI
X
ICP
IVN
MVN
PP
V
VII
CST
C
AP
NG
MAO
CST
D

Cerebellar Cortex

Early studies of cerebellar corticonuclear projections lead to the conclusion that the cerebellar cortex is organized into three longitudinal, rostrocaudal zones that project in mediolateral sequence to the fastigial, interposed, and dentate nuclei [66, 67]. Subsequent degeneration studies based upon silver impregnation techniques indicated that cortical regions of the cerebellar hemisphere projected to one or more deep cerebellar nuclei, but vermal regions of the cortex projected almost entirely to the fastigial and vestibular nuclei [46, 56, 108]. The median cortical zone, constituting the vermis proper, projected to the fastigial nuclei, the two halves of the zone being related respectively to the nucleus on right and left [108]. The projection from the vermis to the fastigial nucleus is strictly unilateral with a topographical distribution of fibers from the cortical lobules of the vermis to the nearest region of the nucleus [39]. Thus, there is a sequential representation of the cerebellar vermis in the fastigial nucleus.

In our own studies of fastigial afferent fibers, based upon the retrograde transport of horseradish peroxidase (HRP) from localized injections into the fastigial nucleus in the cat, retrograde transport of the enzyme to Purkinje cells was seen in a narrow longitudinal band of the ipsilateral vermis in folia of lobules I through X [75, 93]. Retrograde labeling of somata and dendritic expansions of Purkinje cells was impressive and many dendritic profiles extended almost to the pial surface (Figs. 1, 2, 4A). With labeling of nearly the entire fastigial nucleus, maximal retrograde transport to Purkinje cells was seen in folia of lobules VI, VII, V, and X, in that order (Fig. 1). In these animals there was no evidence of retrograde transport of HRP to Purkinje cells in other cortical areas.

In several animals with unilateral HRP injections of the fastigial nucleus a few cells in the contralateral nucleus were labeled, mainly in rostral parts of the nucleus. While it is possible that those cells might give rise to commissural fibers, it seems more likely that retrograde transport occurred via axonal collaterals. Since collaterals of this type were not described in a detailed Golgi study of the fastigial nucleus [80], uptake of the enzyme probably occurred from fibers, or collaterals, of the fastigial nucleus projecting to the cerebellar cortex. Labeling of superficial regions of the cerebellar cortex with HRP has been reported to produce transport of the enzyme to the deep cerebellar nuclei [57, 102]. Labeling of lobules V, VI, and VII of the vermis bilaterally resulted in transport of the HRP marker to neurons along the lateral margins of the fastigial nuclei at rostral levels and in the zone separating the fastigial and interposed nuclei. Both anterograde and retrograde transport studies appear to indicate an orderly projection of fibers, or recurrent collaterals, from the deep nuclei to the cerebellar cortex [102]. There are no data suggesting that the deep cerebellar nuclei exhibit endogenous peroxidase activity.

Brain Stem Nuclei

Degeneration studies have indicated that the fastigial nucleus received afferent inputs from a large number of brain stem nuclei. Nuclei considered to project

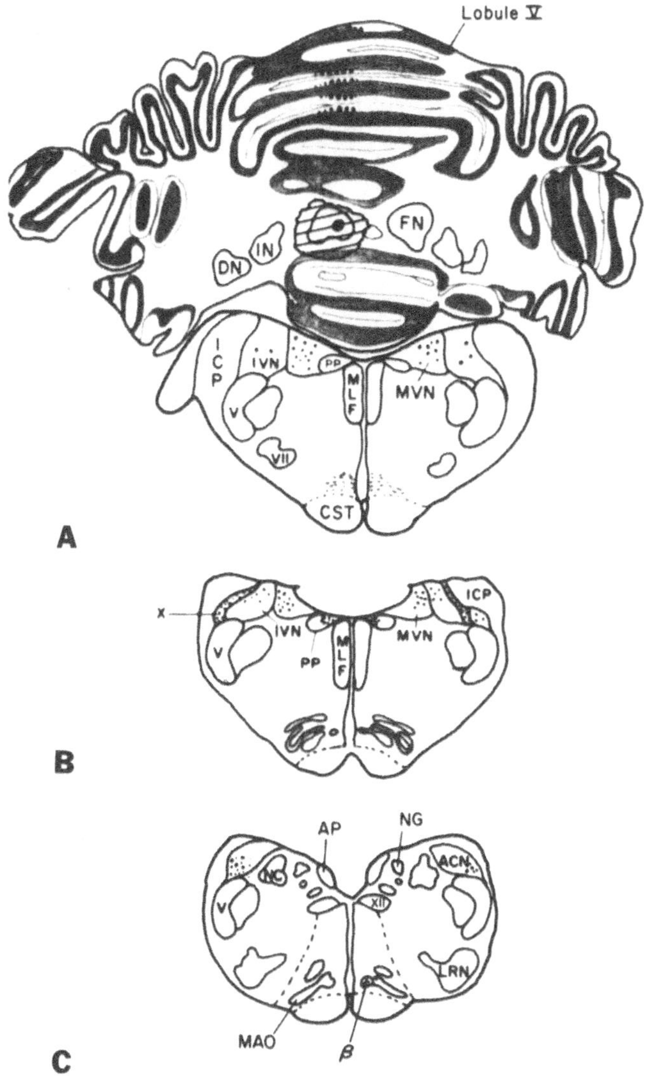

Fig. 2A–C. Cat C-1418. Projection drawings of cerebellum and brain stem demonstrating an HRP injection which labeled the entire left fastigial nucleus (*crosshatched* area in **A**) and basal folia of the pyramis and uvula. Retrograde transport of the enzyme was bilateral to cells in the medial and inferior vestibular nucleus and to cells in group x and the accessory cuneate nuclei. A photomicrograph of the HRP injection site is shown in Fig. 3B. See footnote on p. 252

afferents to the fastigial nucleus included: (a) the inferior and medial vestibular nuclei [24, 28, 31, 44], (b) the paramedian reticular nuclei [23], (c) parts of the perihypoglossal nuclei [103], and (d) certain parts of the contralateral inferior olivary complex [12].

Inferior Olivary Nucleus. In a series of systematic studies of olivocerebellar projections in the cat, Brodal and his colleagues have utilized the HRP retrograde method to map this major cerebellar afferent pathway. These studies indicate that the olivary projection is far more complex than indicated by studies of retrograde cell changes [17, 25, 26, 62, 73]. Observations in one of these studies indicate that the fastigial nucleus in the cat received crossed projections from the dorsomedial cell column and nucleus β of the contralateral medial accessory olivary nucleus [17]. Cells in these small appendages to the medial accessory olivary nucleus also supply lateral parts of the uvula. In our studies of fastigial afferent fibers the principal structure labeled by the enzyme marker was the fastigial nucleus, but in different animals there was diffusion of HRP into surrounding white matter, folia of the pyramis and uvula, and occasionally into basal folia of lobules V and VI. Although it was difficult to define precisely the region of HRP uptake, two criteria were used to support the premise that axon terminals within the fastigial nucleus had taken up the marker, namely: (a) retrograde transport of HRP to the somata and dendritic expansions of Purkinje cells in the ipsilateral vermis, and (b) retrograde transport of the enzyme marker to cells of the dorsomedial cell column and nucleus β of the contralateral medial accessory olivary nucleus (Figs. 1, 2, 4D). Labeling of portions of the cerebellar cortex, either alone, or in addition to the fastigial nucleus, produced a different pattern of retrograde transport to cells of the opposite inferior olivary complex and labeling of cells in other cerebellar relay nuclei.

Vestibular Nuclei. Prior to the widespread use of retrograde enzyme tracing techniques, most information concerning fastigial afferents was derived from studies of secondary vestibulocerebellar projections. The early studies of Dow [44], based upon Marchi degeneration resulting from lesions in the vestibular nuclei, suggested that secondary vestibular fibers terminated in the ipsilateral nodulus, uvula, flocculus, and fastigial nucleus. Silver impregnation methods confirmed these observations but revealed only scant degeneration in rostral parts of the fastigial nuclei following lesions of the inferior vestibular nucleus [28]. Using the modified Gudden technic Brodal and Torvik [24] reported that lesions involving "vestibular parts" of the cerebellum produced retrograde cell changes in three locations: (a) ventrolateral and caudal parts of the inferior vestibular nucleus, including cell group f [21], (b) ventral and caudal parts of the medial vestibular nucleus, and (c) cell group x, situated along the lateral border of the inferior vestibular nucleus. Because these lesions were not restricted to particular parts of the "vestibulo-cerebellum" and most lesions involving the fastigial nucleus also encroached upon uvula and nodulus, these data cannot be regarded as conclusive. These data were confirmed in part by isolated lesions of the fastigial nucleus that produced retrograde cell changes and cell loss in the inferior vestibular nuclei [31]. Secondary vestibular projections to the fastigial nucleus were described as predominantly uncrossed.

Data reported here concerning fastigial afferent projections were based upon the retrograde axonal transport of HRP in the cat and squirrel monkey. Investigations in the cat employed diaminobenzidine as the chromagen [58, 93], while the more sensitive tetramethylbenzidine was used to investigate fastigial afferents in the squirrel monkey [60, 81]. HRP injections in the cat labeled: (a) the entire fastigial nucleus (Figs. 1, 2, 3A, 3B), (b) rostral parts of the fastigial

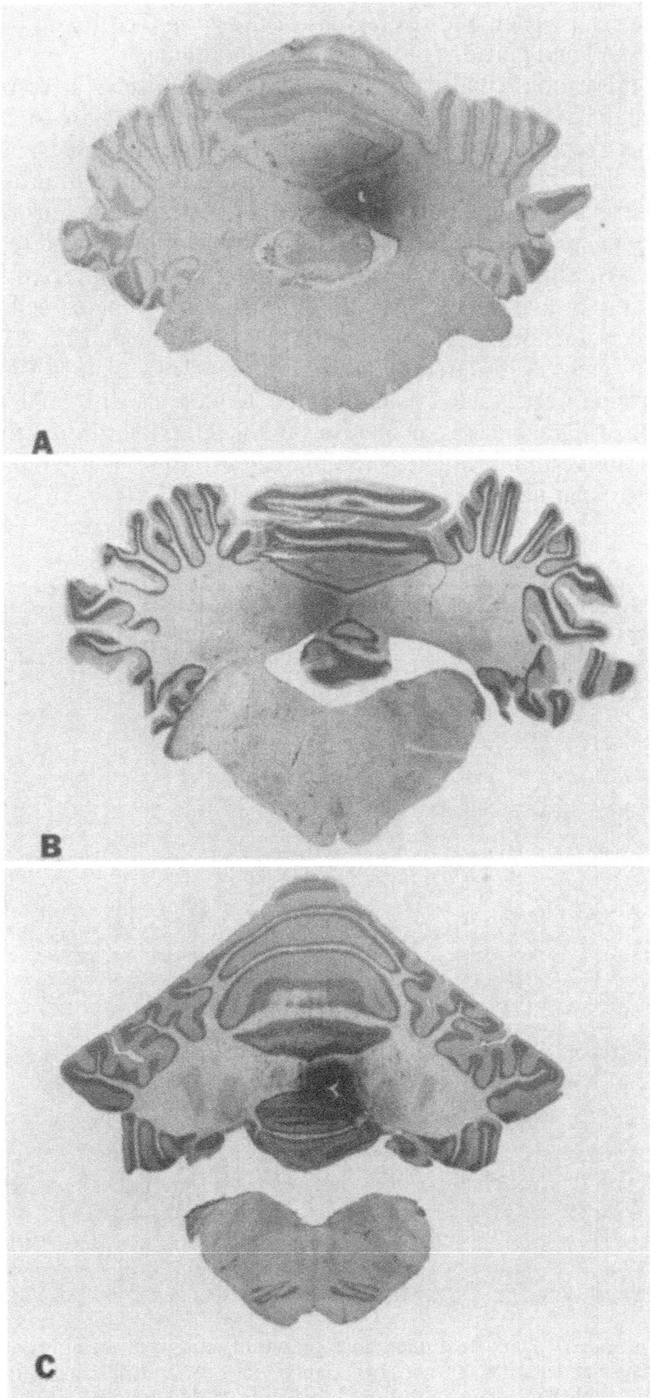

Fig. 3 A–C. Photomicrographs of HRP injections in the fastigial nucleus. **A** cat C-1450; **B** cat C-1418; **C** squirrel monkey U-75. Cresyl violet, × 2.5, × 2.5, × 3

nucleus, (c) caudal parts of the fastigial nucleus, (d) bilateral portions of the fastigial nuclei, and (e) regions of the vermal cortex in basal folia of lobules V and VI and portions of the pyramis and uvula.

Observations concerning the origins of vestibular afferents to the fastigial nucleus based upon retrograde transport of HRP are strikingly different from those reported in degeneration studies. In retrograde transport studies the principal afferents to the fastigial nucleus were found to arise bilaterally from: (a) dorsal and caudal parts of the medial vestibular nucleus (MVN), (b) dorsal and caudal parts of the inferior vestibular nuclei (IVN) and (c) cell group x (Figs. 1, 2, 5A, 5B, 6D). The largest number of fastigial afferent fibers arise from cells in the caudal parts of MVN, although a few labeled cells were seen at all rostrocaudal levels of the nucleus. At all levels the number of labeled cells in MVN was greatest ipsilaterally and more numerous than in IVN. In IVN no cells of group f were labeled on either side. In animals with HRP injections confined to the fastigial nucleus, no neurons in the lateral vestibular nucleus (LVN), the superior vestibular nucleus (SVN), cell group y, or the interstitial nucleus of the vestibular nerve were labeled on either side.

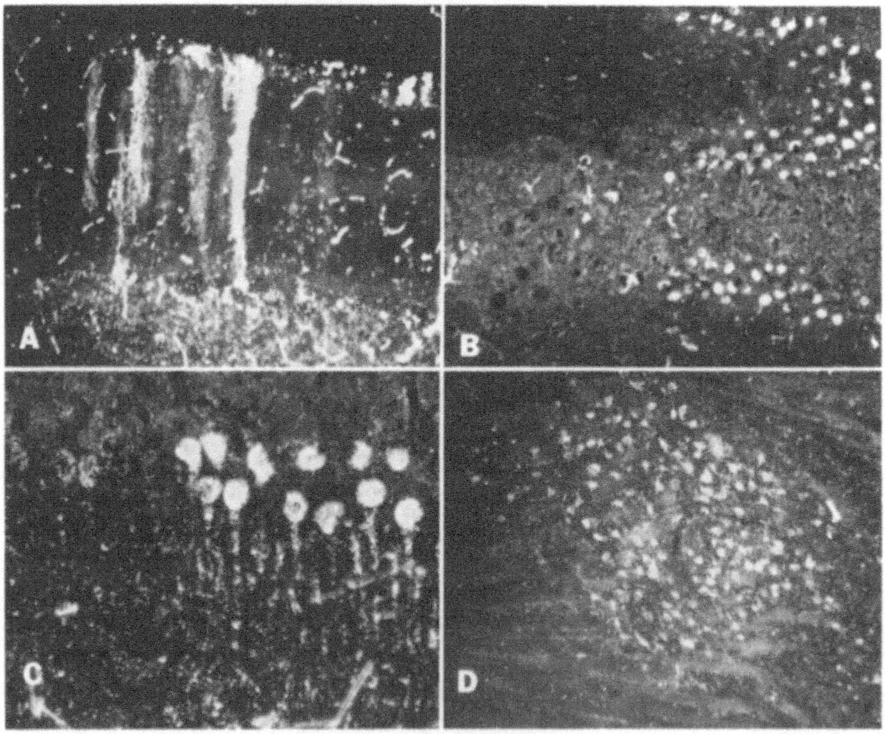

Fig. 4A–D. Dark-field photomicrographs of retrograde transport of HRP to Purkinje cell somata and dendrites. **A** Cat C-1411, cresyl violet, × 52. **B, C** Labeled Purkinje cells in the ipsilateral cerebellar vermis in squirrel monkey U-75. Neutral red, × 25, × 80. **D**, Dark-field photomicrograph of retrograde transport of HRP to cells of nucleus β following injection of the opposite fastigial nucleus in cat C-1417. Cresyl violet, × 52

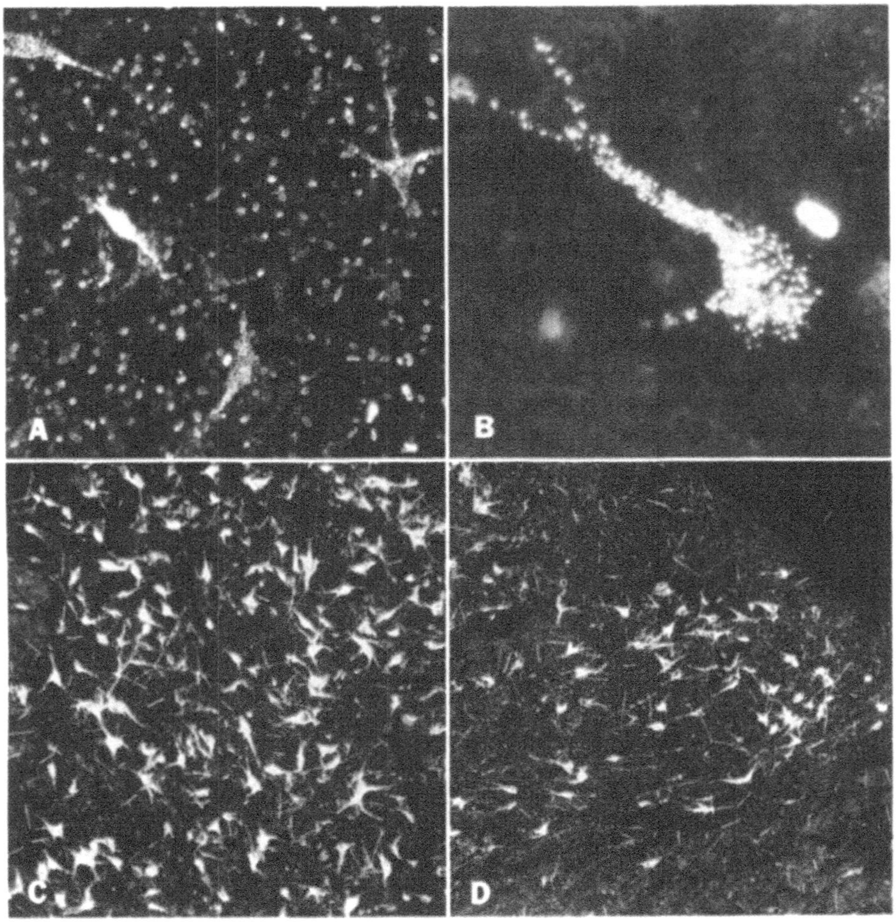

Fig. 5. A, B Dark-field photomicrographs of HRP transported retrograde to cells in dorsal regions of the medial vestibular nucleus in cat C-1411. Cresyl violet, × 63, × 325. Dark-field photomicrographs of HRP transported retrograde to cells in the medial vestibular nucleus **C** and the nucleus prepositus **D** in squirrel monkey U-75; TMB was used as the chromagen. Neutral red, × 25, × 25

Labeling of rostral parts of one fastigial nucleus resulted in more modest retrograde transport of the label to the vestibular nuclei and label in the MVN, although bilateral, was greatest contralaterally. Data from injections of caudal parts of the fastigial nucleus suggested that afferent fibers were derived bilaterally from dorsal regions of MVN, IVN, and cell group x with ipsilateral preponderance. In addition, a small number of cells in peripheral portions of the ipsilateral SVN appeared to project to the fastigial nucleus.

Concomitant labeling of portions of the uvula and the fastigial nucleus resulted in more profuse transport of the enzyme bilaterally to cells in the MVN and IVN than labeling of the fastigial nucleus alone (Fig. 2). Labeled cells were found in dorsal, lateral, and caudal parts of MVN and a greater number of

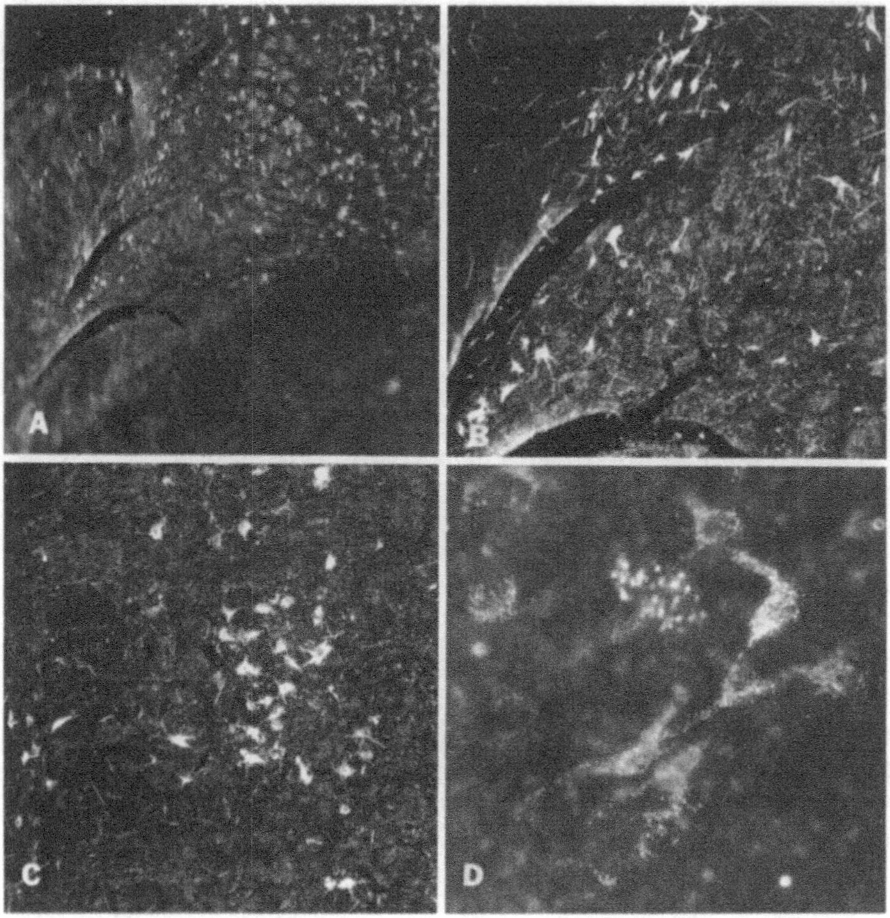

Fig. 6. A, B Dark-field photomicrographs of HRP transported retrograde to cells in the inferior vestibular nucleus and in cell group x in squirel monkey U-75. Few, if any, cells in group f were labeled. Neutral red, × 16, × 25. **C** Dark-field photomicrograph of HRP transported to the contralateral paramedian reticular nucleus in U-75. Neutral red, × 25. **D** Dark-field photomicrograph of HRP transported retrograde to cells of group x contralaterally in cat C-1418. Cresyl violet, × 325

labeled cells were seen ipsilaterally. In the IVN labeled cells were predominantly in dorsal and caudal regions and were more numerous on the side of the injection. None of the large cells of group f were labeled. The small cells of group x were profusely labeled bilaterally (Fig. 6 D). Although none of the cells in the LVN were labeled, some cells in peripheral parts of SVN were labeled bilaterally. A few cells in cell group y and in the interstitial nucleus of the vestibular nerve were labeled ipsilaterally.

Bilateral HRP injections of the fastigial nuclei confirmed all of the above observations and resulted in bilateral, symmetrical, and profuse labeling of cells in: (a) dorsal parts of MVN throughout their rostrocaudal extent, (b) dorsal and caudal parts of the IVN, and (c) group x. No cells of group f were labeled on either side. In addition neurons in SVN were labeled bilaterally in one animal.

These observations concerning fastigial afferent fibers in the cat indicate that: (a) afferent fibers arise bilaterally from parts of the MVN and IVN, (b) the largest number of afferent fibers arise from dorsal and caudal regions of the MVN, (c) the IVN gives rise to a smaller number of afferent fibers derived mainly from dorsal regions, (d) none of the cells of group f project to the fastigial nucleus, (e) cells of group x project bilaterally to the fastigial nucleus, and (f) a small number of cells from the SVN may project to the fastigial nucleus. Evidence from this study also suggests that cells in similar locations within the MVN and IVN and in cell group x also project to basal parts of the uvula. Although neither cell group f nor cell group x receives primary vestibular afferents [107], both receive crossed projections from the fastigial nucleus via the uncinate fasciculus [10, 111]. Cell group f has been considered one of the principal sources of secondary vestibulocerebellar fibers [24], but the present observations indicate that cells of this nucleus do not project to either the fastigial nucleus or to basal folia of the uvula.

More recent studies of cerebellar afferent projections from the vestibular nuclei based upon the retrograde transport of HRP in the cat suggest that secondary vestibulocerebellar fibers project to larger areas of the cerebellum [71]. According to these authors, the MVN and IVN and cell groups f and x project bilaterally to the entire cerebellar vermis, the flocculus, the fastigial nucleus, and the anterior and posterior interposed nuclei. Their evidence suggested a bilateral projection from vestibular nuclei to the cerebellar vermis with a more extensive ipsilateral projection. When large regions of the cerebellar vermis were labeled, retrograde transport of the marker was described in both the superior and lateral vestibular nuclei. It was their interpretation that cerebellar projections from the SVN and LVN to the cerebellar vermis were diffuse, with each folium receiving only a few collaterals of principal axons. This study differs from our own in several respects, namely, projections from cell group f and the LVN. In addition, there appear to be certain quantitative and qualitative differences in the cerebellar projections of the IVN, MVN, and SVN. These differences appeared related largely to more extensive labeling of the vermal cortex and perhaps less labeling of the fastigial nucleus. We concur with these investigators regarding their conclusion that a large number of cells in group x project bilaterally to the uvula.

Perihypoglossal Nuclei. The nuclei grouped under this designation, the nucleus prepositus, the nucleus intercalatus, and the nucleus of Roller, were described in detail by Brodal [13] and considered to project to the cerebellum. In a later study, based upon the modified Gudden method, it was determined that these nuclei projected to the anterior lobe, the pyramis, the uvula, and the fastigial nuclei [103]. Degeneration studies provided data suggesting that crossed fastigial efferent fibers projected to all perihypoglossal nuclei, while uncrossed efferents passed to the dorsal part of the ipsilateral nucleus prepositus [106]. Subsequent HRP studies provided evidence that the perihypoglossal nuclei projected to: (a) the oculomotor nuclear complex [55, 59, 98] and (b) the cerebellar flocculus, nodulus, and lobule VI [3, 57]. The part of the nucleus prepositus projecting to the flocculus appears to be the part most clearly related to eye movements [9, 53]. Studies in the cat indicated that HRP injected into the fastigial nucleus was transported bilaterally to cells in the caudal third of the nucleus prepositus [93]. The largest number of labeled cells in these nuclei was found ipsilaterally, and a few cells with HRP granules were seen in the nucleus of Roller (Figs. 1, 2). Label also was seen in the nuclei prepositus following HRP labeling of posterior vermal cortex, but no HRP-labeled cells were seen in these nuclei when basal folia of lobules V and VI were injected with the enzyme.

It is apparent that the projections of the perihypoglossal nuclei are diverse and incompletely understood. Such data as are available suggest that cells in portions of the nucleus prepositus project to: (a) the oculomotor complex, (b) the flocculus, and (c) the fastigial nuclei. Cells projecting fibers to the fastigial nuclei may also supply portions of the uvula.

Paramedian Reticular Nuclei. These nuclei, originally described by Brodal [14] in the cat, consist of dorsal, ventral, and accessory groups of large cells separated from the median raphe by fibers of the medial longitudinal fasciculus and the medial lemniscus. These cell groups in transverse sections are found at levels through the middle third of the inferior olivary complex, and most, if not all, cells send fibers to the cerebellum. Using the modified Gudden technique it was determined that all three cell groups send fibers to the anterior lobe, the pyramis, and the uvula [23]. It was suggested that certain of the cell groups might project to the fastigial nuclei. Following lesions in various parts of the nervous system, it was determined that afferent fibers to these nuclei: (a) ascend in posterior columns of the spinal cord, (b) descend from frontoparietal cortex, and (c) appear to arise from, or pass through, pontomesencephalic regions of the brain stem [18]. In subsequent studies it was determined that the paramedian reticular nuclei receive projections from the fastigial nucleus [27, 30, 101, 112] and from the dentate nucleus via the descending division of the superior cerebellar peduncle [22, 29]. Most of these fibers from the fastigial nucleus are crossed and end in relationship to cells of the dorsal paramedian reticular nucleus [10]. Projections from the cerebral cortex pass to both dorsal and ventral paramedian reticular nuclei from distinctive regions [97].

Following HRP injections in the fastigial nucleus, only a few cells of the dorsal paramedian reticular nucleus were labeled bilaterally in retrograde fashion [93]. No label was seen in other cell groups of this reticular nucleus. It was our impression that the projection from the dorsal paramedian reticular nucleus to the fastigial nucleus was very modest.

In a comprehensive study of cerebellar afferents from the paramedian reticular nuclei in the cat and monkey, it was concluded that the majority of fibers project to the anterior lobe and the vermis of the posterior lobe [95]. The dorsal nuclear group apparently has broad connections with both the cerebellar cortex and all deep cerebellar nuclei.

Lateral Reticular Nucleus. This nucleus consisting of magnocellular, parvocellular, and subtrigeminal subdivisions receives efferent fibers from rostral parts of the fastigial nucleus which are crossed and mainly end in rostral parts of the magnocellular part [10]. In degeneration studies this fastigial projection was regarded as the smallest to any reticular nucleus [112]. Following well-localized HRP injections of the fastigial nucleus, no retrograde transport of the protein marker was seen in cells of any part of the lateral reticular nucleus [93]. When the enzyme marker labeled caudal parts of the fastigial nucleus and portions of the posterior vermal cortex (i.e., basal folia of the pyramis and uvula), retrograde transport of HRP was seen bilaterally in a few cells in all subdivisions of the lateral reticular nucleus. No labeled cells in the lateral reticular nucleus were seen when HRP injections selectively labeled the rostral half of the fastigial nucleus. These observations suggested that the lateral reticular nucleus may not project specifically to the fastigial nucleus.

In an autoradiographic study in the cat, Künzle [74] traced projections from the lateral reticular nucleus to bilateral terminal fields in the anterior lobe, the paramedian lobule, and vermal lobule VIII, but no fibers were followed into the deep cerebellar nuclei. In another autoradiographic study using [^{35}S] methionine in the rat, fibers from this nucleus were traced to crus I, the paraflocculus, lobules VI and VII, and to the interposed and dentate nuclei [33]. In retrograde transport studies, cells of the lateral reticular nucleus were described as projecting to the entire cerebellar cortex and all cerebellar nuclei [43]. The most impressive projections were to the anterior lobe and lobule VIII of the posterior vermis.

Other Brain Stem Nuclei. In our retrograde transport study of fastigial afferent projections in the cat, labeled cells seen in a number of other brain stem nuclei appeared related to diffusion of HRP into various lobules of the cerebellar cortex [93]. Labeling of basal folia of lobules V and VI was associated with retrograde transport of the enzyme to neurons in the accessory cuneate nucleus as well as contralaterally in parts of the medial and dorsal accessory olivary nuclei. These observations appear consistent with the findings of Rinvik and Walberg [91] concerning the cerebellar projections of the accessory cuneate nucleus. Labeling of various portions of the vermal cortex was in some animals associated with retrograde transport of the enzyme bilaterally to pontine nuclei. Labeled cells in the pontine nuclei were primarily in dorsolateral regions, but sometimes were seen in cells in both medial and lateral cell columns. Occasionally a few labeled cells were found in the reticulotegmental nucleus. Available evidence did not suggest that any of these nuclei project afferents to the fastigial nucleus.

Although our studies of fastigial afferent projections from the brain stem did not reveal a contribution from the locus ceruleus, Somana and Walberg [96] indicate a small projection from this source to both the fastigial and anterior interposed nuclei. When the entire fastigial nucleus was labeled with HRP only three cells of the locus ceruleus contained HRP intracellular granules. These cells were restricted to caudal parts of the locus ceruleus. According to Chu and Bloom [35], cells of the locus ceruleus projecting to the cerebellum lie mainly in dorsolateral parts of the nucleus. Earlier degeneration studies in the cat suggested that the fastigial nucleus may project to the locus ceruleus [94]. Most of these fibers were described as ending in rostral parts of the locus ceruleus. In some control animals with lesions dorsal to the fastigial nucleus, fibers were described as projecting to the locus ceruleus, suggesting direct projections of Purkinje cell axons.

Primary Vestibulocerebellar Fibers

Using the Marchi method some early investigators traced primary vestibular fibers into the ipsilateral nodulus, uvula, and fastigial nucleus [44, 63]. More precise studies based on silver impregnations indicated that most primary vestibulocerebellar fibers ended as mossy fibers in the ipsilateral nodulus, uvula, and flocculus [19]. These authors did not find convincing degeneration in the fastigial nucleus, although degenerated fibers passed through parts of the nucleus. It was pointed out that these studies did not exclude the possibility of primary vestibular fibers ending in the fastigial nucleus. Similar observations were made in a study of degeneration resulting from small lesions in parts of the vestibular ganglion innervating distinctive receptor sites in the labyrinth [32]. However, in both of these studies a small number of primary vestibular fibers were found to end in ventromedial parts of the dentate nucleus. In a retrograde transport study, Kotchabhakdi and Walberg [72] concluded that the majority of vestibular ganglion cells projected to the cerebellar cortex, with indications that these neurons project to virtually the entire vermis. Thus present data concerning projections of vestibular ganglion cells to the fastigial nucleus remain unresolved.

Squirrel Monkey

Attempts were made to confirm the origins of fastigial afferents in two squirrel monkeys (*Saimiri sciureus*) using HRP and a more sensitive chromagen, tetramethylbenzidine (TMB [81]). The enzyme labeled the caudal third of the fastigial nucleus in one animal, while in the other animal the entire nucleus and a small medial part of the opposite fastigial nucleus were labeled (Fig. 3C). In both animals basal folia of the uvula exhibited uptake of the label. Although both injections appeared well localized to the fastigial nucleus in sections reacted with diaminobenzidine (DAB), the area of diffusion appeared larger in sections reacted with TMB. Retrograde transport of the enzyme to Purkinje cells in the ipsilateral vermis was considerable (Figs. 4B, 4C). Labeling of Purkinje cells was maximal in folia of lobules V and VI and relatively sparse in lobules I to IV when the entire nucleus was labeled. Retrograde transport of the enzyme was seen in nucleus β and contralaterally in parts of the medial accessory olivary nucleus.

Retrograde transport of the enzyme to cells in the vestibular nuclei was similar to that described for the cat, but was quantitatively much greater. The largest number of labeled cells were found in dorsal and lateral regions of the caudal half of the MVN.

Labeled cells in the nuclei were bilateral and symmetrical in distribution with only an occasional suggestion of a larger number of labeled cells ipsilateral to the injection (Fig. 5C). Caudal and dorsal portions of the inferior vestibular nuclei contained labeled cells distributed symmetrically, but no cells of group f were labeled (Figs. 6A, B). Cells of group x were labeled bilaterally and part of the labeling undoubtedly was due to involvement of portions of the uvula [93]. This interpretation is consistent with data suggesting that cell group x projects to both the fastigial nucleus and the uvula [17]. Cells in peripheral portions of the SVN were labeled bilaterally in both animals. These data are similar to those reported for the cat in that labeling of portions of the pyramis and uvula along with the fastigial nucleus almost invariably resulted in retrograde transport of the enzyme to cells of the SVN. Although this finding strengthens the possibility that some cells in the SVN may project to the fastigial, this projection, if it exists, is quantitatively less than that from the medial and inferior vestibular nuclei.

Other brain stem nuclei with bilateral retrograde cell label included: (a) the nucleus prepositus (Fig. 5D), (b) the nucleus of Roller, (c) the dorsal paramedian reticular nucleus (Fig. 6C), and (d) the lateral reticular nucleus. Labeled cells of the nuclei prepositus were seen mainly in caudal regions, as described in the cat. While label in the lateral reticular nucleus was not seen in the cat, except when portions of the posterior vermis were concomitantly labeled, the more sensitive chromagen revealed some labeled cells in the magnocellular and subtrigeminal subdivisions that may project to the fastigial nucleus, as reported by Dietrichs and Walberg [43]. On the basis of all data available, it is our impression that relatively few cells of the lateral reticular nucleus project to the fastigial nucleus. The more sensitive TMB technique further suggests that some cells in the dorsal paramedian reticular nucleus and the nucleus of Roller may project to the fastigial nucleus. Only modest retrograde transport to these nuclei was seen in studies of the cat using DAB. Observations with respect to the dorsal paramedian reticular nucleus are consistent with the findings of Somana and Walberg [95], but this nucleus also has strong connections with vermal lobules VII to X.

Summary

Studies of fastigial afferent fibers in the cat and monkey based upon the retrograde transport of HRP indicate that afferent fibers arise bilaterally from fairly symmetrical regions of the vestibular nuclei and from certain medullary cerebellar relay nuclei. These studies emphasize the difficulty in selectively labeling fastigial neurons with HRP. Conclusions drawn from this study and a review of the literature are as follows:

1. The largest number of brain stem efferents to the fastigial nucleus arise bilaterally from fairly symmetrical dorsal and lateral regions of the caudal part of the medial vestibular nucleus.
2. Fastigial afferent fibers arise bilaterally from symmetrical dorsal regions of caudal parts of the inferior vestibular nucleus, but not from cell group f.

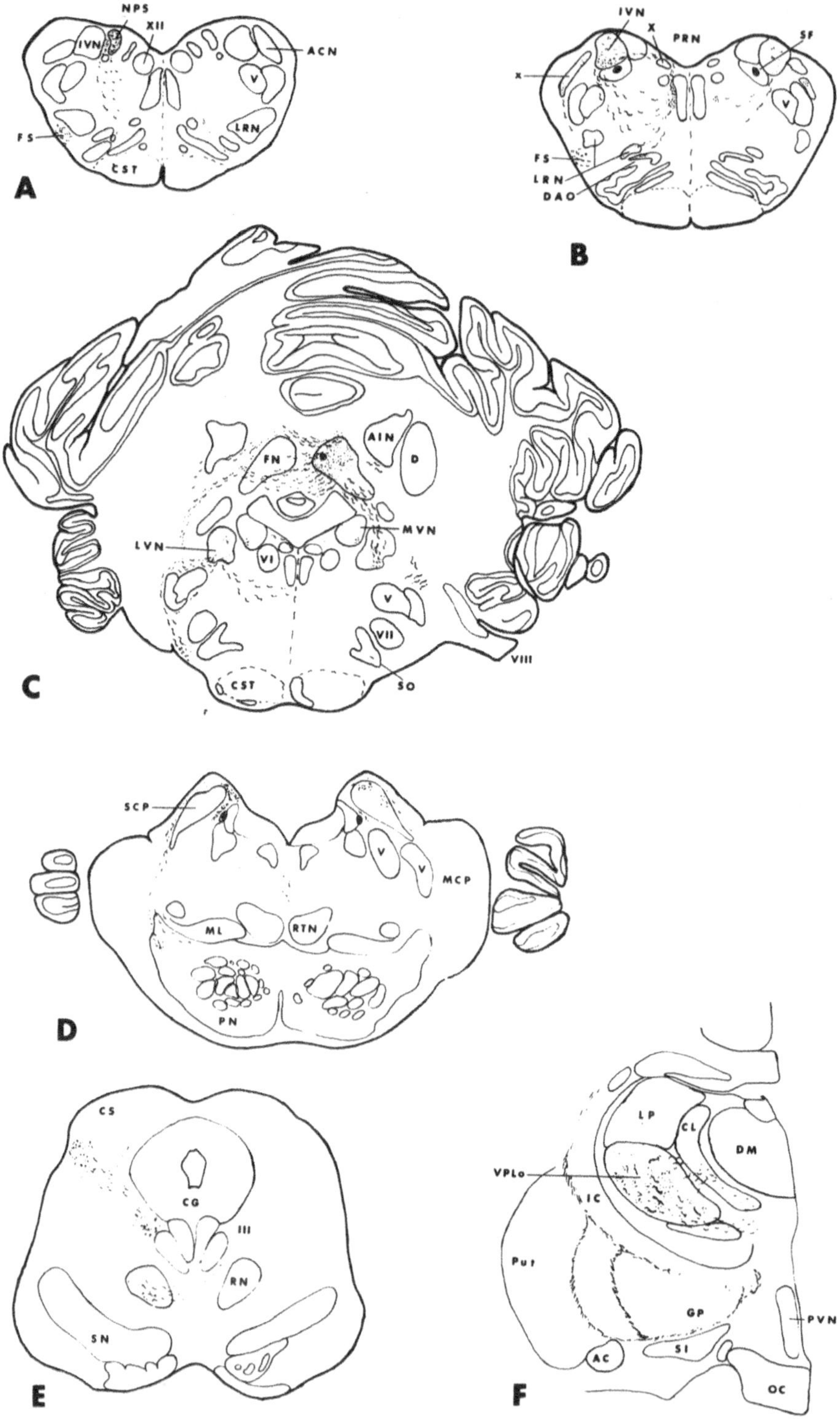
NPS
XII
IVN
ACN
V
LRN
FS
CST
A
IVN
X
PRN
SF
x
V
FS
LRN
DAO
B
AIN
FN
D
MVN
LVN
VI
V
VII
VIII
CST
SO
C
SCP
V
V
MCP
ML
RTN
PN
D
CS
CG
III
RN
SN
E
LP
CL
DM
VPLo
IC
Put
GP
PVN
AC
SI
OC
F

3. Cells of group x of the paravestibular nuclei on each side project to the fastigial nucleus and to basal folia of the uvula.
4. Some cells in peripheral parts of the superior vestibular nuclei may project to the fastigial nucleus, but a larger number of these cells appear to project to posterior portions of the vermal cortex.
5. No cells of the lateral vestibular nucleus project to the fastigial nucleus.
6. The fastigial nucleus receives bilateral projections from: (a) cells in caudal parts of the nucleus prepositus, (b) a few cells in the nucleus of Roller, and (c) cells in the dorsal paramedian reticular nuclei.
7. The fastigial nucleus receives axons of Purkinje cells in the ipsilateral cerebellar vermis, the largest number of which appear to arise from folia of lobules V, VI, and VII.
8. Olivary efferents to the fastigial nucleus arise contralaterally from nucleus β and the dorsomedial cell column.

Fastigial Efferent Projections

Small volumes of tritiated amino acids labeled cells in different parts of the fastigial nucleus in eight rhesus monkeys. Label was taken up by fastigial neurons in: (a) all parts of the nucleus (Figs. 7, 10A, 10B), (b) rostral parts of the nucleus (Figs. 9, 10E) and (c) caudal parts of the nucleus (Figs. 8, 12A). Although many cells within various parts of the fastigial nucleus appear to have common projections to the brain stem nuclei, cells in certain regions appear to have unique connections. An attempt has been made to analyze and synthesize the observations concerning fastigial efferent projections in the monkey based upon anterograde axoplasmic transport.

Efferent Fiber Bundles

It is generally accepted on the basis of degeneration studies that cells of the fastigial nucleus give rise to two distinct efferent bundles: (a) an uncrossed bundle that emerges from the cerebellum via the juxtarestiform body (JRB), and (b) a crossed bundle that forms the uncinate fasciculus (UF). Uncrossed fastigial efferent fibers in the JRB are considered to arise largely from cells in rostral portions of the nucleus, while fibers of the uncinate fasciculus are regarded as

Fig. 7A–F. Rhesus C-1385. Projection drawings of autoradiographs demonstrating transport of isotope from the right fastigial nucleus **C**. Labeled efferent fibers projected to the brain stem via the right juxtarestiform body and the left uncinate fasciculus. Axon terminals in ventral parts of the lateral (*LVN*) and inferior (*IVN*) vestibular nuclei were labeled nearly symmetrically **B, C**. Contralaterally labeled terminals surrounded cells in the dorsal paramedian reticular nucleus (*PRN*), the lateral reticular nucleus (*LRN*), cells in group x and the nucleus parasolitarius (*NPS*) **A, B**. Isotope also was present in fibers and terminals in the medial medullary and pontine reticular formation **B, C, D**. Ascending fastigial efferent fibers projected contralaterally to the superior colliculus **E**, and to the ventral posterior lateral nucleus (*VPLo*) **F** and the ventral lateral (*VLo*) thalamic nuclei. See Fig. 10A

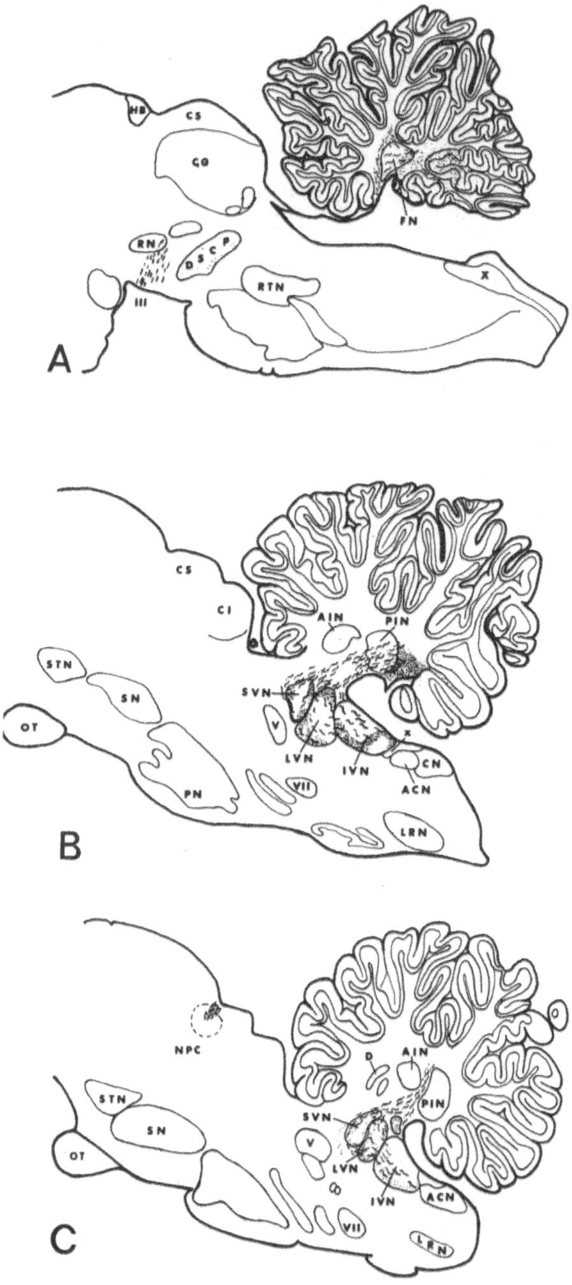

Fig. 8A–F. Cynomolgus C1423. Projection drawing of sagittal autoradiographs illustrating transport of isotope from cells in the caudal half of the right fastigial nucleus (*FN*) and the base of the uvula. **A–C** are ipsilateral to the injection site, while **D–F** are contralateral. Fastigial efferent fibers transported the [^{3}H] amino acid label bilaterally to ventral parts of the lateral (*LVN*) and inferior (*IVN*) vestibular nuclei **B, E**. Terminations in peripheral parts of the

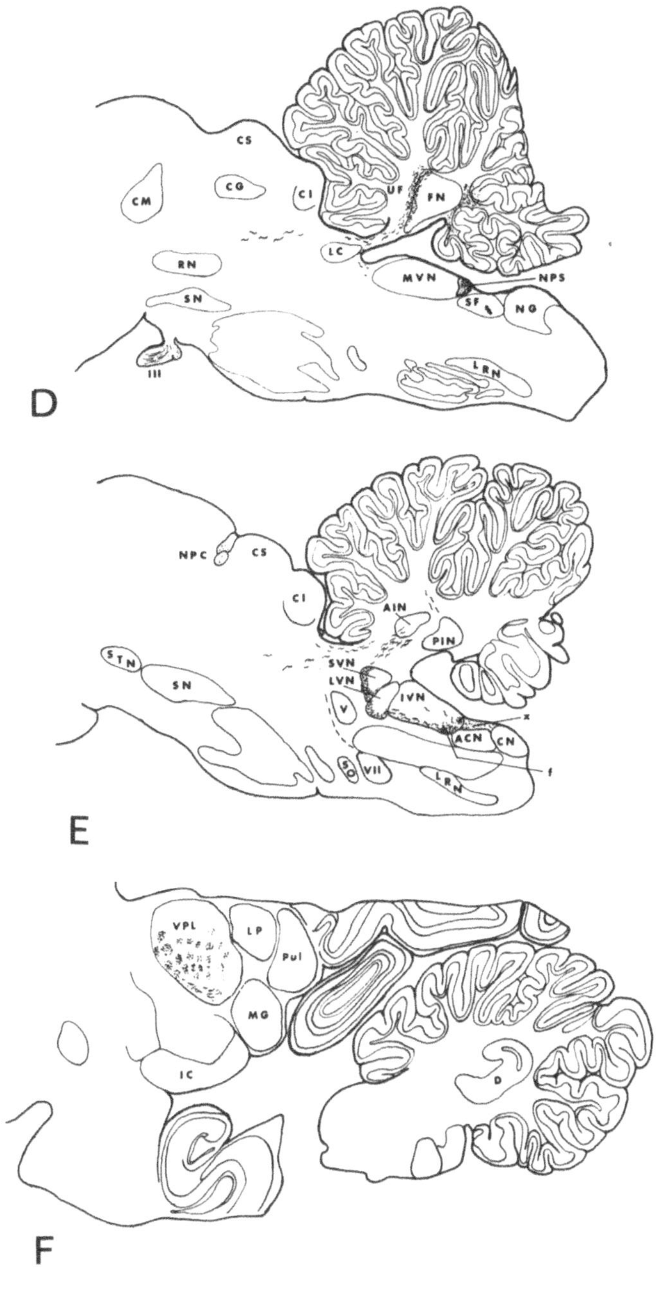

superior vestibular nuclei (*SVN*) were considered to be derived from labeled cortex of the pyramis and uvula **A**. Ascending fibers in the uncinate fasciculus terminated in discrete clusters in the contralateral ventral posterolateral nucleus (*VPLo* and *VPLc*) of the thalamus **F**. See Figs. 12, 13

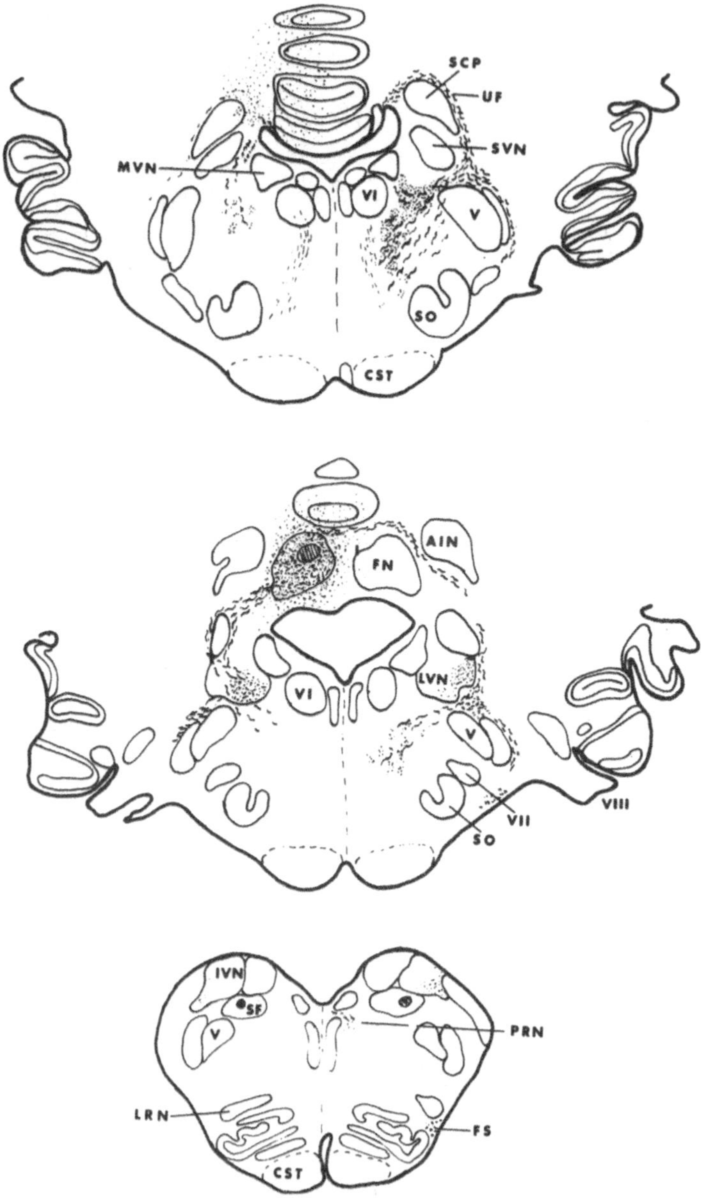

Fig. 9. Rhesus C-1393. Projection drawings of autoradiographs illustrating axoplasmic transport of [^{3}H] amino acid from cells in the rostral part of the left fastigial nucleus (*FN*). Label was transported only to the lower brain stem in the same manner as in rhesus C-1385 (Fig. 7). Descending fastigiospinal fibers (*FS*) were labeled on the right side. No label was transported to midbrain or diencephalic levels. See Fig. 10E

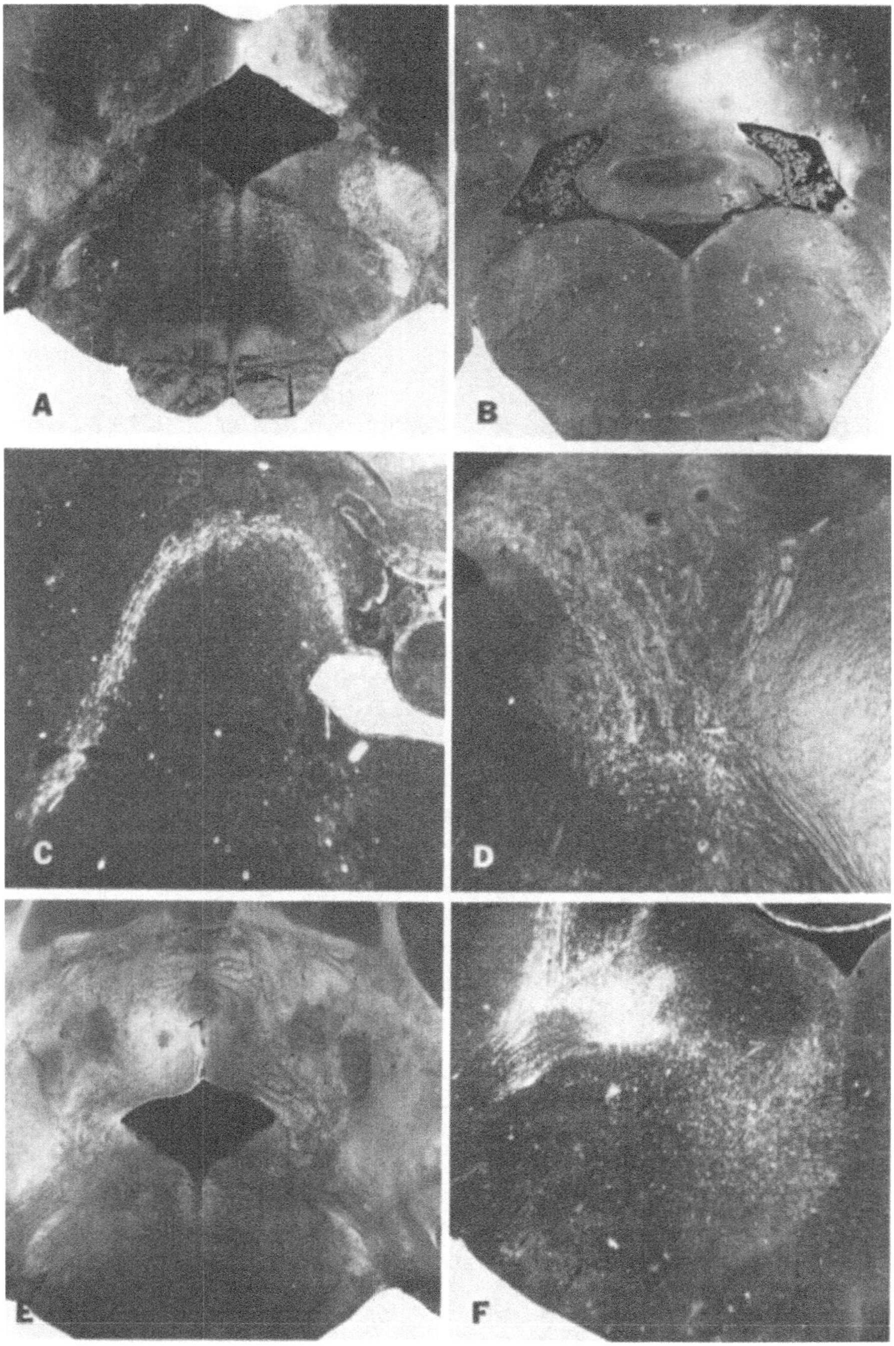

Fig. 10. A, B, E Dark-field photomicrographs of radioactive uptake in the fastigial nucleus in C-1385, U-36, and C-1393. Cresyl violet, ×6, ×10, ×10. Dark-field photomicrographs of isotope transported via the uncinate fasciculus **C** and the juxtarestiform body **D**. Cresyl violet, ×18, ×18. Dark-field photomicrograph of isotope transported to the lateral vestibular nucleus and the medial reticular formation **F**. Cresyl violet, ×12

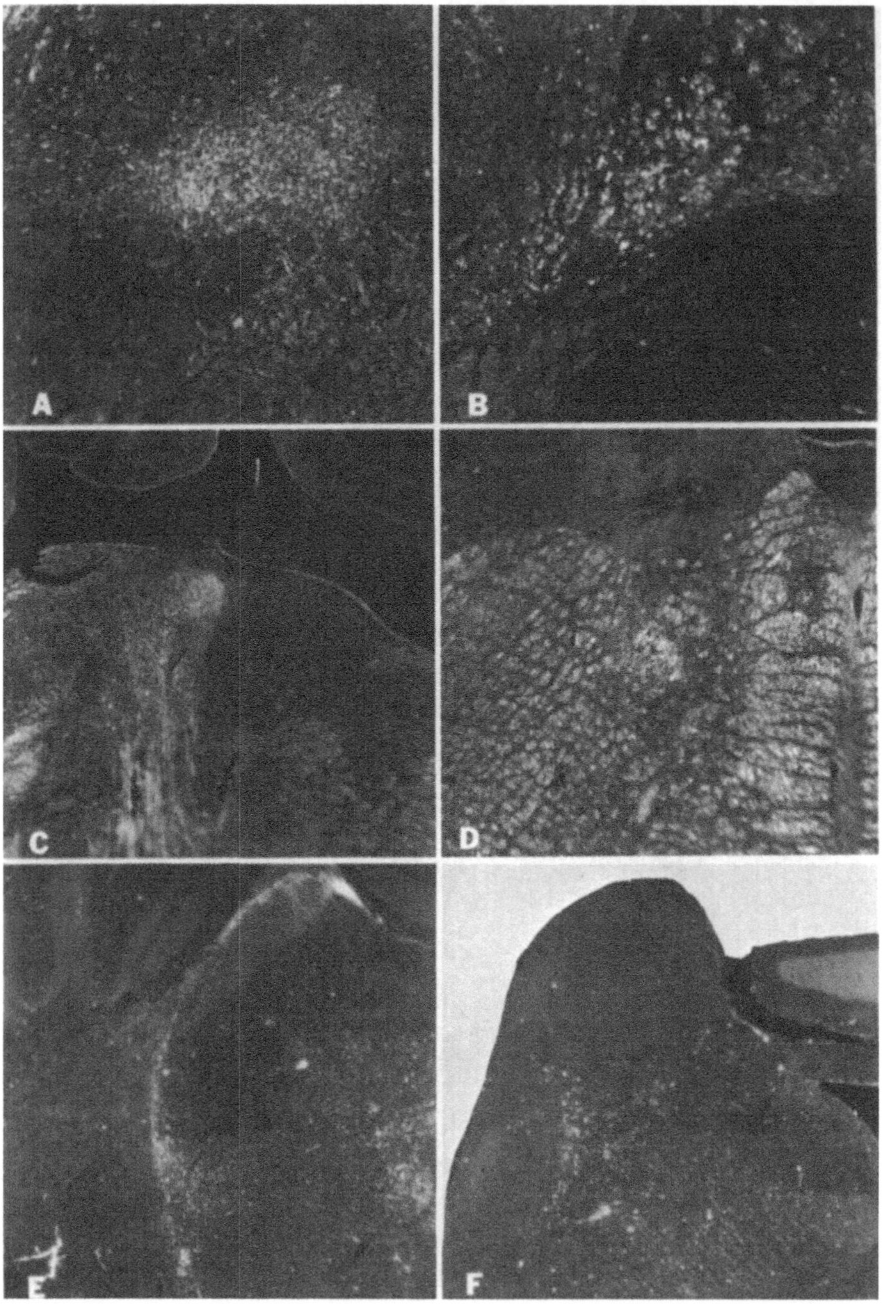

Fig. 11 A–F. Dark-field photomicrographs of isotope transported from the contralateral fastigial nucleus to: **A** the lateral vestibular nucleus; **B** the inferior vestibular nucleus and cell group x; **C** the nucleus parasolitarius; **D** the dorsal paramedian reticular nucleus; **E** the dorsolateral pontine nuclei. Cresyl violet, × 25, × 25, × 18, × 25, × 6. **F** Ascending fibers of the uncinate fasciculus in the dorsolateral tegmentum, ventral to the inferior colliculus and medial to the nucleus of the lateral lemniscus. Cresyl violet, × 12

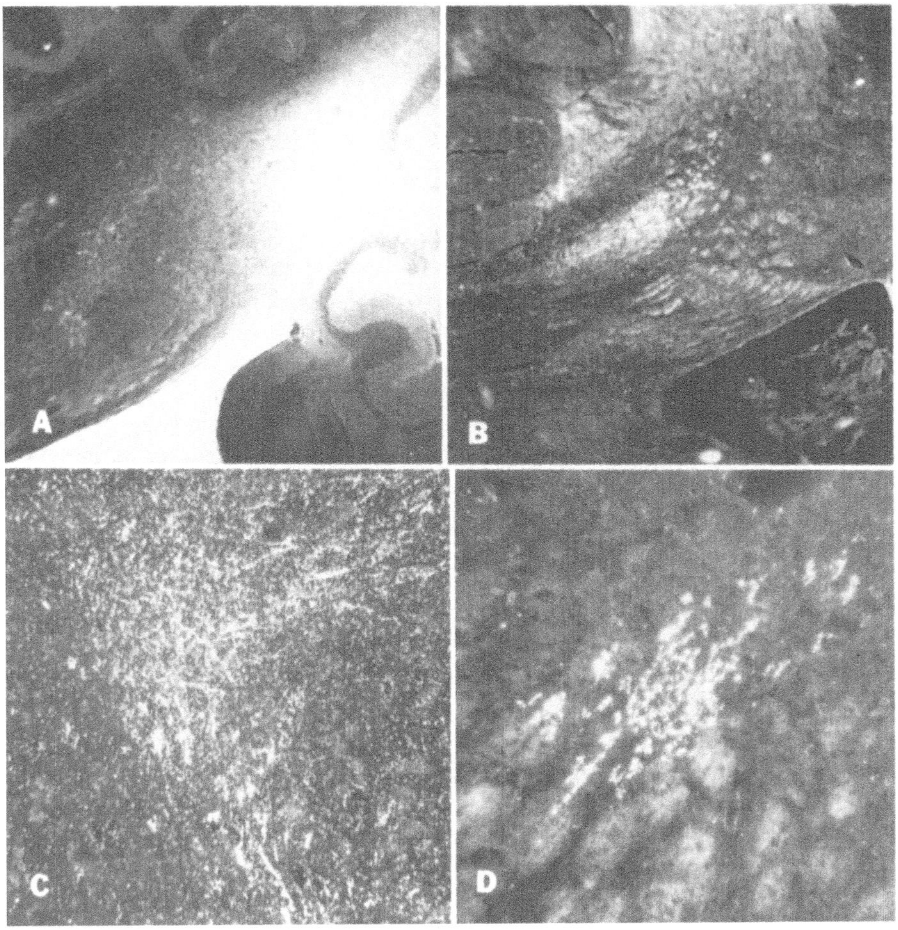

Fig. 12A–D. Cynomolgus C-1423. Dark-field photomicrographs of sagittal autoradiographs. **A** fastigial nucleus showing uptake of isotope in the caudal half of the nucleus and in the uvula; **B** transport of isotope by fibers of the uncinate fasciculus; **C** transport of isotope to cells in peripheral parts of the superior vestibular nucleus due to labeling of portions of the uvula; **D** transport of isotope across the midline in the posterior commissure. Cresyl violet, × 12, × 12, × 52, × 133

arising predominantly from cells in caudal parts of the nucleus [6, 27, 30, 36, 51, 68, 89, 104, 111]. Because lesions of the fastigial nucleus concomitantly interrupt fibers traversing various portions of the nucleus, the resulting patterns of degeneration are difficult to interpret. Observations based upon anterograde transport of [^{3}H] amino acids suggest a different origin of the fibers in these bundles. Fairly selective unilateral labeling of cells in either the rostral or caudal parts of the fastigial nucleus resulted in transport of the isotope via uncrossed fibers in the JRB and crossed fibers in the contralateral UF (Figs. 7, 8, 9, 10C, 10D, 12B). Although transport of isotope via these bundles was not as great as when the entire fastigial nucleus (FN) was labeled, these data suggested that cells at all rostrocaudal levels of the FN give rise to crossed fibers, while axonal collaterals or other cells project fibers ipsilaterally into the brain stem. It is our impression that the crossed fibers greatly exceed those that are uncrossed. It is interesting that in only one degeneration study is the view expressed that the entire FN participates in the formation of the UF [112]. Uncrossed fastigial efferent fibers project largely, but not exclusively, to subdivisions of the ipsilateral vestibular nuclear complex. Although fibers of the UF have been described as crossing through rostral parts of the contralateral FN [27, 36, 84, 101], there is suggestive evidence from degeneration studies [27] and better evidence from axoplasmic transport studies indicating that the majority of fibers crossing to the opposite side pass above, below, or around the rostral pole of the contralateral FN rather than through it [10]. In sagittal sections a large number of fibers of the UF cross to the opposite side rostral to the oral pole of the anterior interposed nucleus (Fig. 12B). In the monkey, fibers of the UF sweep laterally over the dorsal and lateral borders of the superior cerebellar peduncle as a rather broad band. Rostrally fibers descend ventrally to a position dorsal to the trigeminal nuclear complex; caudally the most ventral fibers partially traverse and interdigitate with the root fibers of the vestibular nerve before abruptly arching medially into ventral regions of the lateral vestibular nucleus (Fig. 10F). In the upper pons, a much smaller bundle of crossed fastigial efferent fibers, extending laterally from the superior medullary velum, lies between the anterior spinocerebellar tract and the superior cerebellar peduncle (SCP). No fibers of the UF enter the SCP or pass rostrally with that bundle in the monkey. While the course followed by the UF in the cat is similar, some fastigial efferent fibers traverse dorsal parts of the SCP as this bundle emerges from the cerebellum, but they do not become incorporated within that peduncle [30].

There is no evidence that fibers arising from either the anterior (AIN) or posterior (PIN) interposed nuclei enter either the UF or the JRB [5, 10, 27, 37].

Fastigiovestibular Fibers

Data from degeneration studies suggest that fastigial efferent fibers project bilaterally and differentially to parts of the four vestibular nuclei and to certain paravestibular nuclei [27, 101, 104, 111]. Both crossed and uncrossed projections to the SVN were described as chiefly supplying peripheral regions of nucleus which do not receive terminals from primary vestibular fibers [110, 111].

Particular significance was attached to the FN projection upon the LVN in which crossed fibers were described as projecting to ventral regions of the nucleus, while uncrossed fibers were said to terminate in dorsal regions. Because the cerebellar vermis projects somatotopically in a regular fanlike manner upon the FN [45, 66, 67] and the vestibulospinal projection is somatotopically organized [85], the hypothesis was advanced that a somatotopic linkage existed between the vermal cortex and the spinal cord which involved both the FN and the LVN [111]. While these anatomical data were supported by some physiological findings [86], the authors acknowledged the existence of a number of direct cortical cerebellovestibular fibers that traverse portions of the FN. In the LVN relatively few fastigial efferent fibers are said to establish synaptic contact with giant cells.

Fastigial projections to the IVN in degeneration studies suggested that crossed fibers terminated in ventral regions of the nucleus while uncrossed fibers ended in more dorsal regions. Cells in group f of the IVN and cell group x of the paravestibular nuclei were found to receive projections bilaterally from the FN.

Unlike the other vestibular nuclei, fastigial projections to the MVN were reported to cover the entire nucleus ipsilaterally except for its ventral margin. With certain exceptions like the SVN and cell groups f and x, the general concept proposed was that crossed and uncrossed fastigial efferent fibers projected bilaterally to parts of all four vestibular nuclei and that the ipsilateral projections terminated in regions of LVN, IVN, and MVN that did not receive crossed fibers.

The pattern of fastigial efferent projections upon the vestibular nuclei determined in the monkey by axoplasmic transport techniques [10] were strikingly different from those arrived at from the above-cited degeneration studies. The principal differences evident in axoplasmic transport studies were that fastigial projections to the vestibular nuclei were largely confined to ventral portions of the LVN and IVN, were nearly symmetrical in distribution, and were quantitatively similar on each side (Figs. 7, 8, 9, 10D, 10F, 11A). Labeling of cells in the rostral third of the FN appeared to result in more abundant terminals in lateral regions of the ipsilateral LVN that extended into parts of the IVN. With labeling of cells in all other regions of the FN, isotope was primarily transported bilaterally to ventral regions of LVN; uncrossed fibers appeared to end in slightly more medial and caudal regions of the nucleus. Terminals in LVN surrounded cells of all sizes, but not all large cells in ventral parts of the nucleus appear to receive fastigial efferents. Descending fibers traversing ventral parts of the LVN entered predominantly ventrolateral regions of the IVN on both sides where numerous fibers terminated.

The most notable difference between the two sides concerned the asymmetrical fastigial projections to: (a) cell group f of the IVN, (b) cell group x, and (c) the MVN. Fibers projecting to cell groups f and x arise from all parts of the FN, and are entirely crossed; the largest number of these fibers arise from caudal parts of the FN (Figs. 7, 8, 9, 11B). Labeling of cells in the rostral third of the FN (C-1368) did not result in transport of the label to cells of group f or x on either side. When cells in larger rostral portions of FN (C-1369 and C-1393) or in caudal parts of FN were labeled, silver grains were profuse around cells of group f and x only on the contralateral side. In only one animal were a few terminals seen in cell group f ipsilateral to labeled fastigial neurons (Fig. 9). In none of the animals was label from fastigial neurons transported ipsilaterally to the small cells of cell group x.

Fastigial projections to ipsilateral MVN were seen only in animals in which virtually all cells of the FN were labeled (C-1385 and C-1386); in these animals a modest number of silver grains were seen ventrolaterally in rostral portions of the ipsilateral MVN. A small number of silver grains occasionally were seen about the ventral border of the contralateral MVN, but grains appeared to be mostly in fibers projecting medially and ventrally into the reticular formation. While it is likely that fibers passing to MVN may represent a unique uncrossed fastigiovestibular projection, as postulated by Walberg et al. [111], these fibers are much less numerous than degeneration studies indicate. The possibility remains that part of the fibers described in degeneration studies may arise from the vermal cortex. Although no region of the anterior vermal cortex has been identified as projecting exclusively to MVN [104, 107], portions of lobules IX and X appear to send fibers to some parts of MVN [7, 104].

Crossed fastigial efferent fibers extend nearly to the caudal pole of the IVN, but at levels where the nucleus is quite narrow labeled fibers become concentrated in medial regions. Most of the labeled fibers in this part of the nucleus projected medially to terminate about small cells of the nucleus parasolitarius (Figs. 7, 11 C). Although some authors have considered these fibers to descend in the tractus solitarius, there is no doubt from these studies or those of Walberg et al. [111] or Voogd [104] that large numbers of fibers end immediately lateral and dorsal to the nucleus of the solitary tract, in what is now called the nucleus parasolitarius. Fibers passing to the nucleus parasolitarius (NPS) arise from all parts of the FN and are exclusively crossed. Neither the connections nor the function of NPS are known, but the well-defined nature of terminals in this nucleus suggests that fastigial inputs may influence nuclei concerned with autonomic functions by as yet undisclosed synaptic articulations with vagal nuclei or reticular neurons. A few fibers could be traced caudally beyond the NPS into more caudal parts of the medullary reticular formation.

Transport of label to cells of the superior vestibular nucleus was seen bilaterally in only one animal (Figs. 8, 12C). In this animal (C-1423) primary label was taken up by cells in caudal parts of the FN and in deep folia of the uvula. Terminal label was profuse in peripheral parts of the SVN and corresponded to descriptions based on degenerative technique [111]. This finding was unique in this study in that similar transport was not associated with selective labeling of either rostral fastigial neurons or with labeling of neurons throughout the length of the nucleus. This discrepancy appears due to concomitant labeling of the cortical neurons in deep folia of the uvula. Lesions confined to these portions of the uvula are known to produce degeneration in peripheral portions of the SVN [7, 16, 104]. Since projections from the uvula to the vestibular nuclei pass through parts of the FN, these fibers frequently were interrupted by lesions in that nucleus.

These observations suggest that cells in all parts of the FN project crossed and uncrossed fibers to ventral portions of the LVN and IVN which distributed to nearly symmetrical regions and are quantitatively similar. The ventral regions of termination of fastigial efferent fibers in the LVN, suggest that the excitatory influences relayed by the somatotopically organized vestibulospinal tract probably are restricted to cervical spinal segments. Fastigial efferent fibers projecting to cell group f of the IVN and to cell group x are entirely crossed and while they arise from all parts of the nucleus, the largest number originate from caudal regions (Figs. 7, 8, 11 B). A very small number of uncrossed fastigial efferent fibers terminate ventrolaterally in rostral parts of the ipsilateral MVN. No fastigial neurons project to the SVN or the interstitial nucleus of the vestibular nerve on either side.

Fastigioreticular Fibers

Fastigial efferent fibers projecting to the reticular formation of the pons and medulla have been described by several authors using a variety of degeneration techniques [27, 30, 36, 88, 101, 104, 117]. The largest numbers of these fibers are crossed and appear to end predominantly in dorsal and medial regions of the reticular formation. In the most thorough study of fastigioreticular projections, it was concluded that these fibers: (a) arise from all parts of the FN, (b) largely cross in the cerebellum and emerge via the UF, and (c) are distributed mainly to the nucleus reticularis gigantocellularis (NRG), the reticulotegmental nucleus (NRT) and the paramedian reticular nucleus (PRN). More modest projections listed in decreasing order, were found in the pontine reticular formation, the ventral reticular nucleus, the parvicellular reticular nucleus, the subceruleus nucleus and the lateral reticular nucleus. The authors had difficulty determining whether an ipsilateral fastigioreticular projection existed because: (a) caudal lesions in the FN gave rise to only a few degenerated fibers in the reticular formation, and (b) the intensity and extent of degeneration in the ipsilateral reticular formation could not be correlated with the size of lesions in rostral parts of the FN. Nevertheless, it was their impression that the ipsilateral fastigioreticular projection was modest. No topical arrangement was evident in the fastigal efferent projection to the reticular formation.

Axoplasmic transport studies indicate that fastigioreticular projections: (a) are mainly, but not exclusively, crossed, (b) arise predominantly from rostral parts of the nucleus, and (c) project mainly to three reticular nuclei, the NRG, the dorsal PRN, and the magnocellular part of the lateral reticular nucleus (LRN). These fibers emerge from the cerebellum via the UF, traverse portions of the LVN, IVN, and MVN (Figs. 7, 9, 10 F). At levels of the vestibular nerve root a conspicuous bundle of fibers separates from the UF, arches medially through ventral portions of the LVN and MVN, traverses the facial nerve, and sprays out into a number of small fascicles which project ventromedially into the reticular formation. Other fibers descending in the IVN leave this nucleus at various levels and project ventromedially into the medullary reticular formation. These fibers traverse portions of the spinal trigeminal nucleus and the region medial to it. As described by Walberg, Pompeiano, Brodal, and Jansen [111], a few fibers traverse portions of the NPS and pass ventrolaterally into the LRN. Fibers entering the reticular formation via these diverse routes are distributed to the NRG, the PRN, and the LRN. The most massive reticular projection is to the NRG; terminals and fibers of passage are profuse in medial, rostral, and dorsal regions of the nucleus from levels of the abducens nucleus to caudal olivary levels of the medulla.

Fastigial efferents traversing parts of the NRG project medially to discrete terminations about cells of the dorsal PRN (Figs. 9, 11 D). A few fibers entering this nucleus may pass through or near the NPS. The ventral cell groups of the

PRN only occasionally contained small collections of silver grains. Studies based upon HRP indicate that the fibers from the PRN project to the anterior lobe and to the vermis of the posterior lobe, except for lobules VII B and VIII A [95]; the dorsal nuclear group of PRN appears to be connected with a greater part of the cerebellar cortex and with all deep nuclei.

From medial regions of the NRG fibers projected ventrolaterally and caudally into parts of the LRN. Most of the terminals were found in rostral regions near cells of the magnocellular subdivisions, but occasionally a few silver grains also were seen in the parvocellular and subtrigeminal parts. Transport of label to portions of the LRN was associated with uptake of primary label by cells in rostral fastigial neurons; caudal fastigial neurons showed no transport of label to this nucleus. Thus, fastigial efferent fibers articulate predominantly with cells in the so-called supraspinal part of the LRN, confirming earlier observations from degeneration studies [35, 101, 109, 112]. This is regarded as one of the smallest projections to a specific reticular nucleus and can easily be missed in axoplasmic transport studies if there is a high background of silver grains. The LRN also receives rubrobulbar fibers, but these fibers end in the subtrigeminal division [37, 49, 105]. Both anterograde and retrograde axoplasmic transport studies indicate that the LRN projects bilaterally to nearly the entire cerebellar cortex [43, 74]. Retrograde transport studies further indicate that the cerebellar nuclei receive fibers from all subdivisions of the nucleus, although the majority of these fibers arise from the magnocellular subdivision [43].

In degeneration studies fastigioreticular fibers were described in other reticular nuclei, such as the nucleus reticularis pontis (caudalis and oralis; NRPC, NRPO), and the reticulotegmental nucleus (RTN) [104, 112]. Transport of isotope in relatively small amounts was consistently seen in caudal and medial portions of the pontine reticular formation (NRPC) near its junctions with the NRG. In the RTN only modest transport of isotope was seen in three animals in which caudal fastigial neurons were labeled. Silver grains were present about cells mainly in dorsal regions of the RTN (Fig. 7). Fibers in the pontine reticular formation may project ventrally into the RTN as suggested by Voogd [104], but this was not evident in our material. Isotope seen in these reticular nuclei probably was transported from the opposite FN, since there is no evidence that the AIN or the PIN project to either of these nuclei [5, 36].

In several animals a relatively small number of uncrossed fastigial efferent fibers emerging from the JRB were seen to project ventromedially into the reticular formation ventral to the MVN. These fibers were restricted to dorsal and rostral regions of the NRG, although a few appear to descend in the IVN before passing into the medullary reticular formation. These ipsilateral fastigioreticular fibers were evident in animals with profuse primary label in all parts of the FN. It is our impression that these fibers also arise mainly from rostral parts of the FN.

Thus fastigioreticular fibers arise predominantly from rostral parts of the FN, are mainly crossed and project largely to three reticular nuclei, the NRG, the dorsal PRN, and the magnocellular part of the LRN. Smaller projections pass to the NRPC and the RTN. Three of these nuclei are known to project back to the cerebellum and the dorsal PRN has projections to the FN.

Perihypoglossal Nuclei

Descending fastigiofugal fibers have been traced to the perihypoglossal nuclei, a nuclear complex that becomes increasingly differentiated in higher mammals [2, 101, 105, 106]. Of the degeneraton studies only that of Walberg [106] considered these nuclei in precise detail. According to the latter author, fibers terminating in the nucleus intercalatus (IN), the nucleus of Roller (NR), and the ventral part of the nucleus prepositus (NPP) are derived from caudal regions of the contralateral FN. These crossed fibers were described as passing via the UF. Ipsilateral projections from the FN were described as passing via the JRB to terminations only in dorsal regions of the NPP. These fibers were regarded as arising from rostral parts of the FN. Anterograde axoplasmic transport studies in the monkey failed to confirm these observations. In eight monkeys in which cells in various parts of the FN were labeled, including three animals with label in all parts of the nucleus, no isotope was transported to cells of the perihypoglossal nuclear complex. Even though some fibers projecting to the perihypoglossal nuclei are said to emanate from the region of the nucleus parasolitarius, convincing terminals were not seen in any of the perihypoglossal nuclei. This discrepancy suggests that the FN probably is traversed by fibers from some unidentified source that were interrupted by lesions in the nucleus. Efferent projections from both the uvula and the nodulus enter the FN and some of these fibers pass beyond it to terminate in parts of the SVN and MVN, cell group f and the NPP [7].

Fastigiopontine Fibers

One fastigiofugal pathway apparently not described in degeneration studies is a crossed projection to the pontine nuclei [10]. As previously described, fibers of the UF hook around the superior cerebellar peduncle in a rather broad band that extends from levels of the vestibular nerve root to isthmus levels. Although the majority of fibers in this bundle make an abrupt change of direction near the vestibular root and project into ventral parts of the LVN and the reticular formation, a small distinct part of this bundle continues ventrally between the middle cerebellar peduncle and the spinal trigeminal tract. In some sections it is possible to follow these fibers in continuity from rostral parts of the UF directly to the dorsolateral and rostral pontine nuclei where they terminate in a localized region (Figs. 7D, 11E). In other sections, fibers ventral to the spinal trigeminal tract pass to more rostral regions of the pontine nuclei where they terminate. This is a substantial, totally crossed projection that must constitute part of a feedback system similar to that of the descending division of the superior cerebellar peduncle [22, 29]. Available evidence suggests that the dorsolateral pontine nuclei, which receive fibers from the fastigial nucleus, project chiefly upon the vermal cerebellar cortex [20].

Fastigiospinal Projections

For most of this century, it generally has been accepted that the cerebellum exerted its modulating influences upon segmental levels of the spinal cord indirectly. Older literature describing cerebellar fibers projecting directly to spinal levels was ignored or discredited [78, 83, 99, 100]. These fibers, considered to originate from the dentate nucleus, were described as traversing the vestibular nuclei and descending with the vestibulospinal tract. According to Thomas [100], an ipsilateral cerebellospinal tract descending in the anterolateral region of the spinal cord extended into lumbar segments. A similar tract, said to originate from the dentate and interposed nuclei, was described in silver impregnation studies by Achenbach and Goodman [1], but these uncrossed fibers could be followed only into cervical spinal segments. Crossed projections from cerebellum to spinal cord have been considered to arise from the FN in a number of degeneration studies [1, 101, 104, 113]. These fibers have been considered to terminate in upper cervical spinal segments, except in studies of the rat and tree shrew where they were reported at virtually all spinal levels [1, 113]. The course taken by these fibers in the brain stem through the reticular formation appears quite different from what we have seen.

While our data concerning fastigiospinal projections is limited and incomplete, it provides information relative to the course of these fibers in the brain stem. Further, these data leave no doubt that the system originates within the FN.

Fastigiospinal fibers emerge from the cerebellum with the UF, are entirely crossed, and separate from that bundle near the site where fastigiopontine fibers become distinguishable [10]. As the UF sweeps ventrolaterally around the SCP in the upper pons, part of the fibers continue ventrally in a gentle arc between the middle cerebellar peduncle and the spinal trigeminal tract. Ventral to the spinal trigeminal tract most of these fibers enter the dorsolateral pontine nuclei, either directly or by following a slightly rostral course. A small number of fibers separating from the fastigiopontine bundle ventral to the spinal trigeminal tract descends along the ventrolateral border of the pons and medulla (Figs. 7A, 7B, 9A). These descending fibers are fastigiospinal. In their descent the fibers pass lateral to the facial motor nucleus, enter the retro-olivary region of the medulla, and become intermingled with fibers of the vestibulospinal tract. Rostral to this point the vestibulospinal tract and fastigiospinal fibers are widely separated because the vestibulospinal tract follows a meandering, diffuse course through parts of the reticular formation. Fastigiospinal fibers do not appear to receive additional contributions from the nucleus reticularis gigantocellularis or the lateral reticular nucleus, or the project to these nuclei. Fibers of this small tract are difficult to follow in transverse autoradiographs, but were identified at brain stem levels in five monkeys; these fibers were traced into the C-1 spinal segment in only two monkeys. Silver grains located along the ventrolateral border of the anterior horn could be followed to apparent terminations near anterior horn cells. Because fastigiospinal fibers were identified only in animals where primary label involved cells in rostral parts of the nucleus, it was our impression that most of these fibers originated from that part.

The most precise method to determine the cells of origin of a pathway in the central nervous system is based upon the retrograde transport of HRP. Following HRP injections into the spinal gray of the cat cord at various levels, it was determined that the largest number of retrogradely labeled neurons in the contralateral FN were associated with primary label injected into the C_2-C_3 segments [54, 79]. Horseradish peroxidase injections of the spinal gray at lower cervical spinal levels resulted in retrograde labeling of a smaller number of fastigial neurons and no enzyme was transported to these cells from injections made at lumbar levels. These studies differed in their descriptions of the localization of labeled fastigial neurons. According to Fukushima, Peterson, Uchino, Coulter, and Wilson [54], labeled cells were found throughout the contralateral FN, but were most numerous in rostral parts; in a similar study labeled neurons were distributed primarily in central and caudal parts of the FN and extended ventrolaterally into a zone between the fastigial and the anterior interposed nuclei [79]. Data also suggest that cells in the posterior interposed nucleus give rise to crossed fibers that have a similar termination in the spinal gray at the C_2-C_3 level. An autoradiographic study of spinal projections from the interposed nucleus (not otherwise specified) indicated that these fibers emerge from the cerebellum via the superior cerebellar peduncle, decussate at midbrain levels and descend [8]. These fibers descend into upper cervical segments and apparently end around large neurons in Rexed's lamina VII. None of these fibers appear to terminate around motoneurons. Physiological studies based upon antidromic stimulation of the upper cervical spinal cord and direct stimulation of the fastigial nucleus present strong evidence that axons of fastigiospinal neurons make monosynaptic contacts with motoneurons at the C_2-C_3 level [114]. Stimulation of the rostral fastigial nucleus evoked small EPSPs in some shoulder and dorsal neck motoneurons. Other evidence suggests there is an extensive convergence of impulses on fastigiospinal neurons from both the labyrinth and the periphery (via cutaneous nerves). These excitatory inputs to the FN are modulated by Purkinje cell inhibition [48, 65]. The fastigial output, in turn, exerts excitatory effects upon spinal motoneurons: (a) indirectly via relays in the vestibular nuclei and reticular formation [47, 64, 84], and (b) directly via fastigiospinal projections [114]. While anatomical and physiological results demonstrate a short-latency, monosynaptic, excitatory, fastigiospinal projection to C_2-C_3 motoneurons, this may not be the only connection made by these fibers. As Wilson et al. [114] have pointed out, some fastigiospinal fibers probably extend below cervical spinal segments and those ending in cervical segments could influence neurons at more caudal levels via propriospinal systems. Present anatomical evidence supports the thesis that both direct and indirect fastigial influences upon the spinal cord effect neurons mainly in cervical spinal segments, since fastigiovestibular fibers project to parts of the lateral vestibular nucleus that have connections with the cervical spinal cord [85].

Ascending Fastigial Efferent Projections

In spite of evidence that a considerable number of fastigial efferent fibers project to rostral levels of the brain stem including the thalamus, a clear picture of

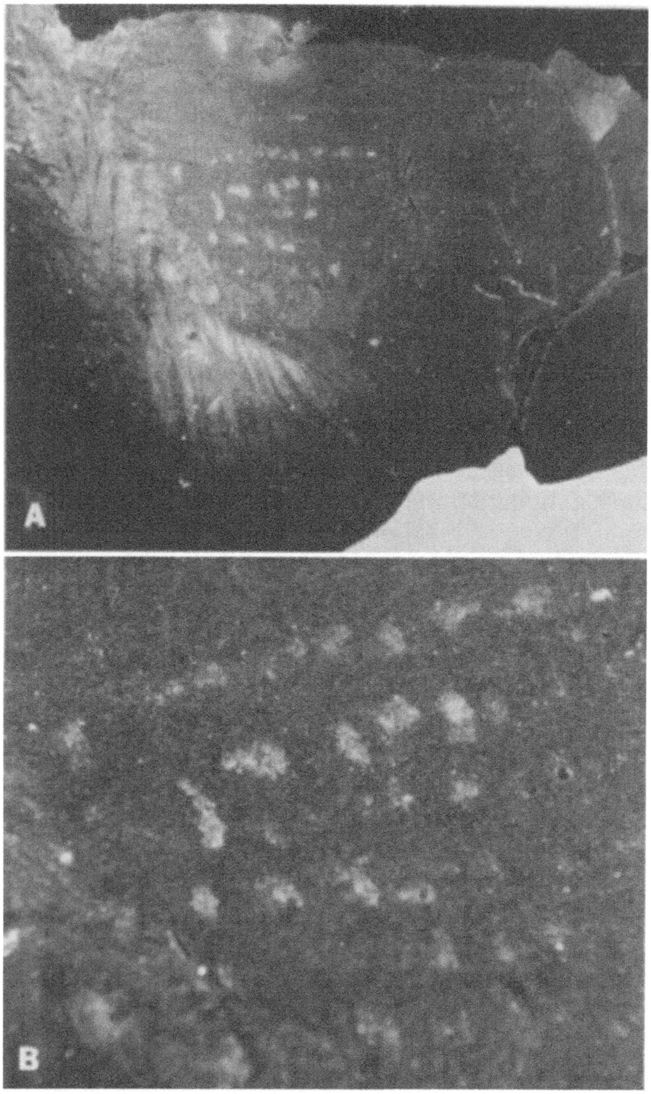

Fig. 13A, B. Cynomolgus C-1423. Dark-field photomicrographs of a sagittal autoradiograph demonstrating transport of isotope to terminal clusters in the ventral posterior lateral thalamic nucleus **A, B.** Cresyl violet, × 6, × 18

this system has not emerged [6, 27, 30, 36, 61, 69, 90, 101, 104]. There is almost universal agreement that ascending fibers are crossed, arise from caudal portions of the FN and constitute a component of the UF [6, 27, 36, 68, 104]. Labeling of cells in caudal parts of the FN resulted in maximum transport of isotope to terminals in midbrain and diencephalic nuclei, while labeling of cells in rostral parts of this nucleus showed no such transport [10]. Even in animals where label was seen throughout the fastigial, contralateral ascending transport was not impressive unless cells in caudal regions were well labeled.

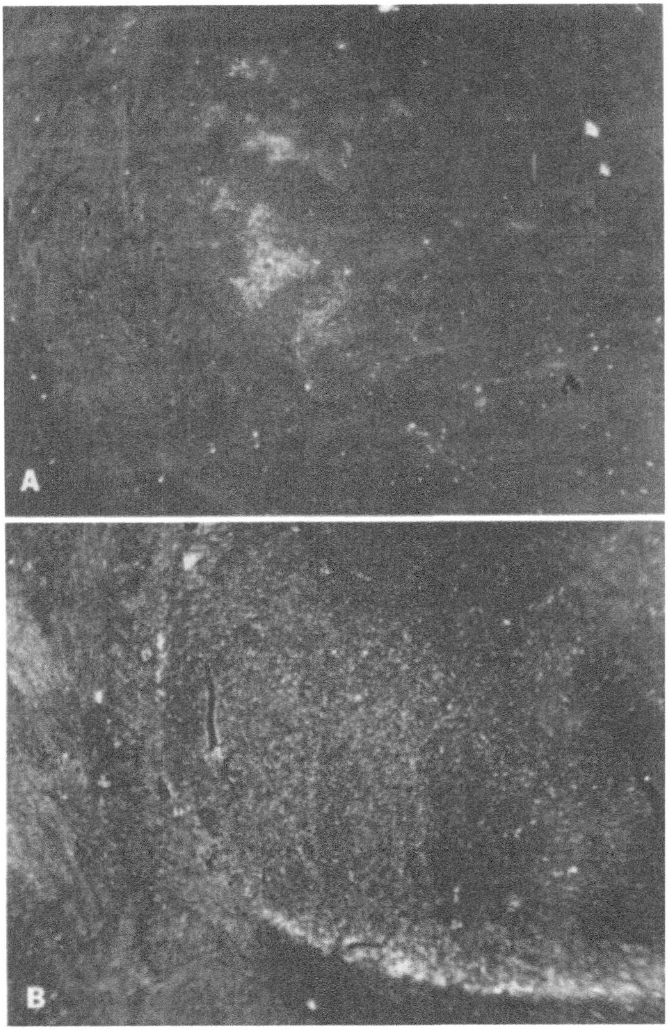

Fig. 14 A, B. Rhesus C-1386. Dark-field photomicrographs of autoradiographs of transverse sections through the thalamus demonstrating regions of termination of fastigial efferent fibers in *VPLo* **B** and *VLo* **A**. Cresyl violet, × 12, × 12

Ascending fibers in the UF cap the superior cerebellar peduncle (SCP) and extend medially into parts of the superior medullary velum. At isthmus levels these fibers are not as numerous as at more caudal pontine levels. As fibers of the SCP begin to migrate ventromedially towards their midbrain decussation, crossed ascending fastigial efferent fibers move into the dorsolateral tegmentum and pass rostrally in an area beneath the inferior colliculus (Figs. 7 D, 11 F). These fibers are dispersed over a broad region between the lateral lemniscus and the central gray. No fibers were seen to enter the inferior colliculus or the nuclei of the lateral lemniscus. At more rostral levels some fibers of this ascending bundle project into deep layers of the superior colliculus (Fig. 7); part of these fibers cross in the commissure of the superior colliculus and terminate in deep layers of the superior colliculus on the opposite side. As described by Angaut [4] most of the terminals end in rostral parts of the superior colliculus. Further rostrally, labeled terminals end in the nuclei of the posterior commissure and some fibers cross via the commissure to end in these same nuclei on the opposite side (Fig. 12D). Most of these connections with the superior colliculus and the nuclei of the posterior commissure have been reported in prior degeneration studies [6, 27, 30, 36, 87, 88, 101, 104]. Although fastigial efferent fibers terminating in the interstitial nucleus of Cajal and the nucleus of Darkschewitch have been described [36, 101, 104], these terminations were not seen in our autoradiographic studies.

Most of the fibers in the ascending limb of the UF projecting to diencephalic nuclei lie in a loosely organized bundle close to the medial geniculate body which traverses parts of the suprageniculate nucleus. These fibers project rostrally and dorsally directly into the ventral posterolateral (VPL) and ventral lateral (VL) thalamic nuclei (Figs. 7, 8, 13A, 13B, 14A, 14B). A smaller number of fibers ascending near the central and periventricular gray abruptly turn ventrolaterally at caudal thalamic levels and pass through parts of the parafascicular, centromedian, and ventral posteromedial thalamic nuclei to enter medial parts of VPL and portions of VLo. Fibers following these different courses projected into broad regions of both caudal and oral parts of VPL (i.e., VPLc and VPLo) where they terminated. While these fibers tend to terminate in prominent localized clusters, this mode of termination was particularly impressive in sagittal sections (Figs. 13A, 13B). This pattern of cerebello-thalamic projections is similar to ones reported by Chan-Palay [34] in dentato-thalamic projections in rhesus monkeys after injections of ^{35}S-methionine autoradiography. Labeled terminations were most profuse throughout VPL, particularly its oral part. Fibers projecting to VLo were less numerous than in VPL and were found mainly in ventral and lateral regions.

Data based upon axoplasmic transport techniques appear quite different than those reported in degeneration studies. Earlier studies in the cat suggested that fastigiothalamic fibers projected diffusely to portions of nearly all ventral tier thalamic nuclei and to significant portions of the intralaminar nuclei [36, 101, 104]. A considerable part of this projection was described as bilateral, suggesting a recrossing of fibers within the thalamus. Angaut and Bowsher [6] concluded that fastigiothalamic projections in the cat traverse portions of the centromedian nucleus in their passage to the ventral medial (VM) and adjacent medial parts of the VL thalamic nuclei. A unilateral lesion in the caudal half of the fastigial nucleus produced bilateral degeneration in VM and VL which was densest contralaterally; degeneration in ipsilateral thalamic nuclei was described as due to a partial recrossing of fibers at thalamic levels in the region of the nucleus reuniens. In spite of fiber recrossings, the principal thalamic projection was regarded as contralateral. Similar degeneration studies in the rat indicated that fastigiothalamic fibers ascend in the dorsal tegmentum of the midbrain, entered the thalamus via the thalamic fasciculus, and established terminations in parts of the parafascicular, the medial part of the VM, and the central part of the VL thalamic nuclei [61]. According to Faull and Carmen [50], the VM-VL complex in the rat is homologous to the ventral anterior-ventral lateral (VA-VL) nuclear complex in the primate. In this study in the rat, a few fastigiothalamic axons crossed the midline to terminate in the dorsal part of VL [50]. It is apparent that fastigiothalamic projections in the rat and cat are not the same as in the primate, an observation also made by Kievit and Kuypers [69].

Studies of fastigiothalamic terminations in the monkey based upon cerebellar bisections destroyed many structures, but because all fibers of the UF cross in the cerebellum they seem appropriate for determination of thalamic projections [69]. Observations based upon silver impregnation techniques revealed that the bulk of the ascending fibers were distributed throughout VPLo (pars oralis) and in parts of VLo (pars oralis). These authors also described ascending fibers as entering VPL by two trajectories, one through the centromedian nucleus and the other directly through lateral parts of nucleus. A much smaller number of fibers projected rostrally into parts of VLo, particularly lateral regions. These observations are in close agreement with findings on our autoradiographic studies [10].

In attempts to identify thalamic neurons relaying vestibular impulses to the cerebral cortex in the cat, based upon injections of HRP into sites where short latency responses to vestibular stimulation were recorded, retrogradely labeled neurons were found mainly in dorsolateral parts of VPL [11]. Although studies in the monkey identify neurons in the ventral posterior inferior (VPI) nucleus as relaying vestibular impulses to the cerebral cortex [42, 52], these data suggest that ascending vestibular and fastigial impulses concerned with equilibrium and modification of muscle tone may impinge upon thalamic neurons receiving inputs from less specialized receptors that also signal information concerning position sense and body movement.

Summary

An analysis of fastigial afferent fibers in the cat and squirrel monkey based upon the retrograde transport of horseradish peroxidase indicates that the fastigial nucleus receives afferents from: (a) Purkinje cells of the ipsilateral cerebellar vermis, (b) nucleus β and the dorsomedial cell column of the contralateral inferior olivary nuclear complex, (c) dorsal, lateral, and caudal regions of the medial and inferior vestibular nuclei on both sides, (d) cell group x on both sides, and (e) portions of the nucleus prepositus, the nucleus of Roller, and the dorsal paramedian reticular nucleus. No cells of the lateral vestibular nucleus or of cell group f of the inferior vestibular nucleus project to the fastigial nucleus. These data suggest that the major inputs to the fastigial nucleus are from the ipsilateral cerebellar vermis and via secondary vestibular fibers arising bilaterally from parts of the medial and inferior vestibular nuclei. Cell group x appears to project to both the fastigial nucleus and the uvula.

Fastigial efferent fibers determined by autoradiographic techniques in the rhesus monkey are distributed widely in the brain stem at all levels. Crossed efferent fibers contained in the uncinate fasciculus arise from cells in all parts of the fastigial nucleus and outnumber uncrossed efferent fibers that emerge from the cerebellum via the juxtarestiform body.

Fastigiovestibular fibers project bilaterally and fairly symmetrically to ventral and lateral portions of the lateral and inferior vestibular nuclei. Fastigial projections to cell group f of the inferior vestibular nucleus and cell group x are entirely crossed, and arise from all parts of the fastigial nucleus, though the greatest number of fibers appear to arise from caudal parts of the nucleus. No fastigial efferent fibers terminate in the superior vestibular nucleus or in dorsal parts of the lateral vestibular nucleus. Some crossed fastigial efferents descending in the inferior vestibular nucleus terminate in the nucleus parasolitarius.

Fastigioreticular fibers arise predominantly from rostral parts of the fastigial nucleus, are mainly crossed, and project to: (a) medial regions of the nucleus reticularis gigantocellularis, (b) parts of the caudal pontine reticular formation, (c) the dorsal paramedian reticular nucleus, and (d) portions of the magnocellular part of the lateral reticular nucleus.

Crossed fastigiopontine fibers separate from the uncinate fasciculus, pass ventrally along the medial border of the middle cerebellar peduncle and terminate in the dorsolateral pontine nuclei. Crossed fastigiospinal fibers separate from the fastigiopontine bundle, descend ventral to the spinal trigeminal tract, and enter the ventral part of the lateral funiculus of the spinal cord in association with fibers of the vestibulospinal tract. Retrograde transport studies and electrophysiological evidence suggests that fastigiospinal fibers project to upper cervical spinal segments and make monosynaptic contacts with motoneurons. Anatomical and physiological data suggest that fastigial efferents exert excitatory effects upon spinal motoneurons: (a) indirectly via relays in the lateral vestibular nucleus, and (b) directly via fastigiospinal projections. Evidence suggests that both direct and indirect fastigial influences effect neurons mainly in cervical spinal segments.

Ascending fastigial projections arise mainly from caudal parts of the nucleus, are entirely crossed, and ascend in dorsal parts of the midbrain tegmentum. These fibers project bilaterally to rostral parts of the superior colliculus and to the nuclei of the posterior commissure. Fastigiothalamic projections terminate in the contralateral ventral posterior lateral (VPLo and VPLc) and in ventral and lateral parts of the ventral lateral (VLo) thalamic nuclei. The largest number of fibers appear to end in VPLo. These data suggest that ascending impulses from the fastigial nucleus probably are relayed to both the primary somesthetic and motor cortex. On the basis of quantitative features, impulses in this ascending system might be expected to influence neurons in the postcentral region concerned with representation of most of the body, except for the head and face.

References

1. Achenbach KE, Goodman DC (1968) Cerebellar projections to pons, medulla and spinal cord in the albino rat. Brain Behav Evol 1:43–57

2. Allen WF (1927) Experimental-anatomical studies on the visceral bulbospinal pathway in the cat and guinea pig. J Comp Neurol 42:393–456
3. Alley KR, Baker R, Simpson JI (1975) Afferents to the vestibulo-cerebellum and the origin of the visual climbing fibers in the rabbit. Brain Res 98:582–589
4. Angaut P (1969) The fastigio-tectal projections: an anatomical-experimental study. Brain Res 13:186–189
5. Angaut P (1970) The ascending projections of the nucleus interpositus posterior of the cat cerebellum: an experimental anatomical study using silver impregnation methods. Brain Res 24:377–394
6. Angaut P, Bowsher D (1970) Ascending projections of the medial cerebellar (fastigial) nucleus. An experimental study in the cat. Brain Res 24:49–68
7. Angaut P, Brodal A (1967) The projection of the "vestibulocerebellum" onto the vestibular nuclei in the cat. Arch Ital Biol 105:441–479
8. Asanuma C, Thach WT, Jones EG (1980) Nucleus interpositus projection to spinal interneurons in monkeys. Brain Res 191:245–248
9. Baker R (1977) Anatomical and physiological organization of brain stem pathways underlying the control of gaze. In: Baker R, Berthoz A (eds) Control of gaze by brain stem neurons. Elsevier/North-Holland Biomedical Press, Amsterdam, pp 207–222
10. Batton RR, Jayaraman A, Ruggiero D, Carpenter MB (1977) Fastigial efferent projections in the monkey: an autoradiographic study. J Comp Neurol 174:281–306
11. Blum PS, Day MJ, Carpenter MB, Gilman S (1979) Thalamic components of the ascending vestibular system. Exp Neurol 64:587–603
12. Brodal A (1940) Experimentelle Untersuchungen über die olivocerebellare Lokalisation. Z Neurol Psychiatr 169:1–153
13. Brodal A (1952) Experimental demonstration of cerebellar connections from the peri-hypoglossal nuclei (nucleus intercalatus, nucleus praepositus hypoglossi and nucleus of Roller) in the cat. J Anat 86:110–128
14. Brodal A (1953) Reticulo-cerebellar connections in the cat. An experimental study. J Comp Neurol 98:113–153
15. Brodal A (1967) Anatomical studies of cerebellar fibre connections with special reference to problems of functional localization. In: Fox CA, Snider RS (eds) Progress in brain research, the cerebellum. Elsevier, Amsterdam, pp 135–173
16. Brodal A (1974) Anatomy of the vestibular nuclei and their connections. In: Kornhuber HH (ed) Handbook of sensory physiology, I. Springer, Berlin Heidelberg New York, pp 239–352
17. Brodal A (1976) The olivocerebellar projection in the cat studied with the method of retrograde axonal transport of horseradish peroxidase. II. The projection to the uvula. J Comp Neurol 166:417–426
18. Brodal A, Gogstad AC (1957) Afferent connections of the paramedian reticular nucleus of the medulla oblongata in the cat. Acta Anat (Basel) 30:133–151
19. Brodal A, Høivik B (1964) Site and mode of termination of primary vestibulocerebellar fibres in the cat. An experimental study with silver impregnation methods. Arch Ital Biol 102:1–21
20. Brodal A, Jansen J (1946) The pontocerebellar projection in the rabbit and cat. Experimental investigation. J Comp Neurol 84:31–118
21. Brodal A, Pompeiano O (1957) The vestibular nuclei in the cat. J Anat 91:438–454
22. Brodal A, Szikla G (1972) The termination of the brachium conjunctivum descendens in the nucleus reticularis tegmenti pontis. An experimental anatomical study in the cat. Brain Res 39:337–351
23. Brodal A, Torvik A (1954) Cerebellar projections of paramedian reticular nucleus of medulla oblongata in cat. J Neurophysiol 17:484–495
24. Brodal A, Torvik A (1957) Über den Ursprung der sekundären vestibulocerebellaren Fasern bei der Katze. Eine experimentell-anatomische Studie. Arch Psychiatr Z Nervenkr 195:550–567
25. Brodal A, Walberg F (1977) The olivocerebellar projection in the cat studied with the method of retrograde axonal transport of horseradish peroxidase. IV. The projection to the anterior lobe. J Comp Neurol 176:281–294

26. Brodal A, Walberg F, Hoddevik GH (1975) The olivocerebellar projection in the cat studied with the method of retrograde axonal transport of horseradish peroxidase. J Comp Neurol 164:449–470
27. Carpenter MB (1959) Lesions of the fastigial nuclei in the rhesus monkey. Am J Anat 104:1–34
28. Carpenter MB (1960) Fiber projections from the descending and lateral vestibular nuclei in the cat. Am J Anat 107:1–22
29. Carpenter MB, Nova HR (1960) Descending division of the brachium conjunctivum in the cat: a cerebello-reticular system. J Comp Neurol 114:295–305
30. Carpenter MB, Brittin GM, Pines J (1958) Isolated lesions of the fastigial nuclei in the cat. J Comp Neurol 109:65–90
31. Carpenter MB, Bard DS, Alling FA (1959) Anatomical connections between the fastigial nuclei, the labyrinth and the vestibular nuclei in the cat. J Comp Neurol 111:1–26
32. Carpenter MB, Stein BM, Peter P (1972) Primary vestibulocerebellar fibers in the monkey: Distribution of fibers arising from distinctive cell groups of the vestibular ganglia. Am J Anat 135:221–250
33. Chan-Palay V, Palay SL, Brown JT, Itallie CV (1977) Sagittal organization of olivocerebellar and reticulocerebellar projections: Autoradiographic studies with ^{35}S-methionine. Exp Brain Res 30:561–576
34. Chan-Palay V (1977) Cerebellar dentate nucleus, organization, cytology and transmitters. Springer, Berlin Heidelberg New York
35. Chu N-S, Bloom FE (1974) The catecholamine-containing neurons in the cat dorsolateral pontine tegmentum: Distribution of cell bodies and some axonal projections. Brain Res 66:1–21
36. Cohen D, Chambers WW, Sprague JM (1958) Experimental study of the efferent projections from the cerebellar nuclei to the brain stem of the cat. J Comp Neurol 109:233–259
37. Courville J (1966) Somatotopical organization of the projection from the nucleus interpositus anterior of the cerebellum to the red nucleus. An experimental study in the cat with silver impregnation methods. Exp Brain Res 2:191–215
38. Courville J, Cooper C (1970) The cerebellar nuclei of Macaca mulatta: a morphological study. J Comp Neurol 140:241–254
39. Courville J, Diakiw N (1976) Cerebellar corticonuclear projection in the cat. The vermis of the anterior and posterior lobes. Brain Res 110:1–20
40. Cowan WM, Cuénod M (1975) The use of axonal transport for the study of neural connections: a retrospective survey. In: Cowan WM, Cuénod M (eds) The use of axonal transport for studies of neuronal connectivity. Elsevier, Amsterdam, 2–23
41. Cowan WM, Gottlieb DI, Hendrickson AE, Price JL, Woolsey TA (1972) The autoradiographic demonstration of axonal connections in the central nervous system. Brain Res 37:21–51
42. Deecke LD, Schwarz DWF, Fredrickson JM (1974) Nucleus ventroposterior inferior (VPI) as the vestibular thalamic relay in the rhesus monkey. I. Field potential investigation. Exp Brain Res 20:88–100
43. Dietrichs E, Walberg F (1979) The cerebellar projection from the lateral reticular nucleus as studied with retrograde transport of horseradish peroxidase. Anat Embryol (Berl) 155:273–290
44. Dow RS (1936) The fiber connections of the posterior parts of the cerebellum in the cat and rat. J Comp Neurol 63:527–548
45. Dow RS, Moruzzi G (1958) The physiology and pathology of the cerebellum. University of Minnesota Press, Minneapolis
46. Eager RP (1963) Efferent cortico-nuclear pathways in the cerebellum of the cat. J Comp Neurol 120:81–104
47. Eccles JC, Nicoll RA, Schwarz DWF, Táboříková H (1974) Cerebellospinal pathway via the fastigial nucleus and medial reticular nucleus. Brain Res 66:525–530
48. Eccles JC, Sabah NH, Táboříková H (1974) The pathways responsible for excitation and inhibition of fastigial neurons. Exp Brain Res 19:78–99

49. Edwards SB (1972) The ascending and descending projections of the red nucleus in the cat: an experimental study using an autoradiographic tracing method. Brain Res 48:45–63
50. Faull RLM, Carman JB (1978) The cerebellofugal projections in the brachium conjunctivum of the rat. I. The contralateral ascending pathway. J Comp Neurol 178:495–518
51. Flood S, Jansen J (1961) On the cerebellar nuclei in the cat. Acta Anat (Basel) 46:52–72
52. Fredrickson JM, Kornhuber HH, Schwarz DWF (1974) Cortical projections of the vestibular nerve. In: Kornhuber HH (ed) Handbook of sensory physiology, vol. 6/I. Springer, Berlin Heidelberg New York, pp 565–582
53. Fuchs A (1977) Role of the vestibular and reticular nuclei in the control of gaze: reticular prepositus and other internuclear neuronal activity. In: Baker R, Berthoz A (eds) Control of gaze by brain stem neurons. Developments in neuroscience. Elsevier/North-Holland Biomedical Press, Amsterdam, pp 341–348
54. Fukushima K, Peterson BW, Uchino Y, Coulter JD, Wilson VJ (1977) Direct fastigiospinal fibers in the cat. Brain Res 126:538–542
55. Gacek RR (1977) Location of brain stem neurons projecting to the oculomotor nucleus in the cat. Exp Neurol 57:725–749
56. Goodman DC, Hallett RE, Welch RB (1963) Patterns of localization in the cerebellar corticonuclear projections of the albino rat. J Comp Neurol 121:51–67
57. Gould BB, Graybiel AB (1976) Afferents to the cerebellar cortex in the cat: evidence for an intrinsic pathway leading from the deep cerebellar nuclei to the cortex. Brain Res 110:601–611
58. Graham RC Jr, Karnovsky MJ (1966) The early stages of absorption of injected horseradish peroxidase in the proximal tubules of mouse kidney. Ultrastructural cytochemistry by a new technique. J Histochem Cytochem 14:291–302
59. Graybiel AB, Hartwieg EA (1974) Some afferent connections of the oculomotor complex in the cat: An experimental study with tracer techniques. Brain Res 81:543–551
60. Hardy H, Heimer L (1977) A safer and more sensitive substitute for diaminobenzidine in the light microscopic demonstration of retrograde and anterograde axonal transport of HRP. Neurosci Lett 5:235
61. Haroian AJ, Massopust LC, Young PA (1981) Cerebellothalamic projections in the rat. An autoradiographic and degeneration study. J Comp Neurol 197:217–236
62. Hoddevik GH, Brodal A, Walberg F (1976) The olivocerebellar projection in the cat studied with the method of retrograde axonal transport of horseradish peroxidase. III. The projection to the vermal visual area. J Comp Neurol 169:155–170
63. Ingvar S (1918) Zur Phylo- und Ontogenese des Kleinhirns. Folia Neuro-biol 11:205–495
64. Ito M, Udo M, Mano N, Kawai N (1970) Synaptic action of the fastigiobulbar impulses upon neurones in the medullary reticular formation and vestibular nuclei. Exp Brain Res 11:29–47
65. Ito M, Yoshida M, Obata K, Kawai N, Udo M (1970) Inhibitory control of intracerebellar nuclei by Purkinje cell axons. Exp Brain Res 10:64–80
66. Jansen J, Brodal A (1940) Experimental studies on the intrinsic fibers of the cerebellum. II. The corticonuclear projection. J Comp Neurol 73:267–321
67. Jansen J, Brodal A (1942) Experimental studies on the intrinsic fibers of the cerebellum. III. The corticonuclear projection in the rabbit and the monkey (*Macacus rhesus*). Nor Vidensk Akad Avh Mat-Naturv 3:1–50
68. Jansen J, Jansen J Jr (1955) On the efferent fibers of the cerebellar nuclei in the cat. J Comp Neurol 102:607–632
69. Kievit J, Kuypers HGJM (1972) Fastigial cerebellar projections to the ventrolateral nucleus of the thalamus and the organization of the descending pathways. In: Frigyesi TL, Rinvik E, Jahr MD (eds) Corticothalamic projections and sensorimotor activities. Raven Press, New York, pp 91–114
70. Korneliussen HK (1968) On the ontogenetic development of the cerebellum (nuclei, fissures, and cortex) of the rat with special reference to regional variations in corticogenesis. J Hirnforsch 10:379–412

71. Kotchabhakdi N, Walberg F (1978a) Cerebellar afferent projections from the vestibular nuclei in the cat: an experimental study with the method of retrograde transport of horseradish peroxidase. Exp Brain Res 31:591–604
72. Kotchabhakdi N, Walberg F (1978b) Primary vestibular afferent projections to the cerebellum as demonstrated by retrograde axonal transport of horseradish peroxidase. Brain Res 142:142–146
73. Kotchabhakdi N, Walberg F, Brodal A (1978) The olivocerebellar projection in the cat studied with the method of retrograde axonal transport of horseradish peroxidase. VIII. The projection to lobulus simplex, crus I and II. J Comp Neurol 182:293–314
74. Künzle H (1975) Autoradiographic tracing of the cerebellar projections from the lateral reticular nucleus in the cat. Exp Brain Res 22:255–266
75. Larsell O (1953) The cerebellum of the cat and the monkey. J Comp Neurol 99:135–200
76. LaVail JH (1975) Retrograde cell degeneration and retrograde transport techniques. In: Cowan WM, Cuénod M (eds) The use of axonal transport for studies of neuronal connectivity. Elsevier, Amsterdam, pp 217–247
77. LaVail JH, LaVail MM (1972) Retrograde axonal transport in the central nervous system. Science 176:1416–1417
78. Marchi V (1981) Sill origine e decorso dei peduncoli cerebellari e sui loro rapporti cogli altri centri nervosi. Riv Sper Freniat 17:357–358
79. Matsushita M, Hosoya Y (1978) The location of spinal projection neurons in the cerebellar nuclei (cerebellospinal tract neurons) of horseradish peroxidase technique. Brain Res 142:237–248
80. Matsushita M, Iwahori N (1971) Structural organization of the fastigial nucleus. I. Dendrites and axonal pathways. Brain Res 25:597–610
81. Mesulam M-M (1978) Tetramethyl benzidine for horseradish peroxidase neurohistochemistry: a non-carcinogenic blue reactionproduct with superior sensitivity for visualizing neural afferents and efferents. J Histochem Cytochem 26:106–117
82. Miale IL, Sidman RL (1961) An autoradiographic analysis of histogenesis in the mouse cerebellum. Exp Neurol 4:277–296
83. Mingazzini G (1894) Sulle degenerationi convecutive alle extirpozioni emicerebellari. Ricerche, Lab Anat Normale, R Univ Roma 4:73–124
84. Pompeiano O (1967) Functional organization of the cerebellar projection to the spinal cord. In: Fox CA, Snider RS (eds) The cerebellum, progress in brain research, Elsevier, Amsterdam, pp. 69–94
85. Pompeiano O, Brodal A (1957) The origin of vestibulospinal fibers in the cat. An experimental-anatomical study, with comments on the descending medial longitudinal fasciculus. Arch Ital Biol 95:166–195
86. Pompeiano O, Cotti E (1959) Analisi microelettrodica delle proiezioni cerebellodeitersiame. Arch Sci Biol (Bologna) 43:57–101
81. Probst M (1902) Zur Anatomie und Physiologie des Kleinhirns. Arch F Psychiatr 35:692–777
88. Rand RW (1954) An anatomical and experimental study of the cerebellar nuclei and their efferent pathways in the monkey. J Comp Neurol 101:167–224
89. Rasmussen AT (1933) Origin and course of the fasciculus uncinatus (Russell) in the cat, with observations on other fiber tracts arising from the cerebellar nuclei. J Comp Neurol 57:165–198
90. Rinvik E, Grofová I (1974) Cerebellar projections to the nuclei ventralis lateralis and ventralis anterior thalami. Anat Embryol (Berl) 146:95–111
91. Rinvik E, Walberg F (1975) Studies on the cerebellar projections from the main and external cuneate nucleus in the cat by means of retrograde axonal transport of horseradish peroxidase. Brain Res 95:371–381
92. Rossum JV (1969) Corticonuclear and corticovestibular projections of the cerebellum. Thesis, State University of Leiden Van Gorcum & Comp. N.V., Assen
93. Ruggiero D, Batton RR, Jayaraman A, Carpenter MB (1977) Brain stem afferents to the fastigial nucleus in the cat demonstrated by transport of horseradish peroxidase. J Comp Neurol 172:189–210
94. Snider RS (1975) A cerebello-ceruleus pathway. Brain Res 88:59–63

95. Somana R, Walberg F (1978a) Cerebellar afferents from the paramedian reticular nucleus studied with retrograde transport of horseradish peroxidase. Anat Embryol (Berl) 154:353–368
96. Somana R, Walberg F (1978b) The cerebellar projection from locus coeruleus as studied with retrograde transport of horseradish peroxidase in the cat. Anat Embryol (Berl) 155:87–94
97. Sousa-Pinto A (1970) The cortical projection onto the paramedian reticular and perihypoglossal nuclei (nucleus praepositus hypoglossi, nucleus intercalatus and nucleus of Roller) on the medulla oblongata of the cat. An experimental anatomical study. Brain Res 18:77–91
98. Steiger H-J, Büttner-Ennever JA (1979) Oculomotor nucleus afferents in the monkey demonstrated with horseradish peroxidase. Brain Res 160:1–15
99. Thomas A (1897) Le faisceau cerebelleux descendant. C R Soc Biol (Paris) 49:36–37
100. Thomas A (1912) Cerebellar functions. J Nerv Ment Dis 12:1–219
101. Thomas DM, Kaufman RP, Sprague JM, Chambers WW (1956) Experimental studies of the vermal cerebellar projections in the brain stem of the cat (fastigiobulbar tract). J Anat 90:371–384
102. Tolberg DL, Bantli H, Bloedel JR (1976) Anatomical and physiological evidence for a cerebellar nucleocortical projection in the cat. Neuroscience 1:205–217
103. Torvik A, Brodal A (1954) The cerebellar projection of the perihypoglossal nuclei (nucleus intercalatus, nucleus praepositus and nucleus of Roller) in the cat. J Neuropathol Exp Neurol 13:515–527
104. Voogd J (1964) The cerebellum of the cat. Structure and fibre connexions. Thesis, Van Gorcum & Comp N.V., Assen
105. Walberg F (1958) Descending connections to the lateral reticular nucleus. An experimental study in the cat. J Comp Neurol 109:363–389
106. Walberg F (1961) Fastigiofugal fibers to the perihypoglossal nuclei. Exp Neurol 3:525–541
107. Walberg F, Jansen J (1961) Cerebellar corticovestibular fibers in the cat. Exp Neurol 3:32–52
108. Walberg F, Jansen J (1964) Cerebellar corticonuclear projection studied experimentally with silver impregnation methods. J Hirnforsch 6:338–354
109. Walberg F, Pompeiano O (1960) Fastigiofugal fibers to the lateral reticular nucleus: an experimental study in the cat. Exp Neurol 2:40–53
110. Walberg F, Bowsher D, Brodal A (1958) The termination of primary vestibular fibers in the vestibular nuclei in the cat. An experimental study with silver methods. J Comp Neurol 110:391–419
111. Walberg F, Pompeiano O, Brodal A, Jansen J (1962a) The fastigiovestibular projection in the cat. An experimental study with silver impregnation methods. J Comp Neurol 118:49–75
112. Walberg F, Pompeiano O, Westrum LE, Hauglie-Hanssen E (1962b) Fastigioreticular fibers in the cat. An experimental study with silver methods. J Comp Neurol 119:187–199
113. Ware CB, Mufson EJ (1979) Spinal cord projections from the medial cerebellar nucleus in tree shrew (*Tupaia glis*). Brain Res 171:383–400
114. Wilson VJ, Uchino Y, Maunz RA, Susswein A, Fukushima K (1978) Properties and connections of cat fastigiospinal neurons. Exp Brain Res 32:1–17

Discussion

Eccles: I've recently seen fastigial stimulation used clinically, for schizophrenia, violence of all kinds, and homicidal tendencies. Stimulators are implanted on the vermis of these patients and the stimulation goes at intermittent periods, and gives amazing control. The pathway you showed from fastigial nucleus to thalamus of course would be a way into the higher centers and it could work that way. Have you any evidence that it might also go through the limbic system?

Carpenter: I know that Bob Heath and co-workers at Tulane [2, 6] have traced pathways to the limbic system and septal area. In neither our transport studies nor our degeneration studies did we see pathways that projected to these structures. I am very skeptical about these connections. I can't say they don't exist, but we have not seen them.

Eccles: Yes, but there could be synapses on the way, then you wouldn't see it. From the thalamus for example.

Carpenter: That could be. I didn't describe the pathway to the thalamus completely. Most of these ascending fastigial fibers project directly to the ventral posterolateral nucleus (VPL) of the thalamus, but there are some fibers that ascend in the periaqueductal and periventricular gray, that reach the ventral lateral nucleus, pars oralis (VLO) and ventral posterolateral nucleus (VPL) nuclei by coursing through ventral posteromedial nuclei (VPM).

Chan-Palay: I was going to ask both you and Dr. Beitz whether or not you had any indication from your horseradish peroxidase (HRP) studies of connections with the raphe. Six years ago, when I began these studies, the first thing that hit me about the serotonin system in the cerebellum was that the fastigial nucleus probably contained the richest serotonin innervation in that part of the brain.

Carpenter: There are a lot of labelled cells in the raphe following HRP injections in fastigial nucleus. When we did our initial experiments in the cat using the diaminobenzidine (DAB) technique we saw nothing in the raphe. But when we did these studies in the squirrel monkey using tetramethylbenzidine (TMB), the whole raphe came alive. There are a great number of retrogradely labeled cells in the raphe, although I did not emphasize these data in my talk.

Martin: Two comments. First of all, I think that the projections from the nuclei fastigius and interpositus posterior to the spinal cord have been underplayed in previous studies and I am pleased that you have been able to define them so nicely in the monkey. I've seen such connections in the opossum and, in collaboration with W. Buck and A. O. Humbertson, in the rat. The other comment I wanted to make is of comparative interest. I think that the projection you found to the basilar pons has been described previously, in a marsupial. In the opossum there's a nucleus referred to by Oswaldo-Cruz and Rocha-Miranda [5] as the nucleus of the pontobulbar body. It lies just medial to the emerging fascicles of the trigeminal nerve and is probably a remnant of the pontobulbar migration. It receives fastigial input as well as projections from the cerebral cortex, the red nucleus, and the spinal cord [4]. It may be that the area of the pons outlined by fastigial projections in the monkey is comparable to the portion of the pontobulbar nucleus receiving fastigial connections in the opossum. In addition, we reported a small fastigial projection to the basilar pons proper in an earlier paper [11]. It is good to know that this projection also exists in the monkey. The question I wanted to ask is whether the particular portion of basilar pons which receives a fastigial input is known by any other of its afferent connections.

Carpenter: This pontine area is very close to that to which we have traced fibers from the superior colliculus. Actually, fastigial fibers emerge in the uncinate fasciculus and go rostrally, so they're really in the rostral dorsolateral part of the pontine nuclei. This area presumably projects back to cerebellar vermis. It may be part of a feedback system.

Marshall: Do you see any indication of projections from the fastigial nucleus to the cerebellar cortex.

Carpenter: Yes, there are projections to the cerebellar cortex. We have seen some labeled cells in the deep cerebellar nuclei, mainly in the fastigial nucleus. I think this is because we have gotten some HRP on the cortex.

Ito: You mentioned that the superior vestibular nucleus receives no projection from the fastigial nucleus. Is this correct?

Carpenter: I know that Kotchabhakdi and Walberg [3] have described projections from the superior vestibular nucleus to the fastigial nucleus and that Walberg et al. [9] have described projections from the fastigial nucleus to the superior vestibular nucleus. In our animals, when isotope or HPR was well localized to the fastigial nucleus, we did not see projections to or from the superior vestibular nucleus. There is a projection to the superior vestibular nucleus that I think comes from the uvula, and in making fastigial lesions you may damage fibers that come from that area. This is why this projection was consistently reported in early degeneration studies.

Ito: The superior nucleus contains relay cells of the vestibuloocular reflex, so it may be heavily involved in eye movements. There is evidence that lobules VI and VII are sites of either smooth pursuit or saccade-related activity. One may imagine that projections from lobules VI and VII to the fastigial nucleus and then to the superior vestibular nucleus may be the pathway responsible for these eye movements.

Carpenter: I think that most of the projections to the superior vestibular nucleus are probably cortical rather than fastigial. These fibers go to the peripheral part of the superior vestibular nucleus, while primary vestibular afferents go to its central part.

Thach: Going along with the lack of projection from fastigial nucleus to superior vestibular nucleus is the work of Gardner and Fuchs [1]. They recorded single-cell activity in the fastigial nucleus, particularly as it related to eye movements. Or, I should say, they looked for it, but were unable to find any. The fastigial nucleus appears to be lacking in oculomotor representation.

Ito: In Ritchie's [7] experiments in monkey, ablation of lobules VI–VII produced serious dysmetria in saccadic eye movements, and I can't think of any structure other than the fastigial nucleus relating to these effects.

Llinás: Yes, but as you know, people in Switzerland have been recording from the fastigial nucleus and have found that there are correlations with given eye movements. So now the real question is: where are these connections? Actually, we're talking about a very specific nucleus and in talking with Gardner, one doesn't really know that all the areas were studied rather than "fastigial nucleus".

Altman: Didn't you mention the praepositus hypoglossi as getting a projection from the fastigial nucleus? Could this be part of the oculomotor loop?

Carpenter: The praepositus projects to the fastigial nucleus and receives fibers from it. However, this is mainly the caudal third of the praepositus. There are also a small number of cells in the nucleus of Roller that project to the fastigial nucleus. I have not seen any fastigial connections with the nucleus intercalatus or rostral parts of the praepositus.

Voogd: In 1964 [8] I made the suggestion that in cat projections to the dorsal part of the lateral vestibular nucleus and the superior vestibular nucleus originated from the cortex. I'm glad to see that when you use other methods it turns out to be true. At that time, I was looking at Haggquist-stained sections. In that material you could distinguish the Purkinje cell axons with equal small caliber fibers from the larger efferents of the fastigial nucleus. In cats which had suffered from a viral infection of the cortex and didn't have any Purkinje cell axons left, you could study the fiber pattern and caliber of the uncinate and direct fastigiobulbar tract directly. It turned out that the fiber pattern of the uncinate tract is different from the direct cerebellobulbar fibers. The latter, the direct fibers, are much larger and have fewer small fibers in between than the uncinate tract. You state that they both originate from the whole fastigial nucleus. I wonder, aren't there any differences?

Carpenter: In most of the literature based on degeneration studies you get the impression that fibers of the uncinate fasciculus originate largely from caudal parts of the fastigial nucleus and that direct fastigiobulbar fibers originate from its rostral pole. I think that an important finding in these studies is that both the crossed and uncrossed fibers come from cells in *all* parts of the nucleus. They are not localized rostrally or caudally. It is true, as Dr. Beitz has said, that rostral parts of the fastigial nucleus give rise to most of the fibers going to reticular formation. In our studies the injection sites which demonstrated the largest number of fastigioreticular fibers always involved the oral pole of the nucleus. With injections in the caudal part of the fastigial nucleus the reticular fibers were very much smaller in number.

Brodal: I have two questions concerning the reticular tegmental nucleus that I don't think you mentioned in the monkey. The first one is: in the cat, Walberg and co-workers [10] have described a projection from the fastigial nucleus to certain parts of this reticular tegmental nucleus. I was particularly interested to hear whether you found evidence of this in the rhesus monkey.

Carpenter: There are a small number of fibers which do go to the reticular tegmental nucleus. But they're really quite small, and in some of our best examples they were scarce.

Brodal: The second question was: from your HRP experiments did you find any labeled cells in this nucleus or in the pontine nuclei?

Carpenter: Yes, there are quite a good number of labeled cells in the pontine nuclei.

References

1. Gardner EP, Fuchs AF (1975) Single unit responses to natural vestibular stimuli and eye movements in deep cerebellar nuclei of the alert rhesus monkey. J Neurophysiol 38:627–649
2. Harper JW, Heath RG (1973) Anatomic connections of the fastigial nucleus to the rostral forebrain in the cat. Exp Neurol 39:285–292
3. Kotchabhakdi N, Walberg F (1978) Cerebellar afferent projections from the vestibular nuclei in the cat: an experimental study with the method of retrograde axonal transport of horseradish peroxidase. Exp Brain Res 31:591–604
4. Martin GF, Linauts M, Walker JM (1977) The nucleus corporis pontobulbaris of the North American opossum. J Comp Neurol 175:345–372
5. Oswaldo-Cruz E, Rocha-Miranda CE (1968) The brain of the opossum (*Didelphis marsupialis*). Instituto de Biofisica, Universidade, Federal do Rio Janeiro, Rio de Janeiro
6. Paul SM, Heath RG, Ellison JP (1973) Histochemical demonstration of a direct pathway from fastigial nucleus to the septal region. Exp Neurol 40:798–805
7. Ritchie, L (1976) Effects of cerebellar lesions on saccadic eye movements. J Neurophysiol 39:1246–1256
8. Voogd J (1964) The cerebellum of the cat. Ph. D. thesis. University of Leiden
9. Walberg F, Pompeiano O, Brodal A, Jansen J (1962) The fastigiovestibular projection in the cat. An experimental study with silver impregnation methods. J Comp Neurol 118:49–76
10. Walberg F, Pompeiano O, Westrum LE, Hauglie-Hanssen E (1962) Fastigioreticular fibers in the cat. An experimental study with silver methods. J Comp Neurol 119:187–199
11. Yuën H, Dom R, Martin GF (1974) Cerebellopontine projections in the American opossum. A study of their origin, distribution, and overlap with fibers from the cerebral cortex. J Comp Neurol 154:257–286

The Cerebellar Nucleocortical Pathway

D. L. Tolbert

Introduction

Evidence for axonal projections from the intracerebellar nuclei to the overlying cortex, until quite recently, was equivocal and a matter of considerable debate. Ramon y Cajal's studies of Golgi impregnated neurons in the rat cerebellar nuclei [18] first suggested the existence of cerebellar nucleocortical projections. Cajal described some fastigial neurons whose axons coursed dorsally from the nucleus into the vermian cortex. In his later studies [19] of the cerebellar nuclei, however, Cajal made no reference to nucleocortical fibers and the existence of this pathway was left in doubt. Subsequent anterograde degeneration experiments by a number of investigators [2, 6, 20] have described degenerating axons in the cortex following lesions of the cerebellar nuclei. Carrea et al. [2] on the basis of their degeneration material proposed that small and large neurons in the cerebellar nuclei send direct or collateral projections to the cortex that end as climbing fibers on Purkinje cells. Thomas et al. [20] and Cohen et al. [6] on the other hand, described the axonal debris in the cortex as being predominantly localized within the granule cell layer after lesions of the deep nuclei. The evidence for a nucleocortical projection obtained from these anterograde degeneration experiments was conjectural, however, because of the inability to distinguish between degenerating nucleocortical fibers *and* the degeneration resulting from interruption of extracerebellar afferents by the lesion in the deep nuclei.

Unitary electrophysiological studies were unable to resolve this issue. Ito et al. [12] originally reported activation of some neurons in the cerebellar nuclei at latencies as short as 0.5 ms following stimulation of the cerebellar cortex, inferring an antidromic activation via a nucleocortical pathway. However, the lack of subsequent anatomical verification for a nucleocortical pathway prompted Ito and colleagues in a later study [13] to suggest that their findings may have been due to current spread from the cortical stimulus, activating the neurons directly or their efferent projections in the brachium conjunctivum.

The Cerebellar Nucleocortical Projection Identified with Intraaxonal Tracers

The application of recently developed orthograde and retrograde intraaxonal tracing techniques to studies of the efferent projections of the cerebellar nuclei have provided new evidence for a cerebellar nucleocortical pathway.

Experimental Brain Research, Suppl. 6

Results from the Retrograde Transport of Horseradish Peroxidase

Experiments utilizing the retrograde transport of horseradish peroxidase (HRP) from injection sites in the cat cerebellar cortex were initially used to demonstrate that neurons in each of the intracerebellar nuclei have nucleocortical projections (Fig. 1A) [9, 23]. Similar experiments have subsequently identified nucleocortical projections in the rhesus monkey [25], tree shrew [10], and pigeon [5]. In addition to providing confirmatory evidence for a cerebellar nucleocortical system, these retrograde labeling experiments also proved useful in identifying some of the general morphological characteristics of the cells of origin of this pathway (Fig. 1). The most common types of neurons retrogradely labeled in the cat were medium-sized, multipolar-shaped cells (Fig. 1C) [9, 23]. Fewer large multipolar- (Fig. 1B) and small spindle-shaped neurons also contained HRP reaction product in each experiment. Measurements of the maximum diameters of neurons in the cat's cerebellar nuclei (Fig. 2) indicated that most of

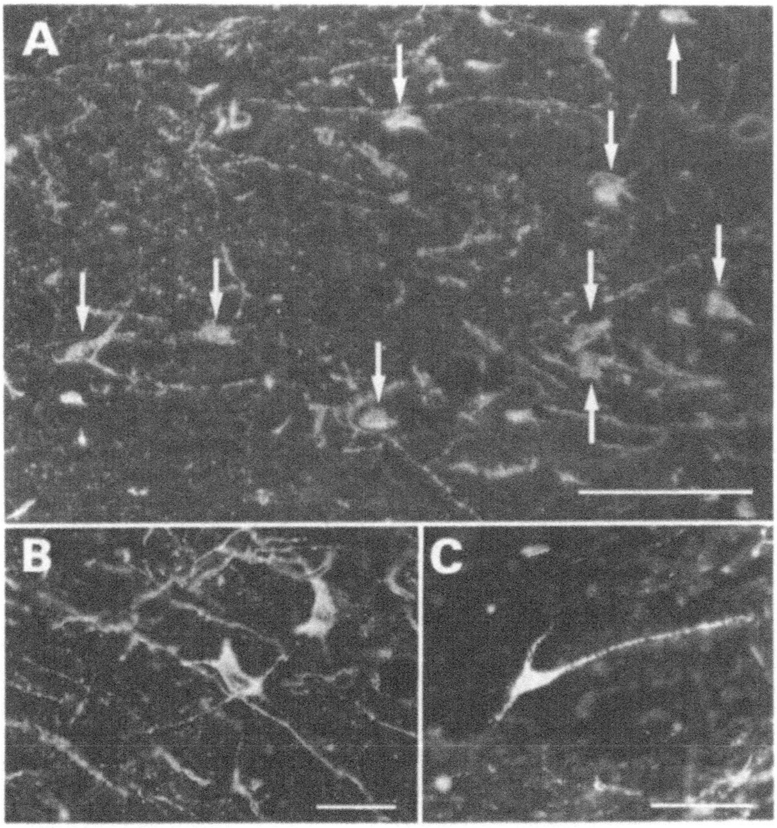

Fig. 1. A Low-power–dark-field photomicrograph of HRP-positive neurons (*arrows*) in the cat fastigial nucleus retrogradely labeled from an injection site in the posterior vermis. **B** and **C** are high-power–dark-field photomicrographs of large **B** and medium **C** sized HRP-positive multipolar cells. *Bar scale* = 200 μm in A and 50 μm in **B** and **C**

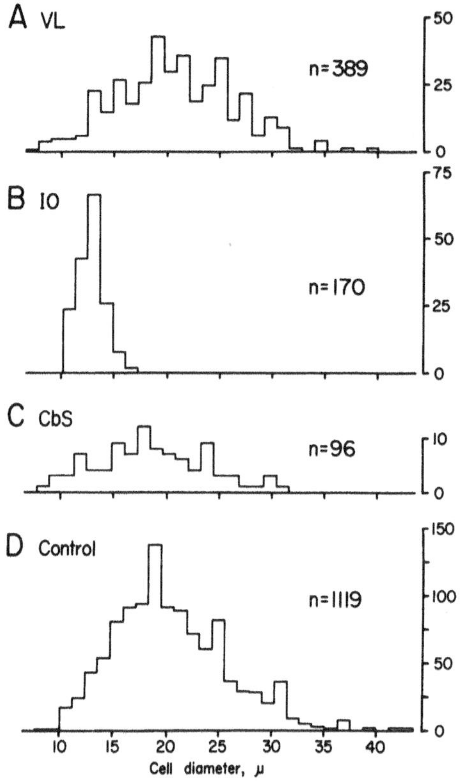

Fig. 2. Histograms of the maximum soma diameters of cerebellar nuclear neurons retrogradely labeled with HRP from injection sites in **A** the thalamus (*VL*), **B** the inferior olive (*IO*), and **C** the cerebellar cortex (*CbS*). **D** is a histogram of the overall size distribution of neurons in the cerebellar nuclei. Note that cerebellothalamic and nucleocortical projections arise from a heterogeneous population of neurons whose diameters correspond to the size spectrum of neurons present in the deep nuclei, whereas the cerebello-olivary pathway arises from a specific population of small neurons. Reprinted with permission from ref. [26]

these somata range from 9 to 40 μm [15, 26], with the largest number being medium-sized, 15–30 μm, multipolar cells [8, 26]. Although Gould [8] has recently shown nucleocortical afferents to the vestibulo-cerebellum arising from a limited population of 20–25 μm diameter neurons, the point to emphasize, however, is that nucleocortical projections to most areas of the cat cortex arise from a heterogenous population of small spindle-shaped and medium and large multipolar neurons with somal diameters corresponding to all sizes of neurons present in the cerebellar nuclei (Fig. 2).

Further morphological characteristics of cells giving rise to nucleocortical projections was recently provided by McCrea et al. [15], who studied intracellularly stained neurons in the cat interpositus nuclei. In addition to showing anatomically the collateral origin of the nucleocortical fibers described later, features of the dendritic arborization of these neurons were also identified. A medium-sized, multipolar stained neuron (20 μm in diameter) supported a dendritic arborization extending 1000 μm anteroposteriorly, 900 μm mediolaterally, and 560 μm dorsoventrally. A larger multipolar neuron (48 by 41 μm) had a more extensive secondary and tertiary dendritic aborization that extended approximately 1100 μm anteroposteriorly, 700 μm mediolaterally, and 610 μm dorsoventrally. The dendrites of both HRP-stained cells bore numerous spines.

In the monkey, Chan-Palay's Golgi studies of the dentate nucleus identified "large neurons" along the lateral boundary of the nucleus and "asymmetrical neurons" within the nucleus proper as the probable cells of origin for nucleocortical projections in this species [3].

Results from Orthograde Labeling with Labeled Amino Acids

Cerebellar nucleocortical axons and their terminal arborizations have also been demonstrated autoradiographically after their orthograde labeling with radioactive amino acids. Following injections in the cat or monkey cerebellar nuclei, a large number of labeled nucleocortical fibers passed directly out of the injected area of the nuclei and projected individually toward the cortex or emerged from fascicules of labeled cerebellofugal axons traveling toward the cerebellar peduncles [23]. These autoradiographic observations have been clarified by McCrea et al. [15], studies which showed nucleocortical axons arising as

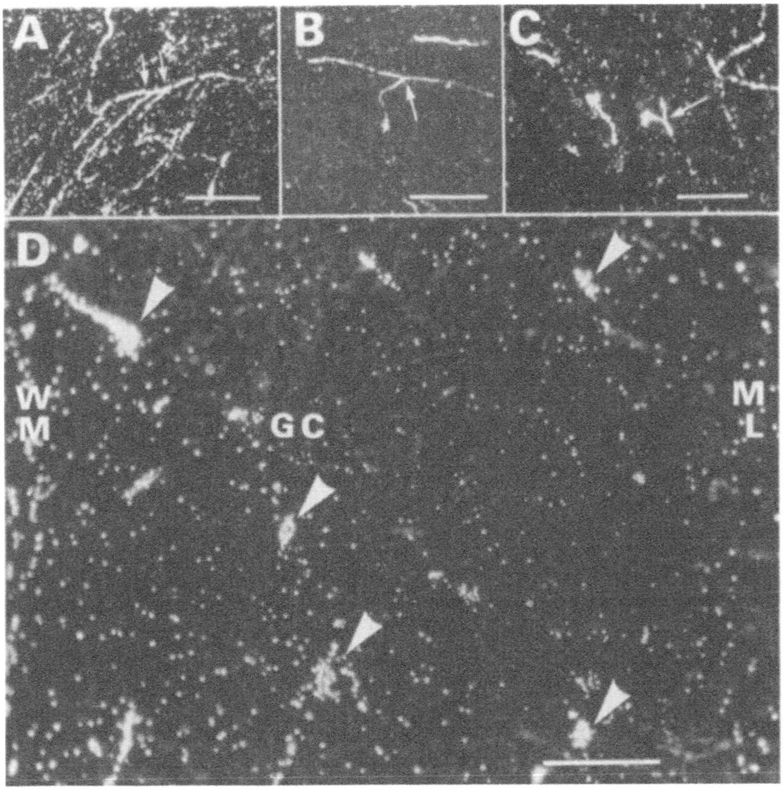

Fig. 3A–C. The linear distribution of autoradiographic silver grains are continuous at branch points (*arrows*) of labeled nucleocortical axons and indicate the fibers give off collaterals in the corpus medullare **A**, folial white matter **B**, and in the granule cell layer **C**. In **D** labeled nucleocortical terminals, as indicated by the clusters of silver grains (*arrowheads*), appear to be uniformly distributed throughout the granule cell layer (*GC*) in this area of cortex. *WM*, folial white matter; *ML*, molecular layer. *Bar scale*=100 μm **A, B** and 50 μm **C, D. A–C** reprinted with permission from ref. [27]

collaterals both within the immediate vicinity of the cell body *and* from more distal segments of the parent fiber as it projected into the brachium conjunctivum.

Labeled nucleocortical axons can be identified in autoradiographs by the dense fiberlike arrays of silver grains overlying longitudinally sectioned fibers. The rows of silver grains over some labeled axons were continuous at apparent points of bifurcation, suggesting that nucleocortical axons continued to branch in the cerebellar white matter deep to the cortex (Fig. 3A), in the folial white matter (Fig. 3B), and within the granule layer itself (Fig. 3C) [27]. In this regard, the nucleocortical projection appears to have characteristics similar to other cerebellar afferent systems [16].

Labeled nucleocortical fibers can be followed from the folial white matter into the granule cell layer of the cortex where many terminate in an ovoid or circular cluster of silver grains (Fig. 3B–D). These silver grain clusters measure 8–16 μm and were usually concentrated over protoplasmic islands between the granule cell perikarya. In these orthograde labeling experiments silver grains were never observed to be above background levels over the molecular or Purkinje cell layers of the cortex. The above findings strongly suggested that the cerebellar nucleocortical pathway was a mossy-fiber type afferent.

This was confirmed in recent experiments where nucleocortical terminals were identified using EM autoradiography [14, 28]. Tritiated leucine injections were made in the cat fastigial or dentate nuclei and all three layers of the cortex and the immediate subgranular white matter analyzed. Labeled nucleocortical axons in the folial white matter were myelinated and appeared identical to other nonlabeled axons in regard to the organization of their internal structure. In the granule cell layer, nucleocortical fibers synapsed at en passant swellings along unmyelinated segments of the axons or, more commonly and numerously, at their terminal arborizations. The en passant swellings can be characterized as a bulbous expansion of the labeled axon where numerous neurofilaments and mitochondria form the central core of the axon and synaptic vesicles localized only within the expanded portion of the axon. These en passant swellings corresponded to the "simple" mossy-fiber rosettes described by Palay and Chan-Palay [16], and made single synaptic contacts with small dendritic profiles or a series of contacts on the shafts of larger dendrites. More commonly, however, the autoradiographic silver grains were present over the coiled, tortuous ends of the mossy fibers (Fig. 4). Depending upon the plane of section there were usually two to five individual labeled profiles intermingled with the terminal dendrites of granule cells. These complex [16] mossy-fiber rosettes probably correspond to the labeled endings observed in light microscopic autoradiographs (Fig. 3B–D). Axon terminals of Golgi cells were not observed within all the glomeruli containing labeled mossy-fiber endings. The synaptic contacts associated with the labeled en passant swellings or the terminal rosettes were of the asymmetric type with clear round synaptic vesicles present in the presynaptic elements (Fig. 4). Profiles of astrocytic processes were located external to the mossy-fiber endings and the postsynaptic granule cell dendrites. Occasionally, labeled nucleocortical axons were also observed closely adjacent to granule cell bodies. These nonglomerular labeled profiles did not synapse di-

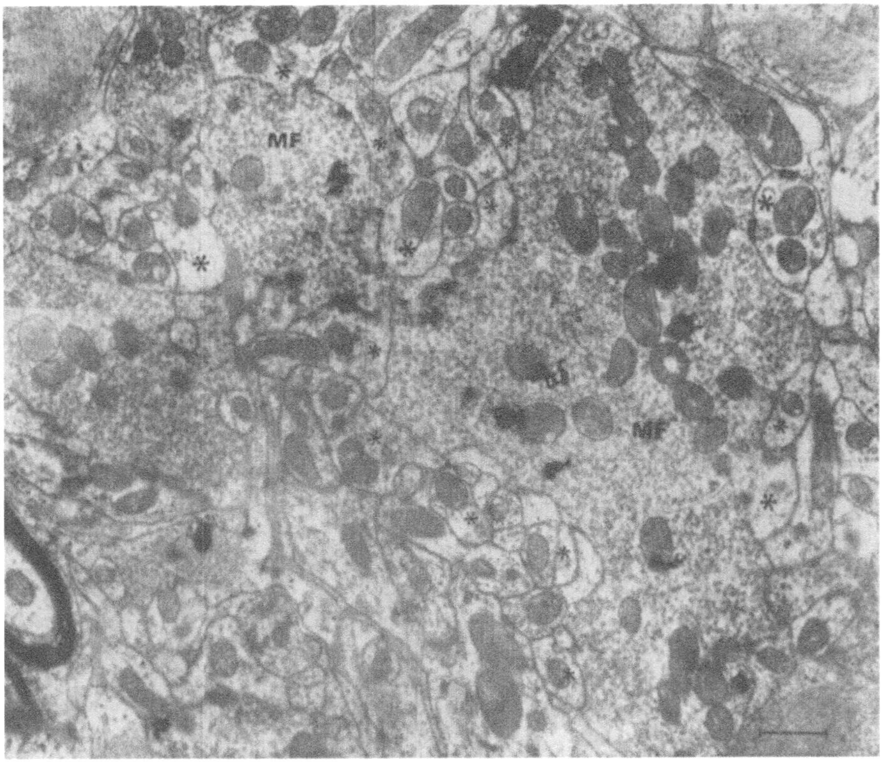

Fig. 4. Photomontage of a labeled complex mossy-fiber rossette (*MF*). This type of terminal ending had a highly irregular shape with two to five profiles of the same bouton usually observed in a single plane of section. These complex rosettes were densely packed with clear, round synaptic vesicles and formed numerous asymmetric type contacts on granule cell dendrites (*). *Scale bar* = 1 μm

rectly on any of the granule cell soma membrane but usually formed asymmetric contacts with large dendritic profiles.

Electrophysiological Evidence for a Cerebellar Nucleocortical Projection

Single unit recordings performed concurrently with some of the studies described above provided electrophysiological evidence for a cerebellar nucleocortical projection [23, 25]. In alpha-chloralose-anesthetized cats and rhesus monkeys (*Macaca mulatta*), stimulating electrodes stereotaxically positioned in the cat brachium conjunctivum or the monkey thalamic ventral lateral nucleus, were used to activate neurons antidromically in the dentate and interpositus nuclei. The ipsilateral cerebellar cortex was stimulated with bipolar surface electrodes. Extracellularly recorded unitary responses which displayed an initial segment (IS)-soma dendritic (SD) inflection on the rising phase of the action potential satisfied the criteria that these recordings were made from the immediate vicinity of a neuronal soma. Stimulation of the cerebellar cortex evoked unitary responses in cat and monkey dentate and interpositus neurons at latencies as short as 0.3 ms [23, 25]. In the cat the mean latency of antidromic activation was 0.6 ms [26]. Figure 5 gives several examples of the types of response evoked in cat cerebellar nuclear neurons to stimulation of the cerebellar surface (CbS) and brachium conjunctivum (BC) at stimulus frequencies of 1/s–100/s. The invariant latency in the onset of the evoked response when the stimulus frequency was increased from 1/s (A, C, E) to 100/s (B, D, G), and when the stimulus intensity was increased from threshold (A, C, E) to suprathreshold levels strongly indicated that these action potentials resulted from the antidromic activation of a cerebellar nucleocortical pathway.

Intracellular recordings from cat cerebellar nuclei were used to confirm that the short latency responses, such as those described in Fig. 5, were not evoked transynaptically through activation of a very efficient excitatory synaptic input. Figure 6 illustrates the responses evoked in a dentate neuron to stimulation of the CbS and the BC before (A) and after (B–E) its penetration by the recording microelectrode. Since no excitatory postsynaptic potentials (EPSPs) were recorded in the neuron immediately following stimulation of CbS it follows that the action potentials recorded in Fig. 6 A–C were evoked by the antidromic invasion of this neuron.

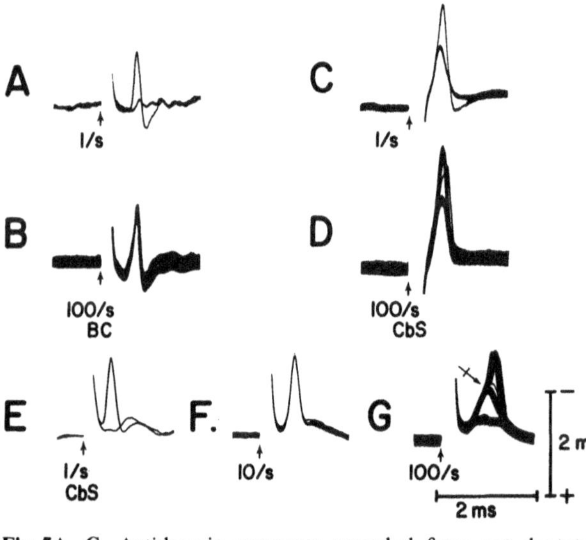

Fig. 5A–G. Antidromic responses recorded from cat dentate neurons to stimulation of the brachium conjunctivum (*BC*) and cerebellar surface (*CbS*). The records in **A** and **B** show the antidromic response of a dentate neuron to threshold stimulation of the *BC* at a frequency of 1/s **A** and suprathreshold stimulation at 100/s **B.** In **C, D** the responses of this neuron to cerebellar surface stimulation (*CbS*) are shown at these same stimulus frequencies. **E–G** are examples of responses recorded from another neuron to stimulation of cerebellar surface at frequencies of 1/s **F,** 10/s **F,** and 100/s **G.** In **G** the decomposition of the action potential into its initial segment-soma dendritic components (*crossed arrow*) can be observed. Reprinted with permission from ref. [23]

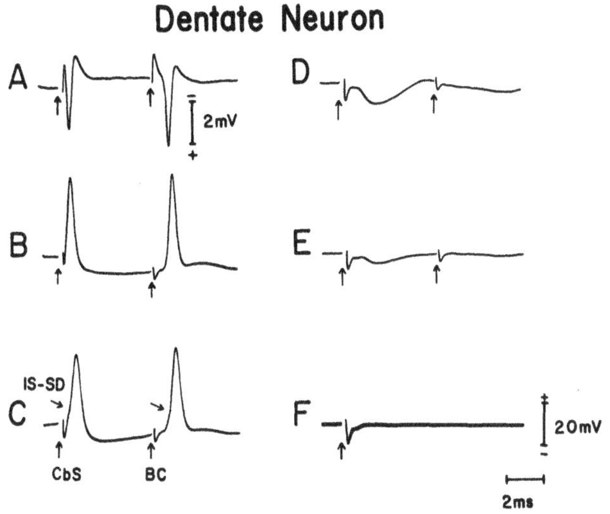

Fig. 6. Recordings from at cat dentate neuron to stimulation of the cerebellar surface (*CbS*) and brachium conjunctivum (*BC*) before **A** and after its penetration by the recording microelectrode **B–E**. As a spike generating mechanism of the cell deteriorated **C**, an *IS-SD* break on the action potentials evoked by these stimuli became apparent (*arrows*). In **D** and **E** when spikes could no longer be evoked, a graded hyperpolarization was observed in response to *CbS* stimulation. The records in **F** are three superimposed traces obtained just outside the cell. Reprinted with permission from ref. [23]

Branching of Cerebellar Efferents

Retrograde labeling experiments have shown that morphological similarities exist between neurons in the cerebellar nuclei projecting to extracerebellar nuclei and to the cerebellar cortex [26]. The longest soma diameters of HRP-positive neurons retrogradely labeled from injection sites in the thalamus (A), inferior olive (B) and cerebellar cortex (C) are given in Fig. 2. Since the size of some of the neurons projecting to brain stem nuclei and cerebellar cortex are comparable, it is suggested that these neurons may have collateral projections to several of these sites [26]. McCrea et al. [15] subsequently demonstrated collateral branching of these axons within the cerebellum. These anatomical findings and the observation that some cerebellar nuclear neurons can be activated antidromically from *both* the BC and the cerebellar cortex in the cat and the ventral lateral nucleus and cortex in the monkey infer that the nucleocortical pathway arises as collaterals of cerebellofugal projections to the brain stem.
The top of Fig. 7 illustrates the experimental paradigm used to test this hypothesis. In chloralose-anesthetized cats stimulating electrodes were positioned at appropriate sites in the ventral lateral thalamic nucleus and inferior olive to activate a large number of ascending cerebellothalamic axons and descending cerebello-olivary fibers [24] respectively. Bipolar stimulating electrodes were positioned directly on the surface of the ipsilateral cerebellar posterior lobe hemisphere. Glass microelectrodes were used to record extracellularly from

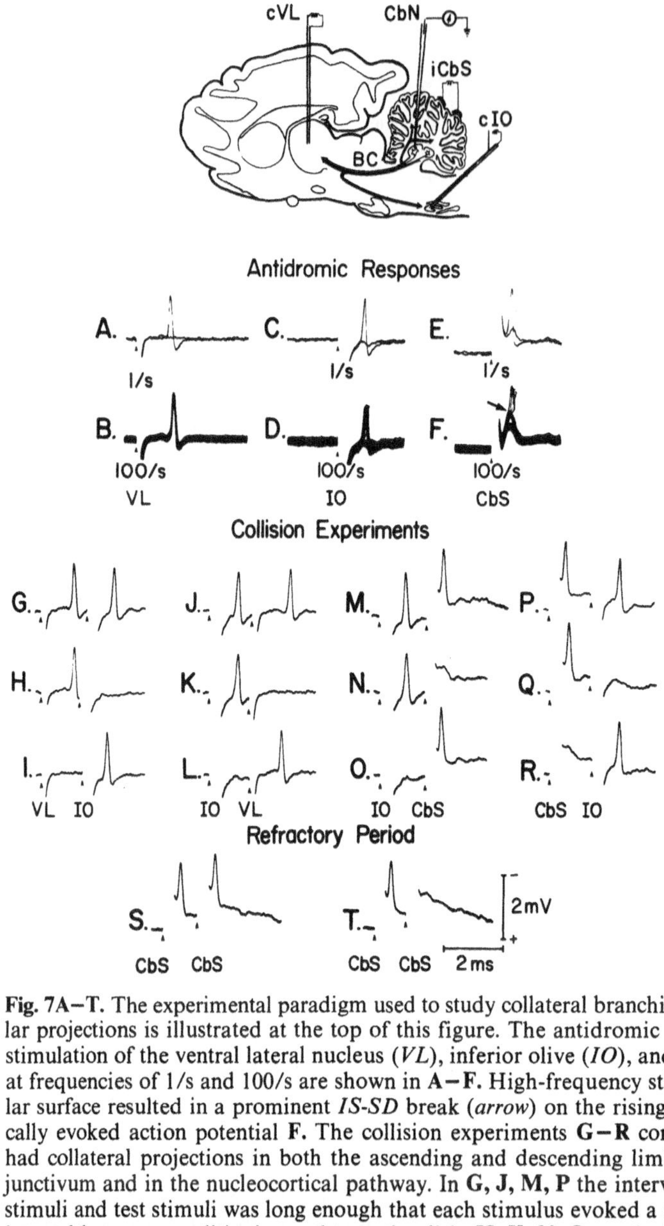

Fig. 7A–T. The experimental paradigm used to study collateral branching of cat efferent cerebellar projections is illustrated at the top of this figure. The antidromic responses of a neuron to stimulation of the ventral lateral nucleus (*VL*), inferior olive (*IO*), and cerebellar cortex (*CbS*) at frequencies of 1/s and 100/s are shown in **A–F**. High-frequency stimulation of the cerebellar surface resulted in a prominent *IS-SD* break (*arrow*) on the rising phase of the antidromically evoked action potential **F**. The collision experiments **G–R** confirmed that this neuron had collateral projections in both the ascending and descending limbs of the brachium conjunctivum and in the nucleocortical pathway. In **G, J, M, P** the interval between conditioning stimuli and test stimuli was long enough that each stimulus evoked a response. Decreasing the interval between conditioning and test stimuli in **H, K, N, Q** resulted in a suppression of the response evoked by the test stimulus. At this critical stimulus interval, when the intensity of the conditioning stimulus was decreased to subthreshold levels the antidromic response evoked by the test stimulus could again be observed **(I, L, O, R)**. In **S, T** paired stimuli were used to determine the refractory period of this neuron. Note that the interval between stimuli in **T** is equal to the refractory period of this neuron and is appreciably shorter than the critical interstimulus interval used above **H, K, N, Q** to demonstrate collision. Reprinted with permission from ref. [26]

dentate and interpositus neurons (CbN). Collision experiments to demonstrate collateral branching were carried out on units antidromically activated from more than one stimulus site. Figure 7A–T illustrates a series of recordings obtained from a neuron activated from all three stimulus sites.

In Fig. 7A–F, the responses evoked by stimulation of the contralateral ventral lateral nucleus (VL), and inferior olive (IO), and the ipsilateral CbS at frequencies of 1/s and 100/s are shown. The invarient latency in the onset of the evoked responses to threshold and suprathreshold stimulation and at low and high frequencies of stimulation indicates that each of these responses were evoked antidromically. Repetitive stimulation of the CbS (Fig. 7F) resulted in a prominent IS-SD break on the rising phase of the action potential, indicating that the recordings were obtained in the vicinity of the soma-dendritic region of the cell.

The collision experiments performed in Fig. 7G–R were used to determine whether the responses recorded in Fig. 7A–F resulted from the activation of collaterals at each of the three stimulus sites. In Fig. 7G, J, M, P the interval between the conditioning and test stimuli was long enough to allow the action potential evoked by the conditioning stimulus to be conducted not only antidromically to the soma but also orthodromically from the branch site past the site of the test stimulus and early enough that the absolute refractory period of the axon at the test stimulus site was over before the test stimulus was applied. Decreasing the interval between the conditioning stimulus to the VL and test stimulus to the IO in Fig. 7H, and between the stimuli to the IO and CbS in Fig. 7N, identified a *critical interstimulus interval* at which collision consistently occurred between the action potential evoked by the conditioning stimulus and the responses evoked by the test stimulus. This *critical interstimulus interval* is a measure of the conduction time for propagation of the action potential from the conditioning stimulus site to the test stimulus site *and* the absolute refractory period of the axon at the test stimulus site. By reversing the order of stimulation in Fig. 7K and Q, a second critical interstimulus interval was similarly determined. At the critical interstimulus interval when the strength of the conditioning stimulus was decreased to subthreshold levels (Fig. 7I, L, O, R) then the response evoked from the test stimulus site was no longer supressed. Since the conduction time for an action potential to propagate between the conditioning and test stimulus sites is independent of the direction of propagation, the critical interstimulus intervals obtained in Fig. 7H, K or Fig. 7N, Q must be identical if the responses were conducted by collaterals of the same neuron. The critical interstimulus intervals were identical and independent of the order of stimulation [26].

Paired stimuli were applied to each of the stimulus sites in order to ensure that the suppression of the response evoked by the test stimulus (Fig. 7H, K, N, Q) did not result from the neuronal soma being in refractory period due to its antidromic activation by the conditioning stimulus. In Fig. 7S, two stimuli were applied to the cerebellar surface at a latency between stimuli long enough that each stimulus evokes an antidromic response. Decreasing the interval between the paired stimuli in Fig. 7T results in the consistent suppression of the second response. The interval between the paired stimuli in Fig. 7T therefore defined the refractory period of the neuron and was considerably less than the critical interstimulus interval obtained in the above collision experiments. These type of experiments, therefore, confirm that there are neurons in the cerebellar dentate and interpositus nuclei which have multiple terminations, via collaterals, in the ventral lateral nucleus, inferior olive, and cerebellar cortex.

Topography of Cerebellar Nucleocortical Projections

The organization of nucleocortical projections to specific cerebellar folia has been mapped using retrograde labeling techniques [8, 9, 11, 27] and the projections of individual intracerebellar nuclei have been studied by the orthograde transport of labeled amino acids [3, 27]. The topography of the nucleocortical pathway has been studied in greatest detail in the cat [8, 9, 23, 27]. These results show that the cat nucleocortical projection is generally organized into three rostrocaudally oriented longitudinal zones [27].

Labeled terminals in the cortex (Fig. 3B–D) were plotted onto drawings of transverse sections of the cerebellum using an X–Y recorder interfaced with the mechanical stage of the microscope (Figs. 8–10).

The distribution of labeled fastigiocortical terminals are illustrated in Fig. 8. In this animal, the largest number of labeled terminals were present in the ipsilateral vermis. This dense projection extended 2.5 mm laterally from the midline in vermian lobules V–X and 1.5 mm from the midline in lobule I–IV. There was a sharp demarcation of the midline vermis by the density of ipsilateral fastigiocortical fibers and terminals. Fewer terminals were observed in the cortex surrounding the dense longitudinal band described above. Ipsilaterally the lighter projection zone extended laterally from the dense area of termination up to 3.5 mm from the midline in lobules V through X and approximately 2.5 mm from the midline in the rostral four lobules (I–IV). A similar density of terminals was also noted within 1.5 mm from the midline in the contralateral vermis [27]. In each autoradiograph a few nucleocortical terminals were also observed in the ipsilateral lobus simplex, ansiform lobule, dorsal and ventral subdivisions of the paraflocculus, and the flocculus. Labeled terminals were occasionally observed in the hemisphere contralateral to the injection site in the fastigial nucleus. Although the injection site in this animal involved only intermediate and rostral levels of the nucleus, the distribution of terminals in the cortex was quite apparent throughout the rostral-caudal extent of the vermis. Injections of HRP in the vermis and the resultant labeling of neurons in the intracerebellar nuclei confirmed the general organization of fastigial nucleocortical projections [8, 27]. In these experiments the greatest number of neurons retrogradely labeled from vermian HRP-injection sites were present in the underlying fastigial nuclei. Appreciably fewer definitively labeled HRP-positive neurons were present in adjoining interpositus nuclei. Gould [8] has noted that these fastigiocortical projections arose from neurons located peripherally within the nucleus.

The distribution of nucleocortical projections from the posterior interpositus nucleus is plotted in Fig. 9 and is representative of the basic organization of nu-

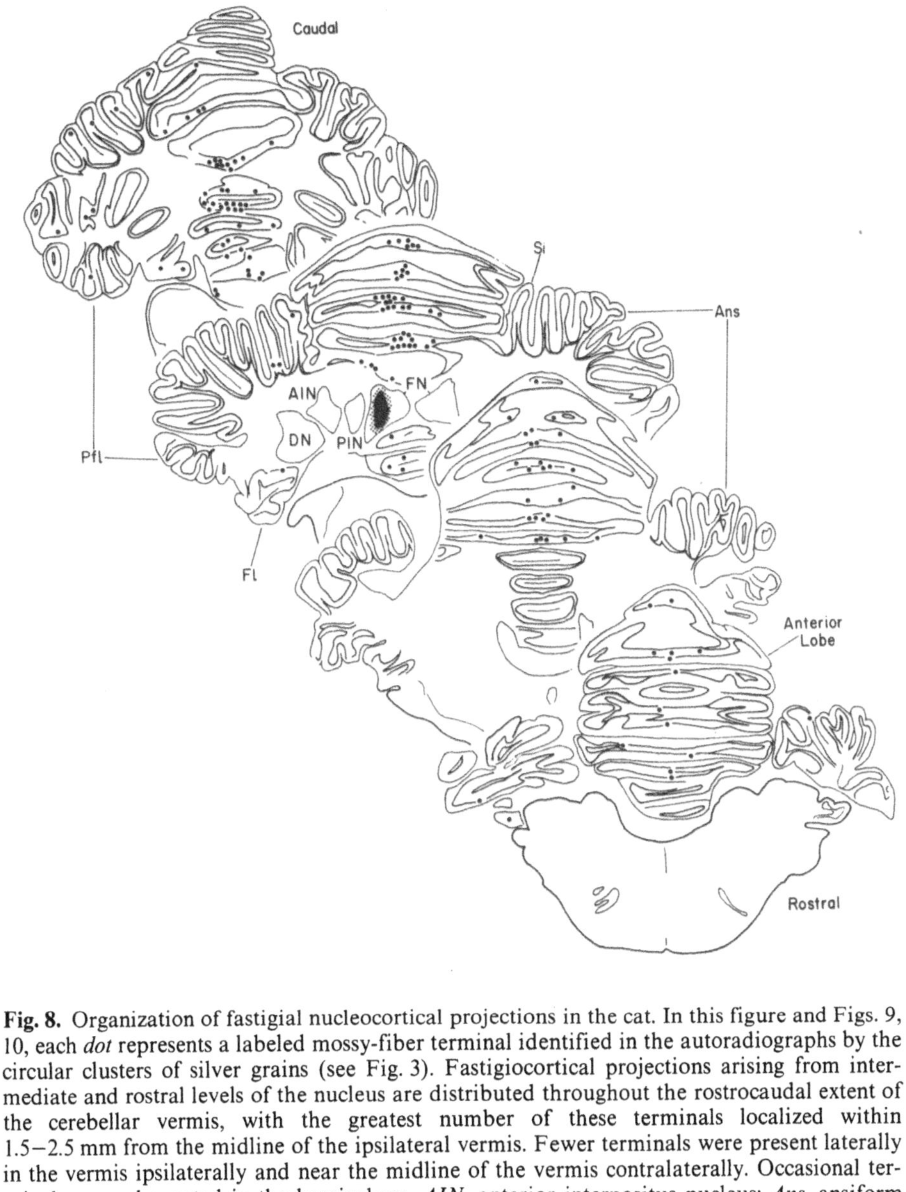

Fig. 8. Organization of fastigial nucleocortical projections in the cat. In this figure and Figs. 9, 10, each *dot* represents a labeled mossy-fiber terminal identified in the autoradiographs by the circular clusters of silver grains (see Fig. 3). Fastigiocortical projections arising from intermediate and rostral levels of the nucleus are distributed throughout the rostrocaudal extent of the cerebellar vermis, with the greatest number of these terminals localized within 1.5–2.5 mm from the midline of the ipsilateral vermis. Fewer terminals were present laterally in the vermis ipsilaterally and near the midline of the vermis contralaterally. Occasional terminals were also noted in the hemisphere. *AIN*, anterior interpositus nucleus; *Ans*, ansiform lobule; *DN*, dentate nucleus; *Fl*, flocculus; *FN*, fastigial nucleus; *Pfl*, paraflocculus; *PIN*, posterior interpositus nucleus; *Pmd*, paramedian lobule; *Si*, simplex lobule

cleocortical projections of both the anterior and posterior nuclei. From an injection site in the posterior interpositus nucleus labeled nucleocortical axons coursed dorsally, laterally, or caudally to terminate in greatest numbers in the paramedian lobule, the paraflocculus, and the caudomedial end of the lobus simplex, Crus I and Crus II. In the paraflocculus, labeled terminals were more

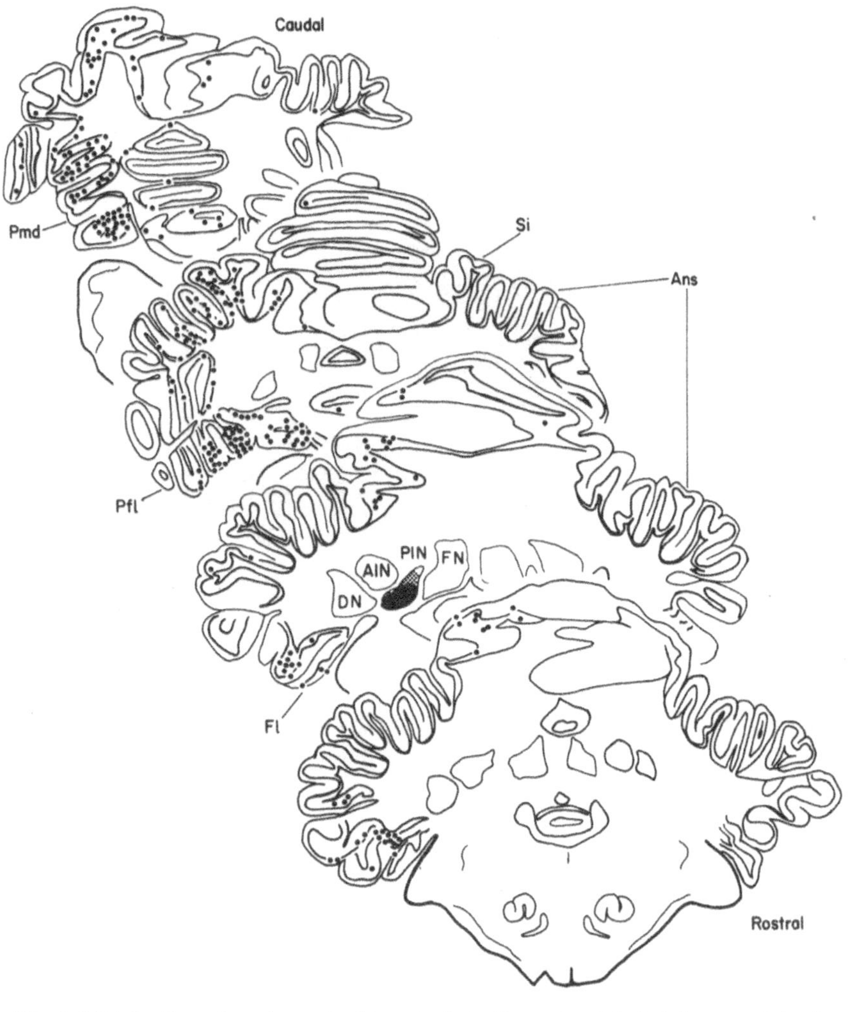

Fig. 9. Distribution of nucleocortical terminals in the cortex labeled from an injection site in the posterior interpositus nucleus. Labeled terminals were primarily localized within the ipsilateral paramedian lobule (*Pmd*), paraflocculus (*Pfl*), and caudal folia of the lobus simplex (*Si*) and medial Crus I. The lateral edge of the vermis, intermediate areas of the hemisphere, and the flocculus (*Fl*) received a lighter projection. Abbreviations see Fig. 8

numerous in the caudal two-thirds of the folia than more rostrally. Significantly fewer terminals were observed in the folia adjacent to those which receive a dense projection. These areas included intermediate regions of the ansiform lobule (Crus I and II), the flocculus, and along the lateral edge of the vermian folia V–X.

Injections of the anterior interpositus nuclei (not illustrated) resulted in a heavier distribution of labeled nucleocortical terminals in more rostral area of

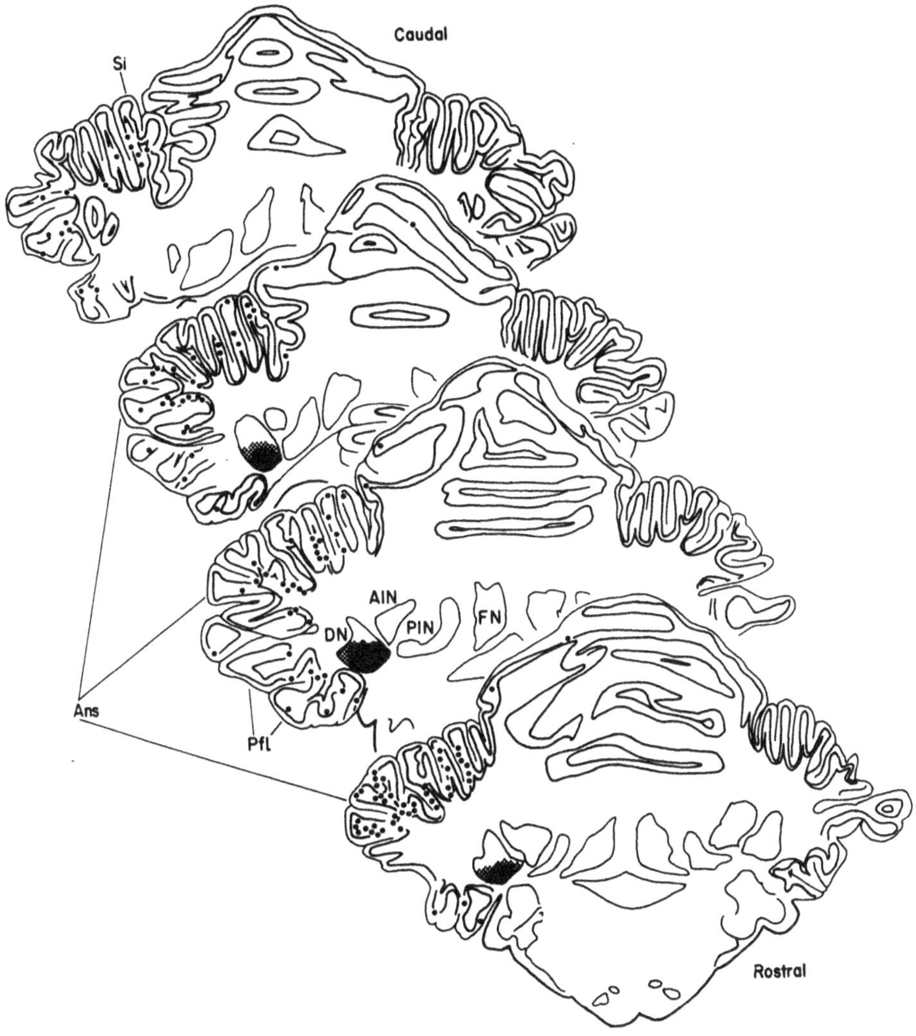

Fig. 10. Distribution of dentatocortical terminals labeled from an injection in the ventral part of the nucleus. Terminals are most heavily localized in Crus II and lateral folial of Crus I of the ansiform lobule (*Ans*). Fewer terminals were present in medial Crus I, the Lobus Simplex (*Si*), and occasionally in midline areas of the cortex. Abbreviations see Fig. 8

the intermediate cortex including the middle half of anterior lobules IV and V, the rostral end of the lobus simplex, and medial folia of Crus I. A significant number of labeled terminals were also present in the granular layer of the dorsal paraflocculus and in the paramedian lobule.

Placements of HRP in those areas of cortex identified in the autoradiographic studies as receiving interpositus-nucleocortical projections confirmed that these nuclei projected upon a rostrocaudal longitudinal zone of intermediate cerebellar cortex. In Gould's [8] studies, HRP injections into the paramedian lobule, resulted in retrograde labeling of neurons primarily in the posterior interpositus nucleus and in adjacent areas of the dentate nucleus. Injections in the paraflocculus labeled neurons localized in ventral and caudal areas of the interpositus nuclei. Interpositus nucleocortical projections to the lateral edge of the vermis were verified in experiments where the enzyme diffused from midline injections into the lateral edge of the vermis [8, 27]. Finally, injections limited to the lobus simplex resulted in characteristic labeling of neurons in both the anterior and posterior interpositus nuclei, with fewer neurons present in adjacent areas of the dentate nucleus [27].

The organization of dentatocortical projections arising from neurons in the ventral half of the nucleus is shown in Fig. 10. In this experiment the majority of labeled terminals were observed throughout Crus II and the more lateral folia of Crus I. Medial to these areas fewer labeled terminals were observed in the medial folia of Crus I, the lobus simplex, the paraflocculus, and occasionally along the lateral edge of the ipsilateral vermis. It was noted [27] in another animal that injections of the dorsal dentate nucleus labeled terminals mainly in lateral Crus I and dorsomedial folia of Crus II.

Injections of HRP into Crus I and II resulted in retrograde labeling of neurons predominantly within the underlying dentate nucleus with occasional HRP-positive neurons also present in the ipsilateral interpositus nuclei [27].

Based on the findings obtained using orthograde and retrograde labeling techniques in the cat, it was concluded that nucleocortical projections from the dentate, interpositus, and fastigial nuclei are principally to the lateral hemisphere, medial hemisphere-paravermis, and vermis respectively. In between these three rostrocaudal longitudinal zones there is an overlap of terminals from adjacent nuclei. Interpositus and dentatocortical projections overlap in the middle region of the hemisphere, interpositus and fastigial nucleocortical terminals overlap along the lateral edge of the vermis, and projections from the fastigial nuclei overlap along the midline of the vermis.

Recent experiments by Dietrichs and Walberg [7], in which HRP injections were localized to one or more of the six longitudinal zones of the cat paramedian lobule, resulted in retrograde labeling of neurons in very circumscribed areas of the deep nuclei. Although these studies imply a more precise level of organization than that described above, the existence of collateral branching of nucleocortical axons, particularly in the subcortical and folial white matter [27], would argue otherwise. Very small placements of radioactive labeled amino acids in the cerebellar nuclei are needed to resolve this.

Although the topography of the monkey nucleocortical projection has not been studied as extensively as in the cat, results from both retrograde and orthograde labeling experiments indicate that the organization of the monkey nucleocortical projection differs markedly from the cat [27].

Chan-Palay's [3] ^{35}S-methionine injections of the macaque dentate nucleus labeled terminals ipsilaterally in lobules V to VIII of the vermis and paravermis, the lobus simplex, ansiform lobule, and rostral areas of the dorsal paraflocculus and flocculus. The topography of dentatocortical terminals corresponded in an anteroposterior and mediolateral fashion with injected areas in

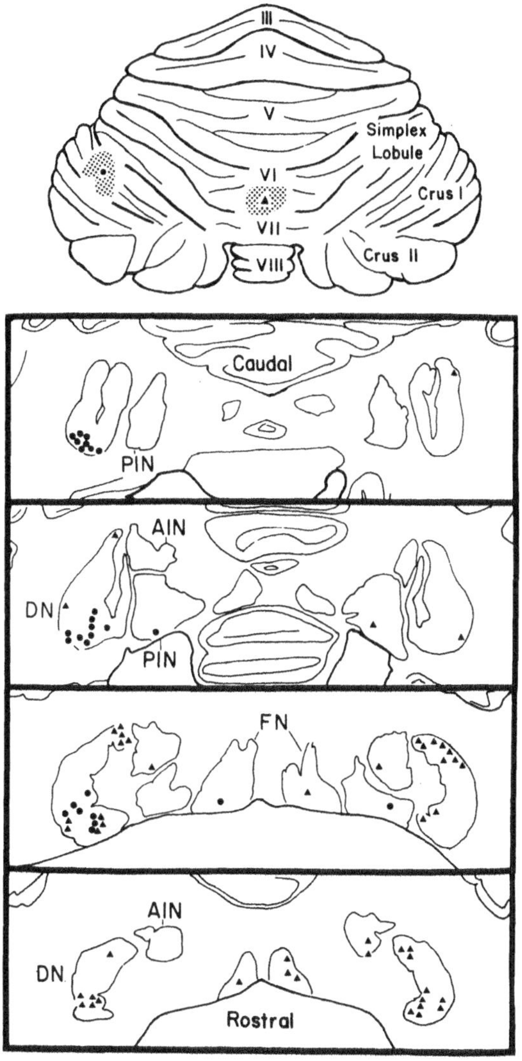

Fig. 11. Distribution of HRP-positive neurons in the monkey cerebellar nuclei retrogradely labeled from enzyme placements (*stippling*) in the lateral hemisphere and midline vermis in two different animals. The results from the animal with the vermal injection were superimposed upon identical levels of the cerebellar nuclei containing neurons retrogradely labeled from Crus I. Neurons projecting to the lateral hemisphere (*dots*) were localized primarily within the ventral area of the ipsilateral dentate nucleus (*DN*). Horseradish peroxidase-positive neurons retrogradely labeled from the midline injection (*triangles*) were present predominantly in dorsomedial and ventral areas of the dentate nuclei bilaterally. In this animal, fewer HRP-positive neurons were present in the fastigial (*FN*) and interpositus nuclei (*AIN, PIN*)

the dentate. The caudal pole of the nucleus projects caudally on the above folia whereas the rostral dentate projects upon more rostral folia. Similar relationships exist between lateral and medial areas of the nucleus and cortex respectively. Projections to the cortex from a single injection site in the nucleus are not "exclusive" [3], however, in that considerable overlap of terminals from neurons in different areas of the nucleus occurs in the cortex. In addition to these projection fields, Chan-Palay noted occasional nucleocortical axons projecting into the vermis and nonspecified areas of the hemisphere contralaterally.

Injections of HRP into the monkey vermis, paravermis, or lateral hemisphere resulted in retrograde labeling of neurons in the dentate nucleus [27], supporting the autoradiographic findings of Chan-Palay [3]. An unexpected observation in these studies, however, was that independent of the location of the HRP placement in medial, intermediate, or lateral cortical zones, the largest number of retrogradely labeled neurons were always present in the ipsilateral dentate nucleus. The results from two animals with injections of the lateral hemisphere and the midline vermis are given in Fig. 11. This figure is a composite in which the results obtained from the animal with a vermis injection were transposed onto diagrams of the cerebellar nuclei at almost identical levels used to plot the distribution neurons labeled from the lateral hemispheral injection. Injections of HRP in lateral Crus I caused a significant number of neurons to be labeled in ventral areas of the ipsilateral dentate nucleus. Occasional HRP-positive neurons were also present in the other ipsilateral cerebellar nuclei and rarely in the contralateral nuclei. Injections in the midline of lobule VI of the vermis resulted in *retrograde* labeling of a large population of neurons localized within dorsomedial and ventral areas of the dentate nuclei bilaterally. Appreciably fewer HRP neurons were observed in the more medial fastigial nuclei. In the dentate nucleus, neurons retrogradely labeled from the injection site in the lateral hemisphere were located more caudally in the nucleus, whereas the HRP-positive neurons labeled from the vermis injection were present more rostrally. There were intermediate levels of the nucleus, however, where it would appear that projections to the lateral hemisphere and to the vermis may arise from a common ventral area in the nucleus.

In another animal with a paravermal-medial hemispherial HRP injection (not illustrated), again the findings were that the labeled neurons were present mainly in the ipsilateral dentate nucleus with fewer in the interpositus nuclei. Although these findings were obtained from a relatively small number of animals the data nevertheless indicates that the organization of macaque nucleocortical projections to the vermis, paravermis, and lateral hemisphere arises principally from the dentate nucleus with secondary projections to the paravermis and vermis arising from the interpositus and fastigial nuclei respectively.

Recently Haines [10] in a study of nucleocortical projections to the paraflocculus of the tree shrew reported findings for a small yet consistent contralateral projection of nucleocortical fibers. Nucleocortical cells retrogradely labeled from the ipsilateral paraflocculus were present mainly in the lateral aspect of the posterior interpositus nucleus and in caudal and ventral areas of the dentate nucleus. Contralateral nucleocortical projection neurons were present in homologous areas of the same nuclei with the ratio of cells labeled in the ipsilateral and contralateral nuclei ranging between 6:1 and 12:1. Although in the cat and rhesus monkey occasional contralateral nucleocortical projections from the dentate and interpositus nuclei were noted [9, 27], the density of these projections was not as extensive as those seen in the tree shrew.

Reciprocal Corticonuclear-Nucleocortical Connections

The question arises as to whether a reciprocal organization exists between the cerebellar corticonuclear and nucleocortical projections. Comparing the results of studies on cerebellar corticonuclear projections with some of the findings described above would indicate that there may be an overlap in the areas of termination and origin of these pathways respectively [27]. Anatomical and electrophysiological evidence support this hypothesis.

One method of examining this interrelationship has been to make combined ^{3}H-amino acid *and* HRP injections into the cerebellar cortex of the cat [8] and monkey [21]. These combined injections resulted in the simultaneous orthograde labeling of Purkinje cell axons and their terminals and the retrograde labeling of neurons in the cerebellar nuclei projecting in the nucleocortical system. Both orthogradely labeled corticonuclear axons and their terminals and HRP-positive neurons were demonstrated together in sections of the cerebellar nuclei processed both histochemically and for autoradiography. In both the cat and monkey cerebellar nuclei, HRP-positive nucleocortical neurons were observed in areas of the nuclei also overlain by a dense plexus of autoradiographic silver grains that resulted from the radioactive labeling of corticonuclear axons and their terminals (Fig. 12). Gould [8] and Haines and Pearson [11] have shown that orthogradely labeled corticonuclear fibers end in a perisomatic-proximal dendritic relationship with the HRP-positive nucleocortical neurons. Experiments by Dietrich and Walberg [7], Haines and Pearson [11], and Chan-Palay [3] using other anatomical methods have provided similar evidence for a

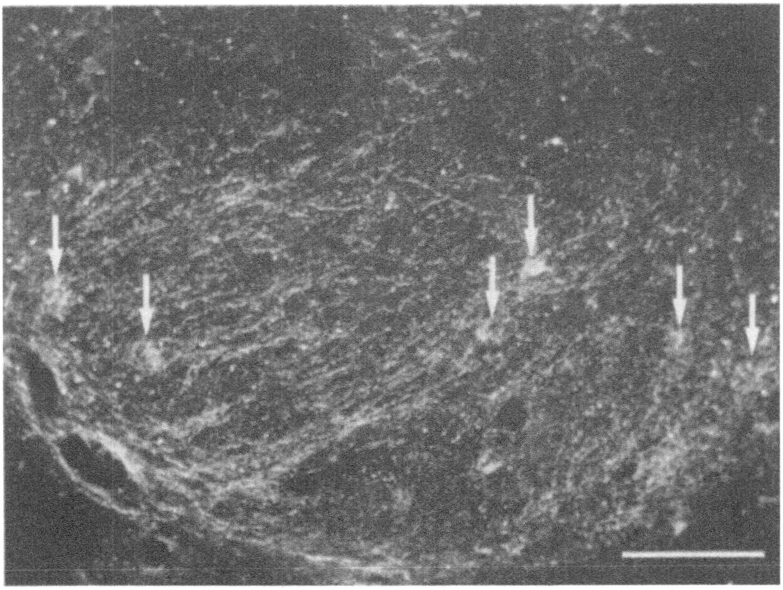

Fig. 12. Low-power–dark-field photomicrograph of the ventral part of a monkey dentate nucleus processed for both autoradiography and histochemically for demonstrating HRP. This animal received a combined HRP-tritiated leucine injection in Crus I. Horseradish peroxidase-positive neurons (*arrows*) are slightly below the plane of focus and are intermingled with autoradiographic silver grains which overlie orthogradely labeled corticonuclear axons and their terminals. *Scale bar* = 300 μm. Reprinted with permission from ref. [21]

reciprocal organization between the cerebellar corticonuclear-nucleocortical system.

In support of these anatomical data are results from intracellular recordings made from nucleocortical neurons [23]. In Fig. 6 the antidromic activation of the neurons from stimulus sites in the cerebellar surface and brachium conjunctivum was confirmed by intracellular recordings (Fig. 6B, C). Once the spike generating mechanism of the cell failed (Fig. 6D, E), stimulation of the cortex (Fig. 6D) at the same stimulus intensity used in Fig. 6A–C evoked a hyperpolarizing potential at approximately 1 ms latency. Lowering the stimulus strength in Fig. 6E resulted in a decrease in the amplitude of this hyperpolarization. Since this membrane hyperpolarization occurs at a latency within the range proposed by Ito et al. [13] to be a monosynaptic evoked inhibitory postsynaptic potential, it was concluded that the neuron sent a nucleocortical projection to the same area of cortex from which it received a corticonuclear input.

Perhaps just as significant as the findings for a reciprocal relationship between the cortex and deep nuclei were the observations that some neurons projecting to an area of the cortex lie outside the zone of termination of orthogradely labeled corticonuclear fibers [3, 7, 8, 11, 21]. This was particularly prominent in an experiment where combined ^{3}H-leucine and HRP injections were made in the posterior lobe vermis of the rhesus monkey [27]. In this case, the majority of neurons retrogradely labeled with HRP were again observed in the ipsilateral dentate nuclei. However, in the same sections there was a clear absence of a corticonuclear projection from this area of cortex to the dentate nucleus.

A stronger argument for nonreciprocal corticonuclear-nucleocortical projections can be made in the case of the tree shrew where a significant contralateral nucleocortical pathway to the paraflocculus exists but where no direct corticonuclear projections from the opposite cortex terminate [11].

Discussion

Although cerebellar nucleocortical projections have been demonstrated in a number of different experimental animal species where specific details concerning the origin, course, pattern of branching, and topographical organization have been identified, other important features concerning this pathway remain unresolved. Recent findings by several investigators have implicated dentatocortical projections as a possible GABAergic pathway. Injections of ^{3}H-gamma aminobutyric acid (GABA) into the cat dentate nucleus results in a conspicuous labeling of axons directed not only toward the cortex but also into the brachium conjunctivum [1, 22]. Since labeled axons entering the brachium conjunctivum or projecting toward the cortex have characteristics similar to axons orthogradely labeled with other amino acids, it can be argued, that the nucleocortical axons were orthogradely labeled with the ^{3}H-GABA [22].

Other evidence suggestive of a GABAergic nucleocortical pathway was obtained in experiments by Chan-Palay et al. [4]. Following injections of anti-glutamic acid decarboxylase (GAD) antibody, in the rat cerebellar cortex or dentate nucleus, Chan-Palay and colleagues demonstrated immunoreactive retrogradely labeled neurons in the deep nuclei and orthogradely labeled mossy-fiber rosettes in the cortex respectively. The presence of GABAergic neurons and terminals in the cerebellar cortex and the inhibitory postsynaptic action of this neurotransmitter is well established [4]. The above anterograde and retrograde labeling studies would therefore infer that the nucleocortical pathway may be inhibitory in nature.

Preliminary observations of nucleocortical terminals identified using EM autoradiography following injections of ^{3}H-leucine in the cat cerebellar nuclei would argue against this possibility [14, 28]. The labeled simple or complex mossy-fiber rosettes always contained clear, spherical synaptic vesicles and, more importantly, these contacts were of the asymmetric type. Since these morphological characteristics are generally equated with excitatory synaptic action [17, 29] in the cerebellar cortex one could argue that cerebellar nucleocortical afferents are excitatory in nature. To resolve this point, further anatomical and electrophysiological studies are required. The anatomical studies are needed to identify more thoroughly and characterize nucleocortical terminals, both in regard to their structure and relationship to postsynaptic elements as well as the identification of possible neurotransmitters used by this pathway. Electrophysiological experiments are required not only to provide substantiation of the anatomical findings but also to study the overall affect of this input on the synaptic circuitry in the cortex.

Any comments as to the function of the nucleocortical pathway, due to the lack of any experimental substantiation, would be purely speculative. However, an obvious and elementary hypothesis is that this pathway functions to modify the local physiological state of the cerebellar cortex. Since it is apparent that many nucleocortical fibers arise as collaterals of cerebellofugal projections to the brain stem, and that there is some degree of reciprocal organization between the nucleocortical and corticonuclear pathways, it is possible that any increase in activity in the cerebellar nuclei, would be reflected in an increase in activity in not only the output of the cerebellum but also in the nucleocortical pathway. These nucleocortical afferents would then, acting through Purkinje cell inhibition, result in a tempering of the output of the cerebellar nuclei. This internal-feedback system could then serve to regulate the output of the cerebellum and tend to modify any fluctuation in cerebellar nuclear activity. It is probable that more complex functions could be ascribed to the cerebellar nucleocortical pathway if they were considered in relation to some specific motor activity. Further electrophysiological studies should clarify this question.

Acknowledgments. Research reported in this review was supported in part by NIH grant NS 09447, NIH contract NS 42332, USPHS grant FR 05388, and NIH fellowship NS 0557. The author acknowledges the collaboration of Drs. Heinrich Bantli and James R. Bloedel, University of Minnesota, and Drs. Kristy Kultas-Ilinsky and Igor Ilinsky at St. Louis University, in some of the studies reported in this review. I wish to acknowledge the helpful comments made by Dr. Young during the preparation of this manuscript. The author is indebted to Mrs. Pat McGavran and Ms. Jill Warhoover for secretarial assistance and especially to Mrs. Connie Marshall for her assistance in preparing the illustrations.

References

1. Bantli H, Tolbert DL (1978) Uptake and transport of ^{3}H-GABA injected extracellularly in the cat dentate nucleus. Neurosci Abstr 4:63
2. Carrea RM, Reissig EM, Mettler FA (1947) The climbing fibers of the simian and feline cerebellum. Experimental inquiry into their origin by lesions of the inferior olives and deep cerebellar nuclei. J Comp Neurol 87:321–365
3. Chan-Palay V (1977) Cerebellar dentate nucleus. Organization, cytology and transmitters. Springer, Berlin Heidelberg New York
4. Chan-Palay V, Palay SL, Wu J-Y (1979) Gamma-aminobutyric acid pathways in the cerebellum studied by retrograde and anterograde transport of glutamic acid decarboxylase antibody after in vivo injections. Anat Embryol (Berl) 157:1–14
5. Clarke PGH (1977) Some visual and other connections to the cerebellum of the pigeon. J Comp Neurol 174:535–552
6. Cohen D, Chambers WW, Sprague JM (1958) Experimental study of efferent projections from the cerebellar nuclei to the brain stem of the cat. J Comp Neurol 109:233–259
7. Dietrichs E, Walberg F (1979) The cerebellar corticonuclear and nucleocortical projections in the cat as studied with anterograde and retrograde transport of horseradish peroxidase I. The paramedian lobule. Anat Embryol (Berl) 158:13–39
8. Gould BB (1979) The organization of afferents to the cerebellar cortex in the cat: projections from the deep cerebellar nuclei. J Comp Neurol 184:27–42
9. Gould BB, Graybiel AM (1976) Afferents to the cerebellar cortex in the cat: evidence for an intrinsic pathway leading from the deep nuclei to the cortex. Brain Res 110:601–611
10. Haines DE (1978) Contralateral nucleocortical cells of the paraflocculus of tree shrew (*Tupaia glis*). Neurosci Lett 8:183–190
11. Haines DE, Pearson JC (1979) Cerebellar corticonuclear-nucleocortical topography: A study of the tree shrew (*Tupaia*) paraflocculus. J Comp Neurol 187:745–758
12. Ito M, Yashida M, Obata K (1964) Monosynaptic inhibition of the intracerebellar nuclei induced from the cerebellar cortex. Experientia 20:575–576
13. Ito M, Yashida M, Obata K, Kawai N, Udo M (1970) Inhibitory control of intracerebellar nuclei by the Purkinje cell axons. Exp Brain Res 10:64–80
14. Kultas-Ilinsky K, Tolbert DL, Ilinsky IA (1979) An autoradiographic ultrastructural identification of terminals of cerebellar nucleocortical fibers in the cat. Neurosci Abstr 5:102
15. McCrea RA, Bishop GA, Kitai ST (1978) Morphological and electrophysiological characteristics of projection neurons in the nucleus interpositus of the cat cerebellum. J Comp Neurol 181:397–419
16. Palay SL, Chan-Palay V (1974) Cerebellar Cortex. Cytology and organization. Springer, Berlin Heidelberg New York
17. Palay SL, Chan-Palay V (1977) General morphology of neurons and neuroglia. In: Kandel E (ed) The nervous system, vol. I. I. Cell biology of neurons, Am Physiol Soc, Bethesda, p 5–37
18. Ramon y Cajal S (1895) Ganglion cerebelleux. Bibl Anat 3:33–42
19. Ramon y Cajal S (1911) Histologie du système nerveux de l'homme et des vertébrés, vol II. Maloine, Paris. Translated by L Azoulay
20. Thomas DM, Kaufman RP, Sprague JM, Chambers WW (1956) Experimental studies of the vermal cerebellar projections in the brainstem of the cat (fastigiobulbar tract). J Anat (Lond) 90:371–385
21. Tolbert DL, Bantli H (1979) HRP and autoradiographic study of cerebellar corticonuclear-nucleocortical reciprocity in the monkey. Exp Brain Res 36:563–571
22. Tolbert DL, Bantli H (1980) Uptake and transport of ^{3}H-GABA injected into the cat dentate nucleus. Exp Neurol 70:525–538
23. Tolbert DL, Bantli H, Bloedel JR (1976) Anatomical and physiological evidence for a cerebellar nucleo-cortical projection in the cat. Neuroscience 1:205–217
24. Tolbert DL, Massopust LC, Murphy MG, Young PA (1976) The anatomical organization of the cerebello-olivary projection in the cat. J Comp Neurol 170:525–544
25. Tolbert DL, Bantli H, Bloedel JR (1977) The intracerebellar nucleocortical projection in a primate. Exp Brain Res 30:425–434

26. Tolbert DL, Bantli H, Bloedel JR (1978a) Multiple branching of cerebellar efferent projections in cats. Exp Brain Res 31:305–316
27. Tolbert DL, Bantli H, Bloedel JR (1978b) Organizational features of the cat and monkey cerebellar nucleocortical projection. J Comp Neurol 182:39–56
28. Tolbert DL, Kultas-Ilinsky K, Ilinsky IA, Warton S (1980) EM-autoradiography of cerebellar nucleocortical terminals in the cat. Anat. Embryol (Berl) 161:215–223
29. Uchizono K (1969) Synaptic organization of the mammalian cerebellum. In: Llinás R (ed) Neurobiology of cerebellar evolution and development. AMF-ERF, Chicago, pp 549–581

Discussion

Beitz: In your slides of cat with isotope injections in the fastigial nucleus you showed anterograde labeling of fibers passing into more lateral parts of the hemispheral cortex and, I think, the intermediate cortex. Yet, when you made injections of horseradish peroxidase (HRP) into that part of cortex, I didn't see any labeled cells in the fastigium. I wondered if you have seen them there, and if you can explain the discrepancy between the results obtained using the one technique versus the other.
Tolbert: In my cases lateral hemispheral injections did result in retrograde labeling of some neurons in the fastigial nuclei, but the number was very small compared to the number present in the dentate nuclei.
Carpenter: In your HRP cases, I noticed that you showed a considerable number of cells that have a preferential location in ventral parts of dentate. Were there any cells that were labeled in cell group y, which is a vestibular nucleus that underlies the dentate? Do these cells have any projections to the cortex?
Tolbert: I really didn't notice at the time. Perhaps Dr. Gould could comment.
Gould: We saw many labeled cells in cell group y in two cases with HRP-injection sites involving the flocculus in the cat. In the case we had with an injection site involving the nodulus, there were neurons in that general area that were labeled, but I can't say for sure that they were in cell group y. They were ventral to the deep nuclei proper, but not clearly in cell group y; that is, overlapping partly with it, but not defining it.
Chan-Palay: Recently we have performed experiments involving injection of antibodies against glutamic acid decarboxylase (GAD) into the cerebellar cortex, then tracing the transport of GAD backwards into the deep cerebellar nuclei. It became clear that there were certain systems which were very much equivalent to the nucleocortical systems, which label with anti-GAD antibody. I think that they're almost equivalent to those neurons, for example, in the dentate, that project upward. Now, that means that certain of those mossy-fiber rosettes and certain of those neurons are GAD immunoreactive. I'd like to interject the possibility that in fact these might belong to a gamma aminobutyric acid (GABA) system which is internally regulated within the cerebellum. I'm not saying that all of the nucleocortical systems may be GAD- or GABA-containing, but that some of them are. There is a figure in one of our recent papers [1] showing, very clearly, equivalent mossy-fiber structures and nucleocortical cells.
Tolbert: When we made injections of tritiated GABA in cat dentate nucleus we saw labeled axons coursing toward the cortex. We have also observed a dif-

ferential uptake of tritiated GABA around the periphery of these injection sites, so we have spent a lot of time thinking about these particular terminals. Perhaps there are two separate populations of neurons projecting to the cortex: one that can be labeled using, for example, tritiated leucine, others that may be labeled more selectively with tritiated GABA. We're pursuing EM-autoradiographic studies of the cortex to see if we can differentiate between the labeled terminals. To date, we haven't seen any difference between labeled and unlabeled mossy-fiber rosettes in the same area of cortex.

Snider: You had a descending axon that went all the way back to olive and one that went to VL, the same axon?

Tolbert: These neurons were relatively numerous, and they projected to all three sites: ventrolateral nucleus, inferior olive, and cerebellar cortex.

Eccles: What's the *population* of these nucleocortical lines as compared with the ordinary normal output of the cerebellum? What fraction is it?

Tolbert: If you make large HRP injections in the cortex you see a corresponding large number of retrogradely labeled neurons in the cerebellar nuclei, not only in cat, but also in monkey and tree shrew. Similarly, in orthograde labeling experiments one can easily find four to six terminals in a relatively small area of cortex (ca. 0.1 mm^2). These findings would indicate a very substantial nucleocortical projection.

Chan-Palay: It probably would not be unlikely that many or most nuclear neurons in the dentate, for example, have some projection upwards.

Eccles: The problem is, what synaptic power have they got in the cortex? Is it really significant or can it all be handled by the local machinery?

Palay: If they're there they have power. It is a question of under what circumstances they show that their vote counts.

Ito: There may be two lines of thought. One is feedback: Purkinje cells inhibit the deep nuclei and the results may be fed back to the cortex. But apparently there is no exact correspondence between the corticonuclear and nucleocortical projections. The nucleocortical projection appears more divergent than the corticonuclear, so possible it may serve a cooperative sort of function between different microzones. This would be, so to speak, an internal path between zones.

Tolbert: It may be just the opposite. If one considers the excitatory input of cerebellar afferent collaterals onto neurons in the deep nuclei, any increase in excitability on these neurons will be fed up to the cortex by way of the nucleocortical fibers as well as fed out of the cerebellum, via collaterals. In turn, the nucleocortical axons may activate the inhibitory corticonuclear pathway, which is then going to suppress some of this activity. Perhaps this is a method for tempering wide variations in the activity of these neurons in the cerebellar nuclei.

Snider: I was hoping that we could come out with some longitudinal zones. Dr. Voogd, would you like to comment on that? Didn't you expect longitudinal zones out of this?

Voogd: No. Since most of these fibers are collaterals from neurons which give rise to efferent pathways, then I'm not surprised that the nucleocortical projection is more diffuse. There are many places to give off collaterals, even a couple on the contralateral side if the uncinate branch is considered. In the

main you see good correspondence, at least in the cat, between the general pattern in the corticonuclear projection and these nucleocortical projections. Then, as you mentioned, in the monkey, it is a much more complicated situation.
Snider: How about those large and small cells? Somehow I got the impression from Gould and Graybiel's [2] paper that it was mostly the large cells that were sending back the collaterals.
Gould: No, we found more medium-sized cells; about twice as many medium-sized cells as small or large.
Tolbert: This is because the medium-sized neurons are the most numerous type of cell in the nuclei.
Snider: The small basal cells that were described earlier here, do they also have collaterals going to the cortex?
Tolbert: These cells can be retrogradely labeled from the cortex and are very similar to the neurons that have descending projections to inferior olive. They are very small spindle-shaped neurons.
Marshall: One of the difficulties in studying this projection electrophysiologically is the confluence of fibers around the deep nuclei. As I pointed out yesterday, we don't have these afferent fibers to content with in our cerebellar explants. In fact we have a group of deep nuclear cells and cortical regions. So we can study this relationship. The responses that we've seen by microstimulation, in the deep nuclear region are mostly an EPSP-IPSP sequence. In fact, in about five cells out of 30 Purkinje cells intracellularly recorded, we saw what appeared to be a monosynaptic inhibition. We attributed this, tentatively, to antidromic activation of Purkinje cell axons and monosynaptic inhibition via recurrent collaterals. We have observed recurrent collaterals of Purkinje cell axons with HRP staining of single neurons. There seems to be a possibility that such a monosynaptic inhibition could also arise from an inhibitory deep nuclear cell projecting to the cortex. It would take more work to define some of these individual interrelationships by stimulation and activation of deep nuclear cells and recording intracellularly from single Purkinje cells, but this is feasible with such preparations.
Chan-Palay: My suspicion, now, is that if a GABA pathway does exist, it does not necessarily follow that it is an inhibitory pathway. There is something very peculiar about this.
Llinás: There is another question that is really quite interesting: we are all considering mossy fibers as being very prominent in the particular function of the cerebellum. There is also a possibility that you require a certain amount of background activity that is not going to be as nicely or as precisely related as activity that is generated by specific input. So I think that there is no need to be alarmed about these relations, because there may be other levels of function.

References

1. Chan-Palay V, Palay SL, Wu J-Y (1979) Gamma-aminobutyric acid pathways in the cerebellum studied by retrograde and anterograde transport of glutamic acid decarboxylase antibody after in vivo injections. Anat Embryol (Berl) 157:1–14
2. Gould BB, Graybiel AM (1976) Afferents to the cerebellar cortex in the cat: evidence for an intrinsic pathway leading from the deep nuclei to the cortex. Brain Res 110:601–611

Organization of Cerebellar Corticonuclear Fiber Systems

D. E. Haines, G. W. Patrick, and P. Satrulee

Introduction

It has been known for many years that Purkinje cells are the efferent neurons of the cerebellar cortex. Axons of these cells arise from the basal aspect of their somata and project primarily into the deep cerebellar nuclei thereby collectively forming the so-called corticonuclear fiber system. Specific regions of the cerebellar cortex, namely flocculonodular lobe and certain lobules of the vermis, in addition to sending fibers into their respective areas of the homolateral deep cerebellar nuclei also project into the ipsilateral vestibular complex. The ensuing discussion will be concerned only with the organization of corticonuclear fibers.

Historical Perspective

The first experimental attempt to elucidate the organization of cerebellar corticonuclear fibers was the detailed Marchi study by Klimoff [53] utilizing the rabbit. This work, which represented the author's doctoral dissertation from the Imperial University of Kazan (Fig. 1), was summarized, without illustrations, in a later publication [54]. Although Clarke and Horsley [13] were apparently unaware of Klimoff's work, since neither the dissertation nor its summarized version were cited by these authors, they arrived at fundamentally similar conclusions. These early investigators [13, 53, 54] concluded that cerebellar corticonuclear fibers projected into those areas of the deep cerebellar nuclei which were closest to the region of cortex from which the efferent fibers arose. In the words of Clarke and Horsley [13] " . . . fibers (pass) to the nearest cerebellar nuclei, whether roof, globose, or dentate but none (go) directly from the cortex

* This research supported by USPHS Grant NS 11327 from NINCDS. The senior author has communicated with, shared ideas and data with, and received many constructive suggestions from a number of colleagues over the years. For all of this stimulating scientific camaraderie he would especially like to thank Dr. J. Voogd (Leiden), Drs. F. Walberg and A. Brodal (Oslo), Dr. J. Courville (Montreal), Dr. G. F. Martin (Ohio State), Dr. E. Lauer (Michigan), Dr. O. Oscarsson (Lund), and Drs. J. Culberson and P. Brown (West Virginia). We also wish to express our appreciation to Dr. V. Chan-Palay and Dr. S. Palay for the opportunity to participate in their Symposium. Personnel of the Biomedical Photography Department (Ms. G. Heard, director) reproduced Figs. 1 and 2. Ms. A. L. Carr was responsible for all histologic preparations and Ms. A. Police conscientiously typed the entire final draft. G. W. P. was a Research Associate supported by Grant NS 11327 and P. S. was supported by a Royal Thai Government Scholarship

Experimental Brain Research, Suppl. 6

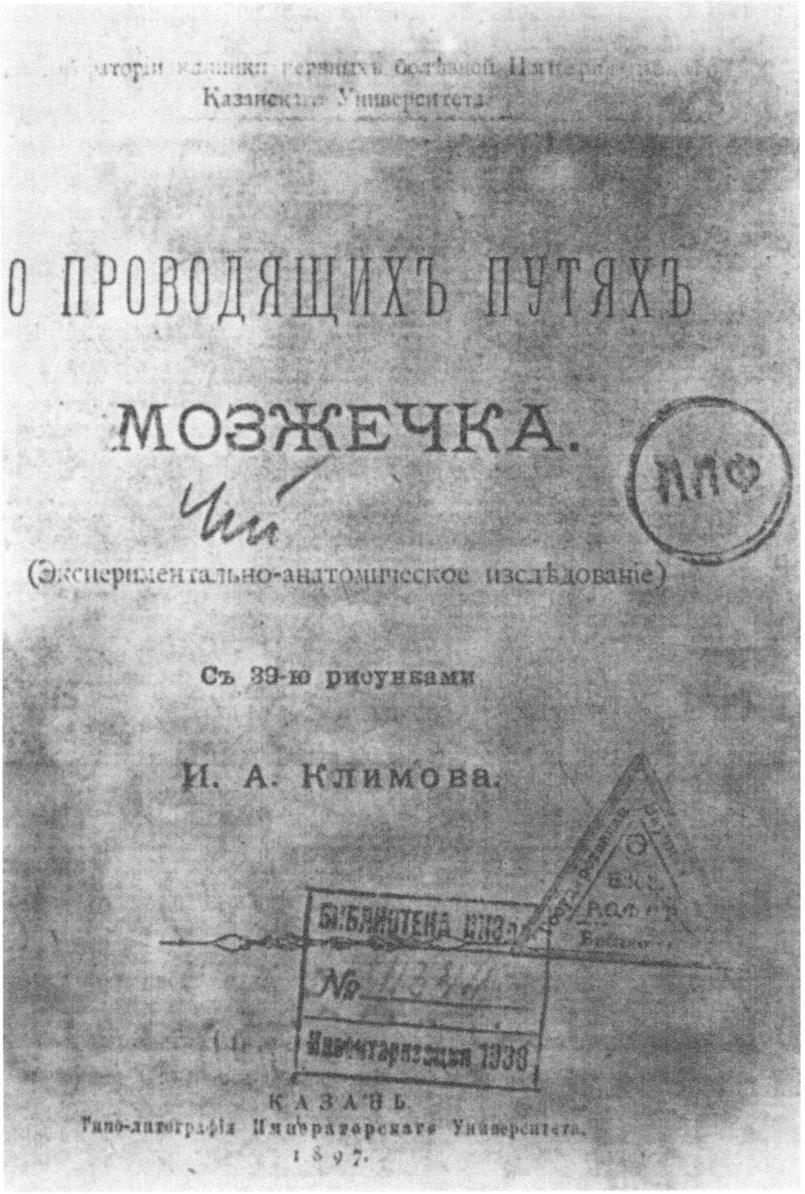

Fig. 1. Title page of the dissertation by Klimoff [53] on efferent fibers of the cerebellar cortex of rabbit. This was the first experimental attempt to detail corticonuclear fibers[1]

---

1 Abbreviations: A, B, C_1, C_2, C_3, D_1, D_2, compartments and zones as designated by Voogd [78]; *caud.*, caudal; *cNL*, caudal NL; *CNX*, crossed corticonuclear fibers; *CN–*, uncrossed corticonuclear fibers; *CVX*, crossed corticovestibular fibers; *CV–*, uncrossed corticovestibular fibers; *dor.*, dorsal; *DPML or dpml*, dorsal paramedian lobule; *f*, flocculus; *h*, hemisphere area; *IC*, intermediate cortex; *lat. or l*, lateral; *LC*, lateral cortex; *lvn*, lateral vestibular nucleus; *l-nia or lNIA*, lateral NIA; *med. or m*, medial; *mNL*, magnocellular NL; *m-nia or mNIA*, medial NIA; *m-nip*, medial NIP; *nia or NIA*, anterior interposed nucleus; *nip or NIP*,

cerebelli to any of the peduncles. Our series of sections also show that all efferent cerebellar cortical fibers in the first instance pass to one or other of the cerebellar nuclei, and principally to the one which is nearest to their origin". Collectively these initial observations showed that corticonuclear fibers were arranged in very general rostral to caudal and medial to lateral patterns. Anterior cortical areas projected into anterior regions of the deep cerebellar nuclei, while posterior cortex was related to their more caudal portions. The roof nucleus (fastigial) received input mainly from medial cortical areas (e.g., vermis) while progressively more lateral cortical regions projected into the interposed and then the dentate nuclei.

Hohman [50] made two important observations which, in retrospect, foreshadowed a more complex organization of cerebellar corticonuclear fibers. First, he provided evidence of a more precise medial to lateral arrangement of cortical efferent fibers. Subsequent to bilateral damage of the anterior lobe "vermis" in the cat Hohman [50] described three ipsilateral fascicles of degenerated fibers each clearly separated from its neighbor by an area of white matter which contained no Marchi granules. The most mesial bundle (his fascicle A-V-F) originated from medial portions of the cortical damage and terminated in the fastigial nucleus. A middle bundle (designated A-V-D) coursed between the fastigial nucleus and the "... intermediate cell mass (globosus and emboliform)..." to enter the lateral vestibular (Deiter's) nucleus, while the lateral most fascicle (his A-V-I) terminated in the intermediate cell mass. Second, Hohman [50] described somewhat more precise relationships (for example, his experiment No. 30) between specific lobules of cerebellar cortex and a particular deep cerebellar nucleus or portion thereof. He [50] also noted that even in cases with bilateral damage of vermis there was no evidence to suggest that the cortex may project bilaterally to any of the deep nuclei.

It remained for Jansen and A. Brodal [51, 52] in a series of elegantly detailed observations on the cat, rabbit, and monkey to provide conclusive proof that cerebellar corticonuclear fibers were arranged into three ipsilateral areas (subsequently called zones) which projected into relatively localized portions of their respective deep nuclei (Fig. 2). A vermal or medial area projected into the medial cerebellar nucleus (NM) and vestibular complex, the paravermal region was related to the interposed nucleus while the most lateral area of cortex projected into the lateral cerebellar nucleus (NL). These authors showed that the interface of two adjacent zones was more easily defined in anterior areas of the

1 Continued: posterior interposed nucleus; *nl or NL*, lateral cerebellar nucleus; *nm or NM*, medial cerebellar nucleus; *Ocf–*, *x*, crossed and uncrossed cerebellofugal fibers; *p*, paravermal area; *pf*, primary fissure; *pNL*, parvicellular NL; *ros.*, rostral; *rNL*, rostral NL; *v*, vermal area; *VC*, vermal cortex (Figs. 4, 5 only); *VC or vc*, vestibular complex (Fig. 10 only); *vent.*, ventral; *vmNL*, ventromedial NL; *vm & lNL*, ventromedial and lateral NL; *VPML or vpml*, ventral paramedian lobule; *x*, zone x of Oscarsson [67, 68]. *Vermis lobules* after Larsell [61]. I, anterior lobe lobule I, the lingula; II, anterior lobe lobule II, the ventral central lobule; III, anterior lobe lobule III, the dorsal central lobule; IV, anterior lobe lobule IV, the ventral culminate lobule; V, anterior lobe lobule V, the dorsal culminate lobule; VI, posterior lobe lobule VI, the decline; VII, posterior lobe lobule VII, the folium and tuber vermis; VIII, posterior lobe lobule VIII, the pyramis; IX, posterior lobe lobule IX, the uvula; X, vermis lobule X, the nodulus

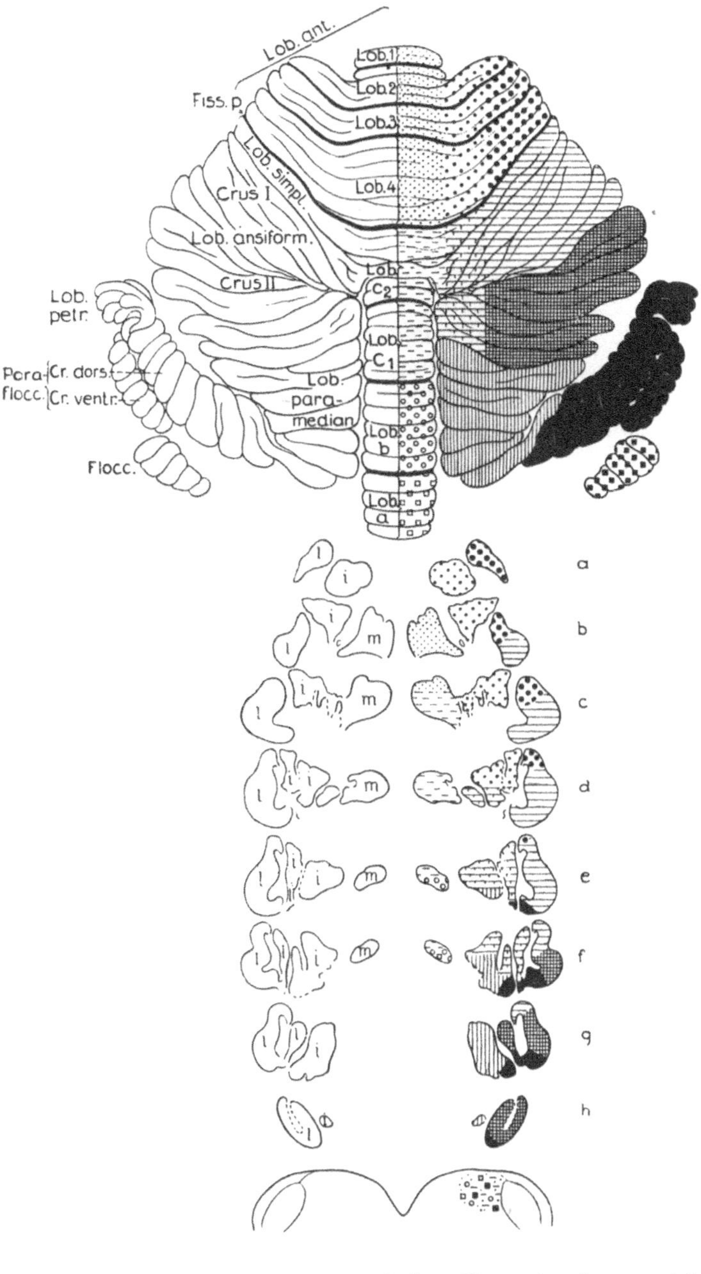

Fig. 2. Topography of corticonuclear fibers of *Macaca* cerebellum illustrating the essential features of the basic three zone plan developed by Jansen and Brodal [51, 52]. This was the first comprehensive description of zones in the cerebellar cortex. Figure 22 from Jansen and Brodal [52]. Abbreviations see p. 321–322

cerebellum, while the complex foldings of the posterior lobe vermis and hemisphere partially obscured the precise relationships of zones in caudal regions. Jansen and Brodal [51, 52] also showed that the cortex of a particular zone projected primarily into its respective nucleus. For example, although most of the vermal cortex (the medial zone) sent some fibers into the vestibular complex, the rostral NM recieved input from only its anterior lobe portion while its posterior region projected into the caudal NM (Fig. 2). Similarly more precise relationships, when compared to earlier studies, were also described for paravermal and lateral cortices with the interposed and lateral nuclei respectively (Fig. 2). Experimental observations on a number of mammalian (rat, cat, monkey, rabbit) and nonmammalian (bird) forms corroborated the essentials of the three ipsilateral cortical zone pattern [11, 12, 21, 22, 27–29, 51, 52, 74, 82]. It has also been suggested that the two zones seen in certain nonmammalian vertebrates (alligator) are homologous to the vermal and paravermal zones of mammals [26, 73].

In his detailed analysis of ferret cerebellum Voogd [78], utilizing the criteria of fiber diameter, described seven ipsilateral compartments (A, B, C_1, C_2, C_3, D_1, and D_2) in the subcortical white matter (Fig. 3). Each compartment, with the exception of B, the fibers of which bypassed the cerebellar nuclei to enter vestibular complex, contained part of or all of a particular deep cerebellar nucleus. The NM was found in A, medial and lateral areas of the anterior interposed nucleus (NIA) were contained in C_1 and C_3 respectively, the posterior interposed nucleus (NIP) was found in compartment C_2, while compartments D_1 and D_2 were related to parvi- and magnocellular portions of NL. This report [78] which represented a refinement of an earlier study [77], implied a markedly more

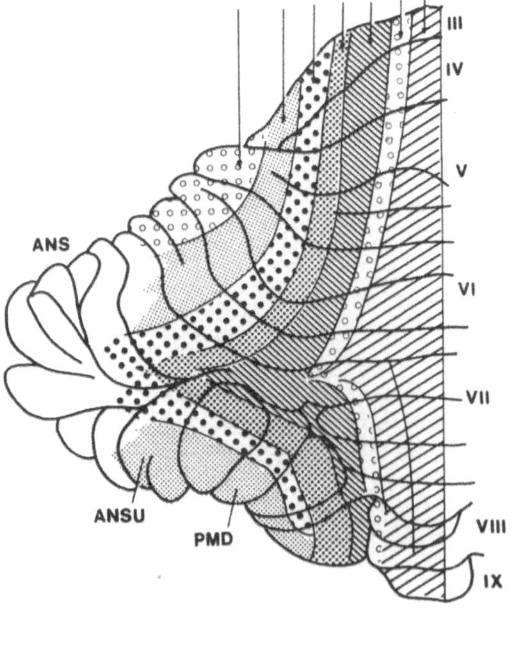

Fig. 3. Semidiagrammatic representation of compartments in the white matter and their potential overlying cortical zones as described by Voogd [78] in the ferret. Figure 7 from Voogd [78]. Abbreviations see p. 321–322

complex and precise organization of the cerebellar cortex and its efferent system than had been previously suspected. For example, the evidence from all earlier studies had suggested that anterior cortex, in general, projected into anterior portions of the deep nuclei. If the cortex overlying the C_2 compartment contained Purkinje cells which projected into its respective nucleus (the NIP), this would indicate that a particular area of anterior lobe may project exclusively to only NIP; a specificity of trajectory not alluded to in any previous investigation. Voogd [78] concluded that, at least in ferret, these compartments in the subcortical white matter may have corresponding overlying zones in the cortex. The implication being that a given cortical zone may have a specific topographical relationship to the nucleus, or portion thereof, located within its respective compartment. Although Oscarsson [64–66] had only recently described more than three ipsilateral zones in the anterior lobe, based on spino-olivocerebellar input, there was essentially no data available to support the contention that there may be more than three ipsilateral zones in the corticonuclear fiber system.

An Approach to the Question of Corticonuclear Organization

The observations of Voogd [78] implied a markedly more complex organization of cerebellar corticonuclear fibers than had been previously thought. Consequently, we elected to address this question from two standpoints. First, we decided to investigate individual lobules in greater detail by placing small overlapping lesions in relatively confined areas of cortex. We reasoned that if there were narrow cortical zones only small lesions would fully elucidate their spatial organization. Second, rather than investigate only one species, thereby acquiring a limited view of the overall complexity of these systems, we felt a comparative approach would yield a proportionately greater amount of data. The representative primate species utilized were the lesser bushbaby (*Galago senegalensis*) and the squirrel monkey (*Saimiri sciureus*). The albino rat was selected because although a commonly used mammal in neuroscience research comparatively little data is available on connections of its cerebellum. The North American opossum (*Didelphis virginiana*) and the tree shrew (*Tupaia glis*) are frequently held to be living representatives of the more generalized mammalian state. For this reason it was considered prudent to include these forms in a comparative investigation.

Protocol

Even though the basic arrangement of the ipsilateral three-zone pattern had been indisputedly proven [e.g., 11, 12, 21, 22, 28, 51, 52, 74, and others] two frequently used methodological approaches complicated the picture. First, it was common to remove overlying bone, then open the dura, thereby exposing a given cortical area prior to making a lesion. The mere act of opening the dura provided the potential for artifactural damage outside the area of intended primary injury. Second, some earlier studies used aspiration or suction techniques to remove a spot of cortex. Although suction will successfully damage a particular point it may also precipitate a peripheral area of diffuse injury resulting from the touching and tugging (especially on blood vessels) of cortex as the lesion is being placed.

In an effort to eliminate these variables we elected to place transdural heat lesions; that is, remove bone and apply the heated tip of a metal teasing needle to previously identified folia through the overlying unopened dura. Thus in one movement a small opening was made in the dura and an equally small lesion placed in the immediately subjacent cortex. In most of the species utilized in our studies individual folia and/or lobules can be identified through the unopened translucent dura. Following survival times of 3–12 days all animals were killed by transcardiac perfusion of heparinized 0.9% saline followed by 10% unbuffered formalin. Cerebelli with brainstems intact were serially sectioned at 40 µm in parasagittal, coronal, and horizontal planes and impregnated with a variation of the Fink and Heimer [25] selective silver method. In every case all sections were kept and stained using one or a combination of the following techniques. In some experiments all sections were impregnated (Fink-Heimer), with every other section being decolored in a 1% solution of potassium ferricyanide then counterstained with cresylviolet acetate. Other cases had every other section impregnated and the intervening sections stained with cresylviolet acetate. In certain situations, once the configuration of the deep nuclei was established, all sections were impregnated with Fink-Heimer.

The ensuing discussion is based on the examination of the trajectory of corticonuclear fibers from over 220 lesions placed in various areas of the cerebellar cortex of the lesser bushbaby (*Galago senegalensis*), squirrel monkey (*Saimiri sciureus*), North American opossum (*Didelphis virginiana*), albino rat, and tree shrew (*Tupaia glis*). Special attention has been given to the anterior lobe, vermis of anterior and posterior lobes, and certain lobules of posterior lobe hemispheres. Data which has been previously published will be so noted and only briefly summarized; the reader is referred to the original papers for additional detail.

Laterality of Cerebellar Cortical Efferents

The laterality of cerebellar corticonuclear (CN) and corticovestibular (CV) fibers has been debated in the literature. Early investigators, utilizing the Marchi method for degenerated myelin (Table 1), arrived at a remarkable uniformity of opinion concerning the ipsilateral nature of both CN and CV fiber systems. The only exceptions being the studies of Bender [7] on the dog, Vachananda [75] on *Macaca* and, to a limited extent, Allen [2] on the guinea pig. Bender [7] described extensive cerebellofugal fibers (Ocf-Table 1) as being distributed bilaterally to a variety of brainstem nuclei subsequent to lesions ascribed to the vermal cortex. However, scrutiny of the illustrations and descriptions of some cases clearly suggest that certain of the deep cerebellar nuclei were undoubtedly involved. Although the point was not specifically addressed,

Table 1. Laterality of cerebellar corticonuclear (CN) and corticovestibular (CV) fibers: marchi method [a]

Author/year	Animal	Laterality
Klimoff, 1897, 1899	Rabbit	CN- CV-
Clarke and Horsley, 1905	Dog, cat, *Macaca*	CN- CV-
Allen, 1924	Guinea pig	CN-(X?) CV-(X?)
Hohman, 1929	Cat	CN- CV-
Bender, 1932	Dog	CN-, (X?) CV-, (X) Ocf-, X
Dow, 1936, 1938	Cat, rat, *Macaca*	CN- CV-
Jansen and Brodal, 1940, 1942	Cat, rabbit, *Macaca*	CN- CV-
Vachananda, 1959	*Macaca*	CN-, X(v)

[a] Abbreviations see p. 321–322

Bender [7] alluded to the fact that there were probably some bilateral CN and CV fibers. Vachananda [75], while describing bilateral CN projections from the vermis, noted that those fibers going to the contralateral NM were markedly fewer than those remaining on the ipsilateral side. Allen [2] commented briefly on only two cases with lesions in the cerebellar cortex. In his series No. 96 "... the lesion involved most of the left cortex..." and Marchi degeneration was distributed to the ipsilateral cerebellar nuclei and contralateral NM. In the second case damage to the vermis, laterality not indicated, produced degeneration in the "... fastigial nuclei". Although not specifically stated the impression is given that Allen [2] saw some bilateral degeneration.

With the advent of more reliable pathway tracing methods (e.g., selective silver techniques and autoradiography) there appeared to be less agreement concerning the laterality of both CN and CV fibers (Table 2). For example, although Walberg and Jansen [81] concluded that CV fibers in the cat were ipsilateral, Eager [21] in a later study described a bilateral CV projection in this species after unilateral damage to the vermal cortex. Voogd [77], in his detailed analysis of the cat cerebellum, essentially corroborated the earlier ipsilateral data of Walberg and Jansen [81]. However, Angaut and Brodal [3] in their study of efferent fibers of the cat 'vestibulocerebellum' indicated that lesions of the flocculus and/or paraflocculus produced "... some..." or "... scattered..." degeneration in the contralateral vestibular complex, chiefly its lateral and spinal nuclei.

Concerning CN fibers there is a voluminous amount of comparative data which strongly supports the contention that this is an exclusively ipsilateral system (Table 2). Although Eager [21] reported bilateral CN fibers following lesions

Table 2. Laterality of cerebellar corticonuclear (CN) and corticovestibular (CV) fibers: Contemporary tracing methods [a]

Author/year	Animal	Laterality
Walberg and Jansen, 1961, 1964	Cat	CN- CV-
Goodman et al., 1963	Rat	CN-, X (v)
Eager, 1963	Cat	CN-, X (v, p) CV-, X (v)
Voogd, 1964, 1969	Cat	*CN- *CV-
Eager, 1966, 1969	Cat, rabbit, *Macaca*	CN- CV-
Angaut and Brodal, 1967	Cat	CN- CV-, X (h)
Achenbach eand Goodman, 1968	Rat	*CV-
van Rossum, 1969	Rabbit	CN- CV-
Brodal and Courville, 1973	Cat	CN-
Courville et al., 1973	Cat	CN-
Sreesai, 1974	Opossum (*Didelphis*)	CN-, X (v, p, h) CV-, X (v, p, h)
Haines, 1975 a, b, 1976, 1977	Lesser bushbaby (*Galago*)	CN- CV-
Courville and Diakiw, 1976	Cat	CN-
Courville and Faraco-Cantin, 1976	Cat	CN- CV-
Haines et al., 1976	Opossum	CN- CV-
Haines and Withworth, 1978	Tree shrew (*Tupaia*)	CN-
Armstrong and Schild, 1978 a, b	Rat	CN-
Haines and Rubertone, 1979	Lesser bushbaby	CN-
Gould, 1977, 1979	Cat	*CN-
Bishop, 1977	Cat	*CN-
Bishop et al., 1979	Cat	*CN-
Haines and Koletar, 1979	Rat	CN-
Satrulee, 1980	Opossum	CN-
Haines and Patrick, 1980	Tree shrew	CN-

The asterisk (*) indicates that while these authors did not specifically discuss laterality, the ipsilateral nature of these systems is self-evident from their results
[a] Abbreviations see p. 321–322

which involved both vermal and paravermal cortices, Walberg and Jansen [82] presented detailed and convincing evidence that CN fibers in the cat were ipsilateral. Indeed, all subsequent studies on the cat (Table 2) have arrived at essentially the same conclusion.

In their study on CN fibers of the rat, Goodman et al. [28] included eight cases with ipsilateral vermal lesions, two of which were restricted to the "... lateral half..." of the vermal cortex. In all eight experiments these authors reported that "... a small amount of degeneration was traced to the ventral half of the contralateral fastigial nucleus...". Goodman et al. [28] described a mediolateral gradient in these ipsilateral vermis-to-contralateral NM fibers; lesions of vermal cortex adjacent to the midline produced greater amounts of debris in contralateral NM while damage to more lateral areas of vermis produced less degeneration in contralateral NM. Subsequent investigators have utilized more contemporary tracing techniques to ascertain the trajectory of CN fibers arising from both vermal [4, 40] and lateral [5] cortices of the rat. These recent reports have failed to substantiate earlier observations [28] that CN fibers of rat vermis are even in a graded fashion, bilateral. To the contrary, these recent data strongly suggests that CN fibers of the rat, like the cat, are ipsilateral.

The only comprehensive report on CN and CV fibers in a more generalized mammal was that of Sreesai [74] on the North American opossum. This author described extensive bilateral projections in both CN and CV systems (Table 2). Following ipsilateral lesions of vermal, paravermal, and hemisphere cortices, degenerated fibers were usually identified in all ipsilateral cerebellar nuclei, the lateral vestibular nucleus (from all zones), and in one or more of the contralateral cerebellar nuclei. Noting that this may represent a unique condition in more generalized mammalian forms, Haines et al. [47] sought to confirm the more diffuse nature of CN and CV systems in the opossum. Their study of the posterior vermis revealed that CN and CV fibers from that particular cortical region were ipsilateral and to a certain extent topographically arranged. More detailed analyses of other areas of the opossum cerebellar cortex (this study, [70, 71]) have shown that, although the topographic distribution of CN and CV fibers may differ somewhat from that seen in other mammals, the evidence clearly indicates that these fiber systems in the opossum are ipsilateral.

Corticonuclear Fibers of the Lesser Bushbaby (*Galago*)

The cerebellum of *Galago*, a prosimian primate, has the structural features seen in higher primates albeit organized at a basic level of complexity. The ten vermis lobules [32, 34] of the bushbaby cerebellum and their corresponding hemisphere portions are homologous to those identified in a variety of other primates [61]. The anterior lobe of *Galago* is well developed especially as regards the hemisphere portions of lobules III–V [32, 34, 45]. This particular feature is in contrast to a variety of nonprimate mammals (e.g., the rat, mouse, cat, tree shrew, opossum), whose anterior lobe, especially its hemispheres, make up proportionately less of the total cerebellar mass [32, 61]. The cerebellar nuclei of the lesser bushbaby [33, 34] consist of four separate and clearly identifiable groups of cells of each side of the midline in a configuration similar to that of *Macaca* [14].

During a series of initial experiments on posterior vermis and certain lobules of the posterior lobe hemisphere [34–36, 39], it became obvious that corticonuclear fibers of the bushbaby were topographically organized in their trajectory into the deep cerebellar nuclei. Although earlier investigators [10, 17] saw little or no evidence of cortical zones (a la Voogd) in the posterior lobe hemisphere of the cat, the data from the posterior vermis of *Galago* [36] indicated that zones were clearly present in this area of primate cerebellum. At about this same time Courville and Diakiw [15], working on the cat, and Haines [36] working on the bushbaby, arrived at similar conclusions concerning a relatively specific topographic relationship between the vermal cortex and the ipsilateral NM. The obvious implication of these studies was that a specific organization of corticonuclear fibers and their arrangement into cortical zones may be features common to many regions of the cerebellar cortex in a variety of mammalian species. In an effort to elucidate the topography of corticonuclear fibers and specifically address the question of cortical zones a series of detailed experiments, summarized below, were conducted on the anterior lobe of *Galago* [37, 44, 45].

Anterior Lobe-Lobule V

Lesions restricted to the most lateral area (Fig. 4, No. 160) of the dorsal culminate lobule precipitated degeneration in two partially overlapping terminal fields in the rostroventral NL. Preterminal debris conspicuously avoided the most ventral regions of the NL where there is a greater concentration of smaller somata. Cortical damage at slightly more medial locations (Fig. 4, No. 154, No. 155) again produced fascicles of degenerated axons which entered the rostroventral NL. There was, however, a newly acquired burst of degeneration in the rostral and lateral NIA at its interface with the NL. This projection into the lateral NIA was especially evident in experiment No. 154 (Fig. 4) which was located at a slightly more medial position when compared to No. 155. This data showed that the so-called lateral zone in *Galago* was relatively narrow and the transition from lateral to intermediate cortices was represented by a line drawn through medial portions of the lesions in cases No. 154 and No. 155. Proof of this supposition was realized from experiment No. 148 (Fig. 4) in which the lesion was placed just medial to this arbitrary line. In this case, an intense concentration of preterminal debris was seen in the lateral NIA and a sparse amount in the NIP, while those portions of the NL directly adjacent to the lateral NIA were completely devoid of degenerated axons. These results showed not only the approximate point at which lateral and intermediate cortices meld, but also that lateral regions of the so-called intermediate area were topographically related primarily to the lateral NIA.

A somewhat unexpected finding, following damage located in what turned out to be approximately the middle of the intermediate cortex (Fig. 4, No. 156), was the presence of preterminal degeneration in only the NIP. Not only was debris confined to the NIP but it was arranged as two dorsoventrally oriented lamina separated by a narrow region which contained no degenerated axons. Essentially identical patterns of degeneration in the NIP were seen in experiment No. 149 (Fig. 4). These observations clearly supported the argument that an identifiable area of anterior lobe cortex projected primarily, if not exclusively, into the NIP.

More medial regions of intermediate cortex, as illustrated by case No. 164 (Fig. 4), were related mainly to medial portions of the NIA. In this experiment, numerous degenerated axons ended in the medial NIA while some fibers of passage coursed through the juxtarestiform body to enter the ipsilateral vestibular complex. In animal No. 157, the lesion of which partially overlapped that seen in No. 164 (Fig. 4), degeneration was again seen in the medial NIA and the juxtarestiform body, however a small amount of debris was found in ventrolateral areas of the lateral NM. In addition there was an obvious projection into the NIP from damage in this area of cortex (Fig. 4, No. 157). A

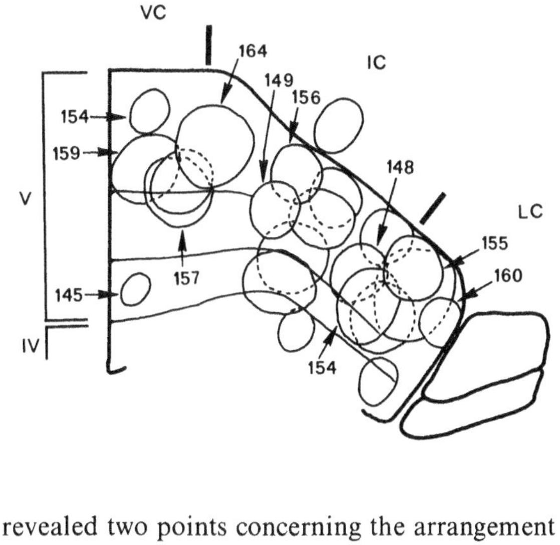

Fig. 4. Semidiagrammatic illustration showing the positions of lesions in lobule V of *Galago*. The trajectory of fibers arising from the numbered cases are described in the text. Abbreviations see p. 321–322

comparison of these two cases revealed two points concerning the arrangement of zones in this region of the cerebellum. First, as seen in No. 164 more medial portions of intermediate cortex project primarily into the medial NIA. Those degenerated fibers of passage which entered the ipsilateral juxtarestiform body arose from more medial portions of the lesion, thus indicating that this part of the injury had invaded the lateral edge of the vermal cortex. Second, the presence of debris in the medial NIA, the juxtarestiform body and *sparse amounts* of degeneration in the NM in case No. 157 showed that this lesion involved medial portions of the intermediate cortex (via projections to the medial NIA) and lateral portions of the vermal cortex (via degeneration in the juxtarestiform body and the NM). Consequently, the approximate interface of intermediate and vermal cortices was interpreted as a line coursing through medial portions of lesion No. 164 and lateral parts of lesion No. 157 (Fig. 4).

Cortical damage close to the midline (Fig. 4, No. 145, No. 154) precipitated debris in a terminal field found in rostrodorsal regions of the ipsilateral NM, with few or no degenerated fibers entering the juxtarestiform body. More extensive injury in the same general area (Fig. 4, No. 159) produced degeneration not only in the rostrodorsal NM (as from the smaller lesions) but also in the juxtarestiform body and, although in sparse amounts, in medial regions of the NIP. These cases illustrated the point that the medial vermal cortex (e.g., No. 145,

No. 154) projected primarily into the NM and, in the case of larger lesions (e.g., No. 159), into the ipsilateral vestibular complex and possibly the NIP. The border between those portions of the vermal cortex related mainly to the NM versus those related primarily to the vestibular complex was represented by a line drawn approximately through the lateral borders of lesions No. 145 and No. 154 (Fig. 4).

Taken collectively, these results from experiments on lobule V of *Galago* (see also ref. [44, 45]) showed that at least six ipsilateral regions of cortex can be

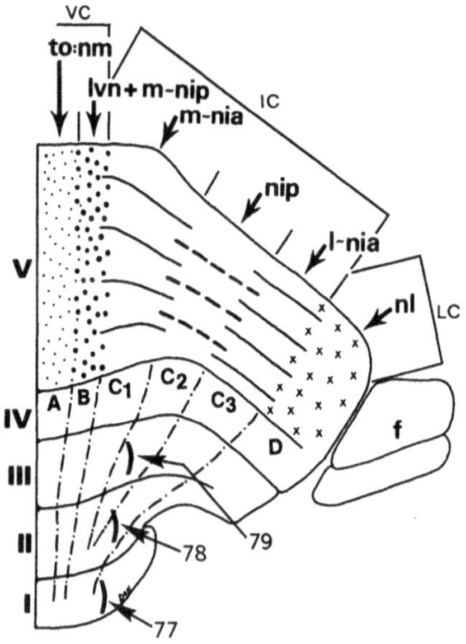

Fig. 5. Semidiagrammatic illustration showing the arrangement of zones and indicating their respective terminal nuclei for the anterior lobe of *Galago*. Designation of zones after Voogd [78]. Note that cortical zones in this primate converge toward the midline in rostral portions of the lobe. Haines and Rubertone [45]. Abbreviations see p. 321–322

identified based on the organization and trajectory of corticonuclear fibers arising therein (Fig. 5). There were distinct similarities between these cortical areas and the compartments in the white matter as described by Voogd [78]. It was therefore appropriate to designate these areas as cortical zones and apply the terminology of Voogd [78]. Based on the organization of corticonuclear fibers, zones A, B, C_1, C_2, C_3, and D were identified in lobule V of this primate (Fig. 5). Each zone is characterized not only by its general position in relation to adjacent zones but primarily by the specific pattern of its efferent projections into the cerebellar nuclei.

Input into the NIP from the B–C_1 Zone Area

A comment needs to be made concerning the persistent, yet somewhat enigmatic, projection into the NIP from the general region of zones B and/or C_1 (Fig. 5). Projections into the NIP which appeared to originate from either the vermis or the vermis-paravermis interface have been described in other mammalian species [9, 15, 22, 28, 50, 52, 74, 82] including *Galago* [36, 37]. Although earlier studies (with the possible exception of Hohman [50] who implied that they may have arose from the lateral vermis – his bundle A-V-I) did not specify the point of origin for these fibers, it was recently suggested that they may originate from the B zone [45].

A reexamination of the data offers another, and perhaps more plausible, explanation. When lesions are placed so as to involve progressively more lateral regions of the contralateral vermis it is possible to determine more precisely when these fibers to the NIP first appear. For example, following a lesion which only slightly crosses the midline preterminal debris is seen only in the contralateral NM in its characteristic terminal field (rostrodorsal NM in the case of lobule V). However, subsequent to a lesion that extends into more lateral portions of the contralateral vermis debris again appears in the NM (as from smaller lesions) and a newly acquired population of degenerated fibers enter the juxtarestiform body. In the same cases where fibers of passage are first seen entering the juxtarestiform body lesser amounts of preterminal debris are present in the medial NIP, obviously implicating zone B as the source. However, it is equally possible that these fibers to the NIP may arise from the narrow x zone, which has been identified by Oscarsson [67, 68] in the cat as being insinuated between zones A and B. Since the x zone is extremely narrow, lesions which cross the midline to involve the contralateral A zone and then the A and B zones would violate the intervening x zone in the latter situation at, or just prior to, the involvement of the B zone. Consequently one would expect to see degeneration in both the contralateral vestibular complex and the NIP at about the same time; and indeed this appears to be the case.

Anterior Lobe In Toto

Data from experiments on lobule V (Fig. 5) provided convincing evidence that corticonuclear fibers from this region of bushbaby cerebellum originated from a series of mediolaterally oriented cortical zones [44, 45]. An earlier study, also on the lesser bushbaby [37], had identified at least two ipsilateral zones in the vermal cortex of lobules I–V and noted that the NIA and NIP appeared to receive a topographically organized input from paravermal regions of lobules I–III and V.

If the results from the anterior vermis [37] are considered in light of the available data for lobule V summarized above (see also refs. [44, 45]), a relatively complete picture is revealed as concerns the spatial arrangement of zones for the entire anterior lobe of this primate (Fig. 5). In experiment No. 77 (from [37]) the cortex of lobule I and ventral lobule II were damaged from the midline lateral to the point indicated in Fig. 5. From this lesion degenerated fibers entered the ipsilateral rostroventral NM and the ipsilateral vestibular complex, indicating involvement of zones A and B respectively. The NIA contained preterminal debris along its rostromedial and rostrolateral borders, however the NIP was devoid of degeneration. This pattern of corticonuclear termination illustrated, as was hypothesized by Voogd [78], that compartments and zones C_1

and C_3 merge in ventral lobule II and obliterate the intervening compartment and zone C_2. An unexpected finding in this case was the sparse number of fibers which coursed laterally to enter the rostroventral NL. This was interpreted as indicating that zone D converges toward the midline sufficiently enough to have been slightly invaded by the lateral edge of the lesion. Projection into the rostroventral NM, the vestibular complex, and the rostral and rostrolateral NIA in experiment No. 78 (from [37]) indicated that zones A, B, and $C_1 + C_3$, respectively, were present in more dorsal regions of lobule II (Fig. 5). In contrast to case No. 77, sparse numbers of degenerated fibers entered the NIP in experiment No. 78. This showed that zone C_2, presumably absent in lobules I and ventral II, was present in more dorsal areas of lobule II. The lack of debris in the NL in case No. 78 indicated that the D zone occupied the relatively narrow region of cortex lateral to the lesion. In experiment No. 79 (from [37]) degenerated fibers entered the rostral and slightly more central NM, the vestibular complex, and only medial portions of the NIA thus signifying involvement of the A, B, and C_1 zones respectively (Fig. 5). The sparse amount of degeneration in the NIP suggested that the edge of the lesion only partially invaded the C_2 zone (Fig. 5). The complete absence of preterminals in the lateral NIA and any area of the NL illustrated the fact that zones C_3 and D were located lateral to the lesion.

The experimental evidence overwhelmingly supports the argument that corticonuclear fibers of the *Galago* anterior lobe originate from at least six (and probably more) ipsilateral cortical zones [44, 45]. Each zone projects not only primarily into its respective nucleus *but* also to a particular region of that nucleus. There is, consequently, a mediolateral zone pattern and, within each zone, a general rostrocaudal topographic projection of corticonuclear fibers into its respective nucleus [36–38, 45]. For example, the A zone of lobules I+II, lobules III, IV, and V project into the rostroventral, rostrocentral, rostrodorsal, and dorsocentral NM, respectively (see also Fig. 19).

Corticonuclear Fibers in the Squirrel Monkey (*Saimiri*)

When it became apparent that corticonuclear fibers arose from a series of rostrocaudally oriented cortical zones in the bushbaby (see above) we thought it appropriate to determine if this arrangement was a feature common to other primates. With the exception of recent observations by Voogd (this volume, p. 134), the report of Eager [22] on *Macaca* and a single comment concerning work in progress on the squirrel monkey [23] constituted the only attempts to analyze the trajectory of corticonuclear fibers in higher primates using contemporary tracing techniques. Eager [22] essentially confirmed the basic three-zone pattern described earlier by Jansen and Brodal [51, 52], however he noted that his data hinted at a more complex, albeit enigmatic, pattern.

The squirrel monkey (*Saimiri sciureus*), a South American primate of the family Cebidae, was selected for a series of preliminary experiments for several strategic reasons. First, the operative procedures developed on the smaller *Galago* (approx. 200–350 gms) could be easily adapted to the slightly larger (approx. 500–800 gms) squirrel monkey. Second, although a detailed description of the gross morphology of the squirrel monkey cerebellum is not available from the literature, a preliminary examination of several specimens revealed that it is markedly similar to that of the bushbaby. Even though the folia pattern is more complex, each lobule of the *Saimiri* cerebellum has a similar position relative to surrounding structures as do the homologous lobules of *Galago*. Third, as the squirrel monkey, along with the rhesus monkey, is one of the more commonly used primates in neuroscience research, it was considered appropriate to investigate the corticonuclear system in a primate that is widely utilized.

Although data on deep cerebellar nuclei of *Saimiri* will appear elsewhere [69], suffice it to say that in general they are similar to those described for *Macaca* by Courville and Cooper [14]. The NM is large, located in the subcortical white matter adjacent to the midline and, through irregular strands of cells, continuous caudolaterally with the NIP (see Fig. 6). The interposed complex consists of the NIA and NIP, these two nuclei having a rostral-caudal relationship to each other. Cerebellar corticovestibular fibers course through lateral aspects of the NM and become concentrated in the area between the NM and the laterally adjacent NIA-NIP complex. The NIA and NIP are separated from each other, as well as from the NL, by thin laminae of fibers. The only exception being a caudolateral continuum of the NIA with the NL. The NL is a medially concave mass of somata with a fairly distinct hilar region (see Fig. 6).

Our studies on *Galago* had revealed a relatively complex arrangement of corticonuclear fibers into zones, with each zone having a topographic relationship with its respective nucleus. Since this data was available in most detail for lobule V, and other areas of anterior lobe, we elected to investigate corticonuclear fibers of lobule V in the squirrel monkey, thus providing a better basis for direct comparison of results between *Galago* and *Saimiri*.

Lobule V

A total of 17 lesions were placed in lobules V (14 cases) and IV (three cases). From this series of unpublished experiments several representative examples from lobule V and one from lobule IV will be discussed. Important points concerning both zonal organization and topography will be emphasized.

Following lesions in lateral areas of lobule V (S194, S197L) preterminal degeneration was localized to rostral areas of the ipsilateral NL (Fig. 6). In case S194, illustrated in the horizontal plane, the damage was located at about the lateral margin of lobule V and its resultant degeneration found in the rostral NL. At more dorsal planes (Fig. 6A, S194) the terminal field appeared to be relatively homogenous. However, at more ventral levels (Fig. 6B, S194) it consisted of two mediolaterally oriented laminae separated by a region completely devoid of preterminal debris. No degenerated axons entered any other of the deep nuclei. Essentially similar results were seen in S197L (Fig. 6) subsequent to a lesion placed at a somewhat more medial position. In this case, traced in the coronal plane, degenerated axons in the rostral pole of the NL (Fig. 6A,

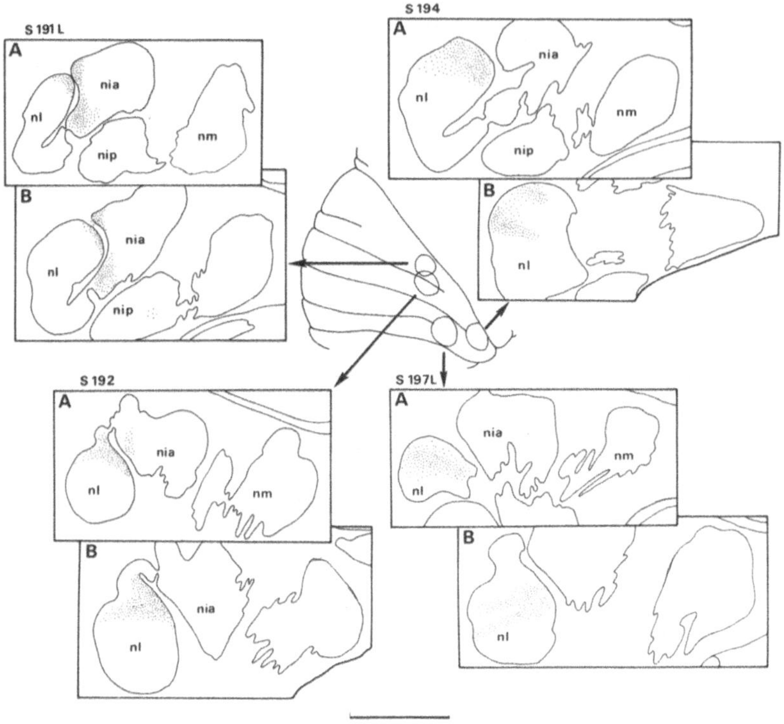

Fig. 6A, B. Tracings of the cerebellar nuclei from four *Saimiri* with lesions in lateral cortex (S194, S197L) and at the lateral-intermediate cortices (S191L, S192) interface. Cases S194 and S191L are shown in horizontal plane and cases S197L and S192 in coronal plane. Tracings are from dorsal **A** to ventral **B** and rostral **A** to caudal **B** respectively. The *fine dots* represent the location of preterminal degeneration. *Scale* = 2.0 mm. Abbreviations see p. 321–322

S197L) occupied a homogeneous area of the nucleus while at more caudal levels (Fig. 6B, S197L) the terminal field consisted of two mediolaterally oriented laminae similar to those seen in S194. These two bands of axonal debris coalesce in medial portions of the NL (Fig. 6, S197L). A remarkable feature of the pattern of degeneration in both of these experiments was the sharp interface between the terminal field and directly adjacent areas of the NL which were essentially devoid of debris (Fig. 7A).

Cortical damage in cases S192 and S191L were located in what was subsequently identified as the junction of lateral and intermediate cortices or, more specifically, the interface of the D_1 and C_3 zones (see also Fig. 9). Subsequent to lesion S192 (Fig. 6) an intense burst of preterminal debris was found in the rostrodorsal NL and a sparse patch in the lateral NIA (Fig. 6A, B, S192). This suggested that while the majority of the lesion in S192 was in the lateral cortical area, as indicated by numerous preterminals in the NL, its medial edge invaded the lateral extreme of the intermediate cortex. The inverse was true for experiment S191L in which the cortical injury was medial to, but overlapped with, that of S192 (Fig. 6). From the lesion in S191L numerous degenerated fibers

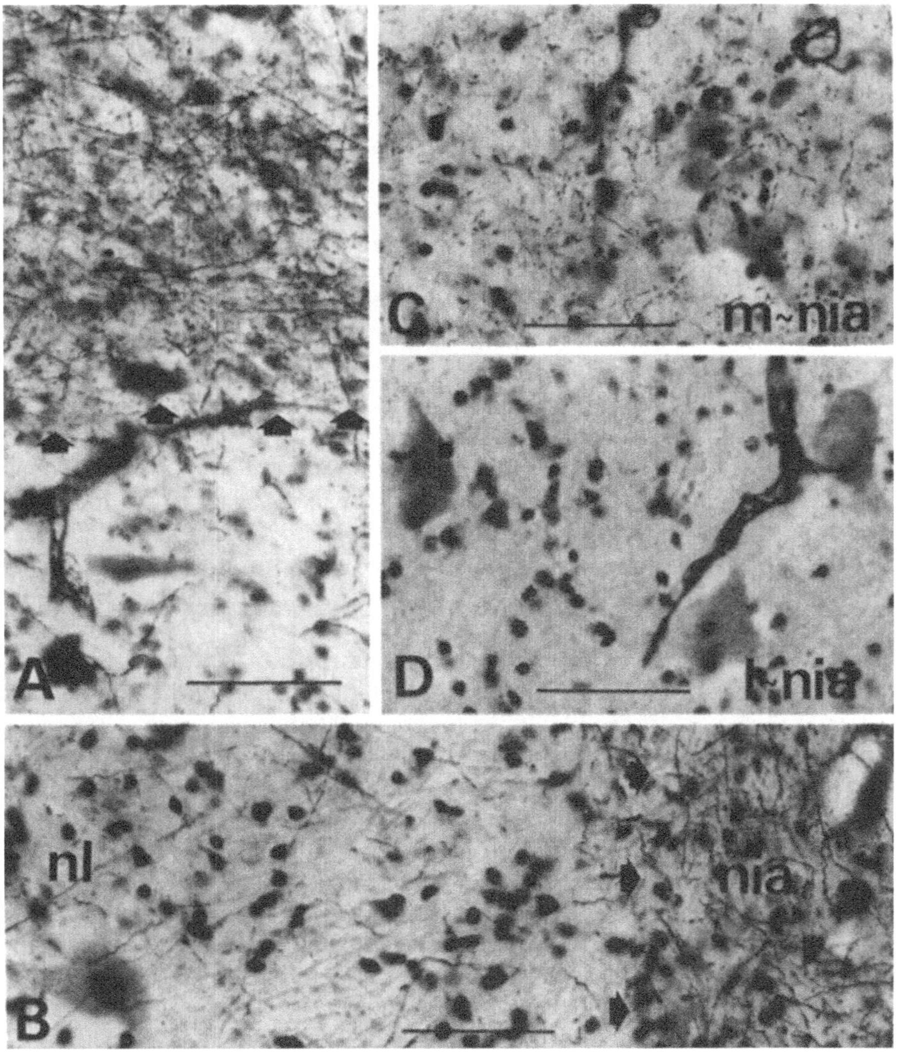

Fig. 7. Photomicrographs of degeneration in *nl* **A**, *nia* **C**, **D**, and at the *nl-nia* interface **B** in *Saimiri*. Note the sharp junction between areas of *nl* which contain debris versus adjacent regions which are free of degeneration (**A** – *block arrows* – detail from case S197L – Fig. 6). After a lesion located primarily in lateral areas of intermediate cortex numerous degenerated fibers are found in lateral *nia*, while rostromedial *nl* is comparatively devoid of debris (**B** – detail from S191L – Fig. 6). Injury to the C_1 area of cortex produced degeneration in medial *nia* (**C**) while lateral areas of the nucleus (**D**) were free of debris. Fink-Heimer method. *Scale*=57 μm. Abbreviations see p. 321–322

entered the lateral NIA while a paucity of debris was present in the rostromedial NL (Fig. 6A, B). A dense concentration of degenerated axons in the lateral NIA contrasted with the sparse amounts of debris in the medial NL (Fig. 7B). These observations indicated that lesion S191L was located primarily in lateral portions of the intermediate cortex as evidenced by its projections into the lateral NIA. It did, however, extend slightly into the medial edge of the lateral cortex (i.e., the D zone). The interface of intermediate and lateral cortices is along a line drawn through lateral aspects of S191L and medial portions of S192 (Fig. 6, see also Fig. 9); this line separates the lateral zone D from lateral portions of the intermediate cortex, the C_3 zone.

There were two interesting features of terminal fields in the NL following lesions in lateral (e.g., S197L) versus more medial (e.g., S192) areas of the D zone (Fig. 6). First, damage to more lateral regions produced a terminal field which, based on the distribution of degeneration in the NL, was divisible into two portions (S194 and S197L – Fig. 6). The terminal field in the NL subsequent to damage in medial areas of zone D, as in S192 (Fig. 6) was not obviously subdivided. Second, the terminal fields in the NL for fibers arising in these two respective areas of cortex are found in slightly different positions in the NL. For example, in S197L debris was located in central and more ventral areas of the rostral NL, while in S192 preterminals were concentrated in rostrodorsal areas of the nucleus. In Fig. 6, cases S192 and S197L are both shown in the coronal plane and one can clearly see the axonal debris was located in two different portions of the rostral NL. In light of the available data from Voogd and Bigaré [79] on the cat, our lesion S192 is presumably located in an area that can be designated D_1, while lesions S197L and S 194 are in regions which represent the D_2 zone.

Projections of the squirrel monkey intermediate cortex are arranged similar to those seen in the lesser bushbaby. Injury to lateral portions of the intermediate cortex, as illustrated from S191L (Fig. 6), precipitated degenerated axons which are largely restricted to the lateral NIA. Following lesions in medial areas of intermediate cortex, preterminal degeneration is located primarily in the medial NIA (Fig. 7C), while lateral portions of the same nucleus (Fig. 7D) contain no axonal debris. In addition to those fibers entering the medial NIA there were also lesser amounts of degeneration in the caudally adjacent NIP. Since this pattern of degeneration was usually accompanied by varying amounts of fibers coursing into the juxtarestiform body, the source of those fibers going to the NIP was not clear. As discussed above for *Galago*, these particular fibers may originate from lateral aspects of the vermis (i.e., zone B), from the narrow x zone, or it is possible that some may originate from medial aspects of the intermediate cortex (i.e., the C_1 zone). Although we had no cases which produced degeneration only in the NIP, the comparative results from several experiments argue strongly that middle portions of the intermediate cortex are related primarily to the NIP (see Fig. 9).

Subsequent to lesions located adjacent to the midline in lobules IV and V preterminal debris was found in the NM while degenerated fibers of passage entered the juxtarestiform body. In experiments S198 and S199 cortical injury was restricted to lobule V and separated from the midline by a very narrow portion of undamaged cortex (Fig. 8). Case 198 is illustrated in cross section and S199 in the parasagittal plane. From this area of cortex degenerated fibers enter the rostrodorsal NM and form a terminal field located just caudal to the rostral pole of the nucleus (S199, Fig. 8). Preterminal debris in both cases is more concentrated in lateral portions of the terminal field (Fig. 8B) than in its medial

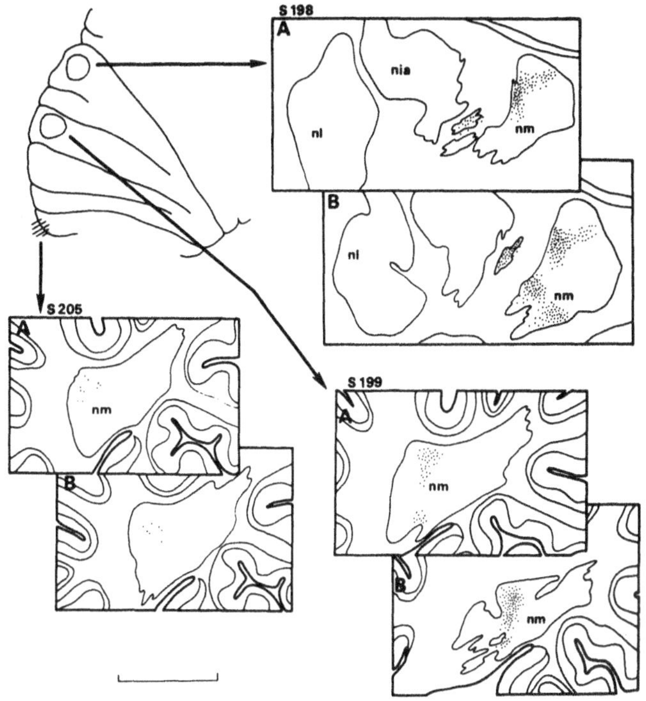

Fig. 8A, B. Tracings of the cerebellar nuclei from three *Saimiri* with lesions in medial cortex of lobules V (S198, S199) and IV (S205). Case S198 is shown in the coronal plane and cases S199 and S205 in parasagittal plane. Tracings are from rostral **A** to caudal **B** and from medial **A** to lateral **B** respectively. *Fine dots* represent the distribution of preterminal degeneration. *Scale* = 2.0 mm. Abbreviations see p. 321–322

area. In addition there is a small burst of degeneration in the ventrolateral NL at rostral levels. These results show that the lobule V vermal cortex of the squirrel monkey projects into both the NM and the vestibular complex. These data corroborate observations made by others (this volume, p. 149) that the A zone may be subdivided. For example, both of these lesions are located, as evidenced by the trajectory of axons arising therein, in the A zone with some involvement of the B zone. There is, however, a narrow portion of undisturbed cortex between the lesion and the midline. This suggests to us that the undamaged cortex is responsible for the sparse amount of degeneration (or lack thereof) in medial parts of the terminal field in the NM, while the dense concentration of debris in its more lateral portions originated from the damage to lateral areas of the A zone (see also ref. [80]).

In animal S205 (Fig. 8), an attempt to make a lesion in the vermal cortex of lobule IV produced a small superficial spot of damage on the midline of this lobule. Although extremely sparse in nature, preterminal debris was located in the rostrodorsal NM, confined to medial portions of the terminal field, and no degenerated axons coursed into the vestibular complex. In the parasagittal plane it is obvious that the terminal field for lobule IV is slightly rostral to that for lobule V (compare S199 with S205, Fig. 8).

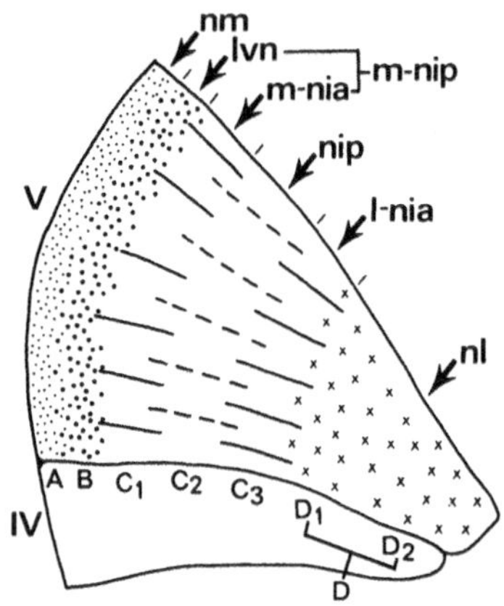

Fig. 9. Semidiagrammatic illustration showing the arrangement of zones and indicating their respective terminal nuclei for lobule V of *Saimiri*. Designation of zones after Voogd [78]. See text for discussion. Abbreviations see p. 321–322

Zones in Lobule V

Taken collectively the data from our series of preliminary experiments on lobule V of the squirrel monkey suggests there are seven ipsilateral areas of cortex whose efferent projections are essentially similar to those described above for the bushbaby. Consequently, it is appropriate to designate these areas as zones A, B, C_1, C_2, C_3, D_1, and D_2 (Fig. 9). There are two general characteristics of zones in lobule V of the squirrel monkey different from that seen in the bushbaby. First, there is an enlargement of the D zone with a clear indication, based on the organization of its corticonuclear fibers, that this region may be divided into a medial D_1 and a lateral D_2 zone (Fig. 9). Second, this enlargement (actually a mediolateral widening) of the D area has apparently taken place at the expense of intermediate and vermal cortices. Consequently, zones A to C_3 are narrower, proportionate to the overall size of lobule V, in the squirrel monkey than in the bushbaby. In the former species, zone D is wider while in the latter it is narrower (see also Fig. 18). When viewed in light of our data on the opossum and Voogd's results on the rhesus monkey (this volume, p. 149), this clearly indicates that as the D zone enlarges the A to C_3 zones become progressively narrower.

Corticonuclear Fibers in the Opossum (*Didelphis*)

Little information is available concerning cerebellar corticonuclear fibers in any of the so-called more generalized mammalian forms such as the North American opossum (*Didelphis virginiana*). As the opossum is held to be representative of the more generalized mammalian state, it was considered prudent to investigate the organization of its corticonuclear system especially as compared to other presumably more advance forms.

The deep cerebellar nuclei of the opossum can be divided into four regions, which, on a comparative basis, are homologous to the NM, NIP, NIA, and NL of other forms (see ref. [62] for review). In general, the NM is large and separated from the interposed complex. The NIA and NIP are smaller, closely apposed to each other, and incompletely separated from the laterally adjacent and rather diminutive NL [62].

Although the morphology of the opossum cerebellum has been known since the early work of Larsell [59, 60] studies concerned with efferent projections from its cortex have only been recently initiated. Henkel [48] and Henkel and Martin [49] commented only briefly on cerebellar corticonuclear fibers of the opossum in their detailed study of its vestibular complex. At about this time, Sreesai [74] made an attempt to analyze the arrangement of opossum corticonuclear fibers subsequent to lesions of areas presumed to represent vermal, paravermal, and hemisphere regions. This author described two diffuse patterns. First, lesions located in what was interpreted to be a zone precipitated degeneration throughout the rostrocaudal extent of its respective nucleus, the NM in cases of vermis, NIA and NIP in cases of the paravermal region, and the NL in experiments of the lateral cortex. Second, Sreesai [74] also described extensive bilateral projections from lesions located on one side of the midline. For example, from lesions in paravermal areas of lobules VI and VII and in lateral areas of crus I of the ansiform lobule, Sreesai [74] found degeneration in all ipsilateral nuclei and in contralateral NL, NIA, and NIP (paravermal case) and NM, NIA, and NIP (lateral case). Noting that this was unique when the opossum was compared to the available data for other species (Table 2), Haines et al. [47] reevaluated projections of the posterior vermis in an attempt to confirm these diffuse patterns. These authors concluded that corticonuclear fibers of the opossum posterior vermis were ipsilateral and, although somewhat different from that seen in other mammals, there was clear indication of a topographical arrangement.

Based on these obvious contradictions between our preliminary observation [47, 70] and the more extensive data of Sreesai [74], and especially between Sreesai's results and what appeared to be an overwhelming consensus from the literature on other species (Table 2), a detailed analysis of corticonuclear fibers in the opossum was undertaken. From a series of 46 unpublished experiments several representative cases in which damage was confined primarily to anterior lobe (Fig. 10A) will be discussed. The data presented addresses two general questions. First, is there any indication that the zonal pattern, seen in the corticonuclear system of other species, is present in this marsupial, and what is its spatial organization? Second, is there evidence that corticonuclear fibers may project in a topographical manner into the deep cerebellar nuclei?

Evidence Concerning Zones

The following results are from 11 representatives cases that had lesions placed in various areas of the anterior lobe (Fig. 10A). Following injury to lobules IV and V on or adjacent to the midline, degenerated fibers entered primarily the NM or, depending on lesion size, the vestibular complex. In experiment 037 (Fig. 10B), where cortical damage was small, numerous degenerated axons entered only the ipsilateral NM. In case 029, the area of cortical damage extended slightly more laterally, and in addition to those fibers in the NM, a small com-

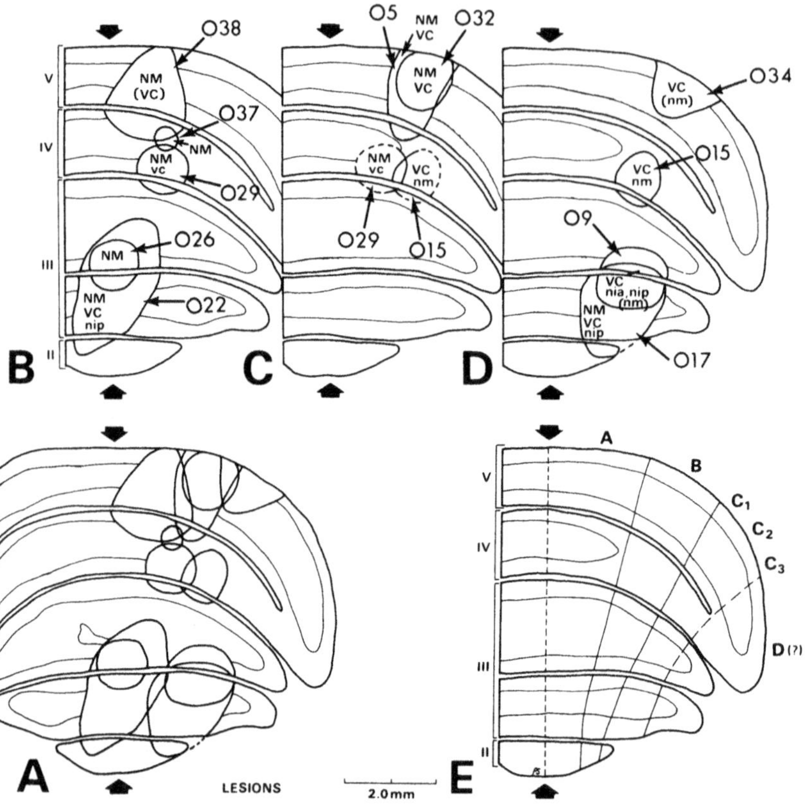

Fig. 10A–E. Drawings of the anterior lobe of *Didelphis* (exclusive of lobule I) showing the positions of 11 representative lesions. *Uppercase letters* (e.g., *NM*) signify that many degenerated fibers from that particular lesion entered that particular terminal nucleus, while *lowercase letters* (e.g., *nm*) indicate a sparser contribution. A composite of all lesions is shown in **A** and the general arrangement of zones in **E**. Abbreviations see p. 321–322

plement of degenerated axons coursed into the vestibular complex (Fig. 10B). From the relatively extensive cortical damage in case 038 (Fig. 10B) many degenerated fibers coursed into both the NM and the vestibular complex; contributions to the latter appeared, subjectively, less than the former. These experiments, plus data from animal 026 in which the lesion straddled the midline of lobule III (Fig. 10B), showed that the cortex adjacent to the midline was related to the NM. As one proceeds laterally, either via a larger lesion (038) or via damage at a slightly more lateral location (029), degeneration is also seen entering the vestibular complex.

Approximately equal amounts of preterminal debris were seen in the ipsilateral NM and vestibular complex subsequent to the lesion in cases 05 and 032 (Fig. 10C). The unexpected finding in these two experiments was the relatively intense degeneration seen in the NM even though these lesions were somewhat removed from the midline. Case 029, as noted above, had numerous degenerated axons in the ipsilateral NM and sparse amounts in the vestibular complex.

However, in animal 015 (Fig. 10C) the lesion was located slightly lateral to, but overlapping with, the area of cortical damage in 029. Many degenerated fibers entered the NM and sparse numbers were seen in the vestibular complex in 029. In contrast, from lesion 015 numerous degenerated axons coursed into the vestibular complex and few found their way into the NM (Fig. 10C). The pattern of degeneration seen in NM versus vestibular complex between these two experiments suggests that in lobule IV a line drawn through the area of overlap of these lesions (Fig. 10C) would represent the approximate border of zones A and B. Substantive proof of this was seen in animal 034 (Fig. 10D), especially when the trajectory of fibers from this lesion were compared with those of 029 and 015. In 034, degenerated fibers were related predominantly to the vestibular complex, indicating that this lesion was located primarily in the B zone of lobule V. The sparse debris in the NM originated from medial aspects of the lesion. The interface of A and B zones in lobule V is represented by an oblique line drawn through medial portions of lesion 034, this also being through lateral parts of lesions 05 and 032 (Fig. 10A, C, D). Cases 05 and 032 are located directly on the junction of A and B zones, therefore their equal contributions to both the NM and vestibular complex are understandable. The relative lack of preterminal debris in the interposed complex (NIA, NIP) in 034 and 015 indicated that zones C_1-C_3 are located lateral to an oblique line drawn along the lateral borders of these lesions (Fig. 10D, E).

Cortical damage in more rostral regions of the anterior lobe provided further evidence concerning the spatial arrangement of zones. Cases 026 and 022 were both midline lesions, the former restricted to lobule III and the latter involving lobule III and caudal lobule II (Fig. 10A, B). From the smaller of these two lesions (026) degenerated fibers entered rostrodorsal NM and no debris was seen in the vestibular complex (Fig. 10B). In experiment 022, the area of cortical damage was not only larger but extended more laterally. In addition to an intense concentration of debris in the NM numerous degenerated axons also entered the juxtarestiform body for subsequent distribution to the vestibular complex. A sparse amount of preterminal debris was also present in the NIP (Fig. 10B). The significant projection to *both* the NM and vestibular complex in case 022 indicated that there is an A zone in this area (projections to the NM) and a B zone, which is a strip of cortex related to vestibular nuclei. The B zone was closer to the midline in lobule III than it was in lobules IV and V (Fig. 10B, E). Damage to slightly more lateral cortex in lobules II and III precipitated degeneration in more lateral areas of the deep nuclei plus the vestibular complex. For example, from lesion 017 (Fig. 10D) degenerated fibers entered the NM and vestibular complex in similar amounts (as in 022), although one could argue that more fibers entered the vestibular area. In addition sparse amounts of debris were found in the NIP. However, from a lesion located in a more lateral position (09, Fig. 10D) extremely sparse numbers of degenerated axons enter the NM, indicating that this lesion is essentially lateral to the A zone. The vestibular complex receives significant input while sparse to moderate amounts of debris were seen in both the NIA and NIP (Fig. 10D).

Collectively, these results indicated that zones are present in the anterior lobe of the opossum and provided data concerning their spatial arrangement. Results from lobules II and III show that zones A and B are not only present in rostral areas of anterior lobe but are closer to the midline than in lobules IV and V (Fig. 10E). Zones C_1-C_3, which are lateral to our lesions in lobules IV and V, as illustrated by the relative lack of debris in the NIA and NIP, are also converging toward the midline in lobules II and III. This interpretation is supported by the fact that both the NIA and NIP receive input from lesions located in intermediate areas of lobules II and III (017, 09). We can not, based on these preliminary studies, specifically suggest a topography for the C_1-C_3 area of cortex. Due to the fact that both the NIA and NIP receive input from lesions in lobules II and III (Fig. 10D) all three zones are undoubtedly represented. No direct data is available at this time, based on corticonuclear fibers, concerning a D zone. However, we feel there is a narrow D region of cortex related to the NL in at least lobules III–V of the anterior lobe, a suggestion also substantiated by the observations of Martin and colleagues [63] on olivocerebellar fibers in the opossum.

Topography

In addition to the above summarized evidence concerning zones in the anterior lobe of the opossum, there is a clear indication that corticonuclear fibers within a given zone may be topographically related to its particular nucleus. Two experiments (05, 017), which had lesions in lobules IV–V and II–III respectively, will serve to illustrate this point (Fig. 11). In both of these cases the cortical damage involved lateral portions of zone A and medial parts of zone B (Fig. 10C, E), consequently, degenerated fibers entered both the NM and vestibular complex on the ipsilateral side. As our goal here is to consider only corticonuclear fibers, those projections into vestibular complex will not be discussed.

In experiment 05 the lesion involved dorsal portions of lobule IV, the width of lobule V, and slightly entered into rostral VI (Fig. 11). Corticonuclear degeneration was concentrated in two regions of the ipsilateral NM. Axonal debris originating from the injury to lobules IV and V entered dorsal aspects of the NM. At more medial planes (Fig. 11A, B, 05), the terminal field was relatively large and occupied the dorsal and central regions of the nucleus. As one proceeds in a lateral direction (Fig. 11C) the terminal field shifts into more caudal and ventral areas of the NM and appears to be somewhat elongated in a dorsocaudal to rostroventral direction. With the exception of large-diameter, degenerated fibers of passage, rostral portions of the NM are largely free of debris (Fig. 11A–C, 05). From the small area of superficial damage to lobule VI degenerated axons were traced, in serial section, into caudoventral areas of NM (Fig. 11B, large arrow). This small terminal area, resulting from damage in lobule VI, melded with the larger field from lobules IV and V at more lateral levels (Fig. 11C, large arrow). In this case there was a conspicious lack of preterminal debris in the rostral and rostrodorsal NM.

In animal 017 the primary lesion damaged upper parts of lobule II and lower portions of lobule III (Fig. 11A, B, 017). Due to a peculiarity of the operative

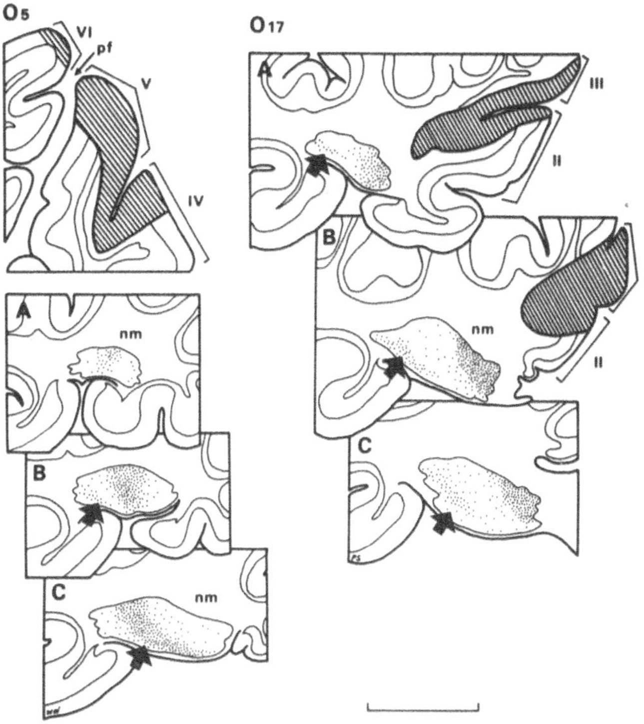

Fig. 11 A–C. Tracings, in parasagittal plane, of lesions and the *nm* of *Didelphis* following lesions in lobules IV, V, and VI (05) and lobules II, III, and VI (017). The large block arrows indicate the terminal field resulting from damage to lobule VI in both cases. Compare the distribution of debris in *nm* and see text for additional discussion. Scale = 2.0 mm. Abbreviations see p. 321–322

procedure a small superficial secondary lesion was also produced in lobule VI just caudal to the primary fissure in case 017. Although this injury is not illustrated it was essentially in the same location as that shown in Fig. 11 for 05. Degenerated fibers that arose from lobule VI were traced, through serial sections, into the caudoventral NM (Fig. 11 A–C, 017 large arrows). This moderate concentration of debris in the caudoventral NM (Fig. 12 A, C) retained its relative position essentially throughout mediolateral extents of the nucleus. From the large area of damage in lobules II and III many degenerated axons coursed into the rostral NM where preterminal debris was concentrated (Fig. 12 A, B). While the terminal field for lobules II and III appeared to occupy the rostral third of the NM at medial levels (Fig. 11 A, 017) it shifts to a more rostrodorsal area at more lateral planes (Fig. 11 B, C, 017). Degenerated fibers of passage coursed through the NM and entered the juxtarestiform body for distribution to vestibular nuclei.

A comparison of these two cases reveals several important points concerning topography in the opossum corticonuclear fiber system. First, this data clearly shows that these fibers are not diffusely distributed throughout the nucleus as was previously reported [74]; specific vermis lobules, in our examples, projected

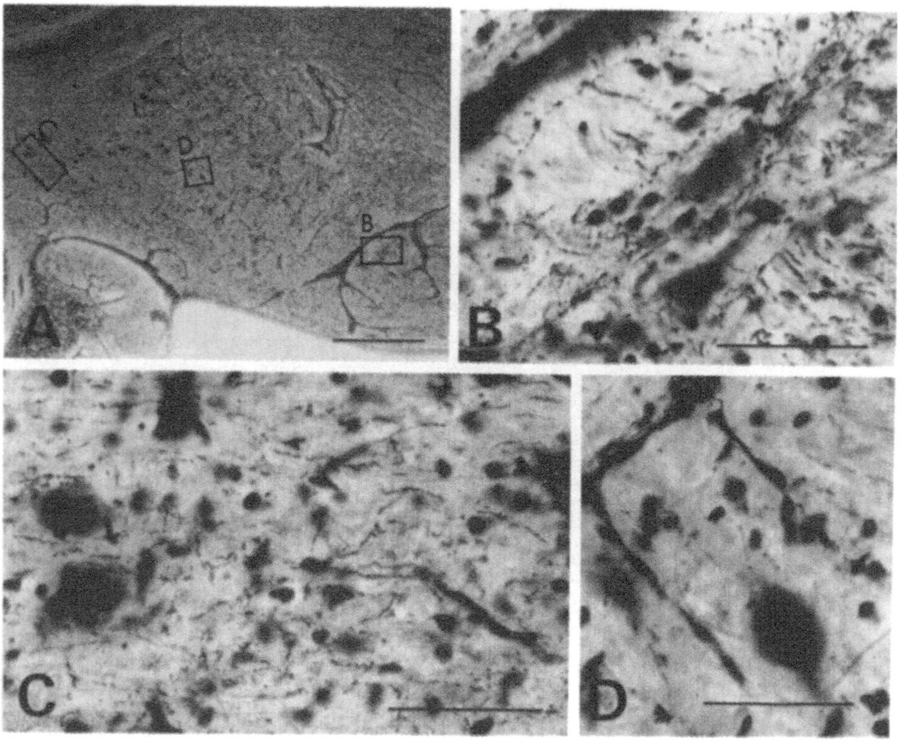

Fig. 12A–D. Photomicrographs of degeneration in NM from case 017 (Fig. 11) of *Didelphis*. The lower-power view **A** is a detail of tracing **B** from Fig. 11, 017. Numerous degenerated axons are found around somata in rostral NM (**B**, detail from **A**) from the damage to lobules II and III. Debris in caudoventral NM (**C**, detail from **A**) originated from the injury to lobule VI while central areas of the nucleus (**D**, detail from **A**) contain essentially no preterminal debris. Compare with Fig. 11, Fink-Heimer method. *Scale*=418.0 μm for A, 57.0 μm for **B–D.** Abbreviations see p. 321–322

into particular regions of the NM. Second, terminal fields in the opossum appear to be larger, that is occupy porportionately more of the nucleus, than those seen in other mammalian species. Although the fields appear larger they are confined to particular regions of the nucleus. In the examples described above, terminal fields arising from different lobules clearly complement each other. At medial planes the field for lobules IV and V is in the dorsocentral NM, leaving rostral regions of the nucleus for lobules II and III (Fig. 11, compare A in both experiments). At more lateral levels the terminal fields for lobules II–III and VI in case 017 are separated by a space largely free of debris (Fig. 12A, D); this area represents the location of the terminal field for lobules IV and V as seen in experiment 05 (Fig. 11, compare B and C in both experiments).

Although preliminary in scope, these results show that even in more generalized mammalian forms the cerebellar cortex is topographically represented in the deep nuclei. The pattern differs in certain respects from that seen in other mammals, however, it clearly exists.

Corticonuclear Fibers of the Albino Rat

The organization of cerebellar corticonuclear fibers in the albino rat has been described using both anterograde degeneration techniques [19, 28, 40] and autoradiography [4, 5]. Goodman and Simpson [27] and Goodman et al. [28] suggested that the three ipsilateral zones described earlier in the cat [11, 12, 51, 52] were also present in the rat cerebellar cortex. Although no effort had been made specifically to address the question of a more complex zonal pattern (a la Voogd) Korneliussen [55–58] provided evidence, based on the embryological development of both cerebellar nuclei and cortex, of a markedly more sophisticated arrangement. Scott [72] in a study of 5′-nucleotidase activity in the mouse cerebellum described a varying number of rostrocaudally oriented bands of enzyme activity in the molecular layer. In general, activity was more intense caudal to lobule VI and less intense rostral to this point.
Concerning the topography of corticonuclear projections in the rat there is some disparity of opinion. Goodman et al. [28], using the Nauta method, concluded that degeneration was distributed rather widely within a given nucleus even from lesions located in individual lobules. For example, damage to the medial (vermal) zone of lobules VI and IX precipitated degeneration essentially throughout rostrocaudal extents of the NM. Injury to areas of cortex in paravermal and lateral zones produced a similarly diffuse pattern of degeneration in their respective nuclei [28]. Subsequent investigators [4, 5, 40] have been unable to corroborate the diffuse nature of corticonuclear fibers in the rat, but instead have provided evidence that these fibers may be organized in a comparatively specific pattern. The following comments concerning corticonuclear fibers from anterior and posterior lobe vermal cortices are summarized from a recent report [40].

Corticonuclear Fibers from the Vermal Cortex

Following lesions of individual lobules of the anterior and posterior vermis, preterminal debris was distributed in a rostroventral to caudoventral circumferential sequence in the ipsilateral NM (Fig. 13). Damage to dorsal portions of lobule I and ventral lobule II in case R 20 precipitated degeneration in the rostroventral NM throughout its mediolateral extent (Fig. 13). Preterminal debris was present around somata and in the neuropil, while degenerated fibers of passage coursed through the rostral NM to enter the juxtarestiform body. In experiment R23 (Fig. 13), a small lesion was placed in the exposed portion of lobule V just rostral to the primary fissure. Preterminal degeneration was located in the dorsal and central NM at medial levels while at lateral planes the amount of degeneration decreased and the remnants of the terminal field shifted to a position just ventral to the so-called dorsolateral protuberance (terminology of Goodman et al. [28]). In addition a sparse burst of degeneration was seen in the ventrolateral NM. Debris was concentrated in the caudodorsal NM in experiment R9 (Fig. 13) following superficial injury to caudal portions of lobule VI. In this case the terminal field retained its relative position

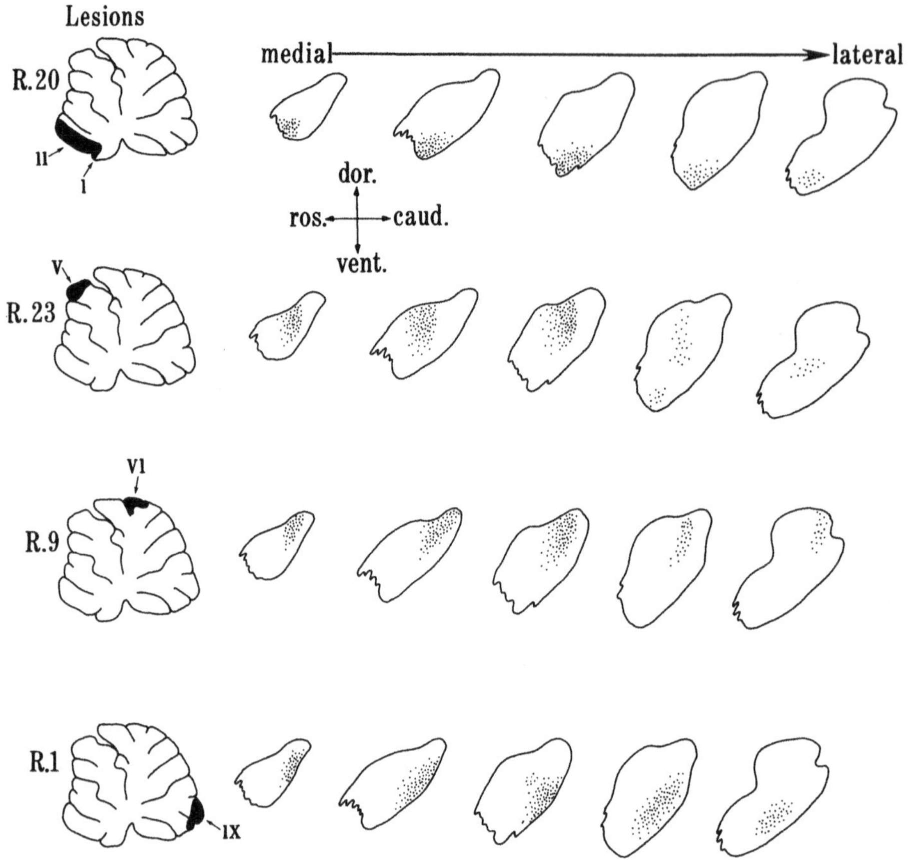

Fig. 13. Tracings, in parasagittal plane, of NM of albino rat from medial to lateral illustrating the distribution of debris following lesions in lobules I and II (*R20*), lobule V (*R23*), lobule VI (*R9*), and lobule IX (*R1*). Abbreviations see p. 321–322

throughout the mediolateral extent of the nucleus. However, at more lateral levels a sparse amount of debris appeared to extend into the so-called dorsolateral protuberance (Fig. 13). In case R1, the lesion was placed in the cortex of lobule IX and the resultant preterminal degeneration distributed to caudoventral areas of the ipsilateral NM essentially throughout its mediolateral extent (Fig. 13). In this experiment, as was seen from lobules I–V, degenerated fibers of passage course through lateral regions of the NM and enter the juxtarestiform body. An overview of these representative cases (Fig. 13) illustrates the topographical arrangement of corticonuclear fibers to the NM arising from individual lobules of the vermal cortex (see also ref. [40]).

Lesions, either purposefully or inadvertently placed, which involve more than one lobule may also reveal important data concerning the specific and orderly arrangement of corticonuclear fibers from the rat vermis. For example, in case R8 (Fig. 14) a large lesion injured caudal lobule VI, superficial portions of lobule VII, and rostral parts of lobule VIII. In this experiment the terminal field in the NM was: (a) larger, (b) contained a greater concentration of debris, and (c) extended slightly more caudal and ventral when compared to case R9 (Fig. 13), in which the lesion was restricted to lobule VI (compare R8 with R9). In case R8, the expansion of the terminal field caudally and ventrally is a reflection of input from lobules VII and VIII. The most ventral region of the NM which was devoid of degeneration in case R8 (Fig. 14) received input from the cortex of caudally adjacent lobule IX (Fig. 13). In another experiment (case R19), a primary lesion was placed in lobule III and, due to inadvertent contact with the cortex during the operation, secondary vascular insufficiency produced a superficial lesion in lobule V and the upper portion of lobule IV (Fig. 14). This experiment, in effect, had a primary lesion in lobule III and a secondary lesion in the upper portion of lobule IV which continued into lobule V. Between these two lesions was an undisturbed strip of cortex on the upper folia of lobule III

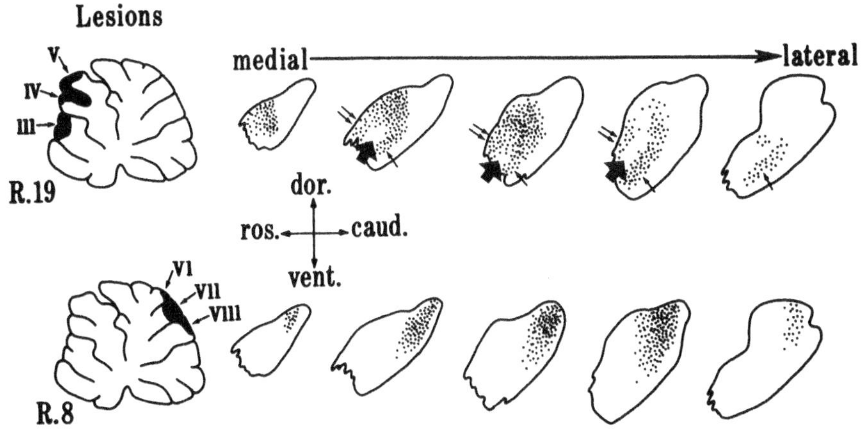

Fig. 14. Tracings, in parasagittal plane, of NM of albino rat from medial to lateral illustrating the distribution of preterminal degeneration following lesions of lobules VI–VIII (*R8*) and a lesion involving portions of lobules III, IV, and V (*R9*). See text for discussion. Abbreviations see p. 321–322

and lower folia of lobule IV (Fig. 14). Preterminal degeneration was found in the entire rostrodorsal NM (Fig. 14), however, a close examination revealed a topographical relationship between the distribution of debris in the nucleus and the cortical damage. From the point of primary injury in lobule III degenerated fibers of passage coursed directly into ventral areas of the rostral NM (Fig. 14, single arrow), where some terminated, while others continued on into the vestibular complex. The most rostroventral region of the NM contained no preterminals in case R19 (Fig. 14) since it was this area of the nucleus that received input from lobules I and II (case R20, Fig. 13). In experiment R19, degenerated fibers arising from the cortical damage in lobules IV and V entered the rostrodorsal and central NM (Fig. 14). It was known from a previous case (R23, Fig. 13) that the dorsal and central NM received input from lobule V. Consequently, the caudal area of the terminal field in case R19 (Fig. 14) was the result of that portion of the lesion restricted to lobule V. Degenerated fibers from the area of secondary damage in lobule IV entered and terminated in the rostrodorsal NM (Fig. 14, double arrows). The somewhat irregularly shaped region in the rostrocentral NM in case R19 (Fig. 14, block arrow), which contained few, if any, preterminals, appeared to be related to the undisturbed cortex bordering on the preculminate fissure; that is, on caudal lobule III (ventral to the fissure) and rostral lobule IV (dorsal to the fissure). This particular case nicely illustrated the fact that corticonuclear fibers of the rat vermal cortex project into the NM in a relatively orderly manner.

These observations on the rat vermis (exclusive of lobule X) show that this region of cortex projects into the NM in a topographical fashion. Although the terminal field of a particular lobule may be larger, proportionate to the overall size of the nucleus, than that seen in the cat or primate [15, 36, 37, 45] it still occupies a similar region of the nucleus. Our data is closely comparable to that of Armstrong and Schild [4] who mapped corticonuclear fibers of the vermis using autoradiography. For example, labeled axons were found in caudoventral regions of the NM in their case CN-12 following an injection which involved lobule IX and parts of lobule X; this is essentially the same area of the NM which contained degeneration subsequent to a lesion in lobule IX in our case R1 (Fig. 13). Equally similar comparisons are possible for other lobules, especially those cut in a parasagittal plane. Armstrong and Schild [4] also described labeled axons in certain areas of the rostral NM after injections in lobules II–V.

The main difference between our results and those of Armstrong and Schild [4] concerns the relative size of the presumed terminal field in the NM. Our results (see also ref. [40]) suggested that corticonuclear debris occupied a relatively specific terminal region of the NM, while Armstrong and Schild [4] found labeled axons in slightly larger regions of the nucleus. It is highly probable that this is simply a reflection of the two different techniques used (lesion and Fink-Heimer versus autoradiography) and does not represent any actual significant differences between these studies.

We have made no firsthand observations on the trajectory of corticonuclear fibers arising from paravermal or hemisphere regions in the rat. However, the observations of Armstrong and Schild [5] on selected regions of the hemisphere suggest that these fibers may also be more complexly arranged than previously reported.

Corticonuclear Fibers of the Tree Shrew (*Tupaia*)

Experimental exploration of the posterior lobe vermis and paraflocculus of the tree shrew [36, 46] revealed evidence of both a topographic and zonal arrangement of corticonuclear fibers. These observations suggested that the posterior lobe, even of more basal mammalian forms, may also share some of the features common to the more sophisticated organization of corticonuclear fibers as seen in other cerebellar regions.

In a series of detailed observations on the efferent fibers from the ansiform lobule crus II and the paramedian lobule, A. Brodal and Courville [10] and Courville et al. [17] concluded that their data did not corroborate the hypothesis of Voogd [78] concerning a mediolateral arrangement of zones in these lobules of the cat. Although these authors did identify terminal fields in the NL, NIA, and NIP subsequent to lesions in both lobules, their data suggested that zones may not be present in certain regions of the posterior lobe. Bishop et al. [9] also failed to confirm a zonal organization of Purkinje cells in the paramedian lobule subsequent to horseradish peroxidase (HRP) injections in the NIA and NIP. These investigators reported that only the most rostral and caudal folia of the paramedian lobule projected into the NIA while the NIP received a topographically organized input from all folia of the lobule. Recent studies by Dietrichs and Walberg [18] and Voogd and Bigaré [79] using HRP have identified a minimum of five ipsilateral corticonuclear zones in the paramedian lobule of the cat. This disparity of opinion prompted an analysis of the paramedian lobule of the tree shrew, *Tupaia glis* (see also ref. [41, 42]).

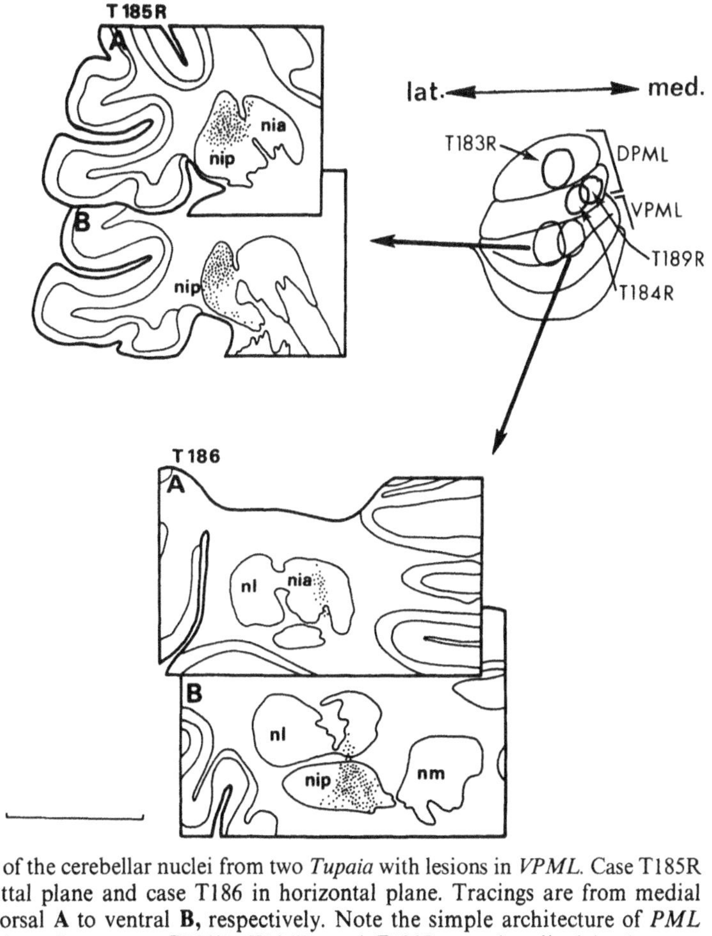

Fig. 15A, B. Tracings of the cerebellar nuclei from two *Tupaia* with lesions in *VPML*. Case T185R is shown in parasagittal plane and case T186 in horizontal plane. Tracings are from medial **A** to lateral **B** and dorsal **A** to ventral **B**, respectively. Note the simple architecture of *PML (upper right)*. Projections from cases T189R, T184R, and T183R are described in the text. *Scale*=2.0 mm. Abbreviations see p. 321–322

Paramedian Lobule (PML)

The paramedian lobule of the tree shrew consists of four to five folia from dorsal to ventral (Fig. 15). The upper two folia represent the dorsal division of the lobule (DPML) and the ventral two to three folia its ventral portion (VPML). It is acknowledged that the lowermost folium of the lobule has been designated as the copula pyramidis in an earlier study [32]. Consequently, the precise and most appropriate terminology for this lower folium awaits further study since, in the present series of experiments, no lesion was placed therein.

Of a total of 16 lesions placed in the DPML and in the upper two folia of the VPML, only representative cases will be summarized here (see also ref. [42]). Injury to medial regions of the DPML precipitated degeneration in only the NIA and NIP. For example, following lesion T184R (Fig. 15) preterminal debris was present in the dorsal and central NIA with a tendency for the terminal field to shift into the lateral NIA at caudal levels. Degeneration was also found although in slightly lesser amounts, in the lateral NIP. Cortical damage at slightly more medial locations (e.g., T189R, Fig. 15) produced a more intense projection into the medial NIA and a corresponding decrease in the amount of debris in the NIP. The inverse was true when lesions were shifted slightly more laterally. In case T183R (Fig. 15), the lesion was placed more toward the central region of the DPML and there was a concurrent decrease in the number of fibers projecting into the medial NIA and a precipitously greater amount of degeneration in the lateral NIP. These data suggested that medial regions of the DPML were related primarily to the medial NIA and as one proceeded laterally (toward central regions of the lobule, Fig. 15) there was a decrease in projections to the medial NIA and corresponding increase in those fibers terminating in the lateral NIP. Confirmation of this general NIA to NIP trend is illustrated by experiments T185R and T186 (Fig. 15) both of which were located in the VPML. From lesion T186, which was located in a slightly more medial portion of the VPML, numerous degenerated fibers entered the medial and central NIP and sparse amounts of debris were found in the dorsal and central NIA (Fig. 15, T186). All other areas of NIA as well as the entire NL and NM were completely devoid of degeneration. However, when the damage was located in a slightly more lateral position (actually in the center of the mediolateral axis of the VPML), as in case T185R, preterminal debris was concentrated exclusively in the medial and central NIP. These results indicated that central regions of both the VPML and DPML were topographically related to the NIP, while more medial areas of these lobules project into the central and medial NIA.

Following lesions located in lateral areas of both the VPML and DPML degenerated fibers were traced primarily into the NL with contributions to the NIA and/or NIP depending on lesion position. To elucidate the trajectory of fibers from lateral regions of the VPML a lesion was placed in its most lateral area in case T187L (Fig. 16). During the surgical procedure, however, inadvertent contact with a slightly more medial spot on the lobule produced a small area of vascular insufficiency (Fig. 16, oblique lines). When sections from this case were examined in serial order it was possible to sort out the trajectory of degenerated fibers arising from each area of damage. Degenerated fibers exited

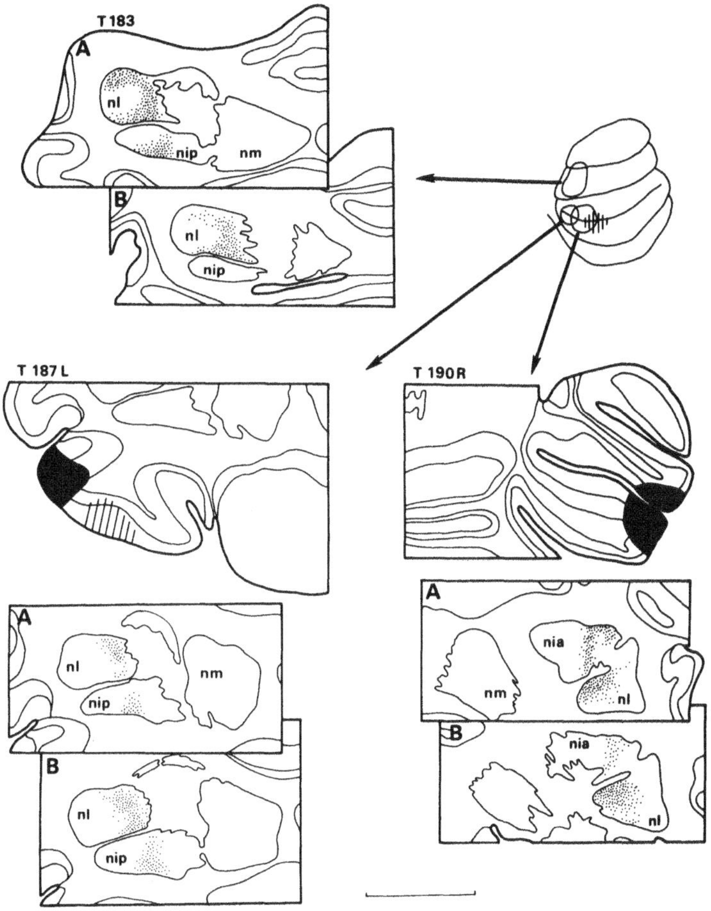

Fig. 16A, B. Tracings of the cerebellar nuclei from three *Tupaia* with lesions in VPML (T190R, T187L), and DPML (T183). Case T190R is shown in coronal plane and cases T183 and T187L in horizontal plane. Tracings are from rostral **A** to caudal **B** and dorsal **A** to ventral **B** respectively. See text for discussion. *Scale* = 2.0 mm. Abbreviations see p. 321–322

from the primary lesion (Fig. 16, T187L solid area), coursed rostrally along the lateral border of the NL, turned medially, and terminated in two areas in the ventromedial NL (Fig. 16). Although there was no actual tissue destruction, degenerated axons from the secondary lesion (Fig. 16, oblique lines) passed rostromedially to enter central areas of the NIP. The NIA and NM in this case contained no debris. In an attempt to clarify further the trajectory of fibers from this area of cortex, a lesion was placed so as to involve medial areas of the primary damage, lateral portions of the secondary injury, and the relatively narrow strip in between in case T187L (Fig. 16). In this latter experiment (T190R, Fig. 16), preterminal debris was found in the medial and ventral NL, essentially in the same locations as in case T187L, and in lesser amounts in the NIP (not illustrated). In addition there was a newly acquired fascicle of degenerated fibers entering the dorsal and more lateral NIA (Fig. 16, T190R); a projection not seen in the previous case. Those fibers entering the NIA were interpreted as arising from the relatively narrow strip of cortex located between the areas of primary and secondary damage in experiment T187L.

Corticonuclear fibers which originated from lateral portions of the DPML also terminated in the NL and portions of the interposed complex. Small lesions in the lateral DPML precipitated degeneration only in the ventromedial NL and in a band which, in cross section, appeared to extend across the rostral pole of the nucleus. Case T183 (Fig. 16) illustrates, in the horizontal plane, the results from a larger lesion in the lateral DPML. In this experiment preterminal debris occupied an area of the ventromedial NL similar to that following lesions in the lateral VPML cortex (compare T183 and T187L, Fig. 16). In addition, the terminal field in the NL extended laterally along the rostral border of the nucleus and, to a lesser extent, laterally along its caudal boundary with the NIP (Fig. 16). This indicated that corticonuclear fibers from the lateral DPML have terminal fields which are partially coextensive with, and partially exclusive from, those of the lateral VPML. Lesions in the lateral DPML produced axonal debris primarily in the NL and NIP. Only damage to the lowermost folium of the DPML, and specifically in its lateral area, precipitated any degeneration in the NIA. In these experiments (not illustrated) debris was confined to a small dorsolateral portion of the NIA. These observations suggest that those portions of cortex related mainly to the lateral NIA are narrow in the VPML and almost nonexistent in the DPML being obliterated by the direct apposition of cortical areas which project to the NL and NIP (Figs. 16, 17).

Taken collectively the data from all paramedian lobule experiments suggests a pattern of zones for this region of tree shrew cerebellum, as well as providing evidence of specific topographic patterns within certain zones (Fig. 17, see also ref. [41, 42]). Based on the organization of its corticonuclear fibers the paramedian lobule of the tree shrew appears to have a minimum of four rostrocaudally oriented zones (Fig. 17). A relatively narrow, lateral zone D, which projects in a topographic manner into the NL, occupies the lateral portions of both lobules. A comparatively broad middle portion of both the DPML and VPML projects primarily into the NIP, and is therefore designated as the C_2 zone. Medial to the C_2 zone is an area of cortex related to the medial NIA and

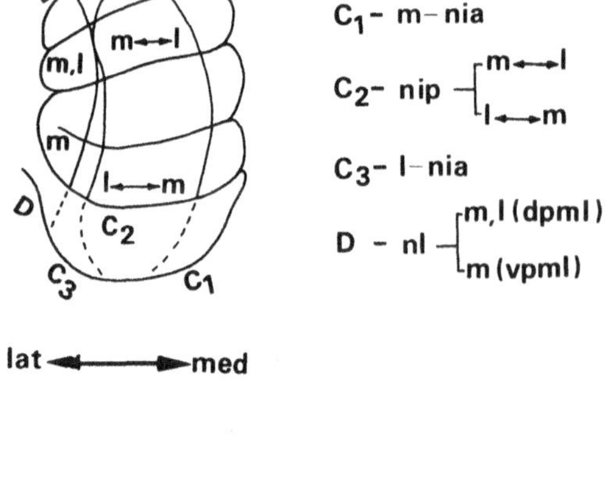

Fig. 17. Semidiagrammatic representation of zones (C_1, C_2, C_3, D) in paramedian lobule of *Tupaia*. The corticonuclear fibers arising from some zones (C_2 and D) appear to project into their respective deep nuclei in a topographic manner described in detail in the text. Abbreviations see p. 321–322

therefore identified as zone C_1. The width of this zone is variable being somewhat wider in the DPML and narrower in the VPML. Lateral to the C_2 zone is a relatively narrow, partially discontinuous region of cortex, the fibers of which enter the lateral NIA. The pattern of degeneration in the deep cerebellar nuclei following a series of lesions in the lateral DPML and VPML suggested that this C_3 region is very narrow in the VPML and obliterated by the direct apposition of the D and C_2 zones in the DPML. Evidence from a detailed analysis described elsewhere [42] suggests that the C_3 zone may appear again in the rostral and rostrolateral DPML (Fig. 17).

There is also tentative evidence of a topographic organization of corticonuclear fibers arising from both the D and C_2 zones (Fig. 17). Lesions in the D zone of the DPML precipitate degeneration in both medial and lateral areas of the NL (see above), while debris is found only in the medial NL subsequent to damage in the D zone of the VPML (Fig. 17). There is also some indication that efferent fibers from the C_2 zone may be specifically organized. Following lesions in the medial area of zone C_2 in the DPML debris was found in the lateral NIP. As lesions were placed in more lateral locations the terminal field in the NIP appeared to shift to a slightly more medial position (Fig. 17). The inverse is true for the VPML. Injury in medial C_2 areas of the VPML precipitated degeneration in the medial NIP, and as the lesions were positioned in progressively more lateral regions the terminal fields in the NIP simply appeared to shift laterally.

Zones in the PML

With the exception of our tree shrew data the recent reports of Dietrichs and Walberg [18], Voogd and Bigaré [79], and Bishop et al. [9] are the only detailed descriptions of corticonuclear fibers of the paramedian lobule: all of these studies being on the cat. Dietrichs and Walberg [18] and Voogd and Bigaré [79] identified five ipsilateral zones in the paramedian lobule, however, certain differences between these two publications and our results, especially as regards the terminology of zones, merits a more detailed comparison.

Voogd [78] in his original study, identified seven ipsilateral compartments and the deep cerebellar nucleus, or portion thereof, which was found in each compartment (see above, Historical Perspective; Table 3). The hypothesis concerning cortical zones [78] stipulated that the cortex overlying a particular compartment may contain a population of Purkinje cells that would project primarily, if not exclusively, into the nucleus, or portion thereof, contained within its respective compartment. Although denied by some for certain areas of cerebellar cortex [9, 10, 17] a number of other studies ([16, 18, 35–38, 41, 42, 45, 46, 76, 78, 79] this volume, p. 139 and others) have shown that the fundamental nature of this pattern is valid. Consequently, the topographic relationship of each cortical zone with its respective nucleus, or portion thereof, essentially constitutes the definition of that particular zone. For example, cortical lesions which produce degeneration in the medial NIA are located, as originally hypothesized [78], in the C_1 zone. The size and/or shape of the zone may vary from species to species or from lobule to lobule within a given species, however, all those cortical areas which project into the medial NIA (in this example) collectively represent the C_1 zone.

In the ferret, Voogd [78] identified at least four compartments and zones in the paramedian lobule (Table 3). He specifically noted "In the paramedian lobule four zones [C_1, C_2, C_3, D_1] are present and in the ventral part of the ansiform lobule a fifth zone [D_2], which just touches the lateral margin of the paramedian lobule" (our brackets). The apposition of the D_2 zone of the ansiform lobule to the lateral paramedian lobule suggested the potential for the D_2 area extending into the latter region (Table 3). Voogd and Bigaré [79], in their HRP study of cat corticonuclear fibers identified a relatively wide C_2 zone after NIP injections, a well developed medial C_1 zone and a small lateral C_3 zone following NIA injections, and D_1 and D_2 zones after caudal and rostral NL injections respectively (Table 3). These authors concluded that, from medial to lateral, the cat paramedian lobule contained zones C_1, C_2, C_3, D_1, D_2. Dietrichs and Walberg [18] utilized HRP as an anterograde tracer to investigate corticonuclear fibers of the paramedian lobule of the cat. They also identified five zones and, although the zone terminology is applied in a modified manner (Table 3), their general results appear comparable to those of Voogd and Bigaré [79] and ours [41, 42]. Dietrichs and Walberg [18] identified a D_2 zone related to the ventral NL, a D_1 zone, which projected to the NL-NIA transition area, but were unable to specify the location of C_3 cortex (Table 3). They further concluded that paramedian projections into the dorsolateral and ventromedial NIP originated from C_2 and C_1 zones, respectively, while input to the dorsomedial NIA arose from a medially located region of cortex in ventral areas of the PML designated by these authors as the B zone (Table 3).

Table 3. A comparison of compartments and cortical zones of the paramedian lobule [a]

Compartments Voogd 1969		Corticonuclear Fibers		
General pattern	Paramedian lobule	Voogd and Bigaré 1980 (cat)	Dietrichs and Walberg 1979 (cat)	Present study [b] (tree shrew)
A-NM				
B-VC			B-dorsomedial NIA	
C_1-mNIA	C_1	C_1-NIA	C_1-ventromedial NIP	C_1-dorsomedial and central NIA
C_2-NIP	C_2	C_2-NIP	C_2-dorsolateral NIP	C_2-NIP [c]
C_3-lNIA	C_3	C_3-NIA	C_3-	C_3-dorsolateral NIA
D_1-pNL	D_1	D_1-cNL	D_1-NL-NIA transition	D-VPML to vmNL
D_2-mNL	(?)D_2	D_2-rNL	D_2-ventral NL	D-DPML to vm & lNL

[a] Abbreviations see p. 321–322
[b] Data also summarized here from Haines and Patrick [41, 42]
[c] Our data suggest that C_2 input into NIP is topographically organized (see text and Fig. 17)

A comparison of these observations is shown on Table 3. It appears that the D regions of cortex are, in their essential elements, comparable in all three studies. Although we have elected not to subdivide the D zone in *Tupaia* there are a number of factors (see [42]) which support the contention that this region of cortex consists of a minimum of two identifiable portions. The D_1 zone of Dietrichts and Walberg [18] projects into both the lateral NIA and medial NL. Subsequent to HRP injection into the NIA Voogd and Bigaré [79] described a narrow discontinuous strip of filled Purkinje cells in the lateral PML (their C_3 zone) and a wider strip of filled somata in the medial PML (their C_1 zone). Our observations on tree shrews essentially corroborate the general features of these two zones (Table 3; see also [42]). Although Dietrichs and Walberg [18] did not specifically identify a C_3 zone it is noteworthy that they did observe projections into the lateral NIA from the presumed C_3-D_1 interface which they attributed to the D_1 zone. These authors stated that if a C_3 zone was present it would be just medial to the D_1 region.
The retrograde HRP study of Voogd and Bigaré [79] and our anterograde Fink-Heimer data [42] indicated that the C_2 zone is a relatively wide middle region of the PML (Table 3; Fig. 17). Dietrichs and Walberg [18] identified a broad C_2 zone related to the dorsolateral NIP, however, those fibers to the ventromedial NIP arose from a narrow medially located strip of cortex designated as C_1 by these authors. It is possible that the C_1 and C_2 zones of Dietrichs and Walberg [18], based on their exclusive relationship to only the NIP, are homologous to the relatively wide C_2 zone as described in other studies on the paramedian lobule [41, 42, 79]. The potential presence of a B zone in medial areas of the ventral PML is partially related to the fact that caudal regions of the contralateral dorsal accessory olive project into the B zone of the anterior lobe and into this medial area of the ventral PML (see [80]). However, cortical lesions in more medial areas of both the DPML and VPML, in our experience to date, precipitated no anterograde degeneration in the ipsilateral vestibular complex. Consequently, we designate this entire medial zone as C_1 due to its predominant relationship with the medial NIA; a convention which not only agrees with the data of Voogd and Bigaré [79] but is consistent with the original concept [78] of what, by definition, constitutes the B zone. Although Dietrichs and Walberg [18] have specified a B zone in medial regions of the ventral PML (see also 81 for olivocerebellar criteria) it appears to be at least partially homologous to the C_1 zone of other studies (Table 3; [41, 42, 79]).

Summary

Ideally one would like to conclude a review of this nature by proposing an all inclusive schema for the particular pathway under consideration. Two factors militate against this option when considering the organization of cerebellar corticonuclear fibers. First, there is the problem of the comparative approach. As briefly illustrated in this paper, there is clear evidence of an overall plan, however, it is modified to varying degrees in all species studied to date. Consequently one specific schema would not be applicable to a broad group of mammalian forms. Second, with the single exception of the cat (the reader is referred to the excellent original contributions [3, 8–12, 15–18, 21, 30, 31, 51, 52, 77, 81, 82] this volume, p. 139 and others), no single species has been completely and exhaustively examined. Although studies are in progress on a number of different mammalian forms, the entire story is not complete. There is, however, adequate comparative data from which certain general points can be made.

Our data presented here as well as that from the literature [18, 35–38, 44–46, 77–79] this volume, p. 139 and others overwhelmingly supports the contention that there are two levels of organizational complexity in the corticonuclear fiber system of all mammals for which data are available. The first level is an overall pattern of cortical zones, these being rostrocaudally oriented strips of cortex, the Purkinje cells of which project into a particular deep cerebellar nucleus or portion thereof. With few exceptions these zones are continuous from lobules I and II through X, faithfully following, in a rostrocaudal direction, all the irregularities of the folia of the various lobules. The second level, which essentially represents a subset of the zonal pattern, shows that corticonuclear fibers arising from different lobules of the same zone will project into different regions of its respective nucleus. Thus, there is the overall zone pattern and within each zone a specific topographic pattern.

Corticonuclear Zones

Although zones may be present in all mammals studied thus far their spatial arrangement may vary markedly from one species to another. In the examples shown for the anterior lobe in Fig. 18 some of these differences are self-evident. An unexpected finding in the opossum was the exceptionally wide area of cortex identified as zones A and B, i.e., vermal cortex. Since A and B zones in the anterior lobe are considerably narrower in the bushbaby, squirrel monkey (Fig. 18), cat ([79] this volume, p. 139), and rhesus monkey (this volume, p. 149) it

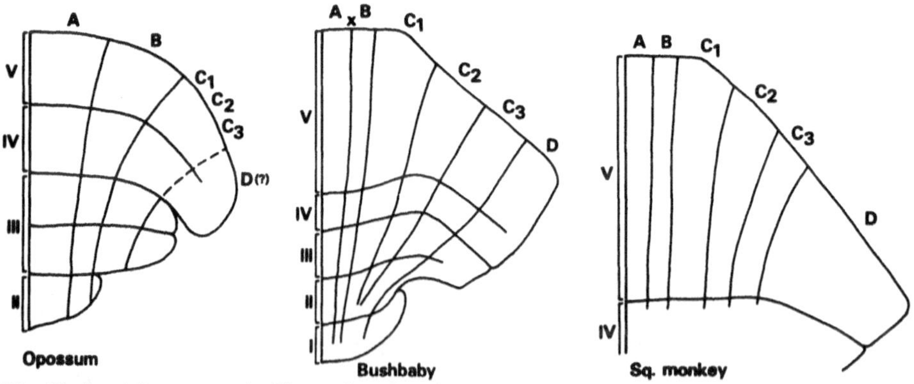

Fig. 18. Semidiagrammatic illustration showing the comparative arrangement of zones for lobules II–V of opossum (*Didelphis*), lobules I–V of bushbaby (*Galago*), and lobule V of squirrel monkey (*Saimiri*). Note the comparative width of vermal, intermediate, and lateral zones in these species. Abbreviations see p. 321–322

may be inferred that a relatively wide vermis may be a characteristic of the more generalized mammalian state. The comparatively small interposed and lateral nuclei in the opossum (see also ref. [62]) and correspondingly modest extents of their respective cortical areas also corroborate this concept. A minimum of six ipsilateral zones are present in the corticonuclear system in all forms, and there is convincing evidence of seven or more zones in some species ([72, 78, 79], and others). It was suggested above that the cortical input to the NIP, which arose from either the B zone or $B-C_1$ interface in the bushbaby, may actually orginate from the narrow x zone insinuated between zones A and B. This suggestion, plus the fact that future studies on the D region in the bushbaby may provide evidence concerning its D_1 and D_2 divisions, shows that the corticonuclear system of *Galago* may consist of a minimum of eight zones. The same is true for the squirrel monkey although at the present time there is little direct evidence concerning efferent projections from the presumed x zone.

There is an obvious tendency for zones of vermal and intermediate cortices to be compressed in a medial direction as the lateral cortex (zone D) enlarges (Fig. 18). This is especially evident as one proceeds from the opossum to rhesus monkey (this volume, p. 152). The D zone, which probably occupies only the most lateral cortex in the opossum, is slightly larger in the bushbaby, considerably wider in the squirrel monkey (Fig. 18), and occupies a large portion of the anterior lobe hemisphere in the rhesus monkey (this volume, p. 152). In all of these mammals the intermediate (C_1, C_2, C_3) and vermal (A, B) cortices become progressively narrower as the lateral cortex expands.

The limited amount of data available indicates that cerebellar cortical zones are a feature common to a wide variety of mammals. It remains for future studies to elucidate the arrangement of these zones in a more comprehensive sample.

Corticonuclear Topography

Within each zone efferent fibers of the cerebellar cortex project in an orderly manner into their respective deep nuclei. Two examples illustrate this point. Lobules I–X of the A zone project into the NM in a circumferential manner from rostroventral (lobules I and II) to caudoventral (lobules IX and X). This pattern, shown in Fig. 19 for *Galago,* is essentially similar to that reported for the rat [4, 40], cat [15] and, based on a less copious sample, is probably similar in other primates ([41, 42], this volume, p. 152). This pattern for the A zone is an orderly arrangement of partially overlapping terminal fields with each field extending throughout the mediolateral aspects of the NM. The fact that the A zone may be subdivided ([6], this volume, p. 149) does not negate the overall uniformity of this pattern.

Other zones also project into their respective terminal areas in an equally specific, albeit less orderly, manner. If we compare the terminal fields in the medial NIA from four lesions located in zone C_1 it is apparent that while C_1 fibers *may terminate* in the medial NIA, their fields are more irregular than those seen in the NM subsequent to lesions of the A zone. A lesion in the C_1 zone of lobule VI (Fig. 20) produced preterminal debris in the caudomedial NIA; these fibers

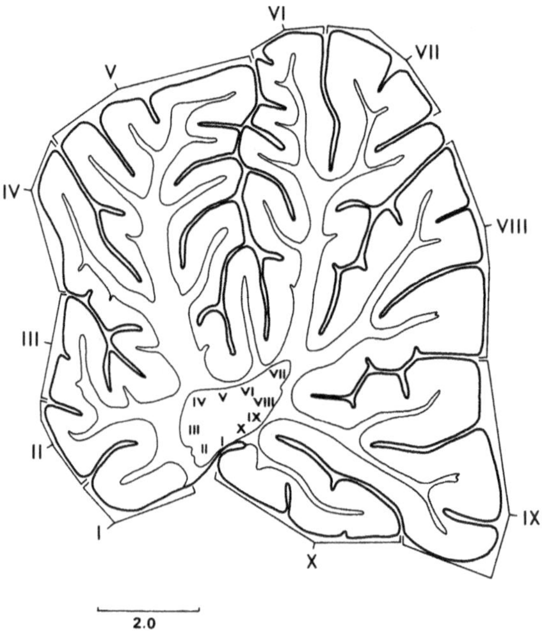

Fig. 19. Tracing of the cerebellum of *Galago* in parasagittal plane through the largest extent of NM. This illustration shows the topographical representation of the various lobules of vermal cortex in NM in a circumferential manner from rostroventral to caudoventral. This plan for *Galago* is essentially similar to that for rat, cat, and other primates. Abbreviations see p. 321–322

conspicuously avoided more rostromedial regions of the nucleus. Two lesions in the C_1 zone of lobule V precipitated degeneration primarily in the rostral and medial NIA. From a lesion in caudal lobule V-C_1 degenerated axons entered the NIA and formed a somewhat oblique terminal field that extended from medial aspects of the nucleus to its rostrocentral area (Fig. 20). This left a conspicuous hole in the rostromedial pole of the NIA which was largely filled by debris subsequent to a lesion in the rostral C_1 zone of lobule V (Fig. 20). Subsequent to damage in the C_1 zone of lobule IV, preterminals were found in a rostrocaudally oriented band in the medial NIA (Fig. 20) in a terminal field which avoided the most medial portions of the nucleus. If all four of these terminal areas are superimposed (Fig. 20, lower left) it is apparent that all are located in the medial NIA, each partially overlaps with the field from the adjacent lobule and each appears to have a portion of the terminal field exclusively to itself.

These examples from zones A and C_1 illustrate the point that each lobule of each zone projects in a topographic manner into its respective portion of the deep cerebellar nuclei. In general terms those zones related to the NM and NL (A, D_1, and D_2) project into their nuclei in a relatively orderly manner (Fig. 19 for NM), while the intermediate cortex (C_1–C_3) is related to the NIA and NIP in a somewhat irregular manner (Fig. 20 for NIA).

Frequent reference has been made to potential species-specific differences in the corticonuclear system. Although the data is somewhat fragmentary there is a clear indication that the location and size of terminal fields arising from homologous lobules may vary from one species to another. We illustrate, as one example, the position and size of the terminal field in the NM subsequent to lesions in lobule V for four different species (Fig. 21). Two features are ap-

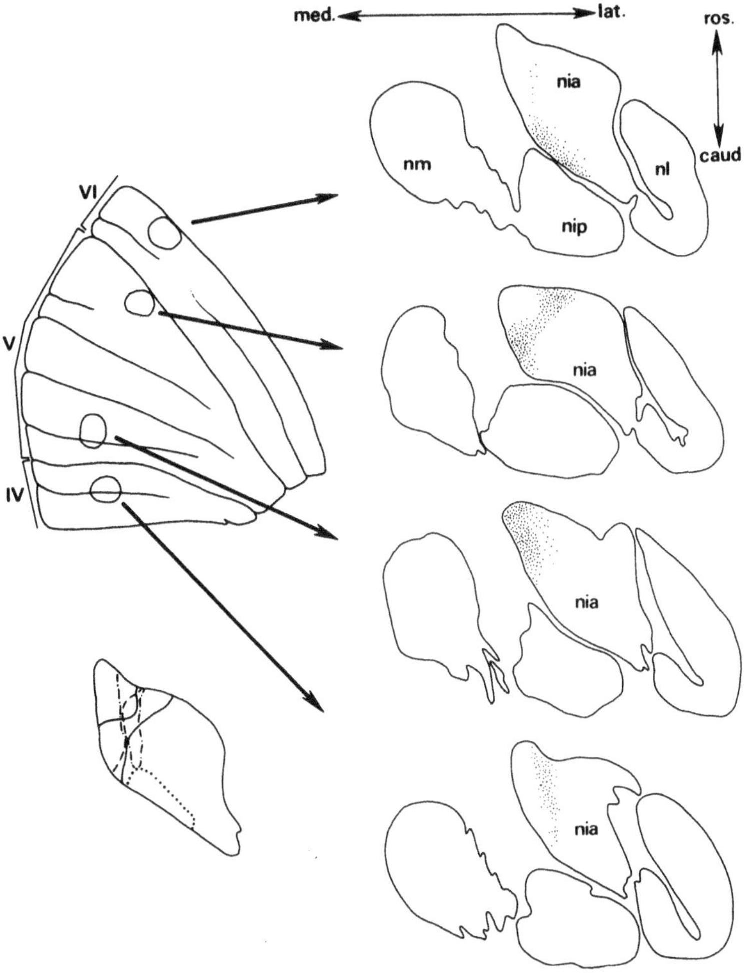

Fig. 20. Tracings in horizontal plane of the cerebellar nuclei of *Saimiri* showing the distribution of degeneration in medial *nia* following lesions in the C_1 zone of lobules IV, V, and VI. Each tracing was made at about the same midhorizontal level. Terminal fields in each case occupy a particular area of medial *nia*, however, when overlapped (*lower left*) each field appears to partially coexist with other fields as well as have some portions of the nucleus to itself. Abbreviations see p. 321–322

parent. First, the terminal field is proportionately larger, compared to the overall size of the nucleus, for the lower species (opossum, rat) and becomes progressively smaller in more advanced forms (bushbaby, squirrel monkey). Second, the position of the terminal field in the NM for lobule V shifts as one progresses from lower to higher forms (Fig. 21). In the opossum, not only is the field larger but it is located in more caudal and ventral regions of the NM, while in the rat the field is slightly smaller and has shifted to a more rostral position. Both the relative decrease in size of the terminal field and its progressive shift to slightly more rostral positions in the NM is further accentuated in the bushbaby and squirrel monkey (Fig. 21).

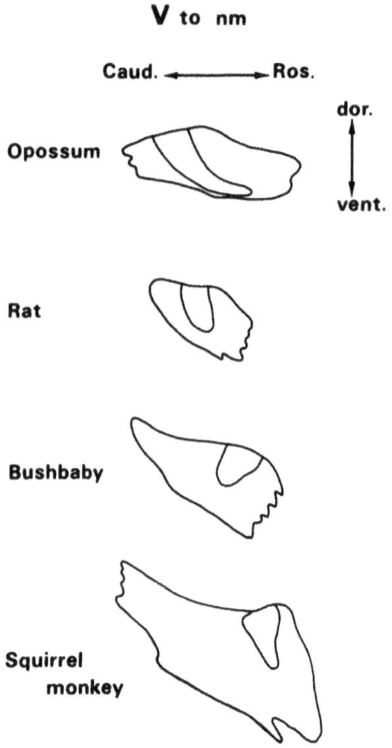

Fig. 21. Tracings in parasagittal plane of *nm* from opossum, albino rat, bushbaby, and squirrel monkey to show the proportionate size and relative position of the terminal field in *nm* following damage to lobule V. Each nucleus was traced at a level through its greatest rostrocaudal and dorsoventral extent and all were traced at the same magnification. Note that as one proceeds from opossum to squirrel monkey the terminal field (a) shifts to a more rostral location, and (b) becomes proportionately smaller relative to the overall size of the nucleus. Additional points are made in the text. Abbreviations see p. 321–322

A Comment on Phylogeny

The comparative observations in our laboratory suggest the following hypothetical model concerning the phylogenetic development of complex corticonuclear fiber systems. This model is illustrated in the parasagittal plane (Fig. 22) for the anterior lobe vermis only, however, its general features are applicable to all regions of cerebellar cortex.

In a hypothetical primitive mammal (Fig. 22A), the cerebellar cortex may have contained interdigitated populations of Purkinje cells, the somata of each population projecting to a particular region of its respective deep nucleus (NM in the example). However, as cells related to one terminal region of the nucleus may have been intermingled with cells projecting to other terminal areas, damage to a specific spot on this hypothetical cortex would produce a large terminal field. Consequently, lesions placed at two spatially separate points on the cortex of this hypothetical form (Fig. 22A, block arrows) would produce degeneration in apparently one large terminal field. This widespread degeneration may actually represent the extensive overlap of several terminal fields.

As the cerebellar cortex became more complex, it expanded in both mediolateral and rostrocaudal directions. In doing so the interdigitated population of Purkinje cells of the hypothetical model would be stretched out as the folial pattern became progressively more complex (Fig. 22B). As this took place populations of like Purkinje cells, that is cells projecting to a common portion of a

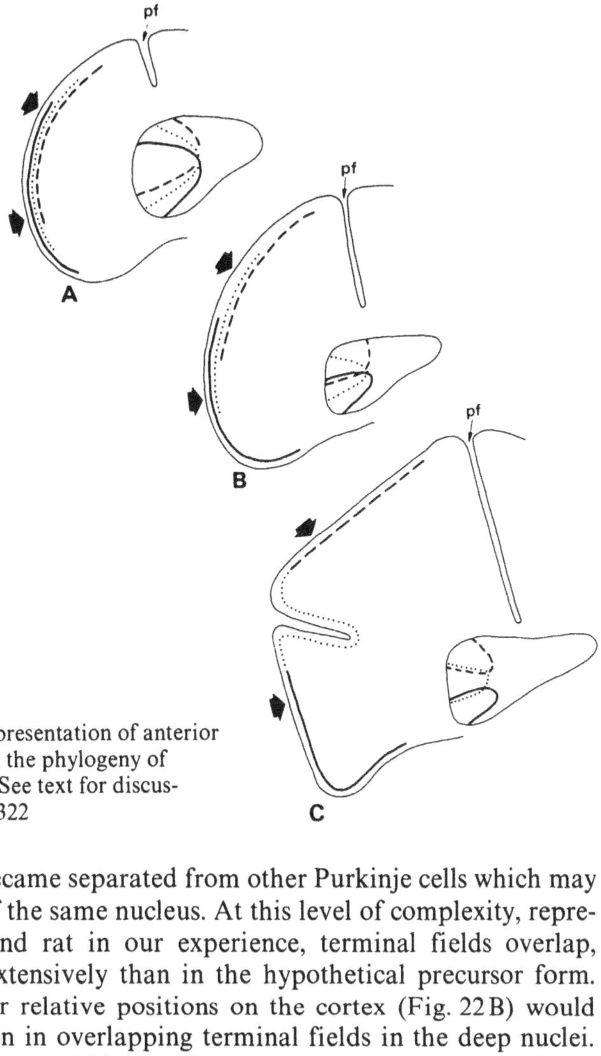

Fig. 22 A–C. Diagrammatic representation of anterior lobe vermis and NM illustrating the phylogeny of the corticonuclear fiber system. See text for discussion. Abbreviations see p. 321–322

particular deep nucleus, became separated from other Purkinje cells which may project to adjacent parts of the same nucleus. At this level of complexity, represented by the opossum and rat in our experience, terminal fields overlap, although somewhat less extensively than in the hypothetical precursor form. Cortical damage at similar relative positions on the cortex (Fig. 22B) would again produce degeneration in overlapping terminal fields in the deep nuclei. However, the terminal zones would be smaller, proportionate to the overall size of the nucleus, and they would overlap less with fields from a more distant point on the cortex (Fig. 22B). It could be said that the expanding population of Purkinje cells are precipitating a concurrent separation of their respective terminal fields in the deep nuclei.

At a higher level of cerebellar development, exemplified by the primates in our studies, the increasing size and complexity of the folia has produced further separation of populations of like Purkinje cells and a parallel separation of their respective terminal fields in the deep nuclei (Fig. 22C). Consequently, in higher forms one finds a population of Purkinje cells which project to a relatively specific area. All cells in this population may not only be terminating in similar regions but they may be responsible for the regulation of more specific tasks. For example, Purkinje cells in zone A of lobule IV by the very nature of their trajectory are undoubtedly modifying different pieces of information than are Purkinje cells in zones C_2 or D_1 of the same lobule. Lesions placed in the cortex in positions similar to those shown in the two previous examples (Fig. 22C, block arrows) now produce preterminal degeneration in smaller terminal fields that are spatially separated by an intervening field which receives input from the undisturbed cortex (Fig. 22). Consequently in higher forms there is the potential circuitry for a more precise and sophisticated relationship between the cortex and the deep nuclei than seen in some lower forms. This would suggest that a given population of Purkinje cells in higher forms may be responsible for the regulation of a specific motor task, or more probably, only a segment of that task. The interdigitated population of Purkinje cells in lower forms may regulate a set or group of motor tasks or perhaps, at best, be responsible for a single complete motor movement.

In recent years we have learned a great deal concerning the organization of corticonuclear fibers. However, no matter how seemingly significant the progress, one is reminded of an old proverb which says "The hurrier I go the behinder I get". Even though some of the complexities of this system have been unraveled numerous new questions have arisen. While the general concepts of zones and topography seem to be clearly established there is little data available concerning the specific functional characteristics of these two interrelated patterns. Are there corticonuclear correlates of the so-called microzones described by Oscarsson [67, 68]? What is the significance of the differences seen in these systems between mammalian forms with markedly different locomotor capabilities? What structural/functional correlates exist between cortical afferent zones (e.g., olivocerebellar, cuneocerebellar) and the efferent corticonuclear zones? It is anticipated that with the fundamental knowledge now available future studies will provide better insight into the organization of this system.

References

1. Achenbach KE, Goodman DC (1968) Cerebellar projections to pons, medulla and spinal cord in the albino rat. Brain Behav Evol 1:43–57
2. Allen WF (1924) Distribution of the fibers originating from the different basal cerebellar nuclei. J Comp Neurol 36:399–439
3. Angaut P, Brodal A (1967) The projection of the "vestibulocerebellum" onto the vestibular nuclei in the cat.E Arch Ital Biol 105:441–479
4. Armstrong DM, Schild RF (1978a) An investigation of the cerebellar cortico-nuclear projections in the rat using an autoradiographic tracing method. I. Projections from the vermis. Brain Res 141:1–19
5. Armstrong DM, Schild RF (1978b) An investigation of the cerebellar corticonuclear projections in the rat using an autoradiographic tracing method. II. Projections from the hemisphere. Brain Res 141:235–249
6. Beitz AJ (1981) Structural organization of the fastigial nucleus. In: Palay SL, Chan-Palay V (eds) The cerebellum: new vistas. Springer, Berlin Heidelberg New York, pp 233–249
7. Bender L (1932) Corticofugal and association fibers arising from the cortex of the vermis of the cerebellum. Arch Neurol Psychiatr 28:1–25
8. Bishop GA (1977) The organization of the projection from the cerebellar cortex to the nucleus interpositus of the cerebellum of the cat. Dissertation, Wayne State University
9. Bishop GA, McCrea RA, Lighthall JW, Kitai ST (1979) An HRP and autoradiographic study of the projection from the cerebellar cortex to the nucleus interpositus anterior and nucleus interpositus posterior of the cat. J Comp Neurol 185:735–756

10. Brodal A, Courville J (1973) Cerebellar corticonuclear projection in the cat. Crus II. An experimental study with silver methods. Brain Res 50:1–23
11. Chambers WW, Sprague JM (1955a) Functional localization in the cerebellum. I. Organization in longitudinal cortico-nuclear zones and their contribution to the control of posture, both pyramidal and extrapyramidal. J Comp Neurol 103:105–129
12. Chambers WW, Sprague JM (1955b) Functional localization in the cerebellum. II. Somatotopic organization in cortex and nuclei. Arch Neurol Psychiatr 74:653–680
13. Clarke RH, Horsley V (1905) On the intrinsic fibers of the cerebellum, its nuclei and its efferent tract. Brain 28:13–29
14. Courville J, Cooper CW (1970) The cerebellar nuclei of *Macaca mulatta:* a morphological study. J Comp Neurol 140:241–254
15. Courville J, Diakiw N (1976) Cerebellar corticonuclear projection in the cat. The vermis of the anterior and posterior lobes. Brain Res 110:1–20
16. Courville J, Faraco-Cantin F (1976) Cerebellar corticonuclear projection demonstrated by the horseradish peroxidase method. Neurosci Abstr 2:108
17. Courville J, Diakiw N, Brodal A (1973) Cerebellar corticonuclear projections in the cat. The paramedian lobule. An experimental study with silver methods. Brain Res 50:25–45
18. Dietrichs E, Walberg F (1979) The cerebellar corticonuclear and nucleocortical projections in the cat as studied with anterograde and retrograde transport of horseradish peroxidase. I. The paramedian lobule. Anat Embryol (Berl) 158:13–39
19. Dow RS (1936) The fiber connections of the posterior parts of the cerebellum in the rat and cat. J Comp Neurol 63:527–548
20. Dow RS (1938) Efferent connections of the flocculonodular lobe in *Macaca mulatta*. J Comp Neurol 68:297–305
21. Eager RP (1963) Efferent corticonuclear pathways in the cerebellum of the cat. J Comp Neurol 120:81–104
22. Eager RP (1966) Patterns and mode of termination of cerebellar corticonuclear pathways in the monkey (*Macaca mulatta*). J Comp Neurol 126:551–566
23. Eager RP (1967) Cerebellar projections to the vestibular nuclei. In: Third Symposium on the role of the vestibular organs in space explorations. NASA SP 152, Pensacola, pp 225–237
24. Eager RP (1969) Modes of termination of Purkinje cell axons in the cerebellum of the cat. In: Llinás R (ed) Neurobiology of cerebellar evolution and development. AMA-ERF Chicago, p 585
25. Fink RP, Heimer L (1967) Two methods for selective silver impregnation of degenerating axons and their synaptic endings in the central nervous system. Brain Res 4:369–374
26. Goodman DC, Simpson JT Jr (1960) Cerebellar stimulation in the unrestrained and unanesthetized alligator. J Comp Neurol 114:127–135
27. Goodman DC, Simpson JT Jr. (1961) Functional localization in the cerebellum of the albino rat. Exp Neurol 3:174–188
28. Goodman DC, Hallett RE, Welch RB (1963) Patterns of localization in the cerebellar cortico-nuclear projections of the albino rat. J Comp Neurol 121:51–67
29. Goodman DC, Horel JA, Freemon FR (1964) Functional localization in the cerebellum of the bird and its bearing on the evolution of cerebellar function. J Comp Neurol 123:45–54
30. Gould BB (1977) The cerebellum of the cat: a study of intrinsic and extrinsic circuitry with neuroanatomical tracer techniques. Dissertation, Massachusetts Institute of Technology
31. Gould BB (1979) The organization of afferents to the cerebellar cortex in the cat: projections from the deep cerebellar nuclei. J Comp Neurol 184:27–42
32. Haines DE (1969) The cerebellum of *Galago* and *Tupaia*. I. Corpus cerebelli and flocculonodular lobe. Brain Behav Evol 2:377–414
33. Haines DE (1971) The morphology of the cerebellar nuclei of *Galago* and *Tupaia*. Am J Phys Anthropol 35:27–42
34. Haines DE (1974) The cerebellum of some lorisidae. In: Martin RD, Doyle GA, Walker AC (eds) Prosimian biology. Duckworth, London, p 725
35. Haines DE (1975a) Cerebellar corticovestibular fibers of the posterior lobe in a prosimian primate, the lesser bushbaby (*Galago senegalensis*). J Comp Neurol 160:363–398

36. Haines DE (1975b) Cerebellar cortical efferents of the posterior lobe vermis in a prosimian primate (*Galago*) and the tree shrew (*Tupaia*). J Comp Neurol 163:21–40
37. Haines DE (1976) Cerebellar corticonuclear and corticovestibular fibers of the anterior lobe vermis in a prosimian primate (*Galago senegalensis*). J Comp Neurol 170:67–95
38. Haines DE (1977) Cerebellar corticonuclear and corticovestibular fibers of the flocculonodular lobe in a prosimian primate (*Galago senegalensis*). J Comp Neurol 174:607–630
39. Haines DE, Culberson JL (1974) Cerebellar corticonuclear projections of the posterior lobe in *Galago* and *Tupaia* (Abstr). Anat Rec 178:368
40. Haines DE, Koletar SL (1979) Topography of cerebellar corticonuclear fibers of the albino rat. Vermis of anterior and posterior lobes. Brain Behav Evol 16:271–292
41. Haines DE, Patrick GW (1980) Cerebellar corticonuclear fibers of the paramedian lobule in the tree shrew, *Tupaia glis*. Anat Rec 196:70 A
42. Haines DE, Patrick GW (to be published) Cerebellar corticonuclear fibers of the paramedian lobule of tree shrew (*Tupaia glis*) with a comment on zones
43. Haines DE, Patrick GW (to be published) The cerebellum of squirrel monkey (*Saimiri sciureus*). II. Corticonuclear fibers of the dorsal culminate lobule (anterior lobe – lobule V)
44. Haines DE, Rubertone JA (1977) Cerebellar corticonuclear fibers: evidence of zones in the primate anterior lobe. Neurosci Lett 6:231–236
45. Haines DE, Rubertone JA (1979) Cerebellar corticonuclear fibers of the dorsal culminate lobule (anterior lobe – lobule V) in a prosimian primate, *Galago senegalensis*. J Comp Neurol 186:321–342
46. Haines DE, Whitworth RH (1978) Cerebellar cortical efferent fibers of the paraflocculus of tree shrew (*Tupaia glis*). J Comp Neurol 182:137–150
47. Haines DE, Culberson JL, Martin GF (1976) Laterality and topography of cerebellar cortical efferents in the opossum (*Didelphis marsupialis virginiana*). Brain Res 106:152–158
48. Henkel CK (1975) The vestibular complex of the American opossum, *Didelphis virginiana* I. Conformation, cytoarchitecture, and primary vestibular afferent distribution. II. Afferent and efferent connections. Dissertation, Ohio State University
49. Henkel CK, Martin GF (1977) The vestibular complex of the American opossum *Didelphis virginiana*. II. Afferent and efferent connections. J Comp Neurol 172:321–348
50. Hohman LB (1929) The efferent connections of the cerebellar cortex; investigations based upon experimental extirpations in the cat. Res Publ Assoc Res Nerv Ment Dis 6:445–460
51. Jansen J, Brodal A (1940) Experimental studies on the intrinsic fibers of the cerebellum. II. The cortico-nuclear projection. J Comp Neurol 73:267–321
52. Jansen J, Brodal A (1942) Experimental studies on the intrinsic fibers of the cerebellum. The corticonuclear projection in the rabbit and the monkey (*Macaca rhesus*). Skr Norske Vidensk, Akad I Math Nat Kl, vol 11, 3:1–50
53. Klimoff J (1897) On the conduction paths of the cerebellum. Experimental-anatomical observations (in Russian). Dissertation, Imperial University of Kazan
54. Klimoff J (1899) Ueber die Leitungsbahnen des Kleinhirns. Arch Anat Physiol Anat Abth:11–27
55. Korneliussen HK (1968a) On the morphology and subdivision of the cerebellar nuclei of the rat. J Hirnforsch 10:109–122
56. Korneliussen HK (1968b) On the ontogenetic development of the cerebellum (nuclei, fissures, and cortex) of the rat, with special reference to regional variations in corticogenesis. J Hirnforsch 10:379–412
57. Korneliussen HK (1969) Cerebellar organization in the light of cerebellar nuclear morphology and cerebellar corticogenesis. In: Llinás R (ed) Neurobiology of cerebellar evolution and development. American Medical Association, Chicago, p 515
58. Korneliussen HK (1972) Histogenesis of the cerebellar cortex and cortical zones. In: Larsell O, Jansen J (eds) The comparative anatomy and histology of the cerebellum: the human cerebellum, cerebellar connections, and cerebellar cortex. University of Minnesota Press, Minneapolis, p 164
59. Larsell O (1935) The development and morphology of the cerebellum in the opossum. Part I. Early development. J Comp Neurol 63:65–94

60. Larsell O (1936) The development and morphology of the cerebellum in the opossum. Part II. Later development and adult. J Comp Neurol 64:275–302
61. Larsell O (1970) The comparative anatomy and histology of the cerebellum from monotremes through apes. Jansen, J (ed). University of Minnesota Press, Minneapolis
62. Martin GF, King JS, Dom R (1974) The projections of the deep cerebellar nuclei of the opossum, *Didelphis marsupialis virginiana*. J Hirnforsch 15:545–573
63. Martin GF, Bishop GA, Culberson JL, King JS, Laxson C, Linauts M, Panneton M (1981) Spino-olivocerebellar circuits in the North American opossum with notes on their development. In: Palay SL, Chan-Palay V (eds) The cerebellum – New vistas. Springer, Berlin Heidelberg New York, pp 162–188
64. Oscarsson O (1968) Termination and functional organization of the ventral spino-olivocerebellar path. J Physiol 196:453–478
65. Oscarsson O (1969) Termination and functional organization of the dorsal spino-olivocerebellar path. J Physiol 200:129–149
66. Oscarsson O (1969) The sagittal organization of the cerebellar anterior lobe as revealed by the projection patterns of the climbing fiber system. In: Llinás R (ed) Neurobiology of cerebellar evolution and development. AMA-ERF, Chicago, p 525
67. Oscarsson O (1979) Functional units of the cerebellum – sagittal zones and microzones. Trends Neurosci 7:143–145
68. Oscarsson O (1980) Functional organization of olivary projection to cerebellar anterior lobe. In: Courville J, de Montigny C, Lamarre Y (eds) The inferior olivary nucleus, anatomy and physiology. Raven, New York
69. Patrick GW, Haines DE (to be published) The cerebellum of squirrel monkey (*Saimiri sciureus*). I. Configuration of the cerebellar nuclei
70. Satrulee P (1980) Cerebellar corticonuclear fibers of the anterior lobe vermis in the North American opossum. Anat Rec 196:166A
71. Satrulee P, Haines DE, Culberson JL (to be published) The organization of cerebellar cortical efferent fibers in North American opossum (*Didelphis virginiana*): I. Laterality and topography of corticonuclear projections from anterior vermis
72. Scott TS (1964) A unique pattern of localization within the cerebellum of the mouse. J Comp Neurol 122:1–7
73. Senn D, Goodman DC (1969) Patterns of localization in the cerebellar corticofugal projections of the alligator (*Caimen sclerops*). In: Llinás R (ed) Neurobiology of cerebellar evolution and development. AMA-ERF, Chicago, p 475
74. Sreesai M (1974) Cerebellar cortical projections of the opossum (*Didelphis marsupialis virginiana*). J Hirnforsch 15:529–544
75. Vachananda B (1959) The major spinal afferent systems to the cerebellum and the cerebellar corticonuclear connections in *Macaca mulatta*. J Comp Neurol 112:303–352
76. van Rossum J (1969) Cortionuclear and corticovestibular projections of the cerebellum. An experimental investigation of the anterior lobe, the simple lobule and the caudal vermis in the rabbit. Dissertation, University of Leiden
77. Voogd J (1964) The cerebellum of the cat. Structure and fibre connexions. Dissertation, University of Leiden
78. Voogd J (1969) The importance of fiber connections in the comparative anatomy of the mammalian cerebellum. In: Llinás R (ed) Neurobiology of cerebellar evolution and development. AMA-ERF, Chicago, p 493
79. Voogd J, Bigaré F (1980) The topographical distribution of olivary and corticonuclear fibers in the cerebellum. A review. In: Courville J, de Montigny C, Lamarre Y (eds) The inferior olivary nucleus, anatomy and physiology. Raven, New York
80. Walberg F, Brodal A (1979) The longitudinal zonal pattern in the paramedian lobule of the cat's cerebellum: an analysis based on a correlation of recent HRP data with results of studies with other methods. J Comp Neurol 187:581–588
81. Walberg F, Jansen J (1961) Cerebellar corticovestibular fibers in the cat. Exp Neurol 3:32–52
82. Walberg F, Jansen J (1964) Cerebellar corticonuclear projection studied experimentally with silver impregnation methods. J Hirnforsch 6:338–354

Discussion

Voogd: When you started these studies I was very glad because at the time no one believed that these zones existed. So you are actually one of the first to provide experimental evidence showing that these cortical zones are really as I described them. Concerning the B zone, which is supposed to project to Deiters nucleus, you mentioned that you also found projections to posterior interposed nucleus. That's interesting, because by injecting HRP into the central nuclei, we found something very similar. When you inject HRP in the junctional region of the fastigial and posterior interposed nuclei, rather caudally, you get filled somata located in what may be the B zone, or perhaps the X zone, I'm not quite sure.

Haines: Yes, as you know that particular projection troubled me a great deal. We repeated the lesion several times and there was a consistent projection from this area of cortex to the posterior interposed nucleus.

Voogd: There may be a relationship between this B zone and the C_2 zone which also projects to the posterior interposed nucleus. In 1964 [2] when I described this zonal system I called this C_2 zone the B′ zone indicating that they could be continuous. From monkey material studied in my laboratory we got the impression that the development of the B and C_2 zones differs from the A, C_1, C_3, and D zones. Initially the Purkinje cell neuroblasts of the future B and C_2 zones form a continuous mass deep in the A, C_1, C_3, and D zones. Subsequently, these Purkinje cell neuroblasts reach their definitive position by penetrating between the superficially located A, C_1, and C_3 zones.

Llinás: Let me ask you, or perhaps Dr. Voogd, a general question, which I think is of interest to physiologists as well as anatomists. You have, grossly, a very beautiful relation in space between the projection of Purkinje cells into the nuclei, with probably a similar kind of orientation of climbing fibers. I wonder if this very strict relationship can be related to the way these things are set down during growth itself and, in addition, I'd like to ask why, this being the case, is there such discrepancy between the ways in which the mossy fibers come in as opposed to climbing fibers and axons of the Purkinje cells.

Voogd: Embryologically it's logical. You have Purkinje cells which develop in a layer which is subdivided into clusters. An embryological cerebellum is very short rostrocaudally. In due time it lengthens from say part of a millimeter to a meter in length and the cells of the clusters are then in a monolayer. The clusters of Purkinje cell neuroblasts which are destined for the cerebellar cortex are embryologically related to certain central nuclei. Then, it's rather simple that these things get interconnected, and when olivary fibers come in they find these Purkinje cells located in clusters related to zones. I thing that's the way the system comes about.

Altman: If you look at the embryonic cerebellum you can see that Purkinje cells form clusters. We have seen it in the rat, and R. Voogd has observed it in the monkey. In the neuroepithelium from which these cells arise you do not see clustering. It is conceivable that this clustering is due to the fact that Purkinje cells first have to migrate through these nuclear zones which are already clustered at an early stage, and it is here that they become separated. In other words, they start off together, then as they migrate through different nuclei they get separated and form these clusters.

Chan-Palay: Let me try and schematize this for you. I think this discussion of corticonuclear-nucleocortical interrelationships has gotten rather complex. It seems to me that we could put all of this together in the following way (Fig. 1). Let's take the dentate nucleus as an example. There exists a peculiar arrangement of cells in which large cells particularly are oriented in columns and other cells, which I thought were interneurons, are oriented perpendicularly to the columns. As corticonuclear projections come in they may very well define a sort of band. In Golgi preparations I have studied the projections of axons of single Purkinje cells. The axon runs along the outside of the nucleus, gives off a branch that enters the nucleus, and may continue further to serve another portion of the nucleus. These are portions of the columns of nuclear neurons. In fact, if a single lesion is made, as Dr. Haines has done, you can get two separate bands of degeneration in the nucleus. Adjacent Purkinje cells would have a similar pattern of projection on the dentate nucleus. The nucleocortical projection is superimposed on this pattern in a larger, less strictly rigid topographic band. A nucleocortical cell serves the broadly defined cortical region from which it receives afferents by giving off mossy fibers which terminate somewhat diffusely in this cortical area. External inputs to the cerebellum also appear to have very precise patterns of termination within the cerebellar cortex and deep nuclei which may be related to these bands. Climbing fibers, for example, give off single fibers in the nuclei that look very much like the terminal fields in the cortex (although they do not terminate exclusively on single neurons here), then continue upward into the same presumed sagittal band, and give off a climbing fiber to the appropriate Purkinje cell within that band. The climbing-fiber afferent system is quite precisely organized in the cortex but slightly less so in the nuclei.

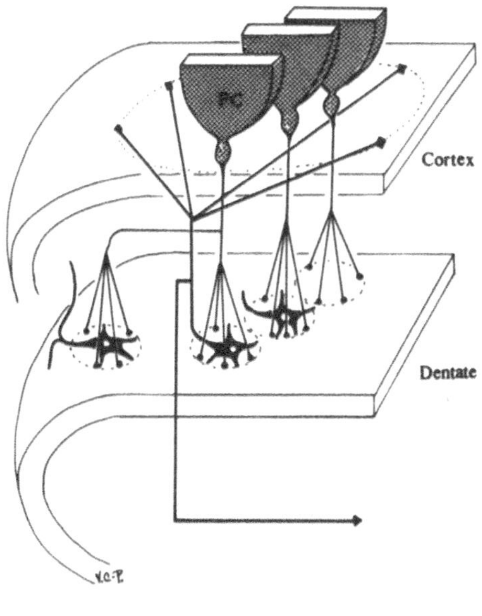

Fig. 1. Comparison of the axonal fields of Purkinje cells and dentate nuclear neurons. The Purkinje cells (*PC*) of the cerebellar cortex project single or multiple conical axon fields upon dentate neurons. Dentatocortical fibers, which are often collaterals of extracerebellar projection axons, have extensive terminal fields in the overlying cortex. Though basically reciprocating the nucleocortical projection, the dentatocortical loop is more diffuse. [From Chan-Palay V (1977) Cerebellar dentate nucleus. Organization, cytology and transmitters. Springer, Berlin Heidelberg New York, p. 359]

Llinás: You are then saying that the climbing fiber is better at recognizing the path of the axon of the Purkinje cell than is the mossy fiber.
Chan-Palay: No, and there is some indication for this, for example, in the pigeon. Visual input from the tectum goes to the pigeon cerebellum in a regulated fashion so that mossy fibers in the granular layer are actually in strata.
Llinás: My question is related to the gross distribution of fibers in the white matter. The feeling that one has, for instance in doing in vitro studies, is that if you can get at the axon of a Purkinje cell you can often get at the climbing fiber that goes to that Purkinje cell, but seldom to the mossy fiber that goes to that Purkinje cell.
Chan-Palay: The problem with mossy fibers is that you would have a *zone* of termination. You would never get a single one-to-one relationship such as you find with climbing fibers. The point here is that there are regions of the cerebellar nuclei that are very strictly related to the overlying cortex in this banded arrangement in terms of corticonuclear and nucleocortical connections as well as the pattern of termination of extracerebellar afferents.
Snider: Did you see any projection that went to the contralateral nuclei so far as you could tell, either directly or by way of collaterals?
Haines: You mean a corticonuclear projection that crossed the midline? No. If the lesions impinged directly on the midline, you would see bilateral corticonuclear projections but we've seen no corticonuclear projections that cross the midline from clear homolateral lesions. I think there may be an interdigitation of these zones. If one assumes that the B and A zone cells interdigitate to a certain degree it would be fairly easy to see that the two A zones may also have an irregular strip along the midline where they interdigitate. This may vary from one lobule to the next. As a whole, however, the corticonuclear system is ipsilateral, at least in the mammals we have examined.
Marshall: If we looked at the scheme of different Purkinje cells with different projections intermixed within a given cortical region, could this equally be explained as Dr. Chan-Palay suggested, by axon collaterals of the same Purkinje cell going to the two different regions?
Haines: Yes, this is possible. The A model in my drawing was purely hypothetical. But if you look at all of the animals we've studied, there are certain consistencies in the relative sizes of terminal fields. In lower forms, using the rat and opossum as representatives, the terminal fields are always bigger, and if you make lesions in individual lobules the terminal fields always appear to overlap more. In my hypothetical models, as the cortex enlarges (becomes more convoluted and complex) there is a concurrent separation and decrease in proportionate size of the respective terminal fields in the associated deep nuclei. But, yes, you're correct. It could be collaterals.
Brodal: Just a comment on the same point. I got the impression that there was evidence of divergence of corticonuclear connections in the monkey. Some of your lesions appeared to produce very small patches of degeneration in different parts of the nuclei. Being rather obsessed with the divergence present whithin the cerebropontocerebellar pathway, it seems interesting that such divergence may exist in the corticonuclear connections as well as in connections from the nuclei to the thalamus, and from the thalamus to the motor cortex.

Haines: Since there are obvious differences when you go from one species to another in the corticonuclear system, I think you may have a difference in the nucleocortical system. There are some cases, for example, where a particular strip of the cortex will have a sort of mosaic representation in its respective nucleus and the adjacent strip will have perhaps just columns, so I think the pattern may change from one zone to the next. It's not a very simple pattern.
Snider: There's a fair amount of electrical evidence to show that there may be dentate-to-dentate connections. Does anybody want to comment on that?
Chan-Palay: We looked but without success even though the experiments were relatively simple because one can inject with HRP or proline or leucine on one side and look on the other.
Snider: And you haven't found fastigial-to-fastigial connections either?
Chan-Palay: Well, fastigial injections are dangerous because the two nuclei are very close, in the midline and spillover of label is a problem.
Martin: Dr. Voogd [2] has reported that there are species differences relative to the distribution of various mossy-fiber projections to the cerebellum and there may be differences relative to his subcortical zones as well. My question is related to zones A–D in the opossum. Is there some question as to the existence of zone D in the opossum?
Haines: In anterior lobe, yes. We have at this time no *direct* corticonuclear evidence for a D zone in the opossum anterior lobe.
Martin: I would like to ask Dr. Voogd if it is fair to use the existence of projections from the principal olive as a means of defining zone D.
Voogd: Yes, it would be correct.
Martin: If that's true, zone D is present in the lateral extreme of the anterior lobe in the opossum [1]. One other comment, with respect to the clear laterality and the lack of diffuseness that you showed in the corticonuclear projection. It is because Dr. Haines has looked for small areas of vascular compromise and recognized them as such that he's been able to do such a clean dissection of these connections.
Haines: I made no comment on materials and methods, but in all of our cases we serial-section every brain and, in most cases, stain and look at every section. Consequently, we can find little mistakes. We are working with fairly small cerebella that lend themselves well to serial study.

References

1. Linauts M, Martin GF (1978) The organization of olivocerebellar projections in the opossum, *Didelphis virginiana*, as revealed by the retrograde transport of horseradish peroxidase. J Comp Neurol 179:355–382
2. Voogd J (1964) The cerebellum of the cat. Med Thesis, University of Leiden

Characteristics of an Isolated Purkinje Cell Fraction *

J. Mallet

Introduction

The nervous system is a highly differentiated system in which the cell patterns and the assembly of synaptic circuits are rigorously organized. Each type of cell is unique in terms of position, synaptic connections, and function. These specificities must be, in part, expressed by means of specific proteins. As a consequence the protein content of an individual class of cells must carry a certain degree of uniqueness.

To study this problem of cell specificity the cerebellum is well suited because of its relative simplicity, the possibility of obtaining a high enrichment of identifiable cells, and the valuable asset of having mutants whose cerebella are altered in a clear cut manner.

We have used two different approaches to search for cell-specific proteins. One is based on the sensitivity of the immune system. Large cells, and therefore mostly Purkinje cells, have been used as antigens. Using an in vitro binding assay and taking advantage of the *Purkinje cell degeneration* (pcd) mouse mutant (which lacks Purkinje cells in the adult state), we have defined a class of antibodies which are directed against antigens specific to the Purkinje cell [1, 2].

A second approach consists of associating the anatomic defect of a given mutant with a defect in its protein pattern. This approach has been used with several cerebellar-mutant mice. We will describe here a protein named P_{400} which is specific for Purkinje cells and which has been identified by making use of Purkinje-cell-defective mutants [3, 4].

Purification of Purkinje Cells

Several methods have been described for the purification of Purkinje cells [5, 6, 7, 8]. We have utilized a method developed by Sellinger et al. [6] in which 12–16-day rat cerebella are homogenized by mincing and sieving through nylon mesh; cells are then fractionated according to their size and shape by centrifugation. A population of large cells devoid of small cells (Fig. 1A) is obtained in about 10% yield. These cells are mostly Purkinje cells but Golgi and

* I am grateful to Drs. J.P. Changeux, A. Privat, and C. Sotelo for their comments on the manuscript

Experimental Brain Research, Suppl. 6

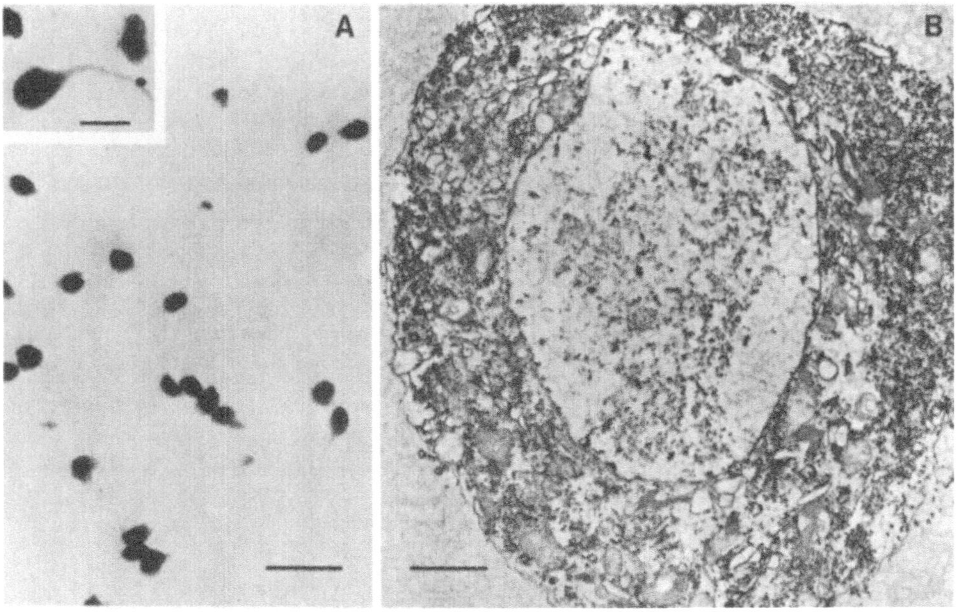

Fig. 1A, B. Purkinje cell fractions purified from rat cerebella used in the biochemical experiments. **A** Purkinje cells after staining by Coomassie brilliant blue. Length of the *bars: main picture,* 50 µm; *insert, 20* µm. **B** thin section of one of the cells in the Purkinje cell fraction. Length of the *bar:* 2 µm

large neurons from the cerebellar deep nuclei might also be present in significant amount.

The homogenization procedure splits axons and dendrites from cells, and the perikarya are not morphologically preserved (Fig. 1 B). However, unlike other methods [8], this one does not include a trypsination step and is therefore expected to preserve surface antigens to a large extent.

Immunological Study of Purkinje Cells

The specificity and the sensitivity of the immune system is well suited to reveal and characterize the antigens, if any, which are specific to a given tissue or cell type. We have analyzed [1, 2] the antibodies raised against a population of Purkinje cells purified as described above. The Purkinje cells account for only a small percentage of the total cell number in the cerebellum. It was thus imperative to immunize with an enriched cell population. Absorption of the sera on various tissues was required to purify cell-specific antibodies. Only $5-10 \times 10^5$ cells were injected in rabbits. Nevertheless, by the Ouchterlony diffusion test, the best serum gave several precipitation lines against cerebellar membranes solubilized by nondenaturing detergents. Quantitative information on the strength and specificity of the anti-Purkinje cell serum was obtained by a direct binding assay. Increasing amounts of cerebellar membranes were added to a

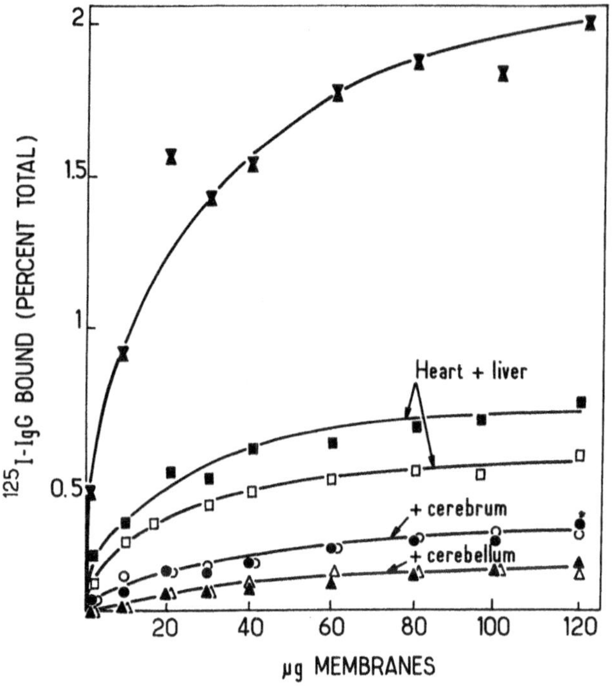

Fig. 2. Binding of ^{125}I-labeled anti-Purkinje cell IgG on rat cerebellar membranes after successive absorptions. Absorptions and binding assays were performed as described [1]. Unabsorbed serum (⧗), serum absorbed once (■) and twice (□) with liver and heart membranes, then once (●) and twice (○) with cerebrum membrane, and finally once (▲) and twice (△) with cerebellum membranes

fixed amount of ^{125}I-labeled IgG. The ^{125}I-labeled IgG which binds to cerebellar membranes was then estimated by Millipore filtration.

This method, combined with absorption experiments, allowed us to test quantitatively the specificity of the IgG with respect to various tissues. About 2% of the antibodies bound to an excess of cerebellar membranes. Of those, 7% were not absorbed by liver, heart, and cerebrum membranes and were specifically directed against cerebellar antigens (Fig. 2).

In order to increase the ratio of specific to nonspecific binding of ^{125}I-labeled IgG, antibodies directed against Purkinje cells were purified by absorption on cerebellar membranes and released at pH 2.9. The released ^{125}I-labeled IgG was then thoroughly absorbed with liver and heart, cerebrum, and cerebellar membranes. The results of these successive absorptions are reported in Fig. 3. After purification about 48% of the total ^{125}I-labeled IgG bound to an excess of cerebellar membranes. Of those, 6.8% were specifically directed against cerebellar antigens. This figure compares well with that obtained from absorption carried out with the total population of IgG. Furthermore, the ratio of specific to nonspecific binding is significantly increased.

The specificity of the anti-Purkinje cell serum toward the Purkinje cell was analyzed by making use of the *pcd* mutant. In the homozygous *pcd*/*pcd* animals

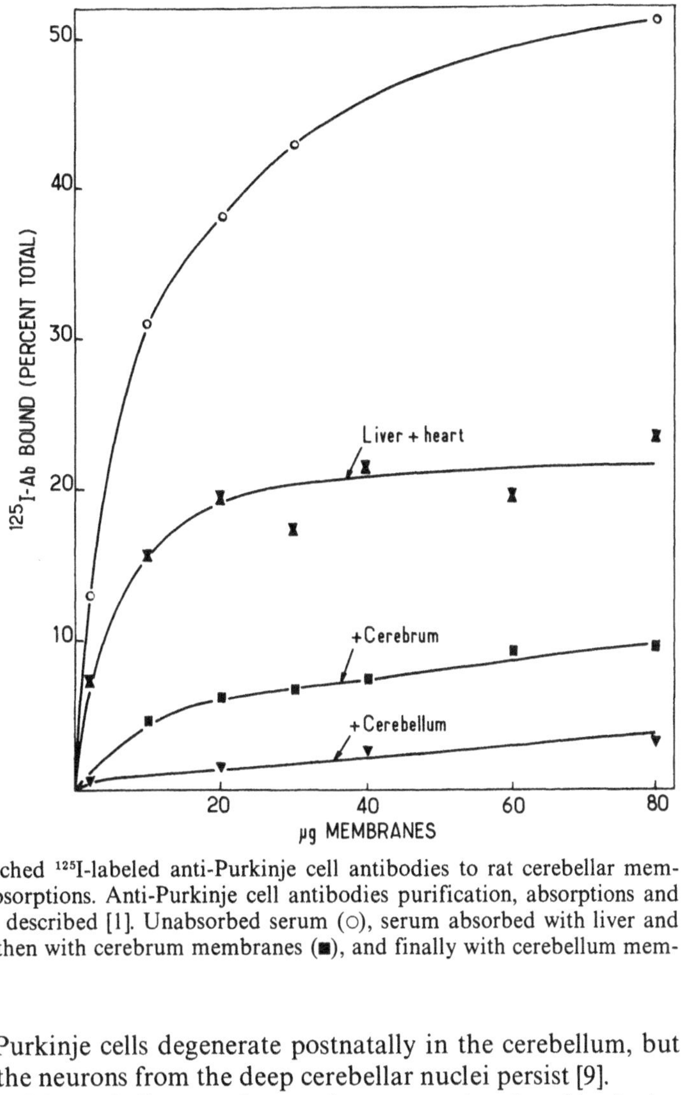

Fig. 3. Binding of enriched ^{125}I-labeled anti-Purkinje cell antibodies to rat cerebellar membranes after various absorptions. Anti-Purkinje cell antibodies purification, absorptions and binding assays were as described [1]. Unabsorbed serum (○), serum absorbed with liver and heart membranes (ẍ), then with cerebrum membranes (■), and finally with cerebellum membranes (▲)

almost 99% of the Purkinje cells degenerate postnatally in the cerebellum, but the Golgi cells and the neurons from the deep cerebellar nuclei persist [9].

The binding curves with cerebellar membranes from normal and *pcd/pcd* mice with unabsorbed and absorbed ^{125}I-labeled anti-Purkinje cell antibodies are compared in Fig. 4. Before absorption (Fig. 4A) a small difference between the two curves was already apparent. After absorption on liver and heart membranes, the difference became more significant. About 17% of the antibodies did not bind to *pcd/pcd* cerebellar membranes (Fig. 2B). Finally, after absorption on cerebrum, this fraction increased up to 75% (Fig. 4C). The binding to *pcd/pcd* cerebellar membranes was nevertheless still significant when compared to the nonspecific binding which was identical with membranes prepared from nomal and mutant cerebella.

The differences observed between *pcd* and normal mouse cerebella unambiguously show that the anti-Purkinje cell serum contains antibodies directed against antigens which are specific to the Purkinje cell. However, about 25% of

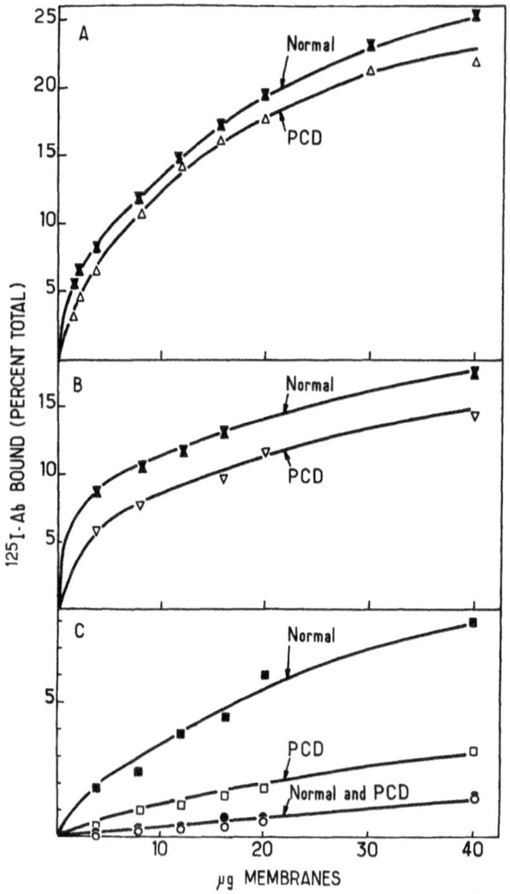

Fig. 4A–C. Comparative binding of enriched ^{125}I-labeled anti-Purkinje cell antibodies to normal and *pcd/pcd* mouse cerebellar membranes. Anti-Purkinje cell antibodies were enriched by selective adsorption and subsequent elution from cerebellar membranes. **A** Unabsorbed antibodies; **B** antibodies were absorbed on heart and liver membranes; **C** antibodies were further absorbed with cerebrum membranes (■ and □) and, finally, in order to determine the nonspecific binding, antibodies were absorbed with cerebellum membranes (● and ○)

the cerebellum-specific antibodies are assumed to correspond to antigens present in other categories of cells in the cerebellum.

Indirect immunofluorescent staining of cerebellar tissue slices confirmed that the cerebrum-absorbed serum contained antibodies directed against the Purkinje cells (Fig. 5). No staining could be detected in the granular layer. However, not surprisingly, analysis of other brain regions revealed that the antiserum also stained large cells in the cerebellar nuclei and brain stem. This finding corroborated and extended the results gained from the comparative binding assays performed with *pcd/pcd* membranes [1].

Interestingly, a further absorption of the serum with brain stem membranes removed the staining not only of the large cells of the brain stem, but also of the deep nuclei while the Purkinje cells were still positive.

The immunohistochemical approach has proved very useful because it allows the site of reaction of the antibody to be localized not only to a particular region of the brain but also to a discrete cell population. However, the specificity of an antibody for a given tissue or cell type cannot be ascertained if only this technique is used. Antigens present in lower amount in some cells than in others may escape detection.

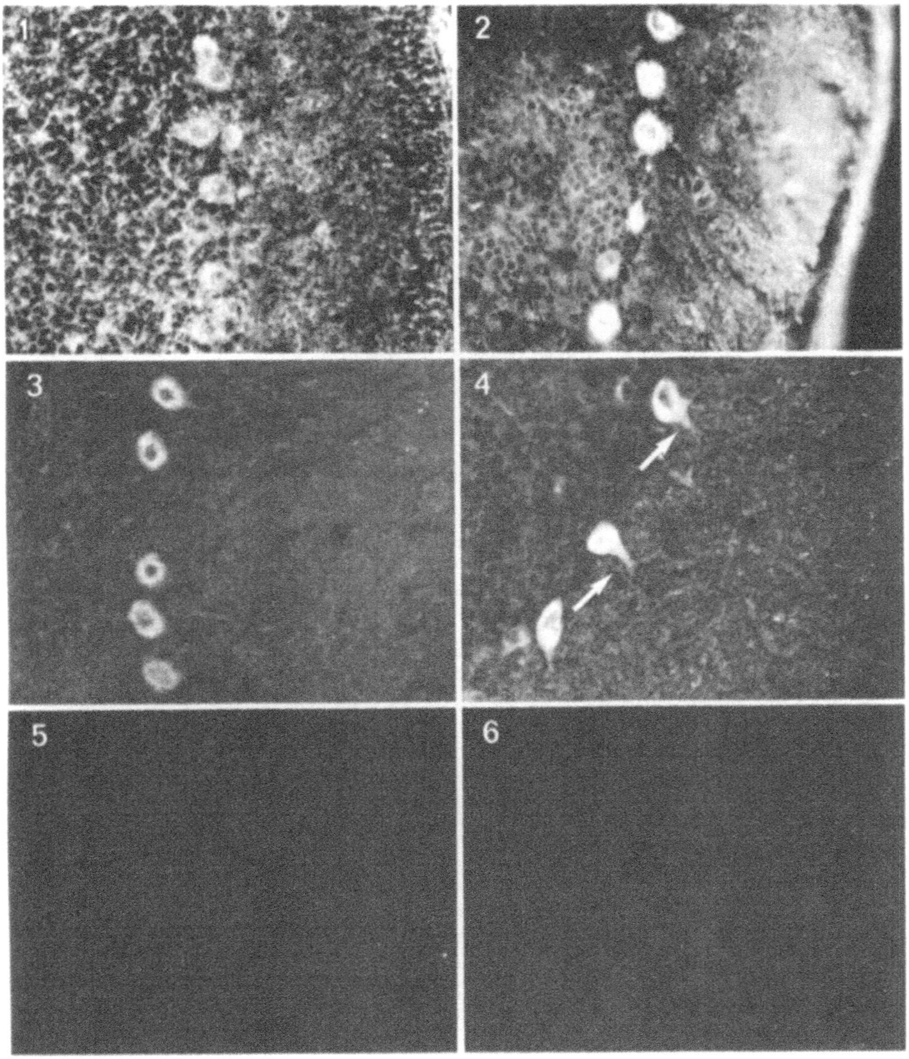

Fig. 5. 1–6. Indirect immunofluorescence staining of transverse sections of 14-day-old rat cerebella. **1** Note the bright fluorescence of the internal granular layer with unabsorbed serum. Progressive absorptions on membranes from heart and liver **2**, forebrain **3**, brain stem **4**, and cerebellum **5**. Purkinje cell dendrites are clearly visible in **4** (*arrows*). Control incubation with preimmune serum is shown in **6**.

The antigens corresponding to the cerebellum and Purkinje-cell-specific antibodies have not yet been identified. The Purkinje-cell-specific antibodies can be of use as cell markers in cultures of explants or dissociated cells [10] and allow one to map the appearance and development of those cells during embryogenesis. The subcellular localization of the cerebellum-specific antigens remains to be established, particularly to see if they are surface antigens.

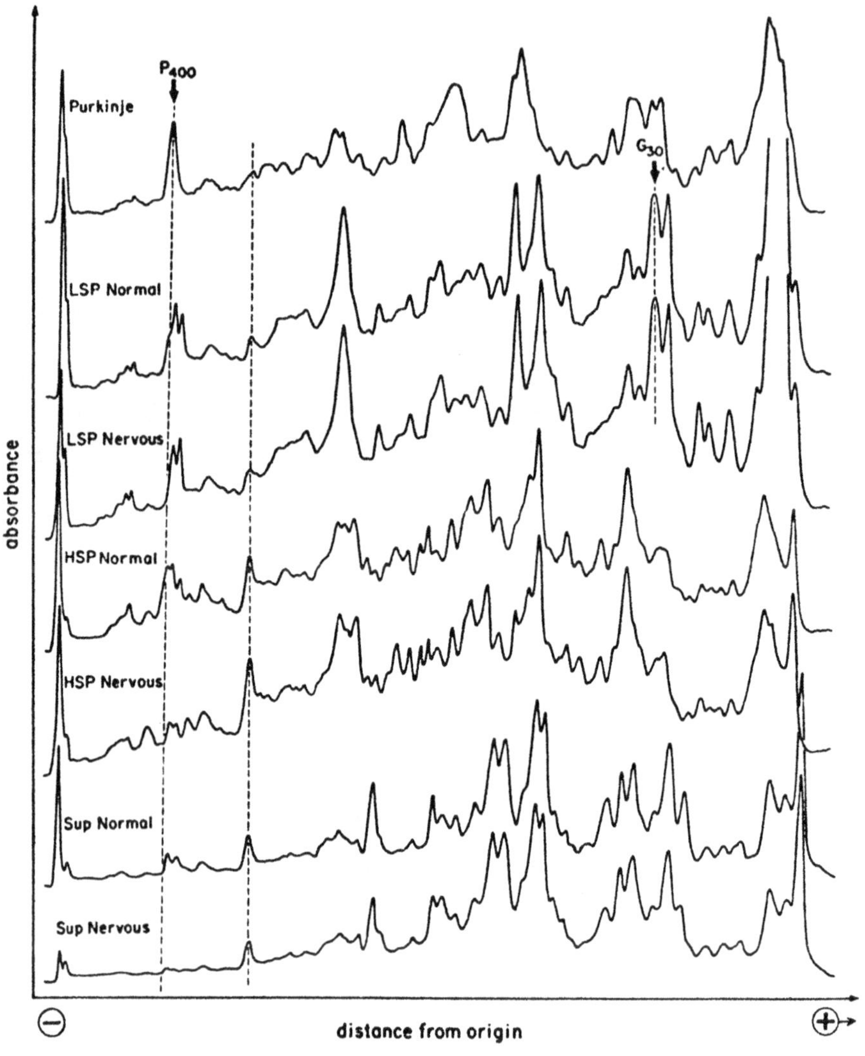

Fig. 6. Densitometric scans of a 10% polyacrylamide gel of nervous and wildtype cerebellar proteins. Three different subcellular fractions were submitted to gel electrophoresis in SDS: a low-speed pellet (*LSP*) which contains nuclei, mitochondria, and various cell debris; a high-speed pellet (*HSP*) in which the microsomes are abundant, and the resulting supernatant (*Sup*) which contains all the soluble proteins. The gel was stained with Coomassie blue. Reproduced with permission from Mallet et al. (1976)

The immunological approach with the aim of obtaining cell-specific antisera has been used in many instances (see [1, 11]). Although each of these studies has provided useful information, none of the antisera that have been analyzed have been shown to be specific for a particular type of cell. This deficiency, for the most part, is due to the fact that heterogeneous tissues have been used for immunization because most cell types cannot be purified to homogeneity in sufficient amount. Several workers have circumvented this hurdle by immunizing with cloned cell lines. However, cloned cell lines suffer from the drawback that the cells may differ in several respects from their normal counterparts.

The need to immunize with a purified cell population has now become less stringent with the advent of the "hybridoma" technique. Clones can be isolated which produce monospecific antibodies in unlimited quantities. This method no longer requires the performance of tedious sequential absorptions. However, statistically, many clones will have to be tested before a specific antibody can be obtained.

The P_{400} Protein

An SDS-gel electrophoresis analysis of the membrane protein pattern of the mutant mouse *nervous* and its control revealed after Coomassie blue staining that a protein of apparent molecular weight 400,000 (P_{400}) failed to appear in this mutant (Fig. 6) [3, 4], which begins to lose its Purkinje cells around day 15 [12, 13]. The P_{400} was present in purified Purkinje cells but was not detected in cerebrum. These first results suggested that P_{400} is characteristic of the Purkinje cell.

The P_{400} protein was found to be a glycoprotein. It has been purified by preparative SDS-gel electrophoresis and its sugar composition has been analyzed. About 43% of its weight is made up of sugars, and among these mannose is preponderant (J.P. Zanetta, personal communication). Mikoshiba et al. [14] took advantage of the high amount of mannose in P_{400} to improve its detection on SDS gels by using ^{125}I-labeled Concanavalin A.

At least 10% of the Purkinje cells remain in *nervous* and, as expected, this very sensitive technique revealed that a small amount of P_{400} was indeed present in this mutant. However, no P_{400} was found in *pcd/pcd* mice in which less than 1% of the Purkinje cells remain. In the agranular mutants *weaver* and *reeler*, the content of P_{400} per milligram of protein increases in the cerebellum [14].

An interesting but rather complex mutation is *staggerer* [15, 16]. As a consequence of the *staggerer* mutation, among other defects, the number of Purkinje cells is reduced, most of the synapses between parallel fibers and dendritic spines on the Purkinje cells are missing, the spiny branchlets are absent, and the arborization of the Purkinje cell becomes abnormally simplified. Also, granule cells die possibly as a consequence of a retrograde transsynaptic degeneration [17]. Despite the loss of granule cells, which should, as it does in *weaver* or *reeler* cerebellum, cause an enrichment in P_{400} protein, a marked deficit in the content of this protein is noticed [4, 14]. Some residual functional [18] and anatomical [19] synapses between parallel fibers and the Purkinje cell are still observed on the main dendritic branches of the Purkinje cell and a direct correlation between the content in P_{400} protein and the number of parallel-fiber–Purkinje-cell synapses is plausible in this mutant.

Such a correlation is supported by the observation that in the course of postnatal development, the P_{400} protein is already present in the cerebellum at birth and increases markedly after the 14th day, at a time when many synapses between parallel fibers and Purkinje cell dendrites are formed [14].

Finally, the ^{125}I-labeled Con A method did not reveal any P_{400} in other tissues such as skeletal muscle, liver, heart muscle, kidney, or cerebrum.
Antibodies have been raised against the P_{400} purified from preparative SDS gels [14]. The indirect fluorescence technique performed on tissue sections showed that the anti-P_{400} antibodies were associated only with the Purkinje cells and their dendritic arborizations. No staining was observed in other large cells of the deep nuclei or of the olfactory bulb. The staining persisted after thorough absorption of the serum on cerebrum membranes, confirming the high specificity of the antibodies. To ascertain fully the specificity of the antibodies quantitative assays with ^{125}I-labeled anti-P_{400} antibodies remain to be performed on cerebellar membranes from *pcd/pcd* mice and their controls, as was described above for the case of anti-Purkinje cell serum. It should also be of interest to test whether the anti-Purkinje cell serum contains antibody against the P_{400}.
The anti-P_{400} serum should allow the localization of the P_{400} protein at the ultrastructural level. Although it is clear that this protein is associated with membranes [14], it is not yet possible to infer whether it is a plasma membrane protein, an intracytoplasmic element, or a component of the glycocalyx. The antibodies may help to elucidate the function of this highly specific protein.

Conclusion

In this study antibodies have been raised against a population of large cells, mostly Purkinje cells, purified in about 10% yield from a suspension resulting from the mechanical dissociation of 12–16-day rat cerebella.
A sensitive binding assay and an immunohistochemical investigation have served as guides for the purification of the serum. After various absorptions on membranes derived from nonneural tissues, the forebrain, and the brainstem, a serum was obtained which reacts exclusively with the Purkinje cells of the cerebellum. Except for this preparation, none has yet been reported which is specific to a single type of neuron.
The use of this purified Purkinje cell fraction and of neurologic mutant mice has also allowed the identification of a protein of an *apparent* molecular weight of 400,000 daltons, which is characteristic of Purkinje cells. This protein has been purified and antibodies have been obtained which should allow its subcellular localization. These results also confirm anatomic and electrophysiological data that the *staggerer* and *nervous* mutations introduce lesion at the level of the Purkinje cell.

References

1. Mallet J, Christen R, Changeux JP (1979) Immunological studies on the Purkinje cells from rat and mouse cerebella. I. Evidence for antibodies characteristic of the Purkinje cells. Dev Biol 72:308–319
2. Woodhams P, Mallet J, Changeux JP, Balàzs R (1979) Immunological studies on the Purkinje cells from rat and mouse cerebella. II. Immunohistochemical specificity of the antiserum to Purkinje cells. Dev Biol 72:320–326

3. Mallet J, Huchet M, Pougeois R, Changeux JP (1975) A protein difference associated with defects of the Purkinje cell in *staggerer* and *nervous* mutant mice. FEBS Lett 52:216–220
4. Mallet J, Huchet M, Pougeois R, Changeux JP (1976) Anatomical, physiological and biochemical studies on the cerebellum from mutant mice. III. Protein differences associated with the *weaver, staggerer* and *nervous* mutations. Brain Res 103:291–312
5. Cohen J, Mares V, Lodin Z (1973) DNA content of purified preparations of mouse Purkinje neurones isolated by a velocity sedimentation technique. J Neurochem 20:651–657
6. Sellinger OZ, Legrand J, Clos J, Ohlsson WG (1974) Unequal pattern of succinate dehydrogenase and acetylcholinesterase in Purkinje cell bodies and granule cells isolated in bulk from the cerebellar cortex of the immature rat. J Neurochem 23:1137–1144
7. Yanagihara T, Hamberger A (1973) A method for separation of Purkinje cell and granular cell enriched fractions from rabbit cerebellum. Brain Res 59:445–448
8. Wilkin GPW, Wilson JE, Balàzs R, Cohen J, Dutton GR (1976) Preparation of cell bodies from the developing cerebellum. Structural and metabolic integrity of the isolated cells. Brain Res 115:181–199
9. Mullen RJ, Eicher EM, Sidman R (1976) Purkinje cell degeneration, a new neurological mutation in the mouse. Proc Nat Acad Sci USA 73:208–212
10. Woodhams PL, Cohen J, Mallet J, Balàzs R (1980) A preparation enriched in Purkinje cells identified by morphological and immunocytochemical criteria. Brain Res 199:435–442
11. Stallcup WB, Cohn M (1979) Cell specific antisera as reagents for studying the nervous system. TINS 2:20–23
12. Sidman RL, Green MC (1970) *"Nervous"*, a new mutant mouse with cerebellar disease (Symposium of the Centre National de la Recherche Scientifique, Orléans-La-Source, France). In: Sabourgy M (ed) Les mutants pathologiques chez l'animal. Leur intérêt dans la recherche biomédicale. CNRS, Paris, pp 69–79
13. Landis S (1973) Ultrastructural changes in the mitochondria of cerebellar Purkinje cells of *nervous* mutant mice. J Cell Biol 57:782–797
14. Mikoshiba K, Huchet M, Changeux JP (1979) Biochemical and immunological studies on the P_{400} protein, a protein characteristic of the Purkinje cell from mouse and rat cerebellum. Dev Neurosci 2:257–275
15. Sidman RL, Lane P, Dickie M (1962) *Staggerer*, a new mutation affecting the cerebellum. Science 137: 610–612
16. Landis DMD, Sidman RL (1978) Electron microscopic analysis of postnatal histogenesis in the cerebellar cortex of staggerer mutant mice. J Comp Neurol 179:831–863
17. Sotelo C, Changeux JP (1974) Trans-synaptic degeneration "en cascade" in the cerebellar cortex of *staggerer* mutant mice. Brain Res 67:519–526
18. Crepel F, Mariani J (1975) Anatomical, physiological and biochemical studies on the cerebellum from mutant mice. I. Electrophysiological analysis of cerebellar cortical neurons in the *staggerer* mouse. Brain Res 98:135–147
19. Sotelo C (1975) Dendritic abnormalities of Purkinje cells in the cerebellum of neurologic mutant mice (*weaver* and *staggerer*). Adv Neurol 12:335–351

Discussion

Palay inquired about localization of the P_{400}, since both soma and dendrites of Purkinje cells showed reaction product. Dr. Mallet replied that he is currently studying this question with electron microscopy and has no answer yet. He also suggested that synthesis of the protein within the cell might result in staining inside as well as on the membrane of the cell.

Sotelo pointed out that in *Staggerer,* not only are spines missing, but also most of the Purkinje cells are absent. Since, under certain conditions some P_{400} can be detected in *Staggerer,* it would appear that P_{400} is not exclusively related to the spines.

In response to Sir John Eccles's concern that the dendrites are missing from the isolated Purkinje cell preparation, Dr. Mallet pointed out that he does get staining of both soma and dendrites with protein from these cells, but admitted the possibility that other dendrite-specific proteins might have been excluded from the preparations.

Fractionation of Cerebellar Cells and Synapses: Certain Properties Related to Neurotransmission

R. Balazs *

Introduction

In order to further the better understanding of the complex biochemical makeup of the brain we have been engaged, over the last few years, in studies aimed at the separation of morphologically defined subcellular fractions and viable identified cell types from the cerebellum. This part of the brain was chosen since it contains only a limited number of neuronal cell types, which are formed in a known sequence during development [1], and its morphology and electrophysiology have been extensively studied [30, 74]. A further attraction was that the mossy-fiber terminals in the cerebellum are among the largest presynaptic structures in the CNS and they form the core of a well-recognizable complex synapse, the glomerulus. These features permit the identification of these structures in the fragmented tissue and thus facilitate their separation.

Separation of Cell Types from the Developing Cerebellum

The techniques developed during the course of these studies have been described previously [21, 22, 90]. Briefly, perikarya (cells) are isolated by mild trypsinization of the tissue and are separated by unit gravity sedimentation. Isotonic conditions and physiological pH are maintained throughout the procedure, and these, together with the avoidance of high centrifugal forces, contribute to the preservation of the structural integrity and metabolic competence of the cells. A high proportion of the cells are viable in tissue culture, and recently we have also been using this technique for obtaining preparations enriched in certain cell types [6] see also [25, 56, 66]).
With respect to the identification of cell types a combination of techniques is used. These include electron microscopy, since the structural appearance of the perikarya of certain cell types is distinct [30, 74], autoradiography, on the basis of established differences in the distribution of certain high-affinity amino-acid carriers in the various classes of cells (e.g., [23, 54, 55]), and immunocytochemistry, as antisera are now available against cell-type-specific antigens. The

* I acknowledge the important contributions of my colleagues to the work reviewed. I am grateful to Dr. J. Garthwaite for his comments on the manuscript and to Drs. A. Csillag, J. Garthwaite, A.J. Johnson, A.J. Patel, G.P. Wilkin, P.L. Woodhams, to Mr. R.D. Gordon, Mr. A. Hunt, Mr. A.N. Patel, and Miss A.E. Kingsbury for many helpful discussions and for providing unpublished material

Experimental Brain Research, Suppl. 6

Table 1. Preparations enriched in various types of cerebellar cells [a]

Preparations	Pretreatment	Dominant cell types in preparations		
		Classification	Means of identification	Purity (%)
B	–	External granule and differentiating granule cells	EM	70
C [b]	–	Replicating cells in the S_1, G_2, and M phase of the cell cycle	^{3}H-thymidine incorporation; autoradiography	30–40
C′	–	Astroglia-like cells	EM (only few cells are GFAP positive)	57
D [c]	HU [d]	Astroglia	EM; immunocytochemistry (GFAP antiserum)	49
E	HU [d]	Purkinje cells	EM; immunocytochemistry (Purkinje cell antiserum)	80

[a] Results from Cohen et al. [21, 22] and Woodhams et al. [94]
[b] Electron microscopy showed that 70%–80% of the cells displayed structural characteristics of external granule and differentiating granule cells (Cohen et al., 21)
[c] The biochemical properties, especially the characteristics of the ^{3}H-GABA transport system, indicated that the proportion of astrocytes is much higher than suggested by the GFAP score (Cohen et al. [23])
[d] Treatment with hydroxyurea (*HU*; see text)

cell types identified by means of the latter technique were as follows (references relating to the immune sera used are given in brackets): astrocytes (glial fibrillary acid protein, GFAP [11, 60]), oligodendroglia (galactocerebrosides [78], fibroblasts (Thy. 1. [6, 67]), Purkinje cells [61, 93, 94], and endothelial cells (immunoglobulins from patients with Chagas' disease, a trypanosomiasis [91 a]. The preparations enriched in the different cell types are listed in Table 1. This shows that from the normal cerebellum, two granule cell-enriched fractions can be obtained, one (B) is enriched in differentiating granule cells and external granule cells in the G_1 phase of the cell cycle, and the other (C) contains a relatively high proportion of neuronal precursor cells in late S and G_2 phase [21]. This latter fraction is especially interesting since it shows a DNA synthesis rate in vitro which is five times higher than that in the original cell suspension. A similar high rate is sustained after 24 h in vitro, thus suggesting that the cells, most of which are morphologically similar to the external granule cells (i.e., they are neuronal precursors), are also able to initiate new rounds of DNA synthesis. However, in order to achieve a high degree of purification of the differentiated cells, it is necessary to eliminate the replicating cells, which show great variation in cell size as they progress through the generation cycle and consequently they distribute throughout the separating gradient. To this end the animals are pretreated in vivo with a DNA synthesis inhibitor, hydroxyurea, and this allows the separation of fractions greatly enriched in GFAP-positive astrocytes and Purkinje cells respectively [22, 94]. Finally, selection by tissue culture techniques has provided two further preparations containing predominantly either astrocytes or differentiated cerebellar interneurons [6].

Properties of the Separated Cells

The metabolic integrity of the isolated cells is attested by the linear, controlled rate of respiration and the rapid reconstitution, during incubation, of physiological ion gradients. The estimated intracellular concentrations of K^+ and Na^+, which are maintained for at least 2 h, are 120 and 20 mEq/l respectively, suggesting that the cells have, on average, normal membrane potentials (−65 to 75 mV) [38, 90]. Finally, the protein composition of the isolated cells, including the newly synthesized proteins, closely resembles that of the whole tissue in vivo in terms of SDS-acrylamide gel electrophoresis profiles.

Characteristic differences in the biochemical properties of the different cell types have also emerged. Thus, although the rate of protein synthesis, in terms of incorporation of ^{14}C-leucine per unit protein, is comparable in the astrocyte and the Purkinje cell fraction, and is incidently of similar magnitude as that observed in vivo [28], the types of protein synthesized by the two fractions, particularly in the molecular weight ranges 18.5–20 K and 25.5–28 K, are significantly different ([38] and N. Patel et al., in preparation).

Amino Acid Transport

It seems that in comparison with most other parts of the CNS, amino acid transmitters are more abundant in the cerebellum. We have therefore investigated certain biochemical properties which are believed to be associated with the transmitter function of these substances, such as high-affinity transport, which is thought to play a role in the removal of the released transmitter, and amino acid receptors.

Considerable effort has been recently devoted towards kinetically defining the characteristics of membrane transport systems in the brain. In many of these studies brain slices have been used and these have the limitation, when formal kinetics based in unidirectional fluxes are applied, that the rate of diffusion through the extracellular space may introduce a bias in the estimated kinetic constants (see e.g., [59]). Synaptosomal preparations, on the other hand, may have the disadvantage of not having a well-defined structural composition. The use of cell suspensions or well-characterized subcellular fractions, such as the glomerulus particles, permitting direct access of known and uniform concentrations of substances, should facilitate a more accurate description of the transport kinetics.

Transport of GABA

The kinetics of ^{3}H-GABA uptake in both the astrocyte and the Purkinje cell preparations display biphasic curves indicating both high- and low-affinity components [23]. The apparent affinity is higher in the astrocytes (1 or 2 μM), while the V_{max} is about six fold greater in the Purkinje cells (4.65 vs 0.76 nmol/10^6 cells per 15 min). Significantly, the uptake rate in the granule cell fractions is very low (see also [17, 29]).

Differences in the properties of the transport carrier have been shown using structural analogues [23]. β-Alanine is a potent inhibitor of ^{3}H-GABA uptake in the astrocytes (IC_{50} = 18 μM), but not in the Purkine cells (where even 1 mM concentration fails to cause 50% inhibition), whereas the reverse applies to D,L-cis-1,3-aminocyclohexane carboxylic acid [13]. In contrast to previous observations, 2,3-diaminobutyric acid is a potent inhibitor in both the glial and neuronal preparations.

High-affinity ^{3}H-GABA uptake is Na^+-dependent in both cell types, neither of which shows cooperativity, the Hill-coefficient being close to 1 [23]. However, the two cell fractions show differential sensitivity to veratridine, which locks open the voltage-dependent Na^+ channels [18], and to ouabain, an inhibitor of Na^+, K^+-AT-Pase. Both agents potently inhibit ^{3}-H-GABA accumulation in the Purkinje cell fraction, but have little effect in astrocytes. The observations on the effect of veratridine also demonstrate the preservation of voltage-dependent Na^+ channels in the plasma membrane of the separated Purkinje cells. The differential effects of ouabain are, however, unexpected in view of the ubiquitous distribution of the Na^+, K^+-ATPase. The results may relate to the low Na^+ permeability of glial cells to Na^+ ions (c.f. [52]), and/or to differences in the properties of the enzyme in nerve cells and astrocytes. In this context, it is worth noting that brain homogenates exhibit two forms of Na^+, K^+-ATPase with respect to ouabain inhibition and the kinetics of ^{3}H-ouabain binding [62]. These effects and the more potent inhibition caused by NaF, a glycolytic inhibitor, in the Purkinje cells than in the astrocytes have therefore revealed significant differences in the mechanisms subserving amino acid transport in these two classes of cells. Furthermore, together with the observed differences in the GABA transport systems (kinetics and effects of structural analogues) the results indicate that the composition of the astrocyte fraction is more homogeneous than suggested by the anti-GFAP labeling (see Table 1).

Transport of Glutamate

The rate of high-affinity uptake of ^{3}H-glutamate is very much higher in the astrocyte preparations than in the other cell fractions (Fig. 1). The rate in the granule cell fractions, especially after corrections are made on the basis of the proportion of GFAP positive astrocytes in these preparations, is very low (see also [29], however, see [17]). This is interesting, since there is evidence suggesting that granule cells operate with glutamate as their transmitter [81, 95], and it is generally believed that nerve cells are endowed with high-affinity transport systems for their transmitters. Further studies have indicated that it is not only the soma of the granule cells where ^{3}H-glutamate uptake is very low. Accumulation of ^{3}H-glutamate in granule cells in culture can virtually not be detected [54, 66], and in recent autoradiographic studies using structurally well-preserved cerebellar slices [40, 41] we have detected massive uptake of labeled acidic amino acids into the glial cells and very little accumulation in the cell bodies, axons, and terminals of the granule cells [91 b].

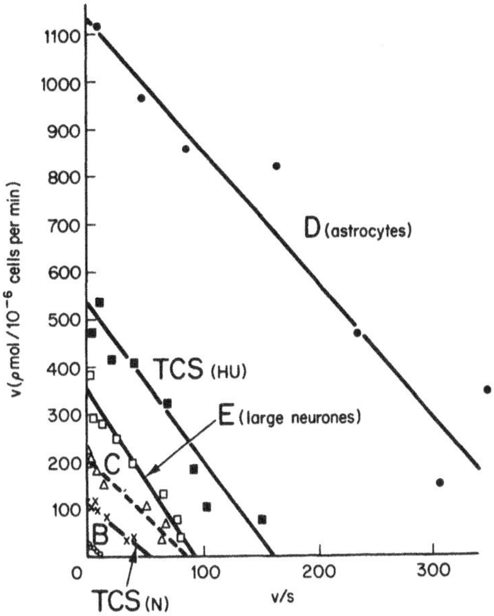

Fig. 1. High-affinity ^{3}H-glutamate uptake by preparations enriched in various cell types. Cells ($0.09 - 1 \times 10^6$/ml) were incubated in Krebs-tris medium, pH 7.4, containing 10 mM glucose, in 100% O_2 atmosphere in the presence of 0.5–100 μM L-^{3}H-glutamate for 4 min. Then, cells were centrifuged and washed and the radioactivity content was determined in the pellet. ^{3}H-Glutamate uptake was calculated after correction for the ^{14}C-inulin space in the pellet. The figure shows representative experiments analyzed in terms of Eadie-Hofstee plots. In three to four separate experiments the apparent affinities were not significantly different in the various cell-type-enriched preparations (the K_t was in the range 2.3 – 3.8 μM), while the maximal velocities, as a percentage of the mean value in the astrocyte fraction (*D*), were as follows: 4% in *B*, 32% in *C* (the characterization of these two granule cell fractions is given in Table 1), and 41% in the Purkinje cell preparations (*E*). The results are from Gordon et al. (unpublished)

Acidic Amino Acid Receptors

There is circumstantial evidence indicating that glutamate may serve as the transmitter of the granule cells, and that aspartate may be associated with the climbing fibers [64, 81, 84, 95]. Stimulation of these pathways in vivo and excitatory amino acids in vitro lead to marked increases in the level of cerebellar cGMP [10, 34, 37, 79]. We have approached the characterization of the receptors, which according to electrophysiological evidence may fall into different categories [88], in terms of cGMP responses, using cerebellar slices in the first instance. Initial studies have shown that the glutamate evoked increase in cGMP concentration changes during development: it is relatively small in the newborn, but increases sharply, reaching a maximum at 8–15 days, after which it declines to the adult level [37]. The experiments have, therefore, been conducted in both 8-day-old and adult tissue, with the aid of different agonists and antagonists for the characterization of the receptor(s) [36, 39].

Dose-response curves have shown that in the immature cerebellum N-methyl-D-aspartate (NMDA) is the most potent agonist ($ED_{50} = 40$ μM), followed by L-aspartate and L-glutamate ($ED_{50} = 300 - 500$ μM) (Fig. 2). The maximal stimulation attained by these agents is similar (from about 0.8 to 160 pmol/mg protein), representing a 200-fold increase over basal cGMP levels. In contrast, the maximal re-

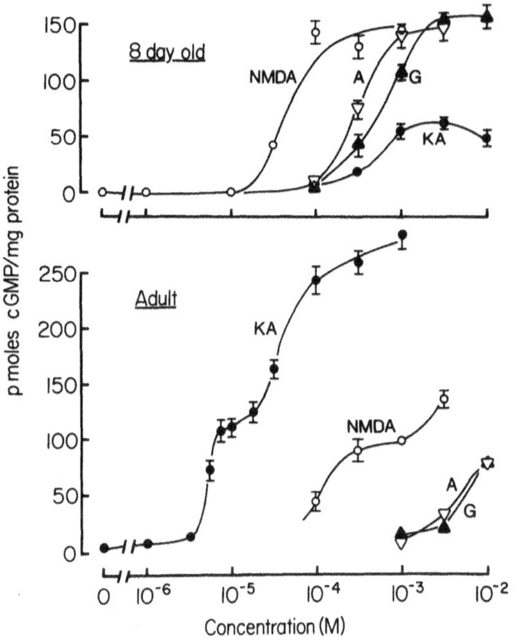

Fig. 2. Dose response curves for cGMP accumulation in cerebellar slices from 8-day-old and adult rats incubated in the presence of *NMDA* (○), L-aspartate (*A*, ▽), L-glutamate (*G*, ▲) and kainate (*KA*, ●). Slices were inactivated at the peak of the responses (in case of 8-day-old or adult tissue 2–5 min or 5–10 min) and cGMP levels measured by radioimmunoassay. (Results from Garthwaite and Balazs [39])

sponse with kainate is lower (70 pmol/mg protein), although its effective concentration is in the same range as for glutamate.

We have observed that the morphological preservation of slices from adult cerebella is a prerequisite for adequate cGMP responses to the acidic amino acids [40]. Chopped slices often used in such studies show extensive structural damage, including degenerating cells and massive glial swelling (Fig. 3), and this is associated with a very poor response to glutamate. In contrast, the structural integrity of handcut slices is comparable with that of the in vivo fixed tissue, and the cGMP responses have therefore been studied in such preparations. The dose-response curves differ both qualitatively and quantitively from those in the immature tissue. The maximal responses are higher (about 280 pmol/mg protein) and the most potent agonist is kainate (ED_{50} about 20 μM), representing an increase in apparent potency of 20-fold. On the other hand, NMDA, L-asparate and L-glutamate are less effective in the adult tissue, the decrease in potency relative to the immature cerebellum being five- to ten fold, but the rank order (NMDA > Asp and Glu) remaining the same.

It has recently been proposed that a group of compounds exemplified by D-*a*-aminoadipate (DAA), as well as low concentrations of Mg^{2+}, selectively antagonize responses at receptors on which NMDA acts preferentially (for review see Watkins [88]). In the 8-day-old cerebellar slices, DAA (250 μM) effectively inhibits NMDA-induced cGMP increases, causing an approximately threefold parallel shift in the dose response curve. However, DAA also antagonizes the effects of kainate. In contrast, in the adult, DAA inhibits the effects of NMDA, but not that of kainate. Furthermore, omission of Mg^{2+} enhances the potency of NMDA, while it has no detectable influence on the kainate-induced cGMP changes. DAA has no effect on the glutamate- or aspartate-evoked cGMP increase in either the 8-day-old or adult slices. On the other hand, at both ages the effect of these amino acids is antagonized

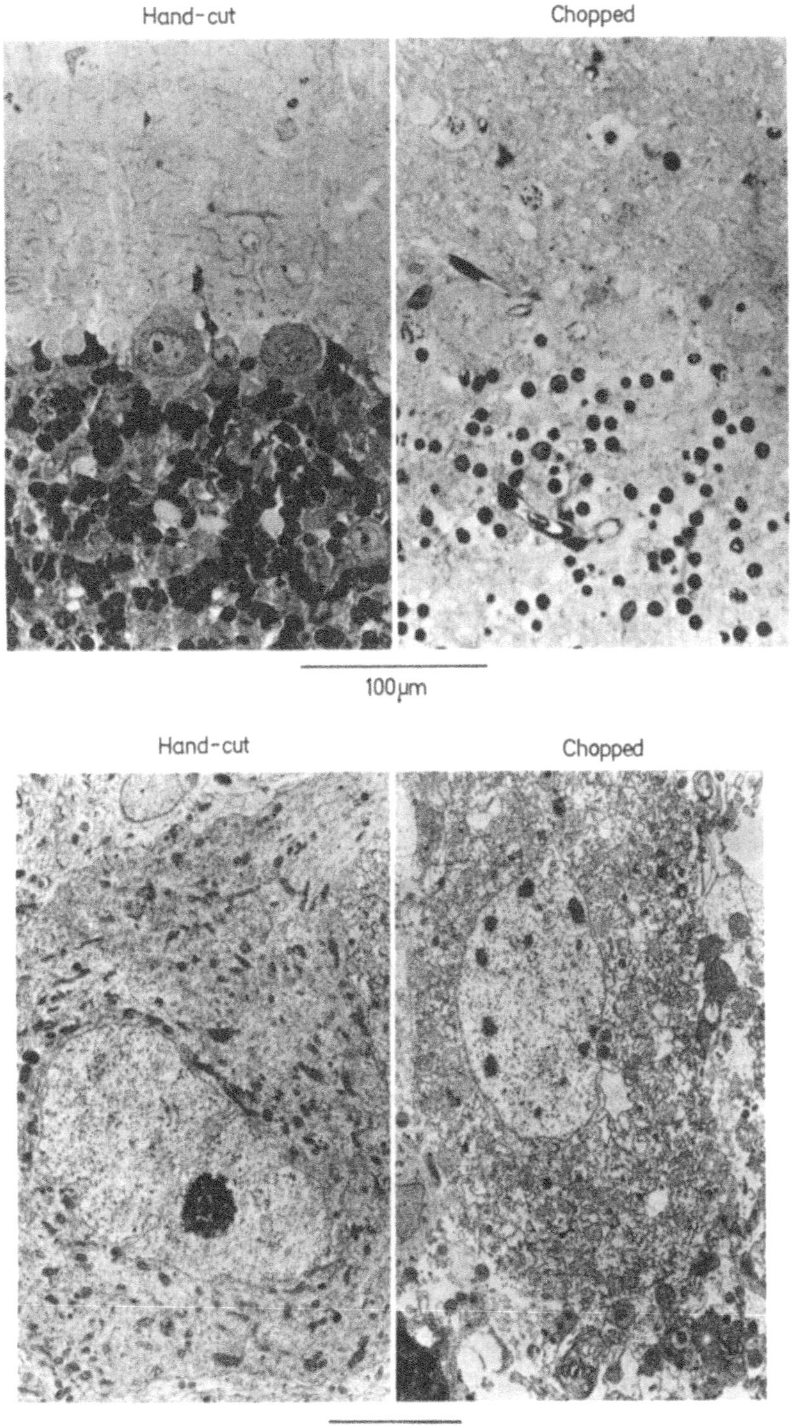

Fig. 3. Appearance of hand-cut and chopped slices from the cerebellar cortex, incubated for 2 h in Krebs-medium, at low magnification (*top*, Garthwaite et al., [40], by permission of Brain Res.). The electron micrographs show representative Purkinje cells in the two preparations (Garthwaite et al., [41], by permission of Dev. Neurosci.)

by glutamate diethylester (GDEE) [43]. Thus, an NMDA-stimulated DAA-sensitive receptor is expressed in both the immature and adult cerebellum. It seems that kainic acid is a weak agonist at this receptor in the young tissue, while in the adult it acts on a receptor that is resistant to both DAA and Mg^{2+}. It would appear that the receptors with which glutamate and aspartate interact are a separate class, since irrespective of the developmental stage they are sensitive to GDEE, but not to DAA (Garthwaite, unpublished observations). The results indicate therefore that the acidic amino-acid-evoked cGMP responses show many similarities to those monitored by electrophysiological methods in other parts of the CNS [44, 88].

In order to attempt the identification of the cell type(s) associated with the acidic amino-acid-evoked cGMP response Garthwaite has studied in our laboratory the effects in isolated cells prepared from 8-day-old cerebella. It has been observed that, under proper conditions, the magnitude of the cGMP increases are fully retained, thus indicating that the cell bodies are the primary site of the effect at this age. There is, however, a striking difference when compared with slices: the apparent potencies of the physiologically occurring amino acids are considerably higher in the isolated cells. Thus, in slices the ED_{50} for glutamate or aspartate is about 450 μM, which is similar to the electrophysiological estimates using brain slices [71], while in the cell suspension the ED_{50} is 5 μM for glutamate and 20 μM for aspartate. On the other hand, the ED_{50} for NMDA is the same in the isolated cells as in brain slices. NMDA is not likely to be significantly accumulated by brain tissue [7, 33, 49], whereas glutamate and aspartate are actively taken up, especially by glial cells (Fig. 1). It has been therefore proposed that the discrepancy in the potencies of the latter amino acids in slices versus isolated cells is due to the significant reduction of their effective concentration while they diffuse through the extracellular space [39]. Cell supension may, therefore, provide more accurate information regarding the potencies of excitatory amino acids on their different receptors.

It has been observed in these studies that high cell concentrations ($> 15 \times 10^6$/ml) are a prerequisite for obtaining opitmal cGMP increase by stimulation with excitant amino acids. A similar dependence on cell density has been recently described in 3T3 cells for plasma-membrane-associated Ca^{2+} fluxes, which are known to be important for cGMP responses. Thus the high cell density requirement of the cGMP response in the isolated neural cells may be related to that of the Ca^{2+} fluxes, and the two functions may have a common underlying mechanism. However, the requirement for such high cell concentrations has imposed severe practical limitations concerning the use of preparations of separated cell types for the determination of the cellular site of the cGMP response. Hitherto, we have obtained evidence that replicating external granule cells are not involved since the cGMP response is, in fact, increased after the elimination of these cells with HU treatment [37, 38]. Furthermore, the response is retained in cell preparations from which the Purkinje cells are excluded (Garthwaite, in preparation), suggesting that these cells do not represent the major site, in contrast to circumstantial evidence obtained in vivo in the adult cerebellum [10]. The cell types which are left for consideration, therefore, are the granule cells, inhibitory interneurons, and glial cells. At the present stage, even the glial cells cannot be excluded from being involved, directly or indirectly, in the response, since it has been observed in our laboratory that astroglial cells have relatively high guanylate cyclase activity (Wilkin et al., in preparation).

Interaction between Different Classes of Cells

In order to approach the question of metabolic interaction between different classes of cells, especially neurons and astrocytes, we have recently investigated the cellular distribution of certain enzymes associated with the metabolism of glutamate [75 a]. Previous kinetic studies on the fate of labeled substances oxidized in the brain have indicated that the metabolism of glutamate and the associated tricarboxylic acid cycles are compartmented in the brain [4, 9, 85]. The first model considering the structural correlates of metabolic compartments was put forward by Garfinkel [35] and it has been further modified on the basis of new information [9, 86]. Studies on the metabolism of labeled GABA in vitro [3] and other substances in vivo [9, 86], as well as the investigation of the influence of metabolic factors on the development of metabolic compartmentation of glutamate [75], permitted the formulation of a hypothesis, in which metabolic compartments were assigned to morphological structures [4]. Briefly, it was proposed that transmitter amino acids released from nerve terminals and taken up by glial cells are converted there to glutamine, which after diffusion into the interstitial space is taken up by the terminals to balance the loss of carbon units in the tricarboxylic acid cycle that occurs as a result of amino acid transmitter release. Certain aspects of this hypothesis have been corroborated by further studies [8, 15, 45, 63, 77]. Significantly it has been shown that glutamine is a better precursor than exogenous glutamate of the 'transmitter' glutamate in vitro [15, 45]. Furthermore, im-

Table 2. The activities in different neural cell types of certain enzymes associated with glutamate metabolism

	Glutamine synthetase (μmol/mg protein per h)	Glutaminase (nmol/mg protein per h)	Glutamate dehydrogenase (μmol/mg protein per h)
Separated cell types			
Astrocytes (D)	1.36 ±0.054	23.7±4.89	14.7 ±0.50
Purkinje cells (E)	0.163±0.010	88.8±4.19	6.69±0.923
Cultures			
Astrocytes	1.33 ±0.141	11± 2.0	6.08±0.31
Interneurons	0.34 ±0.088	131±19	3.65±0.68

Enzyme activities are the mean ±S.E. of 3–4 experiments for each preparation. All the estimates in the Purkinje cell preparations differed significantly from those in astrocytes ($P<0.02$). The assays were based on the following methods (with some modifications): glutamine synthetase – Ward, Bradford [87] (using 1-^{14}C-glutamate as a substrate); glutamate dehydrogenase – Lai, Clark [53]; glutaminase – Kwamme, Olsen [51]. In the last assay glutamine concentration was 0.5 mM (when the rate is linear). Under these conditions in both types of cultures the activity was only about 10% of that obtained with 8 mM glutamine as the substrate. Nevertheless, the ratio of the activity in cultures of interneurons to astrocytes was high (being 17 in this experiment vs 13 assayed at 0.5 mM substrate concentration) Patel et al. [75 a]

munocytochemical studies have indicated that glutamine synthetase is predominantly localized in glial structures [67]. However, in contrast to the general acceptance of the predominantly glial localization of glutamine synthetase, there is less agreement concerning the cellular distribution of glutaminase. It has been reported that in comparison with that in whole brain homogenate, the enzyme activity is high in synaptosomal preparations [15, 87], but it is not significantly lower in forebrain astrocyte cultures [82]. The availability of relatively pure separated cell types has now permitted the direct estimation of some of the enzymes which, according to the above hypothesis, should have selective distributions. The results in Table 2 show that in astrocytes in comparison with nerve cells the activity of glutamine synthetase is about tenfold higher, that of glutaminase much lower, and glutamate dehydrogenase is significantly higher. (It has been proposed that glutamate dehydrogenase is preferentially associated with the compartment utilizing amino acids or fatty acids for glutamine synthesis [85], i.e., with the glial compartment [4].)
Our findings on the differential distribution of these enzymes have been similar in cerebellar cultures of interneurons and astrocytes (however, see [82]). These observations strongly support the hypothesis of metabolic compartmentation and suggest a metabolic interaction between neurons and glial cells.

Glomerulus Particles and the Transmitter(s) of the Golgi Neurons

We have developed previously a method for the isolation in a very pure form of large fragments of the cerebellar glomeruli [5]. These contain the excitatory mossy-fiber terminal core surrounded by the amputated granule cell dendritic digits, which are contacted on their periphery by the axon terminals of Golgi cells. The glomerulus particles exhibit high-affinity transport of ^{3}H-GABA [92], which is selectively accumulated by the Golgi axon terminals [89]. Immunocytochemical studies have demonstrated that glutamate decarboxylase is concentrated in the terminals of the Golgi axons [64]. This is consistent with biochemical observations that in the glomerulus particles both the enzyme activity [5] and GABA-receptor binding[1] [50] are increased about twofold over

1 In the glomerulus particles GABA receptor binding is presumably at the granule cell dendrites which receive the terminals of the Golgi axons. That granule cells in the granular layer are endowed with a relatively high concentration of receptor sites is indicated, besides the observations described above [50], by the finding that GABA receptor binding is high in the dissected granular layer [72], whereas it is low in the agranular cerebellum [72, 83]. In addition, light microscopic autoradiographic studies, in which the endogenous inhibitors of binding were removed, have indicated that GABA receptors are concentrated in the granular layer [73]. On the other hand, Chan-Palay [19] has found that the highest density of ^{3}H muscimol binding occurs in the molecular and Purkinje cell layers, and further electron microscopic studies showed that the baskets surrounding the Purkinje cell soma and initial axon segment, where axo-axonal synapses are rare, are particularly enriched in GABA receptors [20]. This ultrastructural localization may have escaped the resolution of the low-power light microscopic autoradiographic studies [73]. However, in contrast to the preparation of the tissue for the biochemical investigations [31] it is difficult to effect the complete removal of the endogenous inhibitors of GABA receptor binding in the electron microscopic autoradiographic studies, when the aim is to preserve the structural integrity of

that in the whole cerebellum. There is also neurophysiological evidence that GABA is a transmitter of the Golgi neurons [12]. Thus the selective localization of ^{3}H-GABA in the terminals of these cells supports the hypothesis that terminals are specifically endowed with high-affinity transport systems for their transmitter [47, 58].

However, in contrast to observations on preparations from the whole cerebellum [48, 58] glomerulus particles also show high-affinity ^{3}H glycine uptake [92], and electron microscopic autoradiographic studies have now shown that labeled glycine is also predominantly localized over synaptic vesicle-containing structures in the position of the Golgi axon terminals [91].

These results have been unexpected, since it is generally believed that in mammals glycine is not a transmitter in supraspinal regions, including the cerebellum [2, 26, 47], and there is evidence that Golgi cells, in particular, are GABA-ergic [12]. These observations raise the possibility that either the selectivity of the uptake of putative transmitters is limited or there are different populations of Golgi cells. We have approached this question both by kinetic analyses of the influence of one of the relevant amino acids on the uptake of the other and by quantitative electron microscopic autoradiography [91].

The results have shown that glycine is a weak noncompetitive inhibitor of high-affinity ^{3}H-GABA transport (K_i being over 600 μM vs the K_t of about 20 μM), and that GABA is an even weaker inhibitor of ^{3}H-glycine uptake (at 1.5 mM concentration it only decreases ^{3}H-glycine accumulation by 17%). These observations indicate, therefore, that the two substances do not share the same carrier. Nevertheless the different carriers may be on the same structure. This question has been examined by testing the following alternatives using EM autoradiography: if ^{3}H-glycine and ^{3}H-GABA were taken up by the same Golgi axon terminals the grain density per unit area should be the sum of that obtained when glomerulus particles are incubated in the presence of low concentrations (below the K_t) of either labeled amino acid. On the other hand, if the two amino acids were taken up by different populations of terminals the grain density there should be similar to that obtained with the individual amino acids. In these experiments glomerulus particles were exposed to ^{3}H-GABA or ^{3}H-glycine of identical specific radioactivity at concentrations which on the basis of the known kinetic parameters would result in the uptake of similar amounts of the amino acids (concentration ratio 1 μM : 5 μM). The accumulation of the labeled amino acids, in terms of unit protein, was indeed similar, and when the two amino acids were added together the radioactivity content of the glomerulus particles was additive, indicating that at the concentrations used the

1 Continued: the tissue permitting ultrastructural localization. Thus, the discrepancy between the results may reflect differences in the distribution of endogenous inhibitors of GABA receptor binding in the cerebellum. This possibility is supported by observations that around the Purkinje cells, in the basket region, there are very low concentrations of benzodiazepine receptors [96] (thought to be involved with the inhibitory protein, modulin, in the regulation of the GABA receptor [42]), and that the density of benzodiazepine receptors, relative to the GABA receptors is lower in the cerebellum than in other brain regions [76]. There is also evidence for the existence of unusual GABA receptors [14], some of which seem to be extrasynaptic [16], as indeed the receptors in the basket cell axons may also be [20]. Thus it seems possible that in the cerebellum, in terms of regulation, there is more than one population of GABA receptors

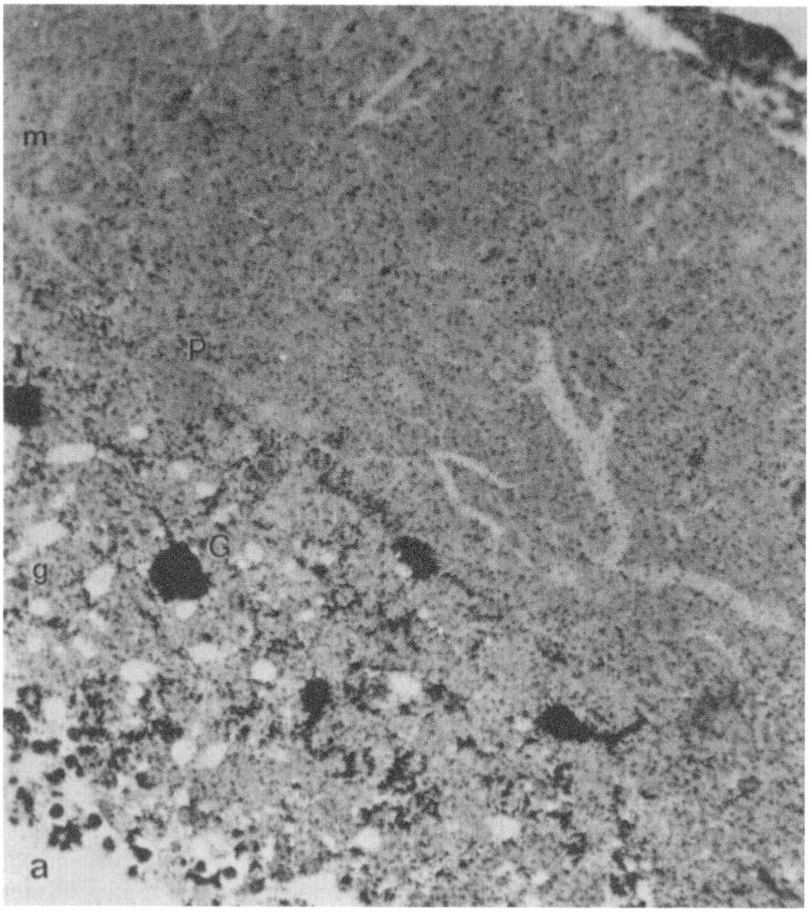

Fig. 4a, b. The localization of the sites of ^{3}H-glycine uptake was studied in adult handcut cerebellar slices preincubated in 10 mM glucose containing Krebs-bicarbonate medium (95% O_2, 5% CO_2, pH 7.4) and further incubated in the presence of 5 μM ^{3}H-glycine (specific radioactivity 4.2 Ci/mmol) for 15 min (50 μg/ml cycloheximide was also added to inhibit amino acid incorporation into proteins). The slices were processed for autoradiography using conventional techniques. **a** Light microscopy of the cerebellar cortex shows heavy accumulation of grains in the granular layer (*g*) over Golgi neuron-like cell bodies (*G*). (*m*, molecular layer; *P*, Purkinje cells). **b** Electron microscopic autoradiography confirms the localization of the heavy concentration of grains over Golgi neurons (*G*) (*gr*, granule cell; *a*, astrocytes). (Results from Wilkin et al. [91])

inhibition of transport of one amino acid by the other is negligible. The autoradiographic studies showed that the number of grains over labeled Golgi axon terminals, expressed as a percentage of the total area surveyed, was not additive, being 58 with ^{3}H-GABA, 42 with ^{3}H-glycine, and 67 (instead of 100) when glomerulus particles were incubated with the two substances together. Thus the results are consistent with the view that ^{3}H-GABA and ^{3}H-glycine are taken up preferentially into separate populations of Golgi axon terminals.

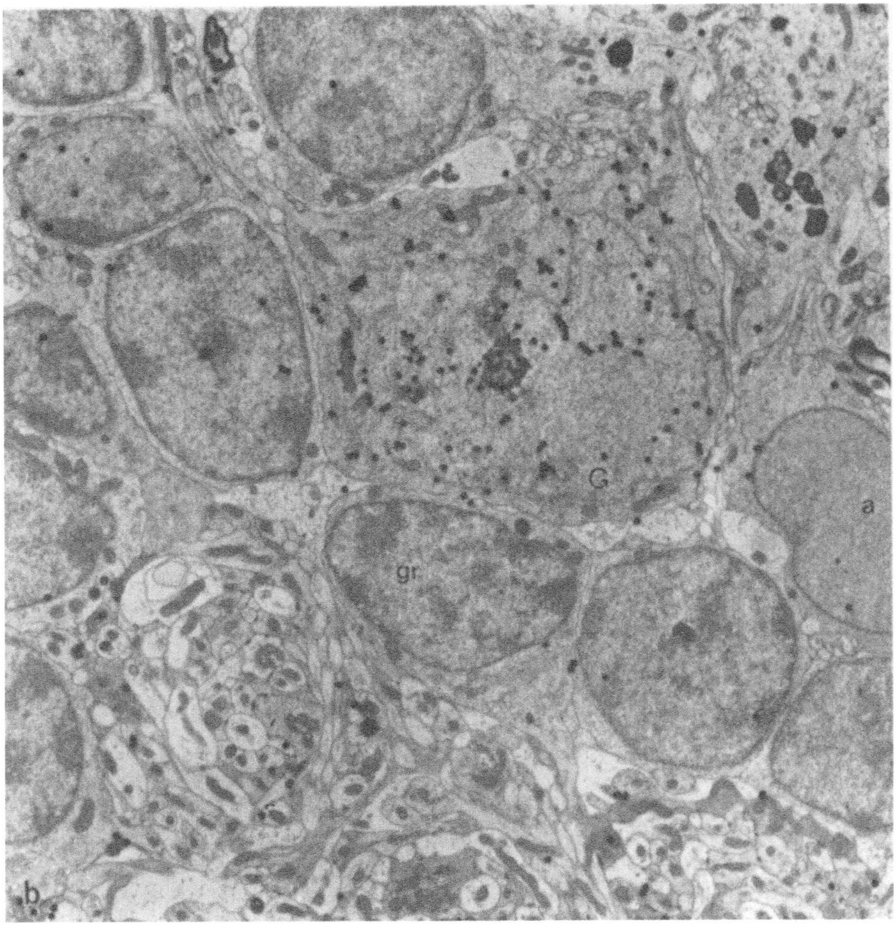

Fig. 4b. Legend see p. 394

Table 3. Localization of ^3H-glycine uptake sites in the cerebellar cortex

	Golgi neurons		Granule cells		Purkinje cells	Glial cells
	Perikarya	Axon terminals	Perikarya	Dendrites	Perikarya	
Grains/10 μm^2	7.8±0.81	7.8±0.89	0.34±0.05	0.63±0.07	0.65±0.10	2.1±0.22

Results are derived from the analysis of 7400 μm^2 area containing recognizable glomeruli in the granular layer and 14 000–34 000 μm^2 area for the perikarya of the different cell types. The estimates for the indicated classes of cells are the mean ±S.E; the rest of the structures gave 1.1±0.13 and 0.79±0.07 grains (per 10 μm^2) in the glomeruli and the molecular layer respectively. The mossy fiber terminals, especially, contained very few grains (0.28±0.10). (Wilkin et al. [91])

Further studies on structurally well preserved handcut slices have confirmed that in the cerebellar glomeruli both ^{3}H-glycine and ^{3}H-GABA are taken up by the Golgi axon terminals, while granule cells and mossy fiber terminals are very lightly labeled, if at all (Table 3). In addition, heavy accumulation of ^{3}H-glycine has been found over the somata, dendrites, and axons of the Golgi cells (Fig. 4). This is in clear contrast to the properties of the other interneurons, which do not accumulate significant amounts of ^{3}H-glycine. In this respect, the labeling patterns obtained with ^{3}H-glycine or ^{3}H-GABA are different, since the latter is markedly concentrated in basket and stellate cells. Both substances, however, also label glial cells, although the grain density after incubation with ^{3}H-glycine is only a quarter of that detected over the somata or terminals of the Golgi neurons (Table 3).

The observations that Golgi cells are unique among neurons of the cerebellar cortex in having high-affinity transport carriers for glycine provides a new addition to our repertoire of cell-specific markers. However, the presence in a nerve cell of a high-affinity uptake system for a substance, although suggestive, is not sufficient evidence for considering this as its transmitter. In the next experiments we therefore investigated whether glycine receptors, in terms of ^{3}H-strychnine binding, are present in the glomerulus particles, where the Golgi axons terminate. Saturable ^{3}H-strychnine binding has been detected, but the apparent affinity is about 100-fold lower than in spinal cord preparations ($K_d = 5 \times 10^{-7}$ M), and the ligand is not displaced by glycine [91].

These observations, however, do not exclude the possibility that glycine may serve as a transmitter of a proportion of the Golgi neurons. Although the case for glycine being a transmitter in the mammalian CNS is most conclusive in the spinal cord and brain stem [2, 26], a great proportion of the nerve cells affected by GABA also respond to microiontophoretic application of glycine in many supraspinal regions. Nevertheless, the potency of glycine in these regions is significantly lower than that of GABA. The inhibition of nerve cells by glycine is usually strychnine-sensitive, but hyperpolarizing strychnine-resistant responses have also been detected, e.g., in the hippocampus [27] and the spinal cord [80]. It would appear that in the frog spinal cord, besides strychnine-sensitive glycine receptors mediating hyperpolarization of nerve cells, there is another class of receptors refractory to strychnine and effecting depolarization [32, 70]. Furthermore, even in parts of the CNS where glycine is a good transmitter candidate, such as the mammalian spinal cord [2, 26], and the pigeon optic tectum [24], a proportion of the ^{3}H-strychnine binding in membrane preparations is not displaced by glycine [46, 57]. Moreover, it has been claimed recently that cerebellar synaptosomal fractions display high-affinity ^{3}H-glycine receptor binding which, in contrast to preparations from other parts of the brain, can virtually not be displaced by strychnine [69]. Finally, it appears that, in contrast to the GABA antagonists, picrotoxine or bicuculline, strychnine does not antagonize inhibition mediated by Golgi interneurons in the cerebellar cortex [12]. These observations by Bisti et al. [12] are consistent with the present findings, which suggest that, besides the GABAergic Golgi axon terminals, there may also be a glycinergic population with associated strychnine-resistant postsynaptic receptors.

References

1. Altman J (1969) DNA metabolism and cell proliferation. In: Lajtha A (ed) Handbook of neurochemistry, vol. II. Plenum Press, New York, pp 137–182
2. Aprison MH, Nadi NS (1978) Glycine: inhibition from the sacrum to the medulla. In: Fonnum F (ed) Amino acids as chemical transmitters, Plenum Press, New York, pp 531–570
3. Balazs R, Machiyama Y, Hammond BJ, Julian T, Richter D (1970) The operation of the γ-aminobutyrate bypath of the tricarboxylic acid cycle in brain tissue in vitro. Biochem J 116:445–467
4. Balazs R, Patel AJ, Richter D (1973) Metabolic compartments in the brain. Their properties and relation to morphological structures. In: Balazs R, Cremer JE (eds) Metabolic compartmentation in the brain. Macmillan, London, pp 167–184
5. Balazs R, Hajos F, Johnson AL, Reynierse GLA, Tapia R, Wilkin GP (1975) Subcellular fractionation of rat cerebellum: an electron microscopic and biochemical investigation. III. Isolation of large fragments of the cerebellar glomeruli. Brain Res 86:17–30
6. Balazs R, Regan C, Meier E, Woodhams PL, Wilkin GP, Patel NJ, Gordon RD (1980) Biochemical properties of neural cell types from rat cerebellum. In: Vernadakis A, Giacobini E (eds) Tissue culture in neurobiology. Raven Press, New York, pp 155–168
7. Balcar VJ, Johnston GAR (1972) The structural specificity of the high affinity uptake of L-glutamate and L-aspartate by rat brain slices. J Neurochem 19:2657–2666
8. Benjamin AM, Quastel JH (1974) Fate of L-glutamate in the brain. J Neurochem 23:457–464
9. Berl S, Clarke DD (1969) Compartmentation of amino acid metabolism. In: Lajtha A (ed) Handbook of neurochemistry. Vol II. Plenum Press, New York, pp 447–472
10. Biggio G, Guidotti A (1976) Climbing fibre activation and 3′,5′-cyclic guanosine monophosphate (cGMP) content in cortex and deep nuclei of cerebellum. Brain Res 107:365–373
11. Bignami A, Eng LF, Dahl D, Uyeda CT (1972) Localization of the glial fibrillary acidic protein in astrocytes by immunofluorescence. Brain Res 14:24–37
12. Bisti S, Iosif G, Marchesi GF, Strata P (1972) Pharmacological properties of inhibitions in the cerebellar cortex. Exp Brain Res 14:24–37
13. Bowery NG, Jones GP, Neal M (1976) Selective inhibition of neuronal GABA uptake by cis-1,3-aminocyclohexane carboxylic acid. Nature 264:97–105
14. Bowery NG, Hill DR, Hudson AL, Doble A, Middlemiss DN, Shaw J, Turnbull M (1980) (−)Baclofen decreases neurotransmitter release in the mammalian CNS by an action at a novel receptor. Nature 283:92–94
15. Bradford HF, de Bellaroche JS, Ward HK (1978) On the metabolism and intrasynaptic origin of amino acid transmitters. In: Fonnum F (ed) Amino acids as chemical transmitters, Plenum Press, New York, pp 367–377
16. Brown DA (1979) Extrasynaptic GABA systems. Trends Neurosci 2:271–273
17. Campbell GleM, Shank RP (1978) Glutamate and GABA uptake by cerebellar granule and glial cell enriched populations. Brain Res 153:618–622
18. Catterall WA, Nirenberg M (1973) Sodium uptake associated with activation of action potential ionophores of cultured neuroblastoma and muscle cells. Proc Natl Acad Sci USA 70:3759–3763
19. Chan-Palay V (1978) Autoradiographic localization of γ-aminobutyric acid receptors in the rat central nervous system by using [^{3}H]muscimol. Proc Natl Acad Sci USA 75:1024–1028
20. Chan-Palay V, Palay S (1978) Ultrastructural localization of γ-aminobutyric acid receptors in the mammalian central nervous system by means of [^{3}H]muscimol binding. Proc Natl Acad Sci USA 75:2977–2980
21. Cohen J, Balazs R, Hajos F, Currie DN, Dutton GR (1978) Separation of cell types from the developing cerebellum. Brain Res 148:313–331
22. Cohen J, Woodhams PL, Balazs R (1979) Preparation of viable astrocytes from the developing cerebellum. Brain Res 161:503–514

23. Cohen, J, Balazs R, Woodhams PL (to be published) Characterization of separated cell types from the developing cerebellum: transport of ^{3}H-GABA by preparation enriched in Purkinje cells and astrocytes. Neurochem Res
24. Cuénod M, Henke H (1978) Neurotransmitters in the avian visual system. In: Fonnum F (ed) Amino acids as chemical transmitters. Plenum Press, New York, pp 221–240
25. Currie DN, Dutton GR, Cohen J (1979) Monolayer cultures of perikerya isolated from postnatal rat cerebellum. Experimentia 35:345–347
26. Curtis DR, Johnston GAR (1974) Amino acid transmitters in the mammalian central nervous system. Ergeb Physiol 69:97–188
27. Curtis DR, Duggan AW, Felix D, Johnston GAR, McLennan H (1971) Antagonism between bicuculline and GABA in the cat brain. Brain Res 33:57–73
28. Dunlop DS, van Elden W, Lajtha A (1974) Measurement of rates of protein synthesis in rat brain slices. J Neurochem 22:821–830
29. East JM, Dutton GR, Currie DN (1980) Transport of GABA, β-alanine and glutamate into perikarya of postnatal rat cerebellum. J Neurochem 34:523–530
30. Eccles JC, Ito M, Szentagothai J (1967) The Cerebellum as a Neuronal Machine. Springer, Berlin Heidelberg New York
31. Enna SJ, Snyder SH (1977) Influences of ions, enzymes and detergents on gamma-aminobutyric acid-receptor binding in synaptic membrane of rat brain. Mol Pharmacol 13:442–453
32. Evans RH, Francis AA, Watkins JC (1976) Bimodal action of glycine on frog spinal motoneurones. Brain Res 118:395–401
33. Evans RH, Francis AA, Hunt K, Oakes DJ, Watkins JC (1979) Antagonism of excitatory amino acid-induced responses and of synaptic excitation in the isolated spinal cord of the frog. Br J Pharmacol 67:591–603
34. Ferrendelli JA, Chang MM, Kinscherf DA (1974) Elevation of cyclic GMP levels in central nervous system by excitatory and inhibitory amino acids. J Neurochem 22:535–540
35. Garfinkel D (1966) A simulation study of the metabolism and compartmentation in brain of glutamate, aspartate, the Krebs cycle and related metabolites. J Biol Chem 241:3918–3929
36. Garthwaite J (1982) Cyclic GMP responses to excitatory amino acids in immature and adult cerebellar slices. Neurosci (in press)
37. Garthwaite J, Balazs R (1978) Supersensitivity to the cyclic GMP response to glutamate during cerebellar maturation. Nature 275:328–329
38. Garthwaite J, Balazs R (1981) Separation of cell types from the cerebellum and their properties. In: Fedoroff S, Hertz L (eds) Advances in cellular neurobiology, vol 2, pp 461–489
39. Garthwaite J, Balazs R (1981) Excitatory amino acid-induced changes in cyclic GMP levels in slices and cell suspensions from the cerebellum. In: Di Chiara G, Gessa GL (eds) Glutamate as a neurotransmitter. Raven Press, New York, pp 317–324
40. Garthwaite J, Woodhams PL, Collins MJ, Balazs R (1980) A morphological study of incubated slices of rat cerebellum in relation to postnatal age. Dev Neurosci 3:90–99
41. Garthwaite J, Woodhams PL, Collins MJ, Balazs R (1979) On the preparation of brain slices: morphology and cyclic nucleotides. Brain Res 173:373–377
42. Guidotti A, Toffano G, Costa E (1978) An endogenous protein modulates the affinity of GABA and benzodiazipine receptors in rat brain. Nature 275:553–555
43. Haldeman S, McLennan H (1972) The antagonistic action of glutamic acid diethylester towards amino acid-induced and synaptic excitations of central neurones. Brain Res 45:393–400
44. Hall JG, Hicks TP, McLennan H, Richardson TL, Wheal HV (1979) The excitation of mammalian central neurones by amino acids. J Physiol 286:29–39
45. Hamberger AC, Chiang GH, Nylén ES, Schiff SW, Cotman CW (1979) Glutamate as a CNS transmitter. I. Evaluation of glucose and glutamine as precursors for the synthesis of preferentially released glutamate. Brakn Res 168:513–530
46. Hunt P, Raynauld J-P (1977) Benzodiazepine activity: is interaction with the glycine receptor, as evidenced by displacement of strychnine binding, a useful criterian? J Pharm Pharmacol 29:142–144

47. Iversen LL, Dick F, Kelly JS, Schon F (1975) Uptake and localization of transmitter amino acids in the nervous system. In: Berl S, Clarke DD, Schneider D (eds) Metabolic compartmentation and neurotransmission. Relation to brain structure and function. Plenum Press, New York, pp 65–89
48. Johnston GAR, Iversen LL (1971) Glycine uptake in rat central nervous system slices and homogenates: evidence for different uptake systems in spinal cord at cerebral cortex. J Neurochem 18:1951–1961
49. Johnston GAR, Kennedy SME, Twitchin B (1979) Action of the neurotoxin kainic acid on high affinity uptake of L-glutamic acid in rat brain slices. J Neurochem 32:121–127
50. Kingsbury AE, Wilkin GP, Patel AJ, Balazs R (1980) Distribution of GABA receptors in the rat cerebellum. J Neurochem 35:739–742
51. Kvamme E, Olsen BE (1980) Substrate mediated regulation of phosphate-activated glutaminase in nervous tissue. Brain Res 181:228–233
52. Kuffler SW, Nicholls JG (1966) The physiology of neuroglial cells. Erg Physiol 57:1–90
53. Lai JCK, Clark JB (1976) Preparation and properties of mitochondria derived from synaptosomes. Biochem J 154:423–432
54. Lasher RS (1974) The uptake of [^{3}H]GABA and differentiation of stellate neurons in culture of dissociated postnatal rat cerebellum. Brain Res 69:235–254
55. Lasher RS (1975) Uptake of GABA by neuronal and non-neuronal cells in dispersed cell cultures of postnatal rat cerebellum. J Neurobiol 6: 597–608
56. Lasher RS, Zagon IS (1972) The effect of potassium on neuronal differentiation in cultures of dissociated newborn rat cerebellum. Brain Res 41:482–488
57. LeFort D, Henke H, Cuénod M (1978) Glycine specific [^{3}H]strychnine binding in the pigeon CNS. J Neurochem 30:1287–1291
58. Logan WJ, Snyder SH (1971) Unique high affinity uptake systems for glycine, glutamic and aspartic acids in central nervous tissue of the rat. Nature 234:297–299
59. Lund-Andersen H, Kjeldsen CS (1976) Uptake of glucose analogues by rat brain cortex slices: a kinetic analysis based upon a model. J Neurochem 27:361–368
60. Ludwin SK, Kosek JC, Eng LF (1976) The topographical distribution of S-100 and GFA proteins in the adult rat brain: an immunohistochemical study using horseradish peroxidase-labelled antibodies. J Comp Neurol 165:197–207
61. Mallet J, Christen R, Changeux J-P (1979) Immunological studies on the Purkinje cells from rat and mouse cerebella. I. Evidence of antibodies characteristic of the Purkinje cells. Dev Biol 72:308–319
62. Marks MJ, Seeds NW (1978) A heterogeneous ouabain-ATPase interaction in mouse brain. Life Sci 23:2735–2744
63. Martinez-Hernandez A, Bell KP, Norenberg MD (1977) Glutamine synthetase: glial localization in brain. Science 195:1356–1358
64. McBride WJ, Rea MA, Nadi NS (1978) Effects of 3-acetylpyridine on the levels of several amino acids in different CNS regions of the rat. Neurochem Res 3:793–801
65. McLaughlin BJ, Wood JG, Saito K, Barber R, Vaughan JE, Roberts E, Wu J-Y (1974) The fine structural localization of glutamate decarboxylase in synaptic terminals of rodent cerebellum. Brain Res 76:377–391
66. Messer A (1977) The maintenance and identification of mouse cerebellar granule cells in monolayer culture. Brain Res 130:1–12
67. Mirsky R, Thompson EJ (1975) Thy-l (theta) antigen on the surface of morphologically distinct brain cell types. Cell 4:95–101
68. Moore L, Pastan I (1979) Effect of cell density on energy-dependent calcium uptake by Balb/c 3T3 membranes is independent of protein synthesis and attachment to substratum. J Cell Physiol 101:109–116
69. Munoz LMO, DeFeudis F, Fando JL (1977) High affinity binding of glycine and beta-alanine to synayptosome enriched fractions of rat CNS regions: effects of strychnine. Gen Pharmacol 8:325–330
70. Nicoll RA, Padjen A, Barker JL (1976) Analysis of amino acid responses of frog motoneurones. Neuropharmacol 15:45–54
71. Okamoto K, Quastel JH (1973) Spontaneous action potential in isolated guinea-pig cerebellar slices: effects of amino acids and conditions affecting sodium and water uptake. Proc R Soc London B 184:83–90

72. Olsen RM, Mikoshiba K (1978) Localization of gamma-aminobutyric acid receptor binding in the mammalian cerebellum: high levels in granule layer and depletion in agranular cerebella of mutant mice. J Neurochem 30:1633–1636
73. Palacinos JM, Scott Young W III, Kuhar MJ (1980) Autoradiographic localization of γ-aminobutyric acid (GABA) receptors in the rat cerebellum. Proc Natl Acad Sci USA 77:670–674
74. Palay S, Chan-Palay V (1974) Cerebellar Cortex–Cytology and Organization. Springer, Berlin Heidelberg New York
75. Patel AJ, Balazs R (1975) Factors affecting the development of metabolic compartmentation in the brain. In: Berl S, Clarke DD, Schneider D (eds) Metabolic compartmentation and neurotransmission. Relation to brain structure and function. Plenum Press, New York pp 363–383
75a. Patel AJ, Hunt A, Gordon RD, Balazs R (1982) The activities in different neuronal cell types of certain enzymes associated with the metabolic compartmentation of glutamate. Dev Brain Res
76. Placheta P, Karobath M (1979) Regional distribution of Na^+-independent GABA and benzodiazepine binding sites in rat CNS. Brain Res 178:590–583
77. Quastel JH (1975) Metabolic Compartmentation in the brain and effects of metabolic inhibitors. In: Berl S, Clarke DD, Schneider D (eds) Metaboli compartmentation and neurotransmission. Relation to brain structure and function. Plenum Press, New York, pp 337–361
78. Raff MC, Mirsky R, Fields KL, Lisak RP, Dorfman SH, Silberberg DH, Gregson NA, Liebowitz S, Kennedy MC (1978) Galactocerebroside is a specific cell surface antigen marker for oligodendroyctes in culture. Nature 274:813–816
79. Rubin EH, Ferrendelli JA (1977) Distribution and regulation of cyclic nucleotide levels in cerebellum in vivo. J Neurochem 29:43–51
80. Ryall RW, Piercey MF, Polosa C (1972) Strychnine-resistant mutual inhibition or Renshaw cells. Brain Res 41:119–129
81. Sandoval ME, Cotman CW (1978) Evaluation of glutamate as a neurotransmitter of cerebellar parallel fibers. Neuroscience 3:199–206
82. Schousboe A, Hertz L, Svenneby G, Kwamme E (1979) Phosphate activated glutaminase activity and glutamine uptake in primary cultures of astrocytes. J Neurochem 32:943–950
83. Simantov R, Oster-Granite ML, Herndon RL, Snyder SH (1976) Gamma-aminobutyric acid (GABA) receptor binding selectively depleted by a viral-induced granule cell loss in hamster cerebellum. Brain Res 105:365–371
84. Stone TW (1979) Glutamate as the neurotransmitter of cerebellar granule cells in the rat: electrophysiological evidence. Br J Pharmacol 66:291–296
85. Van den Berg CJ (1973) A model of compartmentation in mouse brain based on glucose and acetate metabolism. In: Balazs R, Cremer JE (eds) Metabolic compartmentation in the brain. Macmillan, London, pp 137–166
86. Van den Berg CJ, Garfinkel D (1971) A simulation study of brain compartments. Metabolism of glutamate and related substances in mouse brain. Biochem J 123:211–218
87. Ward HK, Bradford HF (1979) Relative activities of glutamine synthetase and glutaminase in mammalian synaptosomes. J Neurochem 33:339–342
88. Watkins JC (1978) Excitatory amino acids. In: McGeer EG, Olney JW, McGeer PL (eds) Kainic acid as a tool in neurobiology, Raven Press, New York, pp 37–69
89. Wilkin GP, Wilson JE, Balazs R, Schon F, Kelly JS (1974) How selective is high affinity uptake of GABA into inhibitory nerve terminals? Nature 252:397–399
90. Wilkin GP, Balazs R, Wilson JE, Cohen J, Dutton GR (1976) Preparation of cell bodies from the developing cerebellum. Structural and metabolic integrity of the isolated 'cells'. Brain Res 115:181–199
91. Wilkin GP, Csillag A, Balazs R, Kingsbury AE, Wilson JE, Johnson AL (1981) Localization of high affinity [^{3}H]glycine transport sites in the cerebellar cortex. Brain Res 216:11–33
91a. Wilkin GP, Woodhams PL, Ribeiro dos Santos R (1981) Rat cerebellar cells in tissue culture. I. An immunological marker for brain endothelial cells (Antibodies from the sera of patients with Chagas' disease). Dev Neurosci 4:296–306

91 b. Wilkin GP, Garthwaite J, Balazs R (1982) Putative amino acid transmitters in the cerebellum. II. Electron microscopic localization of transport sites. Brain Res (in press)
92. Wilson JE, Wilkin GP, Balazs R (1976) Metabolic properties of a purified preparation of large fragments of the cerebellar glomeruli: glucose metabolism and amino acid uptake. J Neurochem 26:957–965
93. Woodhams PL, Mallet J, Changeux J-P, Balazs R (1979) Immunological studies on the Purkinje cells from rat and mouse cerebella. II. Immunohistochemical specificity of the antiserum to Purkinje cells. Dev Biol 72:320–326
94. Woodhams PL, Cohen J, Mallet J, Balazs R (to be published) A preparation enriched in Purkinje cells identified by morphological and immunocytochemical criteria. Brain Res
95. Young AB, Oster-Granite ML, Herndon RM, Snyder SH (1974) Glutamic acid: selective depletion by viral induced granule cell loss in hamster cerebellum. Brain Res 73:1–13
96. Young WS III, Kuhar MJ (1979) Autoradiographic localisation of benzodiazepine receptors in the brains of humans and animals. Nature 280:393–394

Discussion

Krnjevic pointed out that the absence of glutamate uptake into granule cells is consistent with the concept that at glutamate synapses, the glutamate is taken up by glia cells rather than the glutamate releasing neurons. The glia can then convert glutamate to glutamine which in turn is released and taken up by the glutamate-releasing neurons. Dr. Balazs added that the patterns of associated enzyme systems also suggest a glutamate shuttle, since there is considerably more glutamate dehydrogenase and glutamine synthetase in glia than in nerve cells, whereas there is much more glutaminase in neurons than in glia.

Chan-Palay questioned the specificity of the glycine uptake, since in the spinal cord, much glycine seems to be taken up by glia. Dr. Balazs replied that in the slices it is seen that in the molecular layer glycine appears over glial structures, but otherwise the label seems specific for cell bodies, dendrites, and axon terminals of Golgi cells. The results were surprising to Dr. Chan-Palay, since Golgi cells are stained most consistently for glutamic acid decarboxylase, indicating probable use of GABA as a transmitter.

Altman suggested that since both Golgi and Purkinje cells stain for cholinesterase at early developmental stages, it would be interesting to determine whether the glycine uptake mechanism is also present at these stages. Dr. Krnjevic recalled that some Golgi cells also stain for acetylcholinesterase, perhaps suggesting a pluripotentiality for transmitter use by these neurons.

Mallet cautioned against drawing firm conclusions from biochemical studies on Purkinje cell preparations, in view of the inability of these cells to survive alone in culture, and the lack of regeneration of membrane proteins. Dr. Balazs accepted the caution and added that the integrity of the preparations viability was monitored in terms of trypan blue exclusion, sustained respiratory control and the maintenance of ion gradients between the cells and the incubation medium.

Functional Significance of the Climbing Fiber Input to Purkinje Cells: An In Vitro Study in Mammalian Cerebellar Slices *

R. Llinás and M. Sugimori

Introduction

The numerical and spatial organization of the synaptic input to cerebellar Purkinje cells is one of the best understood in the central nervous system today. Purkinje cells are known to receive two classes of excitatory inputs: the climbing fibers and the parallel fibers [25]. These two inputs seem to be present in this cortex throughout the phylogenetic scale in all cases studied to date (cf. [14]). The climbing fiber Purkinje cell junction seems to be a one-to-one relation in which a single climbing fiber (CF) innervates a large portion of the soma-dendritic surface of this neuron except in pathological [11, 17], agranular mutant [7], or developmental [8] conditions. The CF is known to contact the somata and smooth branches of Purkinje cells (PCs) via small stubby spines generally grouped in clusters containing four to five elements [13, 22]. The number of such clusters between a CF and a PC has been calculated for the frog to be 300 [16] and in the alligator to be 180 [12]. The parallel fibers (PFs), on the other hand, range in number from approximately 50,000 in the frog to close to 100,000 in the cat [23], and indeed much higher numbers have been suggested for human PCs [4]. The spatial organization of these two inputs over the PC is such that the CFs cover and maintain possession of the somata and main dendrites while the PFs are restricted to the more peripheral spiny branchlets. This particular distribution only occurs, however, when both fiber types are present. Indeed, damage of the CF input results in an invasion of the parallel fiber (PF) input into the smooth dendrites and the neoformation of spines [3, 26]. In contrast, damage of the PF input results in increased contact by the CF and often in multiple CF innervation [6]. In short, CFs and PFs compete to PC surface.

A point of interest here, however, is that these two excitatory inputs represent, numerically, the two extremes in innervation for any central neuron. Thus, a one-to-one relation such as the CF to the PC is rarely found in the central nervous system. On the other hand, the PFs represent the most numerous single class of input to innervate any neuron. Because of the clarity of this morphological difference, the question of functional significance becomes especially pertinent, not only as relating to PCs but in the context of neurobiology in general. Thus, a study of the electrophysiological properties of PCs following CF activation was recently approached in vitro. The experiments to be described

* Research was supported by U.S.P.H.S. program grant NS13742 from the National Institute of Neurological and Communicative Disorders and Stroke

Experimental Brain Research, Suppl. 6

here were performed in guinea pig cerebellar slices as described by Llinás and Sugimori [19, 20]. In this preparation, activation of CF-PC can be obtained by direct electrical stimulation of the underlying white matter. Because the in vitro approach allows long-term intracellular recordings, the modification of the extracellular ionic milieu, and the addition of drugs, this technique is very useful in characterizing the properties of CF activation of these neurons.

Climbing Fiber Activation of PCs

Examples of CF activation obtained from intrasomatic recording are illustrated in Fig. 1, very much as observed under similar conditions in in vivo preparations [9]. This response consists of a fast action potential of large amplitude followed by a protracted after-depolarization (ADP) consisting of several slower all-or-none spikes and a plateau depolarization which may last for many tens of milliseconds. Direct modification of the extracellular ionic milieu or addition of drugs capable of blocking specific conductances have demonstrated that the initial spike in the CF responses and some of the late action potentials are generated by a voltage-dependent Na conductance probably restricted to the soma-axon level [19]. The rest of the response was demonstrated to be due to Ca-dependent action potentials of dendritic origin. In this preparation the actual mechanism of transmission is, as originally described in vivo [9], the activation of the chemical junction. Following an electrical stimulus to the white matter, a single all-or-none excitatory postsynaptic potential (EPSP) is observed which reflects the all-or-none property of the presynaptic action potential in the particular CF. As in vivo [9, 18], depolarization of the PC membrane potential produces a reversal of the synaptic potential, as shown in Fig. 1 B and C. In short, at the somatic level the set of events which is triggered by the activation of the CF seems to be (a) an excitatory postsynaptic potential capable of activating a Na action potential directly and (b) a large Ca-dependent response of the PC dendrite.

Changes in PC Excitability Following CF Activation: Somatic Recording

While the above records indicate that CF stimulation is accompanied by a complex excitatory response, a more pertinent question is that of the manner in which such response modifies PC excitability. In the slice preparation, the mechanical conditions are such that the electrical properties of intracellularly impaled neurons may be studied in detail for hours. Furthermore, the paring of CF stimulation with direct electrical injection through the recording pipette under such stable electrical conditions permits a high level of reproducibility and, thus, an unambiguous definition of excitability changes that are difficult to obtain in vivo. The study of such interaction reveals that CF activation has two distinct actions on long-term PC excitability and that these two actions relate in an important way to the level of the PC resting potential at the time of the CF activation. Indeed, as shown in Fig. 2A, activation of the CF produces an all-

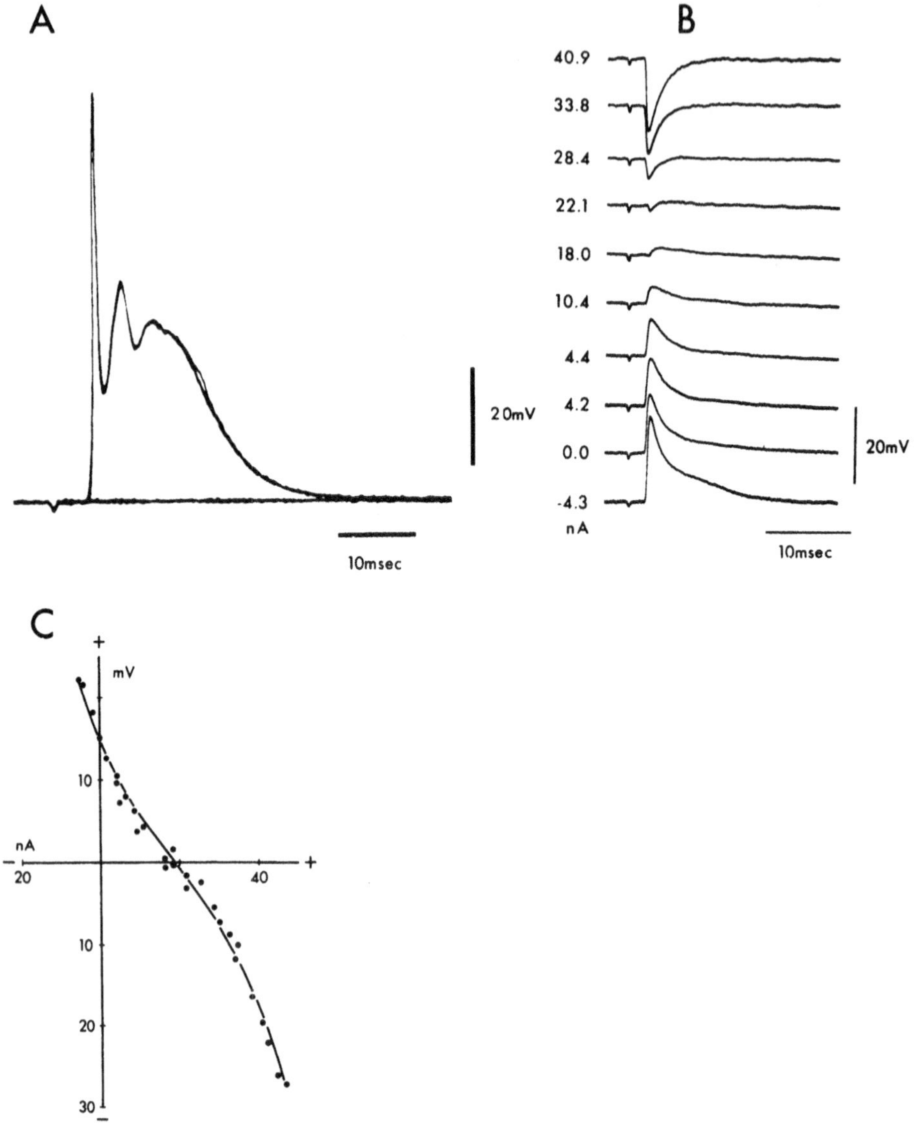

Fig. 1 A–C. Climbing fiber (*CF*) activation of a Purkinje cell (*PC*) from guinea pig cerebellum in vitro. In **A** *PC* response to activation of the *CF*. Note that this all-or-none response consists of a fast action potential followed by a slower after-depolarization (*ADP*) having two peaks. **B** Unitary EPSP produced by activation of the *CF*. Direct current injection (shown in nA to the *left*) in the hyperpolarizing direction produces an increase in EPSP while depolarizing current produces a reduction and then a reversal of the synaptic potential. In this case the reversal is clearly seen at 21.1 nA. **C** Plot of the amplitude of the synaptic potential in mV (*ordinate*) against current injection in the *abscissa*. Llinás and Sugimori [19]

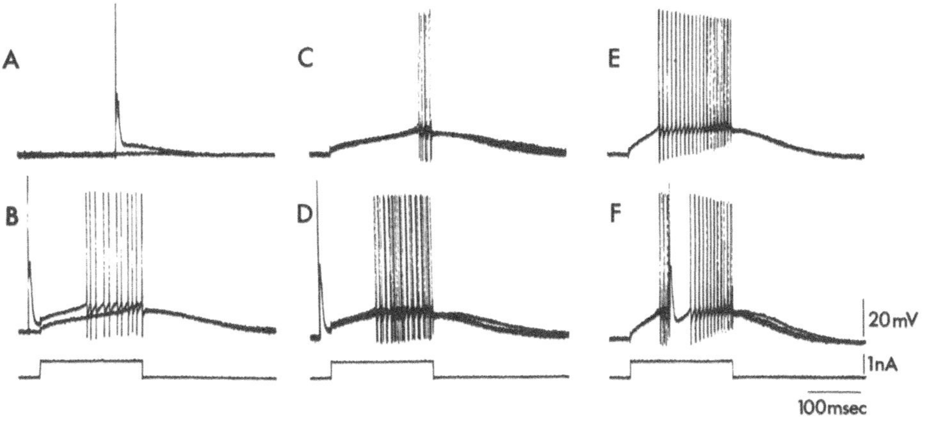

Fig. 2A–F. Interaction between a climbing fiber (*CF*) and direct activation of a Purkinje cell (*PC*) recorded at somatic level. **A** All-or-none response generated in a *PC* by *CF* activation. **B** Direct stimulation of the cell with a square current pulse generates a single action potential. When the pulse is preceded by a *CF* activation, several action potentials are generated by the same current injection. **C** and **D** show the same experiment as in **B.** In **C** square current pulse generates one spike per stimulus; in **D** the increased excitability of the *PC* following *CF* activation is illustrated by the burst of simple spikes which are generated by the same pulse as in **C. E** Increase in the amplitude of the current pulse produces a shower of synchronized action potentials. In **F** *CF* activation during this burst of spikes produces a clear reduction in excitability

or-none complex spike. In Fig. 2B, if the CF activation is followed by a current pulse lasting for 200 ms, which by itself generates one or two spikes at the end of the pulse as shown in Fig. 2C (four superimposed traces), activation of the CF increases the excitability of the PCs such that many action potentials are then generated by the same transmembrane current injection (Fig. 2B, D). The records indicate then that following CF activation of PC cells a delayed increase in excitability is observed for a period of about 100–150 ms from the onset of CF activation, and that such excitability increase may last for several hundreds of milliseconds. It is clear, on the other hand, as seen in Fig. 2A and in the superimposed records of Fig. 2B, that immediately following CF activation there is an ADP which may last 100–150 ms. This prolonged depolarization is often accompanied by a reduction of PC excitability, especially if the resting potential is negative to −65 mV. As the falling phase of the ADP progresses, the aforementioned increase in excitability is encountered, as illustrated in Fig. 2B, where the ADP is followed by rebound activation which reaches threshold for simple spikes.

A direct demonstration of the decreased excitability which follows CF activation can be seen in Fig. 2E and F. In E the trans-somatic current pulse is increased sufficiently to produce trains of simple spikes (three superimposed traces), which have well-defined and reproducible interspike intervals. In F when a CF activation is generated at the center of the simple spike burst, a cessation in firing is seen for a period of approximately 50–100 ms. The duration of this reduction in excitability is related to the amplitude of the stimulating pulse, maximum decrease being observed at threshold depolarization.

Intradendritic Recording

Direct recordings of the type of interactions illustrated above were also obtained following dendritic impalement in the in vitro preparations. In order to determine possible changes in dendritic excitability following CF activation, direct current injection was applied at the dendritic level. In accordance with the finding that full-sized Na-dependent action potentials can only be observed at the somata, in the records shown in Figs. 3 and 4 which were obtained at the dendrite approximately 100 µm from somatic level, Na-dependent spikes are smaller than at the soma [20]. As shown in Fig. 3, following a DC depolarization of the dendrite, a significant modulation of the after-response which follows CF activation may be seen. In this record six traces were superimposed at slightly different levels of depolarization. The initial recording was at −65 mV resting level. The CF activation was initially followed by a depolarization which lasted for about 150 ms and consisted of a plateau and a slowly falling phase. This ADP was followed by a slight hyperpolarization and a return to resting level. With small changes in DC polarization, the amplitude and duration of the ADP increased without generating somatic or dendritic spikes until a slowly rising large dendritic response was generated. This response activated three bursts of somatic spikes and terminated in a full-blown set of dendritic Ca spikes. Such responses may last for 600–800 ms.

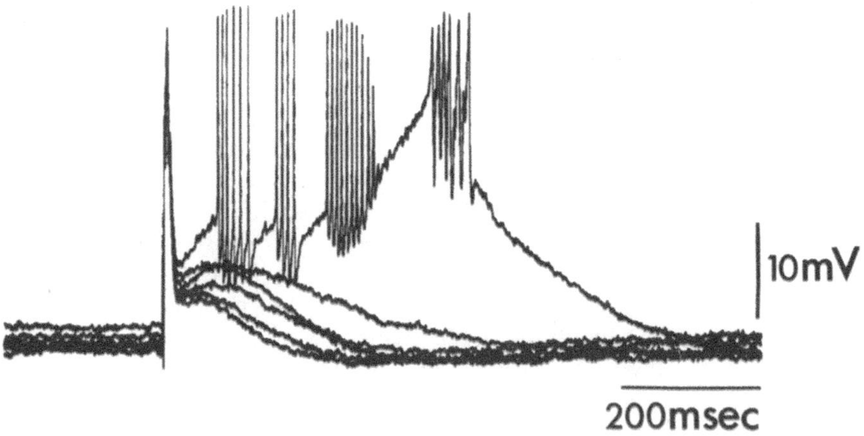

Fig. 3. Intradendritic recording from a Purkinje cell showing climbing fiber (CF) activation. This set of recordings illustrates the effect of depolarizing the cell on the CF response. As the membrane is slowly depolarized, there is a marked increase in the amplitude of the ADP and in the *uppermost* trace a prolonged Ca-dependent response showing both somatic (the three first groups) and a dendritic spike burst (burst to the *right*)

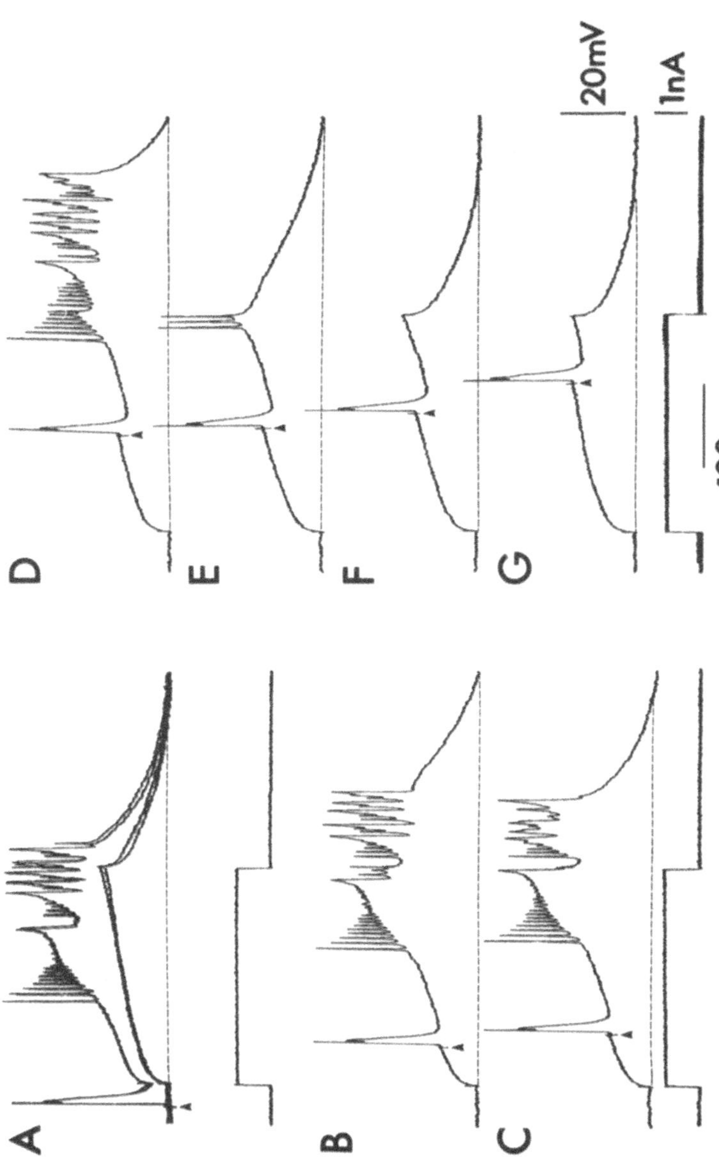

Fig. 4A–G. Changes in excitability produced at dendritic level by climbing fiber (CF) activation. Records obtained by intradendritic recording. In **A** subthreshold depolarization of a dendrite by a square pulse and increased excitability of the dendrite when the square pulse is preceded by CF activation. Note superimposed traces. In **B** to **G** the biphasic excitability change which follows CF activation is illustrated. The CF first decreases excitability and then produces a rebound excitation. This is illustrated by displacing the onset of CF activation (*arrow*) over the square current pulse, which is kept stationary

These records clearly indicate the different responses which may be obtained from PC dendrites when CF activation occurs at different levels of depolarization. Indeed, as demonstrated by direct stimulation at dendritic level [20], two types of Ca-dependent potentials may be obtained in PCs. The plateau type of all-or-none response, which may last for several hundreds of milliseconds and which can generate simple somatic spikes, seems to be produced by the activation of both a voltage- and a Ca-dependent K conductance which generate an equilibrium state represented by the plateau potential [20]. Because of this large conductance change, excitability of the cell at this point may be low.

However, if added to the CF input there is a sufficiently large DC injection to upset this equilibrium, the plateau Ca conductance may be capable of producing a dendritic Ca spike as seen in the uppermost trace of this record. A more direct set of experiments relating to this problem is illustrated for another set of dendritic recordings in Fig. 4. As in Fig. 3, CF activation of this dendrite was generated from a membrane potential such that no secondary Ca spike was generated. Following the CF activation, a subthreshold square wave current pulse was applied across the dendrite. If a CF activation was superimposed on this subthreshold depolarization, a burst of Na spikes followed by a set of dendritic spikes was obtained (Fig. 4 A). Two records were superimposed to show the rather stereotyped nature of this complex response. In Fig. 4 B to G, the stimulus generating CF activation was given at increasing time intervals so that CF activation was generated at different times after the onset of the square pulse. Note that in B and C the rather stereotyped response seen in A was moved to the right but that in B and C the response did not seem to be as sensitive to the exact onset of the CF response. In Fig. 4 D, movement of the stimulus to the right produced a response which outlasted the duration of the direct stimulus. In E, F, and G as the stimulus was further moved to the right, the excitability of the cell was shown to be decreased immediately following CF stimulation, even at a level which previously was capable of activating both somatic and dendritic action potentials.

Discussion

The results illustrated here indicate that CF activation is capable of generating two different types of electroresponsiveness in dendrites and that this electroresponsiveness is deeply related to the level of membrane potential at which CF activation is generated. The first type of response is an ADP whose amplitude and duration may be graded and which is not accompanied by distinct Ca spikes but rather by a plateau-like response. During this response direct activation of the dendrites or soma of the PC may not reach threshold because of the large conductance change which this ADP generates. Indeed this phenomenon may explain the frequently reported "inhibition" of simple spikes which follows CF activation in vivo [1, 2, 10, 21, 27]. The return of PC response to baseline is, on the other hand, accompanied by an increased excitability which may not be observed unless a synaptic input or a direct stimulation is present at the time. In short, the electrophysiological properties of the PC are such that CF activation results in a triphasic excitability change consisting of an early excitation followed by a reduced excitability, itself followed by a rebound excitation. This type of response is, in fact, clearly seen in records such as these shown by ten Bruggencate and colleagues [5] when studying the changes in excitability in Deiters nucleus neurons due to CF activation of PCs. This triphasic excitability is also in accordance with the idea that CFs activate PCs in a rather unique fashion and that such activation is normally quite different from the graded type of PF activation via the PF system. It is, on the other hand, clear that because of the complexities of the electrophysiological responses revealed in these recordings, the precise nature of CF/PF interaction will not be simple to characterize at a given instant since the many variables involved will constantly change the precise nature of the interaction itself. Thus, while the mechanisms for different electrophysiological responses are much clearer now, the final details of the interactions of the two inputs will require a more detailed analysis. At another level of inquiry, several hypotheses have been suggested relating to the ultimate significance of the CF input, ranging from the modifiability of the PF-PC synapse by CF activation to simple short-term interaction between these two systems; this question is still under debate. We believe that ultimately the interaction between these two systems would only be understandable, in a global sense, when taking into account the properties of the cerebellar circuit as a whole [15]. Indeed, in a recent theoretical paper, Pellionisz and Llinás [24] have suggested that the CF system may serve to change a large set of elements in the cerebellar cortex which in geometrical terms may be described as changing the curvature of the n-dimensional vector space represented by the PC firing. If such were to be the case, understanding of the CF-PC junction will require a quite different experimental design from that presently used. Thus, a sufficiently large set of PCs would have to be recorded, simultaneously, in order to make sense of what is in reality a distributed parallel system.

References

1. Bell CC, Grimm RJ (1969) Discharge properties of Purkinje cells recorded on single and double microelectrodes. J Neurophysiol 32:1044–1055
2. Bloedel JR, Roberts WJ (1971) Action of climbing fibers in cerebellar cortex of the cat. J Neurophysiol 34:17–31
3. Bradley P, Berry P (1976) The effects of reduced climbing and parallel fibre input on Purkinje cell dendritic growth. Brain Res 109:133–151
4. Braitenberg V, Atwood RP (1958) Morphological observations on the cerebellar cortex. J Comp Neurol 109:1–34
5. Bruggencate G ten, Teichmann R, Weller E (1972) Neuronal activity in the lateral vestibular nucleus of the cat. III. Inhibitory actions of cerebellar Purkinje cells evoked via mossy and climbing fibre afferents. Pfluegers Arch 337:147–162
6. Crepel F, Delhaye-Bouchaud N (1979) Distribution of climbing fibres on cerebellar Purkinje cells in x-irradiated rats. An electrophysiological study. J Physiol (Lond) 290:97–112
7. Crepel F, Mariani J (1976) Multiple innervation of Purkinje cells by climbing fibres in the cerebellum of the weaver mutant mouse. J Neurobiol 7:579–582
8. Crepel F, Mariani J, Delhaye-Bouchaud N (1976) Evidence for a multiple innervation of Purkinje cells by climbing fibers in the immature rat cerebellum. J Neurobiol 7:567–578
9. Eccles JC, Llinás R, Sasaki K (1966) The excitatory synaptic action of climbing fibres on the Purkinje cells of the cerebellum. J Physiol (Lond) 268–296
10. Granit R, Phillips CG (1956) Excitatory and inhibitory processes acting upon individual Purkinje cells of the cerebellum in cat. J Physiol (Lond) 133:520–547
11. Herndon RM, Oster-Granite ML (1975) Effect of granule cell destruction on development and maintenance of the Purkinje cell dendrite. In: Kreutzberg GW (ed) Physiology and pathology of dendrites, vol. 12. Raven Press, New York, pp 361–371
12. Hillman DE (1969) Neuronal organization of the cerebellar cortex in amphibia and reptilia. In: Llinás R (ed) Neurobiology of cerebellar evolution and development, AMA-ERF, Chicago, pp 279–325
13. Larramendi LMH, Victor T (1967) Synapses on spines of the Purkinje cell of the mouse. An electron microscopic study. Brain Res 5:15–30

14. Llinás R (ed) (1969) Neurobiology of cerebellar evolution and development, AMA-ERF, Chicago
15. Llinás R (1974) 18th Bowditch Lecture: Motor aspects of cerebellar control. Physiologist 17:19–46
16. Llinás R, Bloedel JR, Hillman DE (1969) Functional characterization of the neuronal circuitry of the frog cerebellar cortex. J Neurophysiol 32:847–870
17. Llinás R, Hillman DE, Precht W (1973) Neuronal circuit reorganization in mammalian agranular cerebellar cortex. J Neurobiol 4:69–94
18. Llinás R, Nicholson C (1976) Reversal properties of climbing fiber potential in cat Purkinje cells: An example of a distributed synapse. J Neurophysiol 39:311–323
19. Llinás R, Sugimori M (1980) Electrophysiological properties of *in vitro* Purkinje cell somata in mammalian cerebellar slices. J Physiol (Lond) 305:171–195
20. Llinás R, Sugimori M (1980) Electrophysiological properties of *in vitro* Purkine cell dendrites in mammalian cerebellar slices. J Physiol (Lond) 305:197–213
21. Murphy JT, Sabah NH (1970) Responses of cerebellar Purkinje cells to mossy fiber activation. Brain Res 21:292–296
22. Palay SL, Chan-Palay V (1974) Cerebellar cortex: cytology and organization. Springer-Verlag, Berlin Heidelberg New York
23. Palkovits M, Magyar P, Szentágothai J (1971) Quantitative histological analysis of the cerebellar cortex in the cat. III. Structural organization of the molecular layer. Brain Res 34:1–18
24. Pellionisz A, Llinás R (1979) Brain modeling by tensor network theory and computer simulation. The cerebellum: parallel processor for predictive coordination. Neuroscience 4:323–348
25. Ramón y Cajal S (1911) Histologie du système nerveux de l'homme et des vertébrés, vol II. Maloine, Paris. Translated by L Azoulay
26. Sotelo C, Hillman DE, Zamora AJ, Llinás R (1975) Climbing fiber deafferentation: its action on Purkinje cell dendritic spines. Brain Res 98:574–581
27. Thach WT (1967) Somatosensory receptive fields of single units in cat cerebellar cortex. J Neurophysiol 30:675–696

Discussion

Krnjevic asked why, if the plateau depolarization were generated by a calcium current, the calcium influx did not lead to a potassium efflux which in turn should terminate the plateau depolarization. Dr. Llinás cited evidence from experiments in which sodium was removed from or tetrodotoxin was added to the bathing solution. This evidence indicated that the plateau was calcium mediated and suggested that in fact potassium conductance was increased to some extent by the calcium current. The plateau, which is at a less positive level than the expected calcium equilibrium potential, may result from an equilibrium of increased calcium *and* potassium conductance. This is indicated by the injection of tetraethylammonium into the neuron, which results in plateaus set at much more positive potentials. Such injections also block the phase of high potassium conductance and the cyclical firing following climbing fiber activation.

Chan-Palay inquired whether slices could be taken in the transverse plane to facilitate comparison of electrophysiological properties of Purkinje cells by sampling along the same band. Dr. Llinás replied that in 200 μm slices taken in the transverse plane cells survived poorly. In comparisons from cell to cell of the various ionic conductances described, he finds that the calcium conductance changes are quite similar, and that the greatest difference is seen in the injected current/firing frequency ratio. This difference may be related to variations in amounts of noninactivating sodium current from cell to cell.

Eccles was concerned whether such results as the calcium plateau might be a property of cells in slices, since such observations had not been reported in animal studies. Dr. Llinás responded by showing a slide from some of their earlier animal studies (ref. [9], Fig. 12C–D), showing a prolonged depolarization in a Purkinje cell following climbing fiber activation; he expressed the view that such results had been observed in animal studies though their significance was not appreciated.

Krnjevic mentioned that at least in hippocampal slices, one difference from animal studies is that neuron input resistances are higher in the slices, perhaps reflecting less ongoing inhibitory synaptic activity and thus less maintained chloride conductance. An apparent difference between the hippocampal and Purkinje neurons is that in the hippocampus there is evidence that by far the largest calcium influx is in the cell bodies and not in the dendrites. Dr. Llinás agreed that input resistances are higher in slices and suggested that this might explain the clearer demonstration in slices of the potential changes that he had described.

Ito asked whether, since some of the evidence is based on calcium-free bathing solutions and calcium-current blockers, some of the observed phenomena could be related to calcium-dependent, synaptically transmitted events. Dr. Llinás replied that they had in fact suggested that some of the calcium current could be enhanced by the release of substances from the dendrites.

Palay inquired whether the dendritic branch points might specifically exhibit some of these ionic conductance properties, since these are the most likely points of electrode penetration in the dendritic tree, and since there are special synaptic arrangements of both climbing fibers and basket axons about these joints. Dr. Llinás suggested that a calcium channel marker is required to determine their distribution and to answer such interesting questions.

Field Effect and Chemical Transmission: Dual Inhibitory Action of Basket Cells in the Rat Cerebellar Cortex

H. Axelrad and H. Korn

Introduction

So far, there is perhaps no structure in the mammalian central nervous system which is understood better than the cerebellar cortex, at least at the level of the properties, organization, and performance of its circuitry [10]. In confirmation of R. y. Cajal's predictions [42], the model of the cerebellar organization and networks drawn from morphological and electrophysiological data was shown to be valid in its basic features for the cerebellar cortices of the whole phylum, from the lower forms to higher mammals.

Despite this wealth of information, little is still known about the functioning of the intrinsic cerebellar pathways under conditions other than those of acute experimentation. In fact, some characteristics of the cerebellar basic design remain to be explained, even in these experimental situations. For instance, the inhibitory role of cerebellar interneurons is well established, but the investigations of these cells could not take into consideration the later important finding of Sotelo and Llinás [45] that in the molecular layer of at least some species, these inhibitory cells bear typical dendrosomatic and dendrodendritic gap junctions; in other structures, electrophysiological studies have shown that these specialized junctions may have the role of synchronizing the firing of coupled neurons (for a review see refs. [4–6]). Thus, it can be speculated that in some physiological situations which have not yet been unraveled, gap junctions provide a synchronous activation of, for instance, basket cells which may be quite important in the organization of neuronal subsets in the cerebellum.

Another morphological peculiarity, the physiological significance of which remains to be elucidated, is the so-called pinceau established by basket-cell axon terminals converging on the Purkinje cell initial segment. Numerous descriptions deal with this unusual formation [42] and are summarized by Mugnaini [35], Palay and Chan-Palay [39]. Figure 1 shows its principal characteristics: the descending collaterals of the basket cell axons reach the soma and Purkinje cell initial segment and terminate in groups of digitiform endings, only a few of which contact the surface of the Purkinje cell axon (Somogyi and Hamori, 1976). These few synapses are located at the proximal part of the initital segment and exhibit the typical structure of chemically mediating junctions. The rest of the surface of the initial segment is ensheathed in neuroglial processes [39]. The small number of synaptic terminals indicates that at most only one or two of the numerous collaterals in the pinceau end in this manner, all others ending freely. This whole brushlike region is totally surrounded by

Experimental Brain Research, Suppl. 6

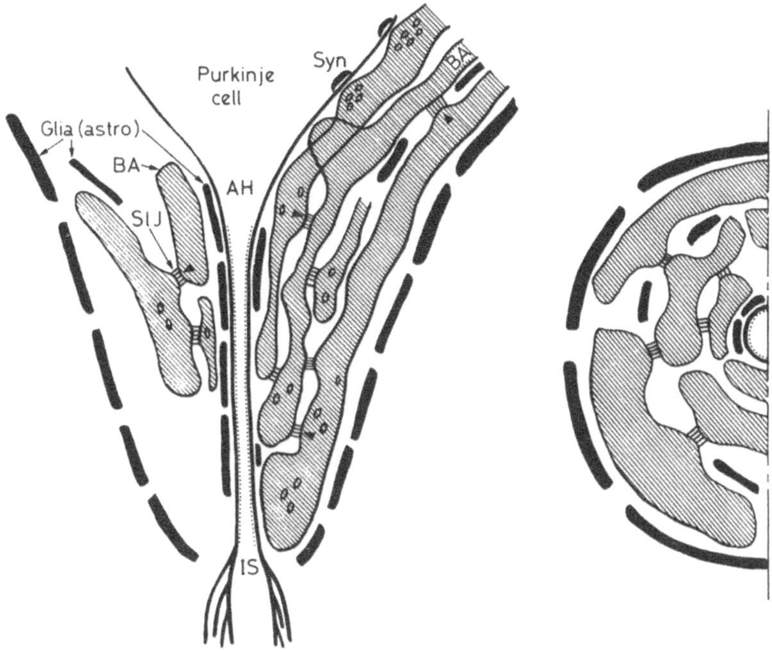

Fig. 1. Diagram showing the relations of a Purkinje cell's initial segment with its associated pinceau. Drawing of axonal pole of a Purkinje cell in the vertical (*left*) and horizontal (*right*) planes. Axons of several basket cells (*BA*) converge around the axon hillock (*AH*) of a Purkinje cell (*PC*), where they form the pericellular basket, after establishing chemical synapses (*Syn*) at the base of the soma. Below this region, the finger-shaped processes of basket axon endings descend along the unmyelinated segment (*IS*) of the Purkinje cell, which receives few, if any, chemical synapses, and they constitute the so-called pinceau around it. The fibers of this brushlike structure produce among themselves axoaxonic septate-like junctions (*triangles*) and they are intermingled with astrocyte processes (*glia*). Neuroglial cells also cover most of the emerging axon and ensheath the entire pericellular nest, thus giving this region a morphology similar to that of the teleostean Mauthner cell axon cap

glia of the astrocytic type and thus appears to be similar in its organization to that of the teleostean Mauthner-cell axon cap.

Inquiry into the functional meaning of this peculiar structure has led to a number of controversies. Its strategic location, close to the cell-spike-initiating zone, appears well adapted for an inhibitory synapse, and Eccles, Ito, and Szentagothai [10] postulated that the prolonged inhibitory action of the basket cells on the Purkinje cells might be accounted for by the accumulation and slow dissipation of transmitter around the initial segment due to this region's encapsulation. This hypothesis does not, however, consider all the aspects of this region's ultrastructure (see [39]). Furthermore, recent evidence indicates that prolonged inhibitory postsynaptic potentials in another vertebrate central neuron may be accounted for by the kinetics of single activated channels [19]. Again, the issue turned out to be more complex when it appeared that axons of the pinceau are bound together by peculiar junctions described both in the cat

[23] and in the cat and rat [39, 45]. These formations are characterized by transverse septa which stretch at regular intervals across the space between axons, like the rungs of a ladder, and contain dense particles arrayed regularly within the interstices, in a honeycomb pattern. Sotelo and Llinás [45] proposed that they be named "septate-like" junctions. This discovery reinforced earlier suggestions by Palay [38] of a similarity of structure and therefore of function of both the pinceau and the teleostean Mauthner-cell axon cap. To illustrate this analogy, which had also been favored by Mugnaini [35], Sotelo and Llinás [45] and Palay and Chan-Palay [39] postulated that the pinceau would distribute the outward action currents of the basket cell end feet as a vertical sleeve around the Purkinje cell axon, thus blocking the latter, but they presented no physiological evidence for this tempting hypothesis.

In order to determine whether Purkinje cells are subjected to an electrical inhibition imposed upon them by basket cell terminals, we have investigated the effects exerted on these neurons by a parallel-fiber volley, which, as shown by a number of authors, monosynaptically excites Purkinje cells and disynaptically inhibits them through cortical inhibitory interneurons [10]. With this procedure we expected to detect an early peak of inhibition preceding the classical chemically mediated (EPSP-IPSP) sequence set up by activation of the parallel fibers. In contrast to the negative findings of Eccles and others and of numerous investigators who, subsequently, explored the cerebellar cortex, we found, using both field potential analysis and extracellular recordings, that a fast mediated peak of inhibition is indeed the first event that can be observed at the level of the Purkinje cells following a parallel-fiber volley. This finding was made possible because, unlike other authors, we used very short increments when progressively delaying conditioning parallel-fiber volleys and testing antidromic activation of Purkinje cells. These first results, which were briefly reported [2], were confirmed and explained satisfactorily by intracellular recordings, which showed [3] that the inhibitory events were correlated both in time and amplitude with passive hyperpolarizing potentials, the properties of which are similar to those observed in the Mauthner cell system [27] and more generally to inhibitory potentials mediated by field effects.

The model for generation of field effects requires that presynaptic elements are passively invaded by action currents and that they behave as an external anode. The best candidates for generation of passive hyperpolarizing potentials in the Purkinje cells would be basket cells since they are the only adjacent presynaptic elements to these neurons at the level of their initial segment, but then a difficult problem has to be faced. Since the passive hyperpolarizing potential (indicating firing of basket cells) evoked by a parallel-fiber volley precedes the EPSP recorded in Purkinje cells, it follows that although both events result from a monosynaptic activation by a common input, basket cells must be activated prior to Purkinje cells by the same stimulus. A comparison of the firing latencies of these two classes of cells was thus performed and gave us indications, not reported previously, that basket cells fire earlier than their postsynaptic targets, their action potentials being well correlated with the early electrically mediated inhibition. These results which were partly reported in a previous note [3] will be described in a more detailed manner in this paper: they are in good agreement with morphological data indicating that parallel fibers in the deep molecular layer are usually thicker than those located superficially and could therefore have a higher conduction velocity [35, 39].

Material and Methods

Experiments were performed on young, adult, male albino rats of 150–180 g body weight, anesthetized with 35 mg/kg sodium pentobarbital injected intraperitoneally, paralyzed with gallamine triethiodide (3.0 mg/kg), and artificially respired. The cerebellar vermis was exposed with care being taken to prevent air embolism, the cisterna magna opened, and the lobules covered with a 4% agar gel in 10% sucrose in order to minimize pulsations. The rectal temperature was maintained constant (37–38 °C) throughout the entire experiment by means of a heating pad, and additional doses of drugs were injected when needed.

The experimental technique was similar to the classical one used in other species [12], and its basic design is illustrated in Fig. 2A. A flat tip, bipolar con-

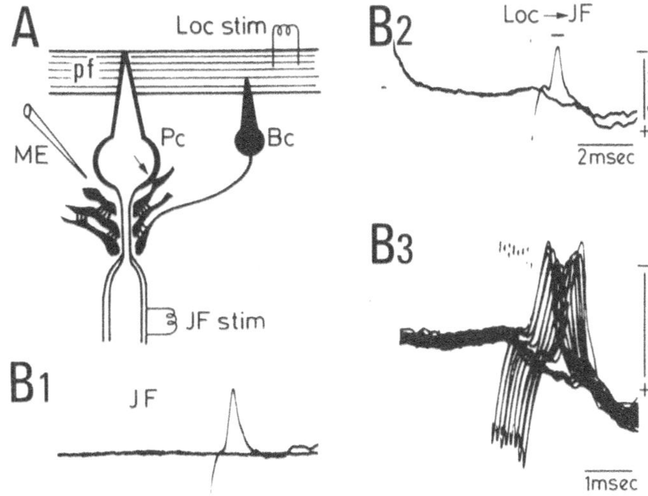

Fig. 2A–B$_3$. Depression of Purkinje cell antidromic field potential following a parallel fiber volley. **A** Diagram of the experimental setup. A concentric bipolar electrode (*Loc stim*) was placed on the surface of the cerebellar cortex to activate a beam of parallel fibers (*pf*) common to a set of basket (*Bc*) and Purkinje (*Pc*) cells, and the latter were antidromically activated through a bipolar electrode placed in the white matter near the fastigial nucleus (*JF stim*). The recording microelectrode, which was positioned near or at the level of the Purkinje cell soma layer, is also illustrated. **B$_1$–B$_3$** Early inhibition of an antidromic field potential, evoked by a juxtafastigial stimulus and by a conditioning Loc stimulus (*Loc →JF*). **B$_1$** Control antidromic field potential (two superimposed traces, with and without a *JF* stimulus). **B$_2$** Reduction in the size of the antidromic spike potential as it was timed to occur at the onset of the positive phase of the conditioning Loc-evoked field potential (two superimposed traces, one with and one without a *JF* stimulus). The *horizontal bar* indicates the amplitude of the control antidromic field, which is illustrated in **B$_1$**. **B$_3$** Expanded sweeps of a series of traces obtained when test *JF* stimuli were successively delayed by intervals of 100 µs from the onset of the Loc stimulus

centric electrode placed at the surface of the cerebellar cortex (Loc stimulus) served to excite a beam of parallel fibers. A pair of silver wires insulated except at their tip and glued 0.4 mm apart was inserted in the cerebellar white matter near the fastigial nucleus (JF stimulus) for antidromically activating Purkinje cells and/or evoking their charcteristic climbing-fiber responses. Rectangular pulses 0.1 ms in duration were delivered through these electrodes by constant-current isolated units. Glass micropipettes filled with 2M NaCl (2–10 MΩ) and 3M KCl (12–30 MΩ) for extra- and intracellular recordings respectively, were driven vertically through the most superficial layers of the cortex in previously determined regions of maximal Loc and JF responses, "on-beam" experiments being defined as those during which the microelectrode was inserted along tracks that passed through the parallel-fiber volley set up by the Loc stimulus. Intracellularly recorded data were stored on magnetic tape for further analysis with a Nicolet 1074 averager.

In some instances, special techniques were used: (a) to discriminate between field effect and chemically mediated inhibitions, picrotoxin (2–4 mg/kg), an antagonist of GABA, the presumed inhibitory transmitter of basket cells [25] was intravenously injected for a series of experiments; (b) in another series, the beam of parallel fibers activated by the Loc stimulus was blocked with xylocaine applied between the stimulating and recording electrodes, by pressure injection through a broken tip micropipette; (c) to avoid complications from stimulus spread to deep mossy or climbing fibers a series of rats were deafferented 1–5 days prior to recording. For this purpose, animals were heavily anesthetized and the technique originally used in cats by Eccles, Llinás and Sasaki [13] was adapted to our experimental material: the head was inclined forward, the occipital bone was completely removed, and the caudal part of the vermis was lifted to visualize the floor of the fourth ventricle. It was thus possible to cut the peduncles bilaterally while reducing bleeding to a minimum. Following the pedunculotomy, a protective muscle flap was created over the craniotomy. Histological verifications performed after experiments showed that in all animals (n=10), both inferior and middle peduncles had been completely cut, whereas the superior ones remained partially undamaged.

Results

The time course of a short latency inhibitory effect upon Purkinje cells was investigated by means of several experimental techniques. For field potential analysis and extracellular recordings conditioning Loc stimuli, at constant stimulus strength and of intensities 1.5–2.5 above threshold for initiating a parallel-fiber volley, were paired with juxtafastigial stimuli above threshold for antidromic activation of Purkinje cells. Recordings were performed in the Purkinje cell soma layer. Test/control curves were obtained by progressively increasing interstimuli intervals by steps of no more than 0.5 ms. Figure 2 B_1–B_3 illustrates the basic finding that led us to believe in the reality of a short latency Loc-evoked inhibitory effect: the field potential generated by antidromic excitation of Purkinje cells was reduced in amplitude by the conditioning stimulus when it was set to occur as early as the onset of the positive-going wave of the Loc-evoked field potential (Fig. 2 B_1, B_2), that is, at the arrival time of the earliest impulses in activated parallel fibers at that depth. This inhibitory action had a short duration, as in some cases the test field potential recovered its control amplitude (Fig. 2 B_3) before the occurrence of the classic phases of facilitation and chemically mediated inhibition described by Eccles and collaborators [13]. Using the same experimental pattern it was confirmed at a unitary level that these phases of depression corresponded to a blockage of Purkinje cell antidromic activation.

Early Inhibitory Effect of a Parallel-Fiber Volley Upon the Purkinje Cell Antidromic Field Potential

Surface stimulation through the Loc electrode results in the excitation of a narrow beam of parallel fibers. When recorded in the first few microns beneath the pial surface, as shown by Fig. 3 A_1, this afferent volley is represented by a triphasic wave and is followed by a slow negativity which, as in the cat [14] is likely to reflect the subsequent postsynaptic activation of Purkinje cells. The arrival of the presynaptic volley under the recording microelectrode is signaled by the peak of the initial positive going potential (Fig. 3 A_1, arrow, and 3 A_2). This positivity was used as a reference to analyze our records and to compare them reliably from one experiment to another, in order to avoid complications introduced by the less reliable method of computing delays from stimulus artifact, this latter interval being proportional to the distance separating stimulation and recording electrodes.

A typical test/control curve obtained as the microelectrode track was placed on-beam for the excited parallel fibers is illustrated in Fig. 3. The conditioning field potential set up by the Loc stimulation and recorded at the depth of the Purkinje cell layer is shown in Fig. 3 A_3; the amplitude of the tested antidromic field potential is plotted at the same time scale in Fig. 3 A_4. The activation of Purkinje cells by the presynaptic volley appears in both the deeply recorded volley and in the histogram of A_4, which was obtained with extracellular recordings from a cell at the same depth as the field potential (not illustrated here). This excitation was followed by an early depression of the juxtafastigial-evoked antidromic field potential (which can be attributed to collision along the axons of the activated Purkinje cells) and by a subsequent phase of depression which reduced the antidromic field potential by as much as 30% of its control value. This peak of inhibition corresponds to the P wave of the deeply recorded Loc-evoked field potential and is brought about by chemically mediated inhibition from cortical interneurons, including basket cells [15]. An early peak of inhibition preceded both excitation and chemical inhibition and manifested itself as a reduction of the antidromic tested field potential by about 8% of its original value (hatched area in Fig. 3 A_4). This phase, which started 0.2 ms after the superficially recorded parallel-fiber volley and lasted about 1 ms, corresponded in time to the early depression obtained in the experiment illustrated by Fig. 2 B_1-B_2. Comparable results were obtained in 15 on-beam

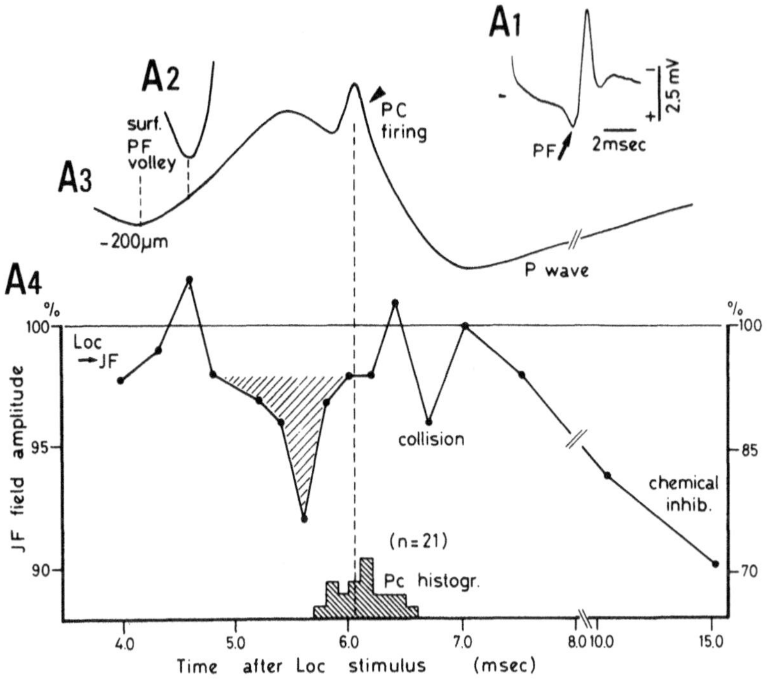

Fig. 3A$_{1-4}$. Inhibitory action of a parallel-fiber volley on the Purkinje cell antidromic invasion. **A$_1$**, **A$_2$**, triphasic field potential recorded on-beam at the surface of a folium after a Loc stimulus. A$_1$, full sweep showing the configuration of this potential; a sharp initial positivity (*arrow*) indicates the time of arrival of the superficial parallel-fiber volley at the recording site. **A$_2$**, this positive peak is illustrated alone at the same magnification as that of **A$_3$**; for this and similar subsequent figures the stimulus artifacts of the two sweeps were aligned along the same *vertical line* (not shown). **A$_3$** field potential evoked by a Loc stimulus of the same intensity as that used for **A$_1$** and **A$_2$**, and recorded along the same track but 200 µm below the cortical surface; Purkinje cell activation (*arrowhead*) is followed by the classic *P wave* generated by action currents underlying the chemically mediated phase of Purkinje cell inhibition by inhibitory interneurons of the molecular layer. Note that at this depth, the parallel-fiber volley (*first dashed line*) has shorter latency than at most superficial levels (*second dashed line* in **A$_2$**). **A$_4$**, inhibitory action of a parallel-fiber volley on the antidromic spike potential of Purkinje cells; interstimuli intervals were progressively delayed by steps of less than 500 µs. The *time scale* is given with respect to the beginning of the stimulus artifact of the Loc stimuls (not shown). Each point of the graph represents the size of the conditioned antidromic field potential expressed as the percentage of the control response (mean of ten trials for each interval). The first event apparent on the plot is an early inhibition (*hatched area*), which occurs after the arrival of the surface presynaptic volley and before the activation of Purkinje cells. The maximum reduction of the antidromic field potential in this experiment was about 10%, and its duration was of the order of 1 ms. It was preceded by a slight facilitation of the antidromic field potential which can be attributed to Purkinje cell excitation via mossy-fiber collaterals by spread of the Loc stimulating current (see text). Following the parallel-fiber-evoked firing of the Purkinje cells, there was a slight depression of the field due to collision between ortho- and antidromically evoked spikes travelling along their axons. Subsequently, the classical chemically mediated inhibition was evidenced by a reduction in the size of the antidromic field to 70% of its control value (same *time scale* for **A$_3$** and **A$_4$**)

experiments, which also confirmed that the early peak of inhibition has a short duration of 0.8–1.5 ms compared to that of 15–25 ms (with often a rebound from 40–70 ms later) for the chemically mediated one; its inhibitory effect was variable, but in all cases, was less powerful: it produced a mean reduction of 12% (SD=8.5; range 5–35%) in the size of the antidromic field in contrast to 38% (SD=16%; range 18–70%) for the chemically mediated phase. Nevertheless, when correctly timed, the antidromic field potential was not only reduced in amplitude by the conditioning stimulus but, in some cases, it was fractionated into several components, thus indicating that this inhibition can either block or delay initiation of spikes depending upon the respective timing of the conditioning and tested responses. Comparable figures were obtained in five experiments where the tip of the recording microelectrode was placed slightly "off-beam" from the activated set of parallel fibers.

Finally, Fig. 3 A_4 shows that a slight facilitation manifested itself as an increase in the antidromic field potential spike height, was produced before or at the time of arrival of the superficial parallel-fiber volley (first vertical dashed line in Fig. 3 A_3–A_4). As we shall see in the next section, this facilitatory effect is brought about by activation of fast conducting mossy fiber branches via current spread to the granular layer and therefore by introducing an axon reflex loop along a pathway illustrated in the diagram of Fig. 5. As a consequence, some Purkinje cells would be depolarized before the arrival of the Loc-evoked

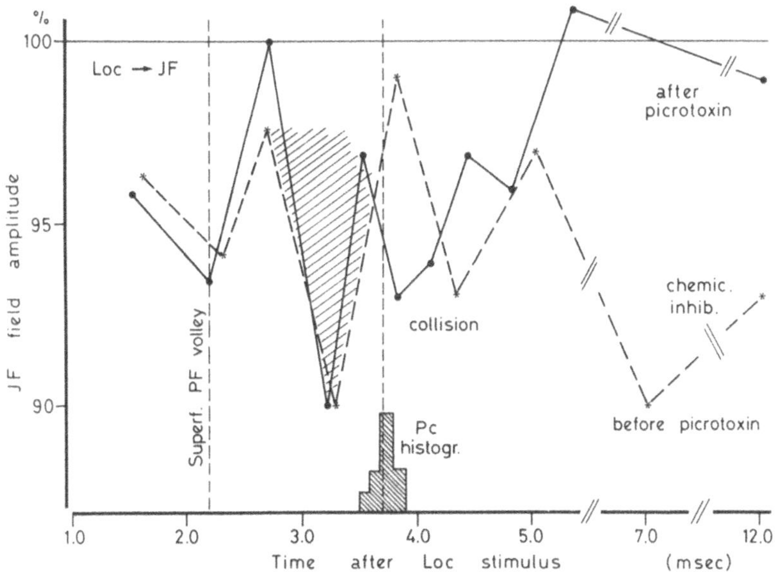

Fig. 4. Lack of effect of picrotoxin on the early Loc-evoked inhibition of Purkinje cells. Two similar plots obtained as for Fig. 3 A_4; one corresponds to control data (*dashed lines*), the other (*solid line*) was computed during the same experiment, after intravenous injection of 3 mg/kg of picrotoxin, the stimulating and recording electrodes remaining at the same site. The main effect of the drug was to suppress the late chemically mediated inhibition; in contrast, the earlier peak of reduction of the conditioned tested antidromic (*hatched area*) response remained undisturbed, in both amplitude and time course

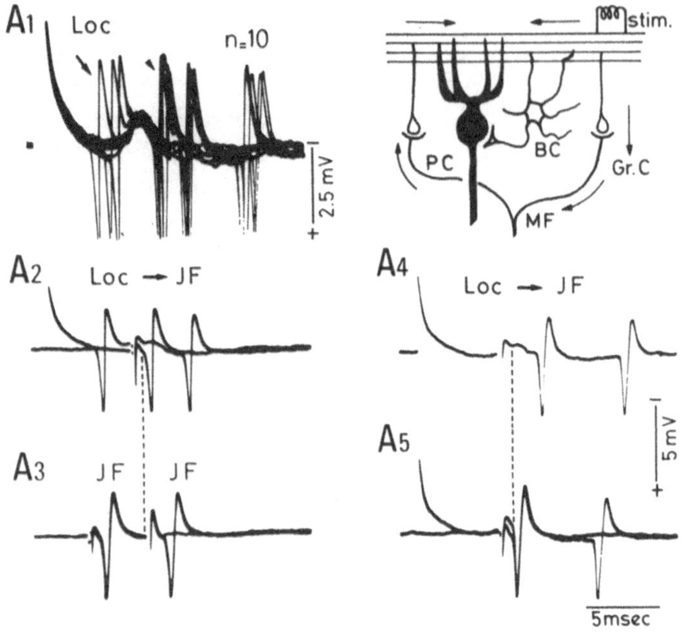

Fig. 5A_{1-5}. Early inhibitory influence produced by a parallel-fiber volley on antidromic spikes of Purkinje cells. $A_1 - A_5$, extracellular recordings obtained from a Purkinje cell. A_1, a Loc stimulus about 2.5 times above threshold for activation of the Purkinje cell evoked in this neuron a train of three orthodromic spiked (a *triangle* indicates the onset of this burst), which were preceded at times by a short-latency action potential (*arrow*). Ten superimposed traces are shown in this series of recordings. The first group of spikes was presumably due to current spread to the fast-conducting mossy fibers situated beneath the stimulating electrode, as indicated in the diagram of the figure, with a consequent activation of the granule-cell–parallel-fiber pathway along an axon reflex-loop (*arrows*), bringing about activation of the Purkinje cells before their subsequent excitation by the more slowly conducting beam of parallel fibers. A_2, A_3, block of antidromic spikes during the refractory period of a Purkinje cell axon. A_2, a juxtafastigial stimulus failed to evoke an antidromic action potential after a spike was produced in the same cell by activation of the fast-conducting, mossy-fiber pathway (two superimposed traces with and without Loc stimulation). A_3, the relative refractory period of this neuron's axon was evidenced by adequately paired juxtafastigial stimulation (two superimposed traces). A comparison of the recordings illustrated in A_2 and A_3 unambiguously shows that in A_2 the antidromic spike fell during the recorded cell's refractory period, when it was preceded by the conditioning action potential (*vertical dashed line*). A_4, A_5, early inhibition of a Purkinje cell by a parallel-fiber volley. A_4, a properly adjusted Loc stimulus could block an antidromic spike, but A_5 this effect was weak and often failed during some trials (one trace with and one without Loc stimulation)

presynaptic volley. Data obtained from single-cell recordings seem to confirm this interpretation as well as those obtained from deafferented animals in which a short latency facilitatory action was abolished.

Although they exhibit different properties, such as their latency and time course, the two peaks of inhibition are likely to be mediated by a common set of interneurons, as already indicated by several lines of evidence. For instance, test/control curves obtained with Loc stimulations of various intensities showed that both types of inhibition varied in parallel. Also, when the beam of activated parallel fibers was blocked with xylocaine, both early and late inhibitions disappeared concomitantly with the Loc-evoked firing of the Purkinje cell; in contrast, there was no change in the amplitude of the control antidromic field after this blockage, thus showing that the observed effects could not be explained by the diffusion of the drug to the electrode recording site (not illustrated).

Field potential analysis suggests that the early Loc-evoked inhibition is generated by a mechanism different from that of the late chemically mediated one. Picrotoxin was intravenously injected and test/control curves were compared before and after injection of the drug. Identical results were obtained in four experiments, one of which is illustrated by Fig. 4. In this case, the control chemical inhibition was rather weak (dashed lines), a fact which may be due to a low level of anesthesia [11]. The injection of picrotoxin totally suppressed this phase of inhibition (solid lines) while the early inhibitory peak remained unchanged but for a slight reduction of its latency. Both the activation of Purkinje cells and the subsequent reduction of the antidromic field due to collision with orthodromic spikes were still present, thus illustrating the specificity of the action of picrotoxin.

Early Inhibition of Antidromic Invasion of Purkinje Cells

Single Purkinje cells were identified at the unitary level by their short latency antidromic spikes produced by JF stimulation and/or their climbing-fiber responses [12]. These cells were orthodromically excited by Loc stimulation, to which they responded with one or two spikes, occasionally followed at higher stimulus strength by a third action potential. Evidence for an early peak of Loc-evoked inhibition was already obtained from the simple procedure of repeated stimulations through the Loc electrode. This finding is illustrated by Fig. 5 A_1 for which ten traces were superimposed. Purkinje cells were first activated with a short and unstable latency (arrow) which corresponded in time to the period of facilitation observed with field potentials (Fig. 3 A_4). These spikes, presumably evoked by a deep mossy-fiber pathway, and those produced directly by parallel fibers (triangle in Fig. 5 A_1) were separated by a silent period 1–2 ms in duration. This interval is concomitant with the early depression disclosed by experiments during which the antidromic field potential was conditioned by a Loc stimulus and with the timing of Loc-evoked block of antidromic invasion to be described below, see also Fig. 9 B_5. Before ascertaining that an antidromic spike was really blocked by a specific inhibitory effect when conditioned by a parallel-fiber volley, it appeared necessary to eliminate those cases in which collision and/or refractoriness following the mossy-fiber-activated responses would bring about a depression of Purkinje cell excitability. For instance, in the experiment of Fig. 5, the antidromic spike illustrated in A_2 was blocked by a conditioning Loc stimulation which also evoked an "early mossy-fiber pathway" action potential just before the juxtafastigial stimulus. In this case, the blocking effect of the Loc stimulus itself was thus masked by the refractory period of the Purkinje cell axon. This is shown by a comparison of A_2 (vertical

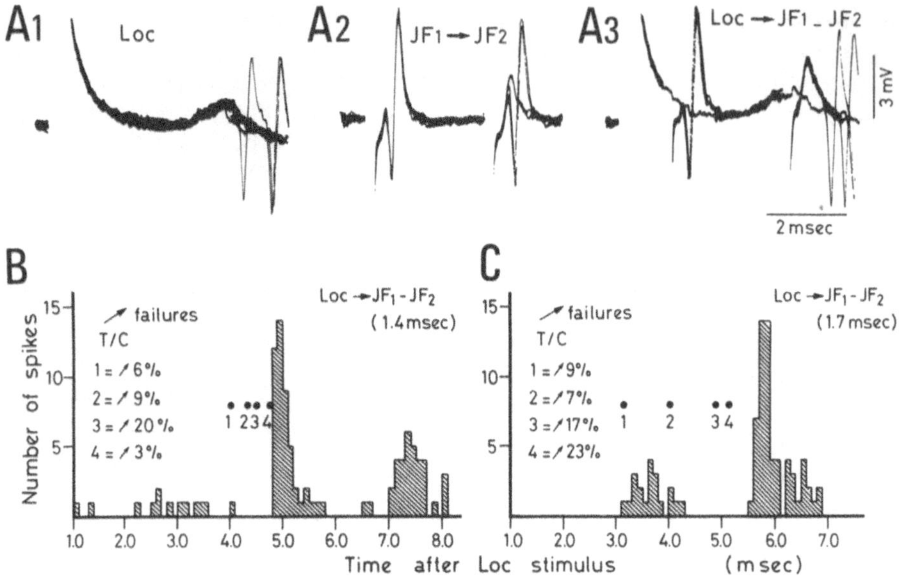

Fig. 6A$_1$–C. Enhancement of the early Loc-evoked inhibition during the relative refractory period of Purkinje cell axons. **A$_1$–A$_3$**, sample extracellular recordings illustrating the method used to unmask the short latency inhibitory effect of a parallel-fiber volley. **A$_1$**, control responses of a Purkinje cell to a Loc stimulation; **A$_2$**, the relative refractory period, as evaluated with adequately paired juxta-fastigial stimulations, was for this neuron, about 2.9 ms; **A$_3$**, the second action potential of paired antidromic spikes was suppressed in all trials when it was timed to occur just before synaptically evoked spikes of the Purkinje cell. **B, C,** diagram of the early suppression of antidromic spikes obtained from two different Purkinje cells under the conditions described above. The latency histograms of their impulse patterns following Loc activation are shown on the *abscissae.* Note that during about 1 ms before the response of the Purkinje cell to the parallel-fiber volley there is a complete silence which is already suggestive of an active inhibitory process occurring at this time. Each *dot* corresponds to a test point where the second spike of *JF–JF* stimuli was timed to fall (the JF stimulus interval is indicated in *brackets* and it falls for each cell within its relative refractory period). The increase in the number of failures (test versus control) at each of the tested points is given on the *left* of the diagrams. It appears that the blocking effect of a parallel-fiber volley is significantly most efficient during the short period preceding activation of the Purkinje cells by the Loc-evoked parallel-fiber volley

dashed line) with Fig. 5A$_3$ which illustrates a block of the second spike during the refractory period of the investigated cell, as determined by paired juxtafastigial stimulations. Nevertheless, blocking effects which were unambiguously due to the Loc stimulation were observed in the absence of a prior Purkinje cell firing, as shown by Fig. 5A$_4$, where a supramaximal juxtafastigial stimulus failed to evoke an antidromic spike when conditioned by activated parallel fibers; as expected from field potential experiments, this Loc-evoked block took place as the antidromic action potential was timed to fall just before the orthodromically evoked Purkinje cell's spike.

A comparison of Fig. 5A$_4$ and A$_5$ demonstrates that the early depression of the Purkinje cell following a Loc stimulus was weak, and repeated trials with single antidromically evoked spikes were necessary to establish its significance statistically. The sensitivity of this test was therefore enhanced by using paired JF stimulations timed adequately to evoke the second antidromic spike during the relative refractory period of the Purkinje cell axon (intervals corresponding to 50% failures were selected for this series of experiments). At this time, the safety factor for impulse transmission from the axon to the initial segment is lowered [9] and any inhibitory action taking place near the region of the Purkinje cell initial segment would be facilitated. Figure 6 demonstrates that such was the case; as shown by the sample records of A_1-A_3, the second of two antidromic spikes separated by 2.9 ms, which was within the relative refractory period of this cell, was easily blocked during the period preceding this neuron's excitation by a conditioning Loc stimulus. We therefore used this technique to study the occurrence, effectiveness, and duration of the early Loc-evoked inhibition; quantitative measurements were obtained by counting the number of failures in the conditioned test situation, taking as a control the number of failures attributable to refractoriness alone.

The results of two such experiments are illustrated in Fig. 6B and C. The graphs represent the poststimulus time histograms of two different Purkinje cells which responded to monosynaptic parallel fiber input with one spike in C and two spikes in B. Each histogram demonstrated that an early and presumably mossy-fiber pathway response was present at times. The already mentioned silent period which separates the two groups of impulses is particularly evident in C. The second spike evoked by paired JF stimulation (each interval used being indicated in brackets) was timed to fall before the Loc-evoked response at different instants which are shown as numbered black dots. The increased percentages of failures relative to the control situations are indicated for each of these intervals and it is obvious that there is a circumscribed inhibitory period in both B and C.

In a series of 15 such experiments, the maximum blocking effect was found to occur during the 0.2–0.8 ms preceding excitation of the Purkinje cell by the parallel-fiber volley and it could be sufficiently effective to increase the number of failures by nearly 50%; intracellular recordings confirmed that for ten of these neurons inhibitory postsynaptic potentials (IPSPs) always started well after the period of depressed excitability.

Passive Hyperpolarizing Potentials in Purkinje Cells

Intracellular recordings were performed in identified Purkinje cells to determine if, as suggested by data from earlier experiments, a transmembrane hyperpolarization underlies the short latency inhibitory action evoked in these neurons by a parallel-fiber volley. Figure 7 is from such an experiment. A Loc stimulus produced a negative-going potential followed by an EPSP-IPSP sequence (A_1-A_4); the excitatory potential was, as in most experiments, below firing level for spike initiation and when impulses were evoked (Fig. 7A_1), it appeared that the action potential generating mechanism deteriorated rapidly (A_2-A_4), although the quality of the impalement remained quite stable, as

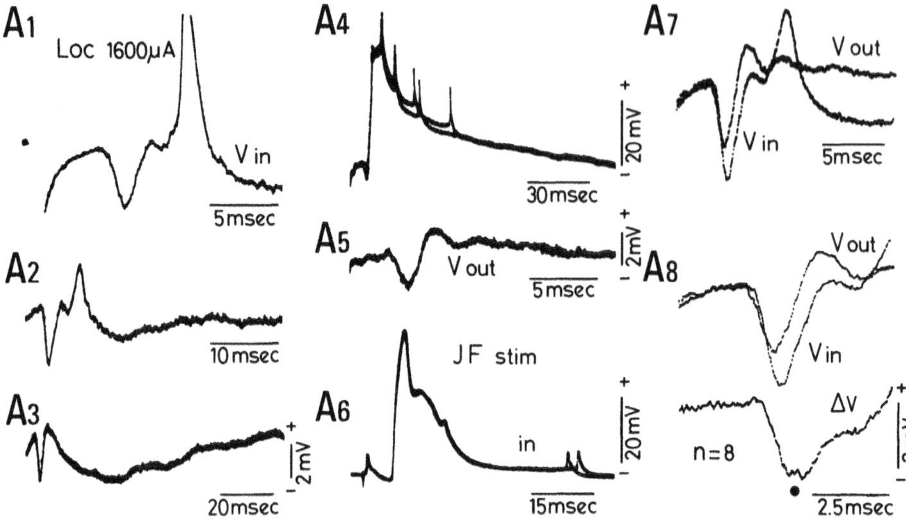

Fig. 7A₁₋₈. Passive hyperpolarizing potentials intracellularly recorded in a Purkinje cell. **A_1–A_4**, intracellular responses (*V in*) evoked by a Loc stimulus and recorded at progressively slower speeds. **A_1**, **A_2**, foot of the orthodromic action potential **A_1** and EPSP-IPSP sequence **A_2**. **A_3**, **A_4**, inhibitory postsynaptic potential, first recorded as a hyperpolarizing potential **A_3** and subsequently converted into a depolarizing potential, which was large enough to initiate partial spikes and was due to Cl^- leakage through the recording microelectrode **A_4**. **A_5**, extracellular potential (*V out*) evoked by the same stimulus outside the cell. **A_6**, climbing-fiber response produced in this neuron by a juxtafastigial stimulus. **A_7**, **A_8**, the earliest negativities evoked outside and inside the Purkinje cell by a Loc stimulus, at the time corresponding to that illustrated in **A_2**, were averaged to determine the net value of the Loc-evoked transmembrane potential difference (n=8). **A_7** superimposed traces of the averaged intra- (*V in*) and extra- (*V out*) cellular potentials. **A_8**, *upper* traces: as in **A_7**, but at faster sweep speed; *lower* trace: computer calculated difference (*ΔV*) demonstrating the net hyperpolarization produced by the parallel fiber volley. The passive hyperpolarizing potential (*dot*) in this case was more than 2 mV and its duration was about 1.5 ms

shown by the persistence of large climbing-fiber responses of more than 35 mV (A_6). As described before, the IPSP was rapidly converted into a depolarizing potential [1, 8, 16] due to leakage of Cl^- ions through the recording microelectrode (A_4). A comparison of the intracellularly recorded initial Loc-evoked negativity illustrated in A_2 with that evoked outside the cell by the same stimulus (A_5) showed clearly that this potential was larger in the recorded cell, thus indicating that a net membrane hyperpolarization was the first event to be initiated in this neuron by the parallel-fiber volley. This conclusion was confirmed by superimposition of a number of averaged intra- and extracellularly recorded sweeps as in Fig. 7 A_7 and A_8 (upper traces), and when the transmembrane potential was computed from these recordings, a hyperpolarization of about 1.3 mV in amplitude and 1.2 ms in duration was found (Fig. 7 A_8, lower trace). A comparable early Loc-evoked hyperpolarization in another Purkinje cell was obtained during the experiment illustrated in Fig. 8. The orthodromically induced firing of this cell was recorded extracellularly (A_1) prior to penetrating it (A_2–A_5). In this case, the early Loc-evoked hyperpolarization, which clearly

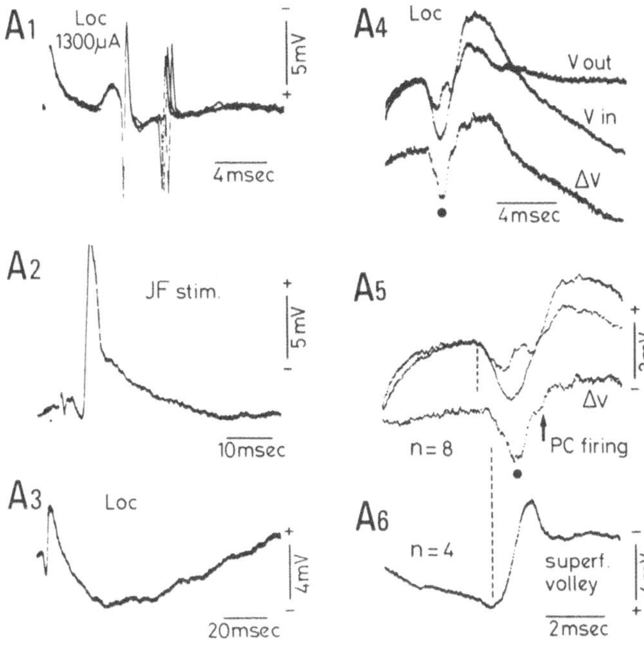

Fig. 8A$_{1-6}$. Time relationship between passive hyperpolarizing potentials and parallel-fiber volleys. **A$_1$**, responses of a Purkinje cell to a Loc stimulus obtained by extracellular recordings, prior to impalement of this neuron (several superimposed sweeps). **A$_2$**, intracellular recording of the same cell's climbing-fiber response following a juxtafastigial stimulus. **A$_3$**, Loc-evoked inhibitory postsynaptic potential (IPSP), the onset of which is obscured by a depolarization presumably representing an excitatory postsynaptic potential (EPSP) mixed with a depolarizing IPSP due to Cl^- leakage through the KCl-filled recording microelectrode (i.e., early component of the IPSP is depolarizing at that time). **A$_4$**, *Upper* two traces: superimposed averaged intracellular (*V in*) and extracellular (*V out*) responses to a Loc stimulus of the same intensity as that used for **A$_3$** (n=8); *Lower* trace: transmembrane potential (ΔV) calculated from the two traces *above*, showing that the EPSP-IPSP sequence is preceded by a passive hyperpolarizing potential (*dot*) of about 2 mV amplitude. **A$_5$**, same as **A$_4$** but displayed at a faster speed. The deep presynaptic volley is indicated by a *vertical dashed line* which was drawn from the earliest positivity recorded in *V out*. The onset of this Purkinje cell's Loc-evoked firing, which was calculated from the extracellular recordings illustrated in A$_1$, is shown by an *arrow*. **A$_6$**, computed triphasic parallel-fiber volley (n=4) recorded at the end of experiment at the pial surface of the cerebellar lobule. The peak of positivity of this potential which is due to the arrival of the superficial presynaptic volley, is signaled by a *vertical dashed line*. Note that the onset of the PHP recorded in the cell followed the deeper parallel-fiber volley by about 0.5 ms

preceded both the EPSP-IPSP sequence (A$_4$, lower trace) and the faster extracellularly recorded action potentials (arrow in A$_5$, lower trace), was about 1.8 mV in amplitude and had a duration of 1.2 ms. At the end of the experiment, the microelectrode was withdrawn to the surface of the investigated folium and recordings at this depth (A$_6$) showed that the onset of the early hyperpolarization coincided in time with the superficial presynaptic volley (vertical dashed line in A$_6$), although it followed the deeply recorded presynaptic volley by about 0.5 ms (vertical dashed line in A$_5$).

Early Loc-evoked hyperpolarizations similar to those shown in Figs. 7 and 8 were found in about half of the 70 investigated cells; they were best seen if the tip of the microelectrode impaled the neuron at the lower border of the Purkinje cell soma layer, as evidenced by the shape of the Loc-evoked field potential along the electrode track. By contrast, when the penetration took place in the molecular layer above the Purkinje cell soma, negative-going potentials were infrequently recorded and it often happened that a slight transmembrane depolarization was recorded at this level, as would be expected from potentials generated by lines of currents associated with electrically mediated inhibition [22, 27, 28].

As detailed elsewhere [26] measurements were obtained from 13 cells with stable resting membrane potentials of 40–60 mV and climbing-fiber responses above 25 mV. The amplitude of the early evoked hyperpolarizations ranged from 0.4 to 3.0 mV ($\bar{m}=1.14$; SD=0.33), their duration ranged from 0.83 to 2.30 ms ($\bar{m}=1.36$; SD=0.37), and the time to peak from 0.61 to 1.31 ms ($\bar{m}=0.85$; SD=0.21), while that of the corresponding IPSPs averaged 57 ms. In two cases, the amplitude of the early responses could be graded by varying the Loc stimulus intensity, thus indicating a mechanism for recruiting the responsible presynaptic elements along the activated pathway. Their termination was followed by the IPSP onset within 0.35–1.20 ms ($\bar{m}=0.8$ ms; SD=0.3), an interval which was generally obscured by an intervening excitatory postsynaptic potential, which, however, required Loc stimulations of higher intensities to reach its maximum amplitude. On average, the onset of the hyperpolarizations followed the deeply recorded parallel-fiber volley by 0.75 ms (SD=0.3), a delay which is just sufficient for activation of a single chemical synapse between parallel fibers and a set of cortical interneurons (see next section). Furthermore, shifts in membrane potential had no effect on the amplitude or time course of the hyperpolarizing potential, both of which were insensitive to Cl^- leakage through the microelectrode. Thus, the characteristics of these hyperpolarizations are similar to those expected from potentials generated by field effects and, more specifically, to the passive hyperpolarizing potentials (PHPs) recorded in the Mauthner cell system [17, 27, 28].

Identification and Firing Properties of Presumed Basket Cells in the Cerebellum of Rat

A study of basket cells was undertaken in order to determine the time relationship between their firing and inhibitory events in their nearby postsynaptic Purkinje cells.

On the basis of some of the criteria established in the cat cerebellum [15], 17 cells exhibiting diphasic spikes of 0.5–1.2 mV amplitude were identified as basket cells. These criteria and the main properties of presumed basket cells are illustrated by Fig. 9. (a) The interneurons were located in the lower half of the molecular layer, i.e., in our experimental series, from 100 to 200 μm beneath the pial surface (Fig. 9 B_1, B_2). (b) In contrast to Purkinje cells, they were not activated antidromically by juxtafastigial stimulations which, however, excited

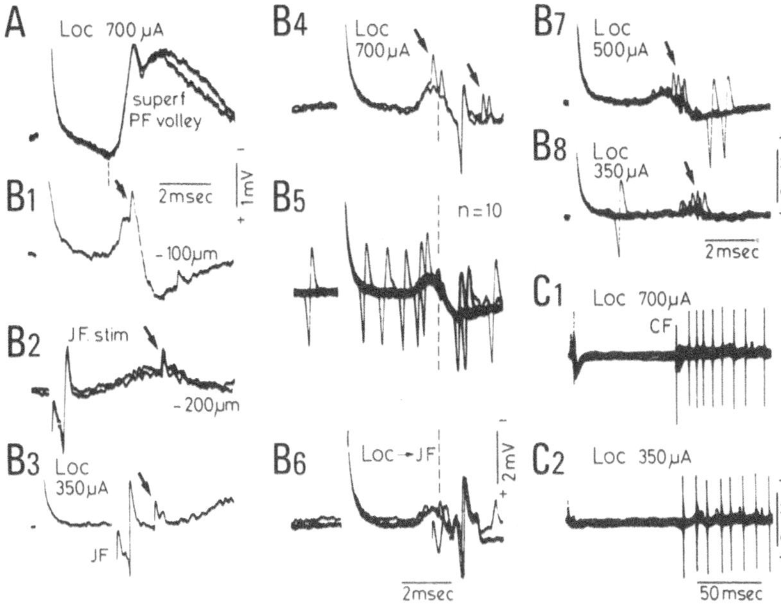

Fig. 9A–C_2. Characterization and properties of presumed basket cells. In this and the next figures, basket cell spikes are signaled by *arrows*. **A**, surface volley produced by a Loc stimulus, the intensity of which was 700 μA. $\mathbf{B_1}$, spikes were evoked in a presumed basket cell with the same stimulus intensity and were recorded as soon as the tip of the microelectrode reached the lower half of the molecular layer, i.e., 100 μm beneath the pial surface. Note the short latency of these action potentials with respect to the superficial parallel-fiber volley, the arrival of which is signaled in **A** by a *vertical dashed line*. $\mathbf{B_2}$, $\mathbf{B_3}$, firing of the same basket cell as that of $\mathbf{B_2}$, recorded at the level of the Purkinje cell layer, i.e., 200 μm below the cortical surface. $\mathbf{B_2}$ a *JF* stimulus produced an antidromic spike in a nearby Purkinje cell, whereas the presumed basket cell responses occurred with a longer latency on the subsequent mossy fiber-evoked synaptic field potential. $\mathbf{B_3}$ a Loc stimulus, the intensity of which was lowered to 350 μA, still evoked action potentials in the presumed basket cells; these spikes showed no collision with a preceding supramaximal Purkinje cell antidromic field potential and spike. $\mathbf{B_4}$–$\mathbf{B_6}$, responses of Purkinje and basket cells recorded simultaneously, following a Loc stimulus of 700 μA; a *vertical dashed line* is drawn along this *column* at the time of the basket cell excitation. $\mathbf{B_4}$, the presumed interneuron fired repetitively whereas the Purkinje cell responded with a single action potential. Note that firing of the interneuron began after a shorter latency than that of the nearby Purkinje cell. $\mathbf{B_5}$, superimposed traces (n=10) showing that a silent period occurred in the Purkinje cell at a time corresponding to that of basket cell firing. $\mathbf{B_6}$, failure of a juxtafastigial stimulus to evoke an antidromic spike in the Purkinje cell during this silent period (superimposed traces with and without a *JF* stimulus). $\mathbf{B_7}$, $\mathbf{B_8}$, evidence that the recorded Purkinje and basket cells had a different threshold for activation by Loc stimulations. $\mathbf{B_7}$, at a lowered stimulus intensity of 500 μA, spikes often failed in the Purkinje cell, while firing remained unaffected in the presumed basket cell. $\mathbf{B_8}$, action potentials began to fail in the basket cell as the stimulus strength was reduced to 350 μA. $\mathbf{C_1}$, $\mathbf{C_2}$, correlation of chemically mediated inhibition of the Purkinje cell with firing in the nearby presumed interneuron. $\mathbf{C_1}$, a Loc stimulus of 700 μA evoked a Purkinje cell response and was followed by a suppression of this cell's spontaneous activity for more than 70 ms (a climbing-fiber complex spike is visible as the neuron resumed firing). $\mathbf{C_2}$, this inhibition was still produced by a Loc stimulation at a strength of 350 μA, which also induced basket cell excitation

them at longer latencies during the late mossy-fiber-induced field potential (Fig. 9 B_2). Spikes evoked in this manner were produced by neurons other than Purkinje cells since they showed no collision with the antidromic responses and the field potential evoked by a supramaximal juxtafastigial stimulation (Fig. 9 B_3). (c) Presumed basket cells responded to a Loc stimulus with a high-frequency train of one to five spikes (Fig. 9 B_4), the latency of which increased when the stimulus intensity was reduced (Fig. 9 B_7, B_8). (d) The long lasting chemically mediated inhibition of Purkinje cells evoked by parallel-fiber volleys and attributed to activation of interneurons in the molecular layer, including basket cells [13], was present at the same weak stimulus strength with still evoked firing of presumed basket cells (Fig. 9 C_1, C_2).

Basket and Purkinje cells encountered along the same track responded with different characteristics to a given Loc stimulus. First, the lowest stimulus strength for activating one or the other type of cell was lower for the basket cells. For instance, in the experiment of Fig. 9, the stimulus intensity required for firing the Purkinje cell was 500 μA (B_7), while the nearby basket cell was still excited at times by Loc stimulations of 350 μA (B_8). In four preliminary experiments, the threshold current i for excitation of both types of neurons was measured: the mean ratio $\bar{m}$ of iBc/iPc was 0.7 within ranges of 0.67–0.74. Second, basket cells were excited earlier than Purkinje cells by a given parallel-fiber volley. This finding, which is already evident on the records of Fig. 9 B_4 and B_7, was studied in detail by systematically comparing the latency of the first spikes evoked in these two classes of cells at depths allowing simultaneous recordings from them. The four different pairs of basket and Purkinje cells illustrated in Fig. 10 exhibited a clear delay in their onset of firing in both the sample records and the computed histograms; this delay averaged 1.14 ms (SD=0.28) for 15 groups of cells studied in this manner. This result seemed somewhat surprising since both cells type are monosynaptically activated by parallel fibers. However, morphological data [35, 39] show that in mammals: (a) there is a constant gradient of increasing parallel-fiber diameter from the surface to deeper levels of the molecular layer, and (b) the spatial distribution of basket and Purkinje cell somata and dendrites is different, which suggests that the former neurons are activated by different sets of parallel fibers than those impinging upon the corresponding Purkinje cells. This hypothesis was verified by computing the firing latencies of basket and Purkinje cells from the deeply and superficially recorded parallel-fiber volleys, respectively. The two presynaptic volleys were determined in each series of experiments in a manner illustrated in Figs. 8 A_5, A_6 and 12 B. These records show that the earlier positivity signaling the impulse arrival time of the fastest-activated parallel fibers was always recorded with a shorter delay in the lower depths of the molecular layer. When the time of occurrence of each presynaptic volley was compared with that of their postulated postsynaptic respective cells, as for each of the neurons studied in Fig. 10, the latency differential was reduced to only 0.49 ms (SD=0.33; n=15 pairs of neurons). This value is compatible with the hypothesis that basket cells are activated monosynaptically by parallel fibers, more numerous, deeper, and faster conducting than those exciting Purkinje cells; it suggests that the EPSPs reach firing level faster in the inhibitory interneurons than in Purkinje cells.

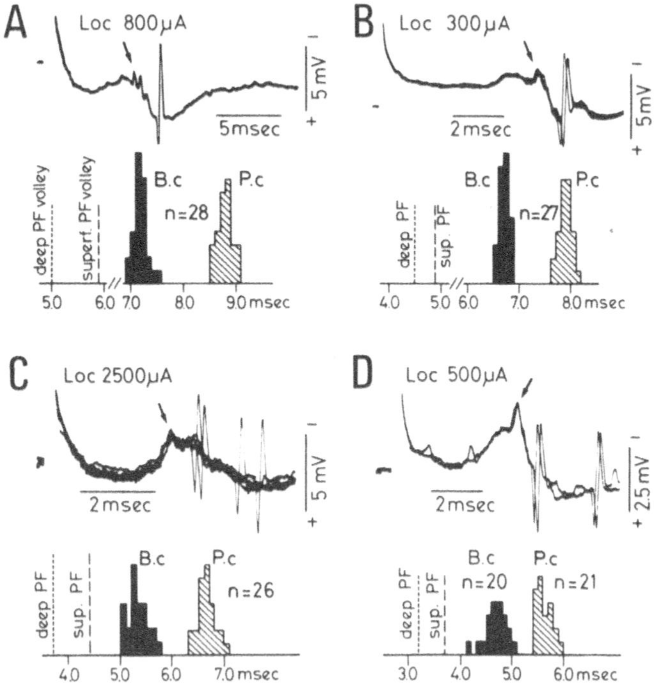

Fig. 10A–D. Respective timing of presumed interneuron and Purkinje cell excitation relative to the time of arrival of the deep and superficial parallel-fiber volleys. **A–D,** *upper* traces: sample traces of extracellularly recorded field potentials and spikes following a Loc stimulation at indicated stimulus intensities. Spikes from presumed basket cells (indicated by *arrows*) and from adjacent Purkinje cells were recorded simultaneously by the microelectrode. Each series corresponds to a different experiment (several superimposed sweeps in **B, C, D**). *Lower* diagrams: computed poststimulus time histograms for the first Loc-evoked spikes in each of the presumed interneurons (*B.c, black area*) and in Purkinje cells (*oblique lines*); the time of arrival of the deep and superficial parallel-fiber volleys (which were determined in a way similar to that illustrated by Fig. **9** $\mathbf{A_5}$, $\mathbf{A_6}$) is indicated by *vertical dashed lines.* The time of origin on the *abscissae* corresponds to the onset of the Loc stimulus artifact and is not shown; note that the *histograms* are drawn with a time scale different from that of their corresponding sample records. Taking into account morphological characteristics of the investigated classes of cells, the above data strongly suggest that basket cells are preferentially activated by a different set of parallel fibers from those exciting Purkinje cells (see also text)

Time Relationship Between Basket Cell's Firing and Passive Hyperpolarizing Potentials (PHPs)

The model for the generation of field effect inhibition (see Discussion) implies that if PHPs were produced in Purkinje cells by the same mechanism as in the Mauthner cell system, the basket cells should fire at the onset of or during the intracellularly recorded postsynaptic PHP. That such is the case is already suggested by the comparison of the extracellular recording of Fig. 9 B_5–B_6: the Purkinje cell's antidromic spike shown in B_3 was blocked (B_6) during the nearby basket cell's firing (B_5). Final proof that such is the case, was conclusively ob-

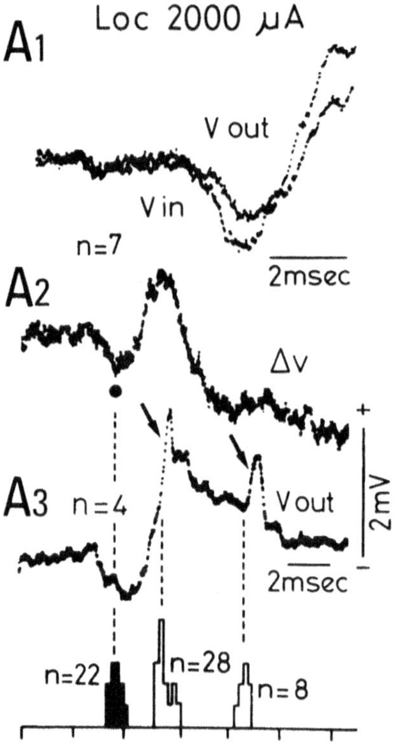

Fig. 11 A_{1-9}. Correspondence between the passive hyperpolarizing potential and the firing of basket cells. A_1, averaged superimposed responses (n=7) recorded intracellularly (*V in*) and extracellularly (*V out*) from a Purkinje cell after a Loc stimulation. A_2, calculated difference (*ΔV*) of the two traces *above*, indicating a net transmembrane difference of about −0.7 mV; this passive hyperpolarizing potential (indicated by a *black dot*) was followed by an EPSP-IPSP sequence. A_3, averaged extracellular responses (n=4) shown at a slower speed than in A_1; the tip of the microelectrode which was positioned in the lower part of the Purkinje cell layer, also recorded action potentials (*arrows*) evoked by the Loc stimulus in a Purkinje cell adjacent to the previously impaled one. *Lower* part of the figure: latency distribution of the earliest spikes evoked by the Loc stimulus in a presumed basket cell (*black histogram*) from which recordings were obtained along the same track, prior to penetration of the Purkinje cell from which A_1, A_2 were obtained and of the first and second Loc-evoked series of spikes illustrated in A_3 (*white histograms*). Note that the peak of the passive hyperpolarizing potential and the basket cell spikes occur near by simultaneously (*first vertical dashed line*)

tained by comparing the latency of action potentials of presumed basket cells with that of PHPs intracellularly recorded along the same tracks and in the immediate vicinity of these inhibitory interneurons. The results of one such experiment is illustrated by Fig. 11. The earlier negativities evoked inside (V in) and outside (V out) a Purkinje cell by a Loc stimulus are superimposed at a fast sweep in Fig. 11 A_1, and the computed net transmembrane potential (ΔV) shown in Fig. 11 A_2 indicates that the stimulation evoked a PHP in this neuron followed by an EPSP-IPSP sequence. The first histogram (shaded) which was obtained from a basket cell encountered above the impaled Purkinje cell, indicates that this interneuron fired its first spike (sample records not shown) as the PHP reached its maximum amplitude. The second histogram (unshaded) is of spikes which were evoked by the Loc stimulus in a nearby Purkinje cell and which were recorded as the microelectrode was withdrawn from the impaled cell; these spikes appear on the traces of Fig. 11 A_3. They correspond in time to intracellularly recorded depolarizing potentials (second and third vertical dashed lines), the first of which is clearly the excitatory postsynaptic potential illustrated in Fig. 11 A_2. Comparable results were obtained in four experiments, with the mean basket cell firing following the onset of the PHP by only 0.1, 0.4, 0.6, and 0.7 ms respectively.

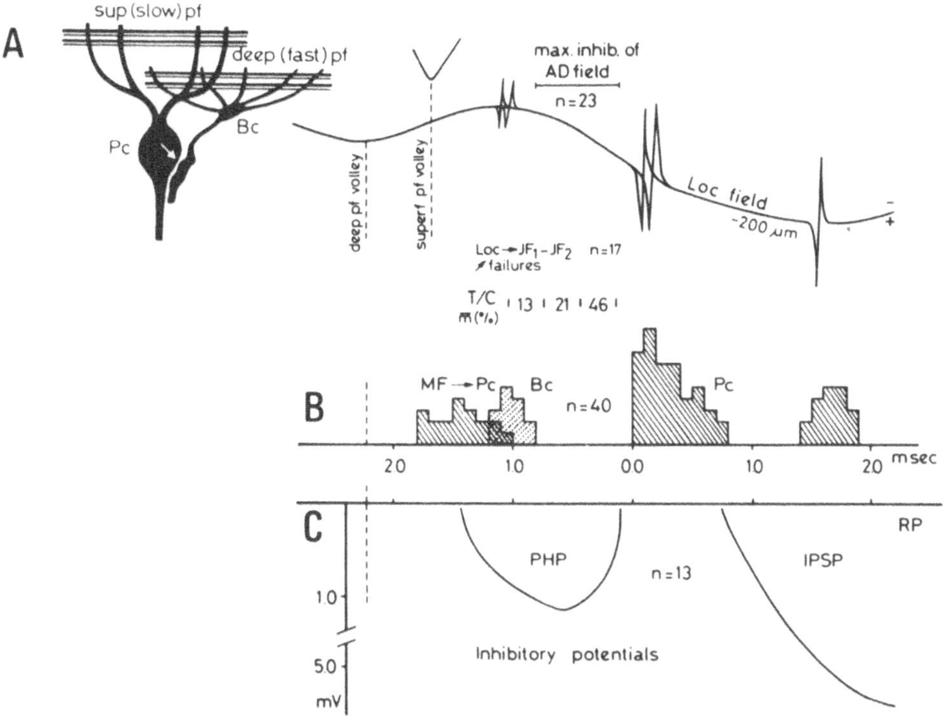

Fig. 12A–C. Diagrams summarizing experimental evidence that the early inhibition of Purkinje cells evoked by a parallel-fiber volley is underlain by a passive hyperpolarizing potential which can be correlated with firing in presynaptic basket cells. **A** Schematic representation of the spatial relationship between a Purkinje cell (*Pc*) and a basket cell (*Bc*) in the cerebellar cortex, showing that both neurons are monosynaptically activated by parallel fibers. In agreement with morphological data it is postulated that a statistically larger number of deeply located and faster conducting parallel fibers are in contact with basket cell dendrites than with those of Purkinje cells. A basket cell axon, which synapses on the Purkinje cell soma (*arrow*) and terminates as a digitiform process in the region of the paint-brush tip, is also illustrated. **B** Extracellularly recorded evidence for a brief and short latency Loc-evoked inhibition of Purkinje cells. In the *upper* part of the figure, the top of the positivity which signals the superficial parallel-fiber volley (*superf. pf. volley*) following a Loc stimulus is drawn and a *vertical dashed line* designates its peak time. The field potential recorded 200 μm beneath the pial surface after the same stimulation is shown *below*, with *schematic spikes* indicating excitation of basket and Purkinje cells respectively. The deeply recorded parallel-fiber volley is also signaled by a *vertical dashed line*. The time of occurrence and the duration of the maximum earlier inhibitory action exerted by a parallel fiber upon the antidromic field potential of Purkinje cells is given at the *top* of the figure (from 23 experiments). The latency histograms are respectively pertinent to spikes produced by excitation of Purkinje cells through the fast mossy-fiber pathway (*MF* → *PC*) and to the earliest spikes due to synaptic activation of basket (*Bc*) and Purkinje (*Pc*) cells (data from 40 experiments). The blocking effect of a parallel-fiber volley upon the second antidromic spike produced by adequately paired *JF* stimulations ($JF_1 \rightarrow JF_2$), which was investigated in 17 cells, is also indicated (see legend of Fig. 7 for explanations). **C** Schematic drawing of the passive hyperpolarizing potentials (*PHP*) and inhibitory postsynaptic potentials (*IPSP*) recorded intracellularly in 13 cells. Note that although the mean values of data obtained from different experiments are arbitrarily represented together in both **B** and **C**, a good correlation is observed between the earliest inhibitory effects of a parallel fiber upon antidromic invasion of the Purkinje cells and the *PHP*. Basket cells appear to start generating action potentials at the onset of the *PHP*

Correlation of Extra- and Intracellular Events Brought About at the Purkinje Cell Level by a Loc Stimulation

Figure 12 represents an attempt to summarize the main results obtained with different techniques throughout this work. Most of the data have been put together in a somewhat arbitrary manner, since they are not from the same experiments. However, a quite satisfactory comparison between the extra- and intracellularly recorded Loc-evoked potentials can be made by taking for a time reference the onset of Purkinje cell firing. Figure 12A is a schematic drawing of the spatial orientation of the soma and dendrites of one Purkinje cell with one of the adjacent basket cells. The corresponding set of presynaptic parallel fibers which is postulated to be activated by a Loc stimulus is also shown: the deeper and presumably more rapidly conducting presynaptic fibers are preferentially connected with basket cells, which are therefore excited prior to the Purkinje cells. The interval between the activation of these two classes of target cells can account for the timing of the successive phases of inhibition and excitation recorded at the level of Purkinje cells.

The field potential evoked at the Purkinje cell layer, i.e., 200 µm below the pial surface is illustrated in Fig. 12B, and a temporal comparison between the superficial and the deep parallel-fiber volleys (first and second vertical dashed lines respectively) indicates that in our experiments the former preceded the latter by about 0.5 ms. The deeply recorded Loc-evoked field potential is represented with small and large spikes aligned with the histograms of basket and Purkinje cell impulses and it exhibits the classical P wave generated by the inhibitory currents flowing during the chemically mediated postsynaptic inhibition of Purkinje cells [13]. The onset and termination of the early Loc-evoked inhibitory phase appears in this figure as determined in 23 experiments utilizing field potential analysis and as evaluated in 17 extracellularly recorded cells (using paired juxtafastigial stimulations). With both these methods, the early inhibition corresponded in time to the silent period observed between the two peaks of the Purkinje cell histogram, which represent respectively the action potentials set up in 40 cells by the deep mossy-fiber axon reflex loop (MF → PC), and the earlier orthodromic spikes evoked by the directly activated parallel fibers (PC). Finally, the mean value and time course of the intracellular inhibitory potentials obtained in 13 cells after Loc stimulation are displayed in Fig. 12C, with the same time coordinates as in Fig. 12B. Early inhibitory potentials were recorded well before any IPSP and their onset showed little delay relative to the histogram of basket cell firings shown in Fig. 12B. These hyperpolarizations, which exhibit the properties expected of potentials mediated by field effects can clearly account for the early Loc-evoked inhibitory action revealed by extracellular recordings and illustrated in Fig. 12B.

Discussion

As discussed elsewhere (Korn and Faber, 1979) electrical interactions mediated by extracellular currents can be separated into two different categories based on possible distinctions between the affected pre- and postsynaptic neurons: (a) Instances in which fields generated by synchronous activation of a homogenous population of neurons enhance the synchronization of those neurons, for example, the field-generated depolarizations of cat and frog spinal motoneurons associated with their antidromic invasion [34, 37]. Theoretically, however, such synchronous activity could result, in some structures, in an inhibition of a second population of cells [41]. (b) Instances in which impulse activity in a presynaptic neuron produces, without synaptic delay, either monophasic excitation [47] or inhibition of the postsynaptic cells. The electrical inhibition mediated by cerebellar interneurons upon Purkinje cells falls into the second category. It has been studied under the assumption that it is generated in the same way as the electrical inhibition in the Mauthner system, the analysis of which has led to the most complete understanding of the mechanisms underlying the production of field effects (for a review, see [19]). In any case, the passive hyperpolarizing potentials described in the Purkinje cells of the rat cerebellum represent the first example of electrical inhibition to be reported in the mammalian central nervous system.

Generation of Passive Hyperpolarizing Potentials by Terminals of Basket Cells

In the teleostean Mauthner-cell system there is a failure of impulse conduction in afferent fibers comprising the axon cap. These terminals, thus, serve as passive extracellular current sources to the more distal active sinks and they behave as an external anode which imposes a positivity on the outside surface of the Mauthner cell membrane. This positivity, named the "extrinsic hyperpolarizing potential" [22] generates an inward current which hyperpolarizes the initial segment of the Mauthner cell and which is quite effective in inhibiting this cell's spike discharges. In turn, impulses in the Mauthner cell also produce an electrical inhibition in the neurons of origin of these fibers which is intracellularly recorded as a hyperpolarization called "passive hyperpolarizing potential" or PHP [19, 27]. A crucial requirement for this mutual field-effect inhibition is the high resistivity of the axon cap relative to the surrounding tissue, which is critical for the intracellular channeling of currents flowing from the adjacent inactive terminals into the postsynaptic cell.

It should be pointed out that, as illustrated by Fig. 13A, B_1-B_3, the original hypothesis of Furukawa and Furshpan [22] that neurons which electrically inhibit the Mauthner cell also mediate the chemical component of this neuron's collateral inhibition was directly proven by experiments using double simultaneous intracellular recordings [29]. The relevance of that work to this paper derives from the unequivocal demonstration that one presynaptic neuron can mediate both inhibitions, thus giving strong support to the postulate that such is also the case for basket cells. For obvious technical reasons, more indirect approaches had to be used to verify this concept for neurons of a structure such as the cerebellum.

The model for one neuron generating both electrical and chemical inhibitions is shown in Fig. 13C; it has been conceptualized for the Mauthner cell system but

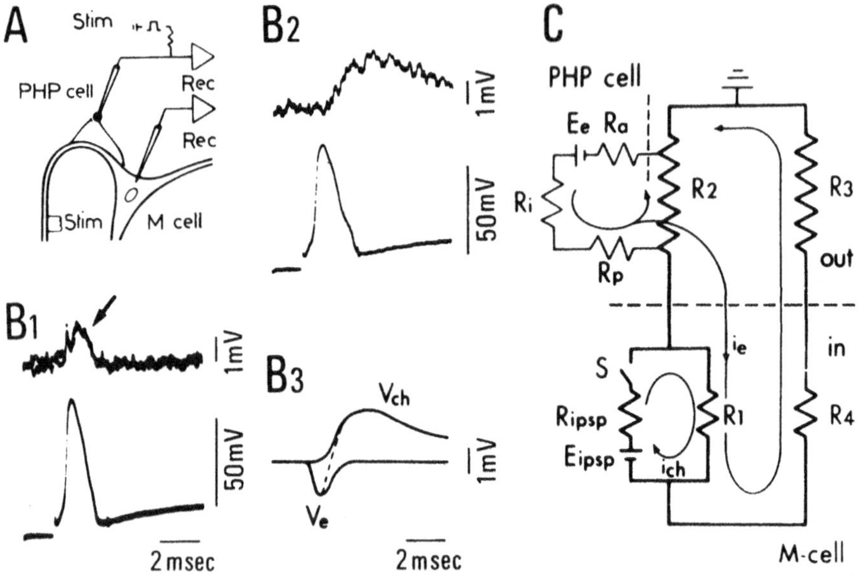

Fig. 13A–C. Unitary electrically and chemically mediated postsynaptic inhibitions produced in the Mauthner cell (M cell) system by a single PHP neuron. Diagram of the experimental setup for simultaneous recording and stimulation of a PHP neuron and the postsynaptic cell. $\mathbf{B_1}$, $\mathbf{B_2}$ Comparison of the potentials evoked outside and inside the M cell (*upper* traces) by a directly evoked presynaptic spike (*lower* traces). $\mathbf{B_1}$ A unitary positivity or EHP (extrinsic hyperpolarizing potential) (*arrow*) was recorded in the axon cap. $\mathbf{B_2}$ The electrode was advanced into the M cell and recordings were made after intracellular injection of Cl^-; the presynaptic spike produced a monosynaptic depolarizing IPSP in the M cell. $\mathbf{B_3}$ Superposition of the potential changes recorded in the upper traces of $\mathbf{B_1}$ and $\mathbf{B_2}$. The electrical component, *Ve*, is inverted with respect to the observed extracellular recording, since external positivity represents a hyperpolarization of the M cell; the chemical IPSP (*Vch*) is left in the depolarizing direction. The net transmembrane potential change is therefore biphasic, with the electrically mediated component being curtailed by the rising phase of the chemical one (*dashed line*). **C** Model for the generation of the two inhibitory components. The *lower* half of the diagram represents the M cell. The equivalent network for the *PHP cell* is to the *left* of the *vertical dashed line*. Abbreviations: *Ra, Ri, Rp:* resistances of the PHP cell's active spike generating membrane, of its internal component and of its noninvaded terminal. R_1 and R_4: resistance of the Mauthner cell soma and axon hillock and of its lateral dendrite. R_2 and R_3: extracellular resistances of the axon cap and of the distal region of the medulla; i_e symbolizes the portion of the action current that flows inward across the M-cell axon hillock and somatic membranes, thereby producing the electrical inhibition. In addition, the release of transmitter by the *PHP cell* produces an inhibitory Cl^- dependent current, i_{ch} in the M cell (E_{ipsp}, driving force for i_{ch}; R_{ipsp}, resistance of the activated inhibitory channels; *S*, switch illustrating the opening of these channels). Faber and Korn, 1978

with few modifications is valid for the Purkinje cell system as well [26]. As already stated, it postulates that terminal processes involved in the generation of the PHPs should lie, at least in part, in a region of increased extracellular resistivity (R_2 in the diagram of Fig. 13C), which seems to be therefore the case for basket cells. The specific causes of this elevated extracellular resistance have not yet been established in the case of the axon cap but they might derive from some of the morphological peculiarities that characterize this region [36], and are also present around the initial segment of the Purkinje cell within the pinceau formed by basket cells [24, 38, 39, 42]. A recent description of axoglial septate junctions at the periphery and within the axon cap [46] further reinforces the concept that the two structures have many similar histological features. Although they have not yet been investigated with all the required care, the electrophysiological properties of the PHPs recorded in Purkinje cells are those expected of potentials produced by field effects and their time course is well correlated with the firing of basket cells, which therefore appear according to both morphological and electrophysiological criteria to be candidates for their generation. In confirmation, the PHPs were found to increase in amplitude in parallel with the intensity of the Loc stimulus; this graded effect is in good agreement with the fact that in the rat, the pericellular basket and the appended paint brush tip of a Purkinje cell are formed by the conjunction of axons from at least three to seven basket cells [39].

Activation of Basket and Purkinje Cells by Their Presynaptic Inputs

Morphological studies support our physiological results indicating that basket cells are activated by more of the deeper and more rapidly conducting parallel fibers than Purkinje cells: (a) There is a constant gradient of increased parallel fiber thickness from the surface to deeper levels of the molecular layer [20, 21, 35, 39, 40, 43]; (b) the fanlike dendritic tree of the basket cell – the soma of which lies exclusively in the lower half of the molecular layer – extends in the same vertical plane as that of Purkinje cells but generally does not extend as far upwards and has, overall, the greater part of its dendrites situated in the deeper part of the molecular layer [39, 42], (c) in most species, parallel fibers establish synapses upon both the cell body and dendrites of basket cells [31, 33], whereas they mainly contact Purkinje cells upon their dendritic branchlet and, to a lesser extent, upon the spines of secondary dendrites [31]; (d) the length of parallel fibers appears to be greater than previously assumed in both the cat and rat [7, 32], and the deeper parallel fibers are about half the length of the more superficial ones. As a consequence, information arriving via mossy fibers to the deeper granule cells should travel to the entire group of postsynaptic cells contacted by their emerging parallel fibers in less time than that needed for information transmitted through more superficial granule cells and their parallel fibers. These differences necessarily imply that more deeper and thicker (in some species even myelinated) parallel fibers contact basket cells than Purkinje cells. Hence, it proved necessary, as stated above, to compute latencies of each cell type with respect to its own corresponding presynaptic volley, although, because of its smooth time course, it is, in fact, difficult to ascertain the peak time of the maximum positivity signaling the arrival of the presynaptic volley in the deeper regions of the molecular layer. In our experiments, the mean difference in latency between Purkinje and basket cell firing, which amounted to 1.14 ms if measured from the onset of the superficial presynaptic volley, was reduced to 0.49 ms if computed according to the input to each cell class. This time lag could be attributed to measurement error and/or to possible differences in synaptic transmission properties, including the rise time of Loc-induced EPSPs.

Possible Role of Electrical Inhibition in Purkinje Cells

In the Mauthner cell system, electrically mediated inhibition can serve two functions: inhibition and/or synchronization [28, 29]. The first alternative appears to be relevant for one group of PHP-exhibiting cells such as second order vestibular neurons, but even in this case the inhibitory effect of the PHP is weak compared to that of the chemically mediated postsynaptic inhibition. Similarly, the effectiveness of inhibition of the Loc-evoked PHPs in blocking antidromic invasion of Purkinje cells was inconsistent, and techniques such as double juxtafastigial stimulation were necessary in order to unmask it. One cannot rule out, however, that in specific conditions such as during high-frequency discharges a suppression of neuronal excitability could be required without delay, presynaptic basket cells being then unable to operate so quickly with a longer latency, chemically mediated transmission alone. Furthermore, our experimental procedures induced a rather artificial massive presynaptic volley and it is not unlikely that in physiological situations activation of basket cells by parallel-fiber volleys below threshold for excitation of Purkinje cells may produce a longer lasting PHP, the inhibitory effect of which would be accordingly prolonged and enhanced. It should be pointed out that PHPs were not found in all the recorded cells, and this finding may indicate that several classes of Purkinje cells exist, which would be determined by the weightings of their inputs from molecular layer interneurons, only one group of which contributes to the formation of the pinceau. Also, the model for electrical inhibition indicates a reciprocal effect between the concerned adjacent neurons; basket cells are therefore subjected to a field-effect inhibition during the time of Purkinje cell firing, but evidence for the existence of this mutual negative feedback and its role are still missing.

The second alternative, that of a synchronizing effect of PHPs, finds strong support from studies in the Mauthner cell network [27]. The electrical inhibition of the Mauthner cell is brought about by simultaneous discharges of numerous cells and clearly the PHP contributes significantly to their synchronization: it functions to reset the activity of the inhibitory interneurons and to increase the probability that they would be activated by their excitatory input, especially in those cells which otherwise would not be brought to their firing level by collateral input from the Mauthner cell. Similarly, PHPs could contribute to the synchronization of Purkinje cell discharges by maximizing during the subsequent rebound the effectiveness of EPSPs produced by parallel fibers. Intracellular recordings confirm that EPSPs start before the termination of PHPs and that their onset can be confused with the termination phase of the PHP, these two events generally overlapping in time. It thus appears that excitatory potentials in Purkinje cells are both preceded and followed by inhibitory processes which could ensure on the one hand their effectiveness through an anodal break rebound mechanism and on the other hand that excitation would not fire the cells repetitively, because of the subsequent postsynaptic, chemically mediated inhibition.

Firing of basket cells might be furthermore synchronized by gap junctions between them [39, 45]. Consequently, excitatory potentials, the onset and termination of which are determined by the same inhibitory influences, would be time-locked in all Purkinje cells receiving their inhibitory inputs from a common pool of basket cells. It is furthermore interesting that the basket cells are the site of electrically mediated transmission at both ends, indicating that speed is one of the major operational features of these inhibitory interneurons.

References

1. Andersen P, Eccles JC, Voorhoeve PE (1964) Postsynaptic inhibition of cerebellar Purkinje cells. J Neurophysiol 27:1138–1153
2. Axelrad H, Korn H (1979) Short latency inhibitory action of a parallel fiber volley upon activation of Purkinje cells in the rat cerebellum: indirect evidence for a field effect inhibition (Abstr) Soc Neurosc 5:97
3. Axelrad H, Korn H (1980) Cerebellar cortex of the rat: presumed inhibitory interneurons are activated earlier than Purkinje cells by a parallel fiber volley (Abstr) Soc Neurosc 6:611
4. Bennett MVL (1966) Physiology of electrotonic junctions. Ann NY Acad Sci 137:509–539
5. Bennett MVL (1972) A comparison of electrically and chemically mediated transmission. In: Pappas GD, Purpura DP (eds) Structure and Function of Synapses. New York, Raven Press, pp 221–256
6. Bennett MVL (1978) Electrical transmission: a functional analysis and comparison to chemical transmission. Ann Physiol Soc:357–416
7. Brand S, Dahl AL, Mugnaini E (1976) The length of parallel fibers in the cat cerebellar cortex. An experimental light and electron microscopic study. Exp Brain Res 26:39–58
8. Crepel F, Delhaye-Bouchaud N (1978) Intracellular analyses of synaptic potentials in cerebellar Purkinje cells of the rat. Brain Res 155:176–181
9. Eccles JC (1957) The physiology of nerve cells. John Hopkins Press, Baltimore, p 270
10. Eccles JC, Ito M, Szentagothai J (1967) The cerebellum as a neuronal machine. Springer, Berlin Heidelberg New York, p 316
11. Eccles JC, Faber DS, Taborikova H (1971) The action of a parallel fiber volley on the antidromic invasion of Purkinje cells of cat cerebellum. Brain Res 25:335–356
12. Eccles JC, Llinás R, Sasaki K (1966a) The excitatory synaptic action of climbing fibres on the Purkinje cells of the cerebellum. J Physiol 182:268–296
13. Eccles JC, Llinás R, Sasaki K (1966b) The action of antidromic impulses on the cerebellar Purkinje cell. J Physiol 182:316–345
14. Eccles JC, Llinás R, Sasaki K (1966c) Parallel fiber stimulation and the responses induced thereby in the Purkinje cells of the cerebellum. Exp Brain Res 1:17–39
15. Eccles JC, Llinás R, Sasaki K (1966d) The inhibitory interneurons within the cerebellar cortex. Exp Brain Res 1:1–16
16. Eccles JC, Llinás R, Sasaki K (1966e) Intracellularly recorded responses of the cerebellar Purkinje cells. Exp Brain Res 1:161–183
17. Faber DS, Korn H (1973) A neuronal inhibition mediated electrically. Science 179:577–578
18. Faber DS, Korn H (1978) Electrophysiology of the Mauthner cell: basic properties, synaptic mechanisms and associated networks. In: Faber DS, Korn H (eds) Neurobiology of the Mauthner Cell. Raven Press, New York, pp 47–131
19. Faber DS, Korn H (1980) Single shot channel activation accounts for duration of inhibitory postsynaptic potentials. Science 208:612–615
20. Fox CA, Barnard JW (1957) A quantitative study of the Purkinje cell dendritic branchlets and their relationship to afferent fibres. J Anat 91:299–313
21. Fox CA, Hillman DE, Siegesmund KA, Dutta CR (1967) The primate cerebellar cortex: a golgi and electron microscopy study. Prog Brain Res 25:174–225
22. Furukawa T, Furshpan EJ (1963) Two inhibitory mechanisms in the Mauthner neurons of goldfish. J Neurophysiol 26:140–176

23. Gobel S (1971) Axo-axonic septate junctions in the basket formations of the cat cerebellar cortex. J Cell Biol 51:328–333
24. Hamori J, Szentágothai J (1965) The Purkinje cell baskets: ultrastructure of an inhibitory synapse. Acta Biol Acad Sci Hung 15:465–476
25. Kawamura H, Provini L (1970) Depression of cerebellar Purkinje cells by microionphoretic application of GABA and related amino acids. Brain Res 24:293–304
26. Korn H, Axelrad H (1980) Electrical inhibition of Purkinje cells in the cerebellum of the rat. Proc Natl Acad Sci USA 77:6244–6247
27. Korn H, Faber DS (1975a) An electrically mediated inhibition in goldfish medulla. J Neurophysiol 38:452–471
28. Korn H, Faber DS (1975b) Mechanisms and functions of electrically mediated inhibition in the vertebrate central nervous system. In: Galun R, Hillman P, Werman R (eds) Sensory Physiology and Behavior. Plenum, New York, pp 289–305
29. Korn H, Faber DS (1976) Vertebrate central nervous system: same neurons mediate both electrical and chemical inhibitions. Science 194:1166–1169
30. Korn H, Faber DS (1979) Electrical interactions between vertebrate neurons: field effects and electrotonic coupling: In: Schmitt FO, Worden FG (eds) The neurosciences: 4th Study Program. MIT Press, Cambridge, pp 333–358
31. Larramendi LMH, Victor T (1967) Synapses on the Purkinje cell spines in the mouse. An electronmicroscopic study. Brain Res 5:15–30
32. Lauder J (1978) Effects of early hypo- and hyperthyroidism on development of rat cerebellar cortex. IV: The parallel fibers. Brain Res 142:25–39
33. Lemkey-Johnston N, Larramendi LMH (1968) Types and distribution of synapses upon basket and stellate cells of the mouse cerebellum. J Comp Neurol 134:73–112
34. Magherini PC, Precht W, Schwindt PC (1976) Evidence for electrotonic coupling between frog motoneurons in the in situ spinal cord. J Neurophysiol 39:474–483
35. Mugnaini E (1972) The histology and cytology of the cerebellar cortex. In: Larsell O, Jansen J (eds) The comparative anatomy and histology of the cerebellum: the human cerebellum, cerebellar connections and cerebellar cortex. University of Minnesota Press, Minneapolis, pp 201–265
36. Nakajima Y, Kohno K (1978) Fine structure of the Mauthner cell: synaptic topography and comparative study. In: Faber DS, Korn H (eds) Neurobiology of the Mauthner Cell. Raven Press, New York, pp 133–166
37. Nelson PG (1966) Interaction between spinal motoneurons of the cat. J Neurophysiol 29:275–287
35. Palay SL (1964) The structural basis for neural action. In: Brazier MAB (ed) Brain function, Vol. II: RNA and brain function; memory and learning. UCLA Forum Med Sci 2:69–108
39. Palay SL, Chan-Palay V (1974) Cerebellar cortex: cytology and organization. Springer, Berlin Heidelberg New York
40. Palkovits M, Magyar P, Szentágothai J (1971) Quantitative histological analysis of the cerebellar cortex in the cat. III: Structural organization of the molecular layer. Brain Res 34:1–18
41. Rall W, Shepherd GM (1968) Theoretical reconstruction of field potentials and dendrodendritic synaptic interactions in olfactory bulb. J Neurophysiol 31:884–915
42. Ramon y Cajal S (1911) Histologie du système nerveux de l'homme et des vertébrés, vol II. Maloine, Paris. Translated by L Azoulay
43. Smolyaninov VU (1971) Some special features of organization of the cerebellar cortex. In: Gelfand IM, Gurfinkel VS, Fomin SV, Tsetlin ML (eds) Models of the structural-functional organization of certain biological systems. MIT Press, Cambridge, pp 250–423
44. Somogyi P, Hamori J (1976) A quantitative electron microscopic study of the Purkinje cell axon initial segment. Neuroscience 1:361–365
45. Sotelo C, Llinás R (1972) Specialized membrane junctions between neurons in the vertebrate cerebellar cortex. J Cell Biol 53:271–289
46. Triller A, Korn H (1980) Glio-axonic junctional like complexes at the Mauthner cell's axon cap of teleosts: a possible morphological basis for field effect inhibitions. Neurosci Lett 18:275–281
47. Werman R, Carlen PL (1976) Unusual behavior of the IaEPSP in cat spinal motoneurons. Brain Res 112:395–401

Discussion

Palay commented on the novelty of the observation of basket-cell firing preceding Purkinje cell activation and observed that in the rat there are some myelinated parallel fibers in the deeper layers. This, together with larger diameter fibers might explain the earlier activation of basket cells, since they should be preferentially influenced by the deeper layers of parallel fibers.

Llinás observed that surface stimulation of the cerebellar cortex can activate mossy-fiber terminals and a resulting "mossy-fiber reflex", which might simulate some of the observed results. Dr. Korn had dealt with this by using surface stimuli that were subthreshold for mossy-fiber activation and by doing some experiments in animals which had undergone transection of the inferior and middle cerebellar peduncles 3 days earlier. Though some mossy fibers would remain, most would be degenerated, and major differences were not observed in the potentials studied.

Chan-Palay noted that the heaviest binding of tritiated muscimol or GABA receptor sites is found at the basket to Purkinje cell junctions, and suggested that another effect of the specialized anatomic arrangement at that site might be to prolong the effects of synaptically released GABA. Dr. Korn replied that there also appear to be many GABA and glycine receptors around the initial segment of Mauthner cells.

Eccles found it curious that there was a temporal separation of the electrical and chemical phases of the basket cell inhibition, leaving a period of noninhibition between them.

Cerebellar Output: Body Maps and Muscle Spindles

W. T. Thach, J. G. Perry, and M. H. Schieber

In an effort to learn how the cerebellar circuitry controls movement, the activity of single nuclear and Purkinje cells has been studied with microelectrodes in the monkey during trained motor performance. These studies have shown the following: (a) The cells normally maintain a high discharge frequency (50–100 spikes/s) even in the absence of movement [26, 27, 28, 29]. (b) The discharge frequency modulates up and down over an extreme range (0–500 spikes/s) in stable relation to rapid alternating movements [26, 29]. (c) The time of change in discharge frequency occurs before or at the onset of movement [21, 27, 28, 29, 30]. These timing data, together with (d) the coding patterns, suggest a hierarchical scheme of motor control in which the earlier changing cells bear an abstract relation to the features of the forthcoming movement and the later cells code for and presumably control the muscle pattern and the force used to move [31]. Finally, (e) the changes in cell activity during the adaptation of a movement support the Albus model of a cerebellar role in motor learning [8, 32]. The present report describes two experiments that further define the relationship of cell discharge to motor behavior. The first reveals that cells controlling different parts of the body are arranged within the cerebellar nuclei in a somatotopic pattern [21]. The second suggests that, for some kinds of movement, cerebellar output is more concerned with control of gamma motor neurons than with alphas [23].

When attempting to correlate a neuron's firing with behavior, it is essential to know if the neuron is connected to a particular part of the body. Yet, how the body is mapped within the cerebellar nuclei is controversial [1, 2, 3, 5, 11, 13, 14, 18, 22, 24, 25, 31, 34], and it was impossible to know where to direct a microelectrode in order to study nuclear cell relation to movement of the arm. For this reason, a direct approach was planned, and a monkey was trained to make rapid alternating movements of different parts of the body, in return for a fruit juice reward (Fig. 1). The arm was placed in a fiberglass-epoxy jointed cast, in which sensors were placed to detect the adduction-abduction of the thumb, the flexion-extension of the wrist, the flexion-extension of the elbow, and the adduction-abduction of the shoulder. The foot clenched repeatedly to close a switch, and rapid movements of the mouth and tongue were made in drinking the fruit juice reward. The limb movements were performed in the sequence of 8–16 alternating movements at any one joint before going on to the next movement; reward was contingent on movement at the one joint and on nonmovement of all but the one joint, and the mouth moved upon delivery of the reward.

Experimental Brain Research, Suppl. 6

When the monkey had been fully trained, the electromyographic (EMG) activity was recorded between Teflon-covered stainless steel wires bared 1 mm at the tip and fish-hooked 1 cm apart in one of a number of different muscles. The EMG study showed that each muscle was active when its joint was moving, and was relatively quiet during movement of the other joints. The EMG activity was rectified and passed through a voltage-to-frequency converter, where the frequency of pulses put out was proportionate to the amplitude of the EMG put in. The frequency coded EMG was then displayed as rasters in which the spacing of dots in a line represented discharge frequency during a cycle of movement, and discharge during the many cycles were shown as lines of dots, with each cycle/line aligned at the time of the flexor or extensor contact. Figure 2a shows the activity of the pollicis brevis during movement of the thumb: the muscle was intensely active during the rapid thumb movement, and much less so during movement of the wrist, elbow, shoulder, or leg. While the rasters give a good visual impression as to how well (or poorly) the muscle's activity correlates with the task, a quantitative measure was developed in order to make more effective comparisons. A period of 75 ms (a vertical time bin across all trials) was selected from the raster in which the frequency was judged by eye to be the highest; the mean frequency within that period and its standard deviation were then computed across all trials. The same operation was performed for a 75-ms period during the least EMG activity. The graphs below the raster display show in arbitrary units the mean high and low frequencies and their standard deviation from trial to trial. A neuron's discharge was thus "well-related" to a movement if the means were far apart and the standard variation small. This corresponds to the criterion implicit in judging a raster by the eye; a unit is judged to be well related to an alternating movement if it modulates greatly between high and low frequency, and if the pattern is the same every

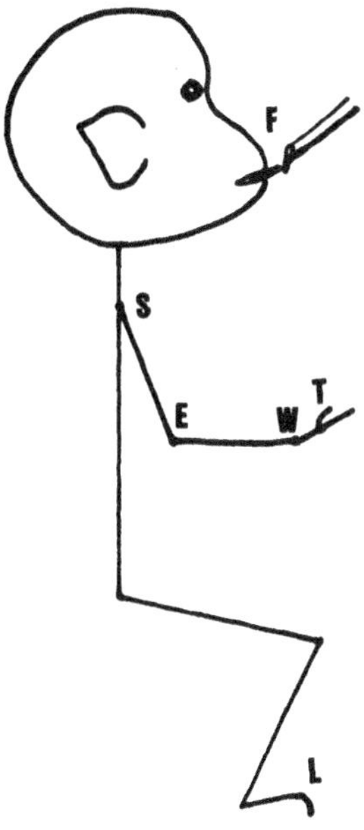

Fig. 1. Sketch of monkey showing the parts of the body that moved under experimental control for single neuron motor mapping in deep cerebellar nuclei. *F*, face; *S*, shoulder; *E*, elbow; *W*, wrist; *T*, thumb; *L*, leg

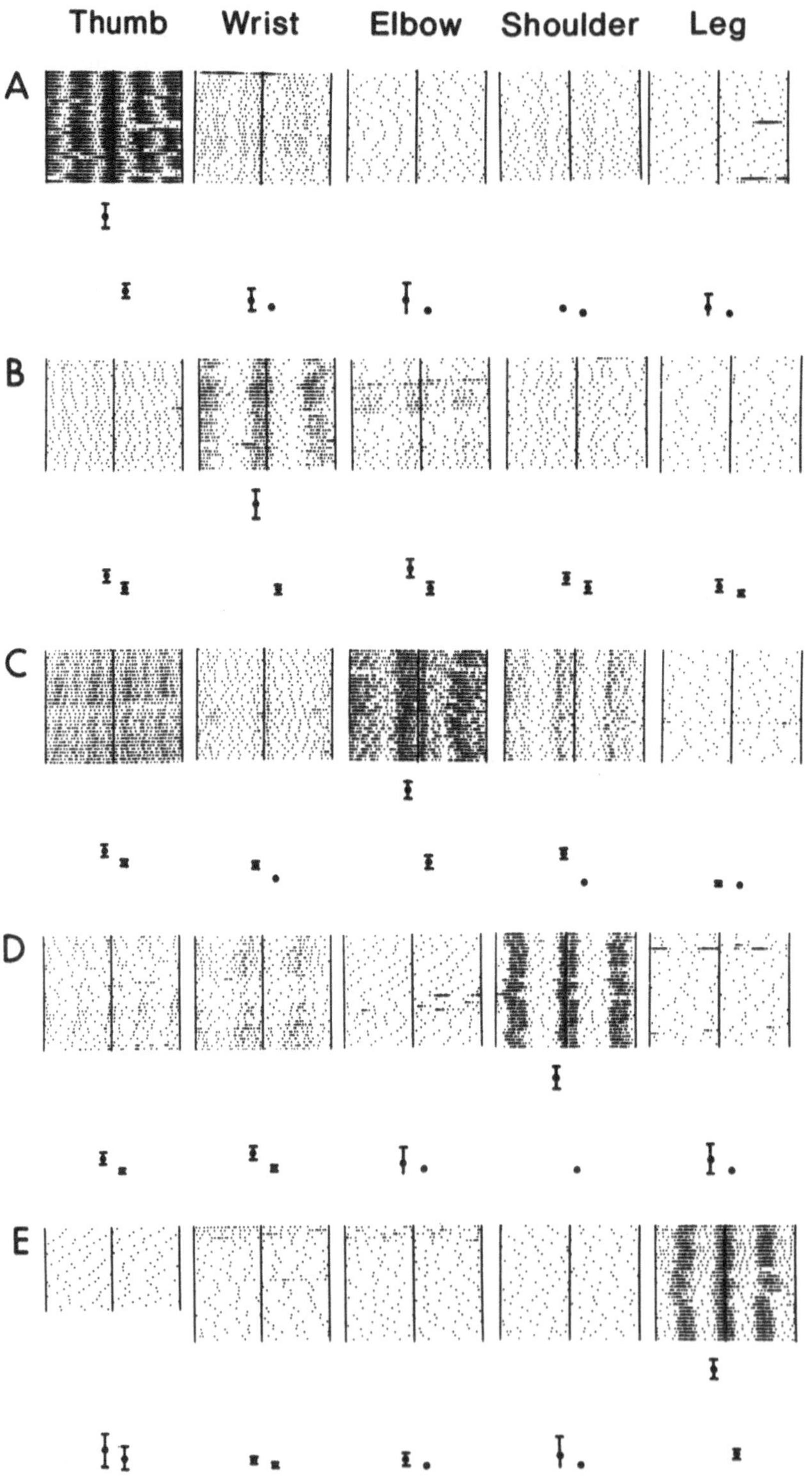
Thumb
Wrist
Elbow
Shoulder
Leg
A
B
C
D
E

trial. Thus, from the graph in Fig. 2a, one can see that the opponens pollicis was active during thumb movement much more than during any other movement. Figures 2B, C, D, E show EMG activity of four other muscles operating wrist, elbow, shoulder, and leg (foot) joints, respectively. In the rasters and the graphs, the muscle is active primarily in relation to movement of the one joint. A study of these and other muscles confirmed the visual impression that each movement was relatively discrete; each movement involved one joint more than others, and the muscle activity was fairly restricted to the muscles acting at that one joint. Having met these criteria, the monkey was a good candidate for mapping the deep nuclei with respect to the topographic representation of bodily movement.

After completion of EMG recording, the monkey was anesthetized, and bolts were affixed to the head to restrain head movement during cerebellar recording [7]. A hole was then cut through the skull over the deep cerebellar nuclei, ipsilateral to the trained arm and leg, and a stainless steel recording cylinder was mounted over the hole. When the monkey recovered from surgery, it was placed in its primate chair, and extracellular recordings were made with glass-covered, platinum-iridium microelectrodes from single neurons in the interposed and dentate nuclei as the monkey performed the movements.

Examples of the neural discharge during the five movements are shown in Fig. 3 for each of six neurons in the dentate nucleus. Each dot represents an action potential, each horizontal row of dots the discharge during one cycle of movement. The discharge during the many cycles is aligned on the time of the flexor or extensor contact (Fig. 3A). The first raster shows that the discharge frequency modulates up and down in relation to the wrist and the thumb movement. The mean frequencies of highest and lowest discharge are plotted below the rasters, and they also show that the discharge frequency modulates most for thumb and wrist movements, and, of the two, more so for the thumb. Figures 3B, C, D, E show discharge of each of four other neurons, each changing frequency preferentially in relation to movement at wrist, elbow, shoulder, and leg, respectively. The last raster (Fig. 3F) shows the discharge of a sixth dentate neuron that underwent extreme modulation in frequency, but without any relation to any of the five trained movements. Instead, the bursts and pauses were easily appreciated by eye to be occurring in relation to movements of the face, tongue, or jaw (or all three), which the monkey made in drinking the fruit juice from the reward spigot.

Figure 4 labels each penetration according to which movements most engaged the activity of the recorded neurons. A penetration was given letter names, the

Fig. 2A–E. Single muscle EMGs acting at each of the five joints during each joint movement. The EMG is full-wave rectified, integrated, and converted to pulse traces whose frequency is proportionate to EMG amplitude. Each *line* of a raster represents EMG during a trial. The different trials are aligned on the time of occurrence of flexor or extensor contacts. *Below* the raster are graphs of mean discharge ± S.D. (arbitrary units) of highest and lowest frequencies in each raster. The figure shows that each muscle might be active during several joint movements but was most active during movement of the joint it spanned. Muscles (labeled according to joint moved) are: *A*, thumb; *B*, wrist; *C*, elbow; *D*, shoulder; *E*, leg

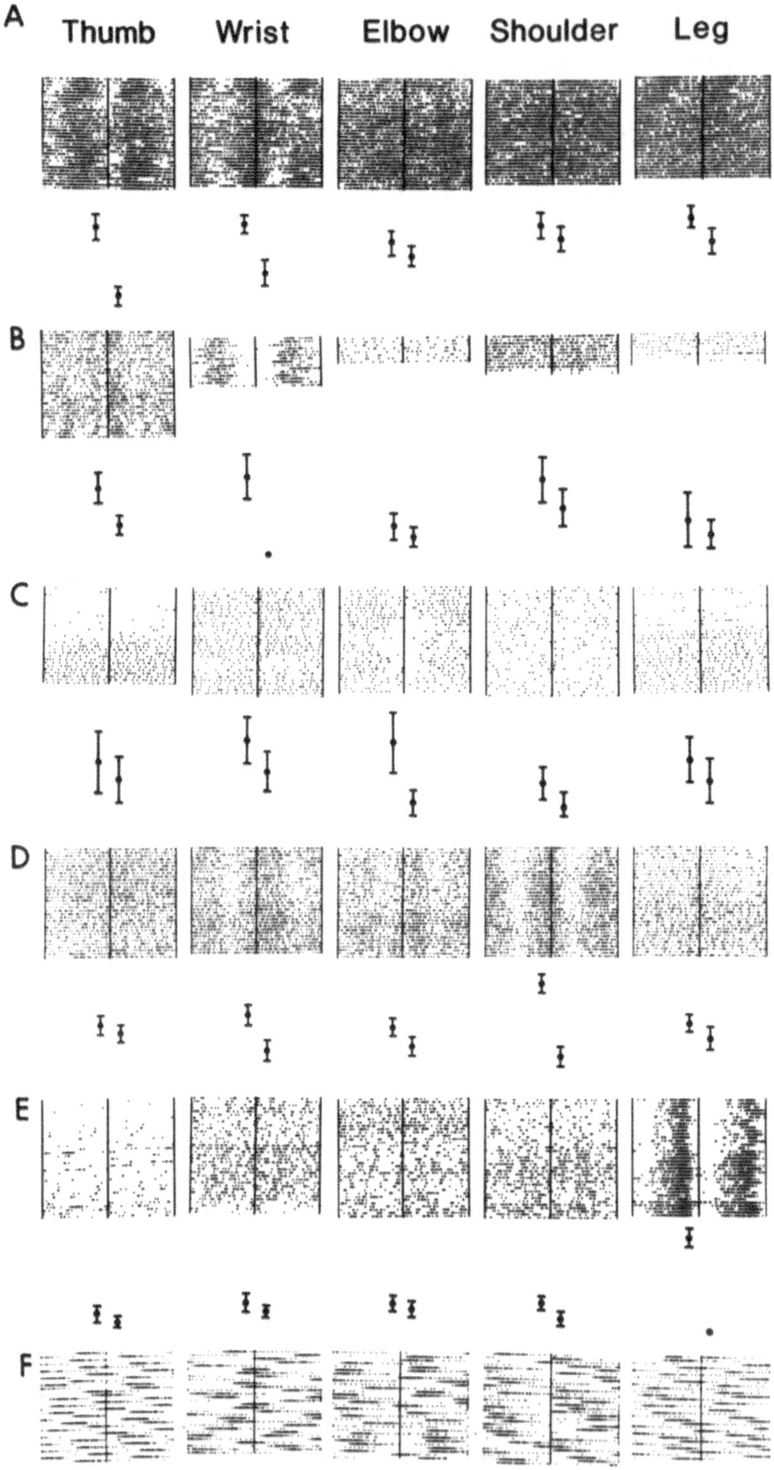
A
Thumb
Wrist
Elbow
Shoulder
Leg
B
C
D
E
F

Fig. 3A–F. Discharge of six neurons in the dentate nucleus during the five trained movements. Each *dot* represents one spike potential; the conventions are otherwise the same as in Fig. 2. The figure shows that the discharge of a neuron might be related to several movements but was appreciably best related to one of the movements. The discharge of neuron *F* was not related to any of the trained movements, but was observed by eye to occur in relation to drinking movements of the face

sizes of which were proportionate to the number of neurons and to the degree to which each modulated in relation to each of the five limb movements. Several formulae were used to make the generalization so as to avoid bias, but the results were generally the same: the most posterior neurons discharged in relation to movement of the face, those in the middle, the arm, and those most anterior, the leg. This was true for both the dentate and interpositus. While the generalization of "somatotopy" would seem valid, Fig. 4 emphasizes a fact that may be just as important: Within each penetration there was variation from one cell to the next as to a neuron's "preferred" movement. A posterior penetration might encounter some cells best relating to movements of the face, and others to the arm, an anterior penetration, to the arm and leg, and a middle penetration, to the face, arm, and leg. Posterior penetrations encountered no leg units, and anterior penetrations no face units. Within the "arm" area, neurons that were

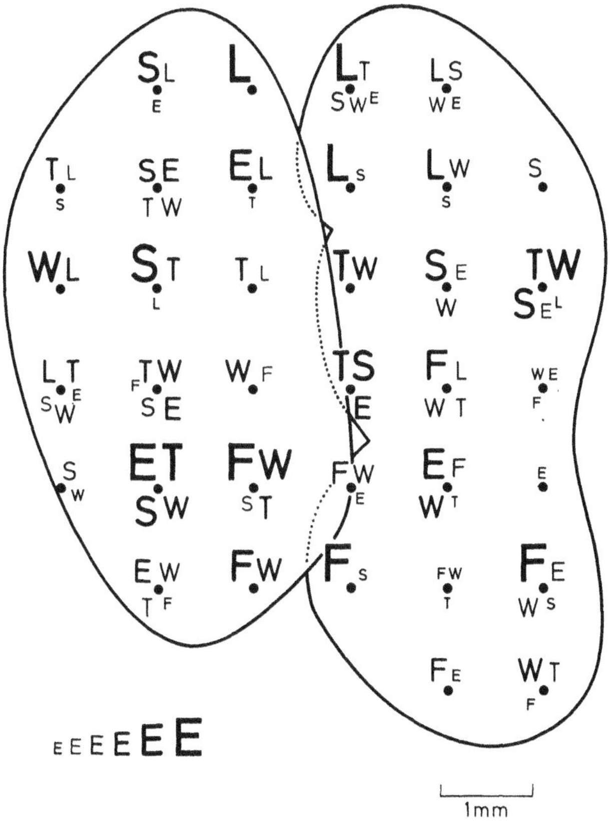

Fig. 4. Horizontal section through interposed (*left*) and dentate (*right*) nucleus, with penetration sites labeled according to movements. For this map, the movement to which a neuron was best related gave each cell a movement name, and the degree of the relationship was quantified using the means and variance of the highest and lowest discharge frequencies (discharge modulation index, DMI). Only the highest DMI (for the best related movement) was used for each neuron. These highest DMIs were then added together within each penetration in each movement. The size of the letter is scaled to the size of the sum. The map is biased toward penetrations with many cells related to a single movement, since DMIs are added instead of averaged, but other methods of display gave similar results

related to thumb, wrist, elbow, or shoulder were mingled in such confusion as to reveal no proximodistal topographic ordering whatsoever. This kind of topography may be the cerebellar nuclear counterpart of what Welker and associates have called in the cerebellar cortex "fractured somatotopy". We do not as yet know whether focal lesions confined to one of the anterior/posterior thirds will affect movement of one part of the body and spare others. We do know now that to find units in the dentate and interpositus that relate to arm movements the electrode should best be directed to their middle region. This knowledge is crucial to the interpretation of the next experiment.

Experiments on coding of cerebellar neurons had got to the point of showing that some cells fire discretely in relation to some parameters of movement and not to others [31]. These parameters included the muscular force, the joint position, the velocity, the direction, the direction of intended subsequent movement (directional set), the start, the stop, and the duration of movement [31]. Since the neurons changed their activity before the onset of movement, we thought that they might discretely control these variables. In an attempt to define these parametric relationships further, monkeys were trained in a task where all the above mentioned variables were included, but so dissociated that we might optimize our ability to appreciate whether a neuron's discharge might be related to one but not the other variables. To do this, the monkeys were trained to follow a slowly moving target beam on an oscilloscope with a smooth pursuit tracking movement of the wrist (Fig. 5). While the neurons did show parametric relationships, the main result came as a surprise. The principal finding

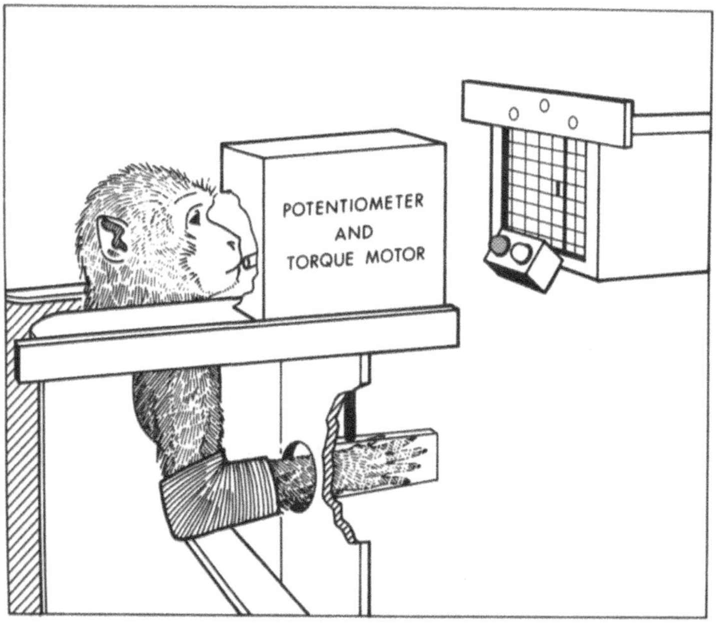

Fig. 5. Sketch of monkey and apparatus used for slow pursuit tracking of a visual stimulus by movement at the wrist

concerns the direction of modulated unit discharge frequency (up or down), and the direction of the wrist movement (right of left). The findings are summarized in Fig. 6. Figure 6A shows the EMG discharge of a long flexor muscle of the wrist and the fingers that was located in the forearm. At the top left of Fig. 6A is the stimulus trajectory that the monkey followed during wrist extension, and below it are three graphs showing the muscle EMG during extension. At the top right of Fig. 6A is the target stimulus trajectory that the monkey followed during flexion, and below it are three graphs showing the EMG discharge of the forearm flexor muscle during flexion. The middle two graphs of Fig. 6A show the EMG discharge during flexion and extension under no load, the upper two graphs under flexor load, and the bottom two under extensor load. When flexing under no load (Fig. 6A, middle right graph), the flexor muscle increases discharge as flexion proceeds. When flexing under flexor load (Fig. 6A, right upper graph), the discharge is greatly increased; when flexing under extensor load (Fig. 6A, lower right graph), the flexor muscle is virtually silent, as the loaded extensors do all the work even during slow flexor movements. When extending under no load (Fig. 6A, middle left graph), the extensor muscle again does the work, and the flexor muscle is mainly silent. This is true also when extending under extensor load (Fig. 6A, lower left graph). But when extending under flexor load (Fig. 6A, upper left graph), the loaded flexor muscle does the work (the extensor muscles are silent), and the EMG of the flexor muscle slowly lowers to let the load carry the hand and manipulandum in an extensor movement. This is the expected relationship of a muscle's activity for the two directions of movement and for the three different load states, and all the muscles in the forelimb that were used in the task behaved in this way (or the reverse pattern for extensors).

The discharge of a neuron in motor cortex is shown in Fig. 6B. When flexing under no load (Fig. 6B, middle right graph), the discharge frequency increased; the frequency increased even higher when flexing under flexor load (Fig. 6B, upper right graph), but was nil when flexing under extensor load (Fig. 6B, lower right graph). When extending, the neuron was active under flexor load (Fig. 6B, upper left); discharge was slight when extending under no load (Fig. 6B, middle left graph) and nil under extensor load (Fig. 6B, lower left graph). This neuron, therefore, had a discharge pattern during the two directions of movement and the two directions of load exactly like that of the flexor muscle (6) (Fig. 6A). Of all the neurons in motor cortex, half discharged in a pattern that resembled activity in a flexor (like this one) or an extensor muscle. We have called this pattern unidirectional or reciprocal.

By contrast, the other half of motor cortex neurons behaved in a distinctly different pattern, an example of which is shown in Fig. 6C. The conventions are the same as in Fig. 6a, b. What is at once apparent is that the pattern of discharge is remarkably the same, regardless of the direction of the movement and the load condition. At the onset of movement there is an abrupt increase of discharge frequency to a peak, which then gradually lowers as the movement progresses. Under conditions which call for marked changes in discharge frequency in muscle (Fig. 6A), and neurons behaving like muscle (Fig. 6B), the pattern is remarkably constant. We call this pattern of discharge, which is constant for the

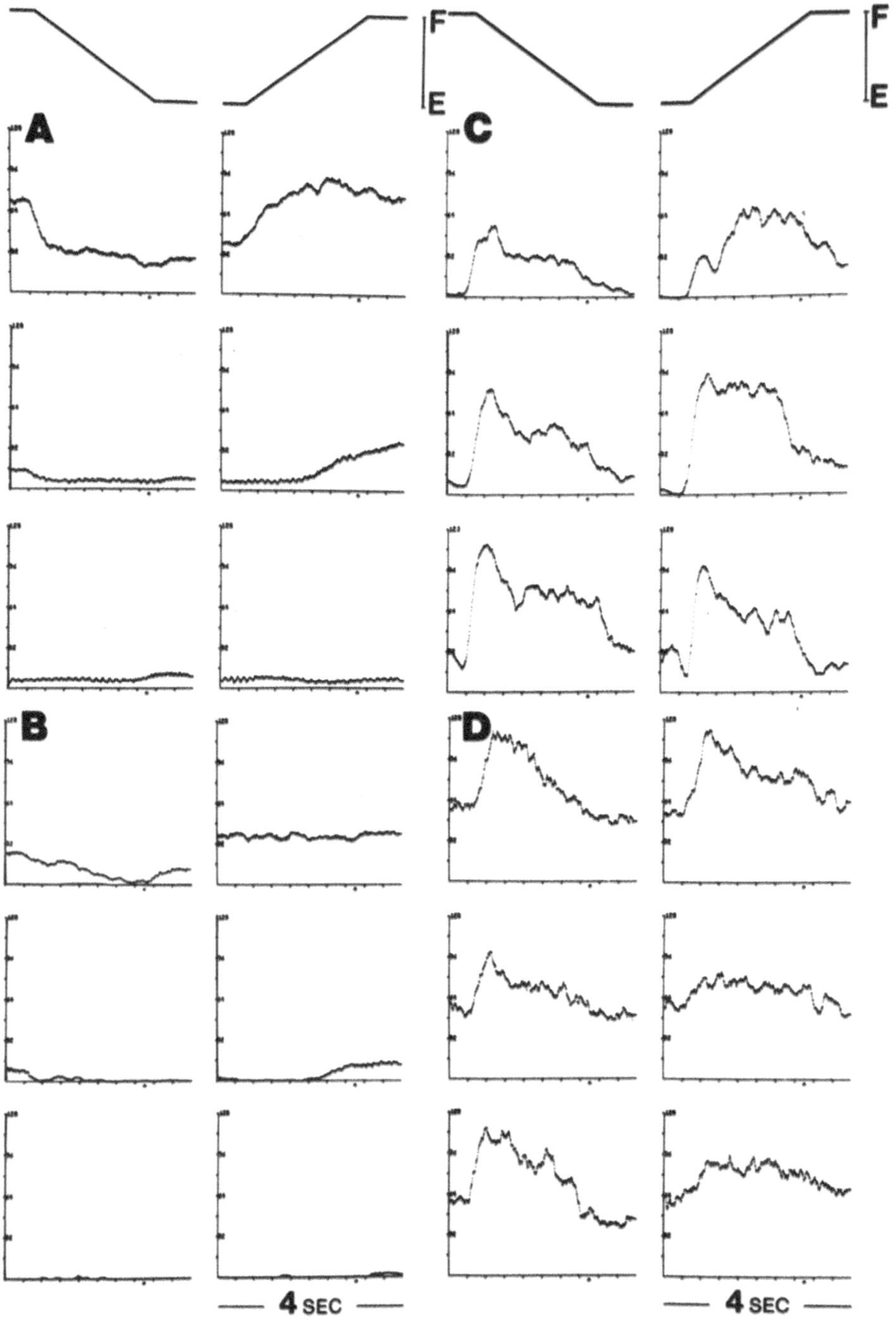

Fig. 6A–D. Legend see p. 449

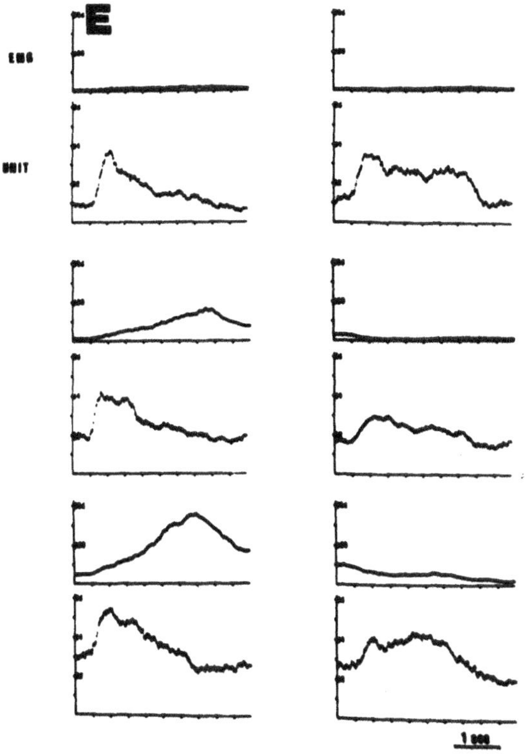

Fig. 6A–E. Discharge of muscle (EMG) and neurons during slow hold-ramp-hold tracking movements in different directions under different loads. **A** Flexor muscle; **B** neuron in precentral cortex; **C** another neuron in the precentral cortex; **D** neuron in dentate nucleus; **E** EMG of extensor muscle and discharge of primary spindle afferent in extensor muscle. **A** *Top left:* hold-ramp-hold stimulus trajectory during extension; *below* are EMG traces during extension. At *top right* of A is stimulus trajectory during flexion; *below* are EMG traces during flexion. On the six graphs, the *top* row is under flexor load, the *middle* row under no load, and the *bottom* row under extensor load. Conventions are the same for B–E. The graphs that: the pattern of discharge for muscle in A and E (*top*) and the type I precentral cortical neuron in B are reciprocal; the pattern of discharge for the type II precentral cortical neuron in C, the dentate neuron in D, and the primary muscle spindle afferent in E are bidirectional

two directions of movement and the two directions of load, "bidirectional" [7]. In the cerebellar nuclei, to our great surprise, most of the neurons discharged like that in Fig. 6d: the pattern was bidirectional. Indeed, we initially did not think that there were *any* neurons in the cerebellar nuclei that were reciprocal. Because of this, we thought that we had directed the electrode to the wrong parts of the dentate and the interposed nuclei – that we were recording from cells that were concerned with parts of the body *other* than the arm, and that the opposing muscles in these other parts were *cocontracting* to help keep the rest of the body still. But this was not the case, for several reasons: (a) the neurons undergoing the greatest changes in discharge frequency (and the most concerned with task performance) were in the middle portion of the interpositus and dentate, and this portion we had just shown to contain the greatest numbers of neurons preferentially related to movements of the arm; (b) there were only a few cerebellar neurons that fired in a reciprocal pattern, and these were weakly correlated; (c) the bidirectional neurons whose discharge best correlated with performance of this task also correlated well with other movements of the arm–rapid alternating movements, response to flexor and extensor torque pulses, and even to physiological tremor of the arm; and (d) in all these other movements, the pattern of discharge was reciprocal. For these reasons, we suspected that under the conditions of this task, many cerebellar neurons were concerned with some aspect of the task, or some component of the body, where a premium was set on *constancy* of pattern. We wondered if this could possibly involve the discharge of gamma motor neurons (which the cerebellum is known to control), or the activity of muscle receptors (which are known to influence the cerebellum). This led us to see if we could record from the dorsal root ganglion cells innervating the muscle spindles of the forearm to see if they might also fire in a bidirectional pattern – possibly the cause or the effect (or both) of bidirectional motor cortex and cerebellar activity.

The same monkey in which we had recorded the EMG and the discharge of neurons in motor cortex and cerebellar nuclei was anesthetized, and a standard recording chamber was implanted over the exposed C 7–8 dorsal root ganglia (DRG). Single neuron recordings were identified [4, 14, 15, 19, 34] as being those of spindle afferents from forelimb muscles if they had: (a) a receptive field in the muscle belly (and not skin); (b) a spontaneous maintained discharge that (c) could be driven by brief taps to the receptive field; (d) a response to a tuning fork of 128/s frequency applied to the receptive field, with discharge following at 128 or a subharmonic of 64 cps; (e) reciprocal responses to flexor and extensor torque pulses and (f) to rapid alternating movements; and finally (g) a pause in firing when the muscle in which it lay was made to contract by direct electrical shock so as to unload the spindle. One neuron satisfied all of the criteria, and four others, most of the criteria, and these were identified as muscle spindle afferents. The discharge of one of these is shown in Fig. 6 E, along with the EMG of the extensor muscle in which it lay. One can see that the extensor muscle behaved in a pattern just the opposite of that shown for the flexor muscle in Fig. 6 A. Under no load (Fig. 6 E, middle graphs), the muscle is active during extension (left), and not flexion (right). Under extensor load (Fig. 6 E, bottom graphs), the muscle is active during both flexion (right) and extension (left); and under flexor load (top graphs), inactive during both flexion (right) and extension (left). By contrast, the spindle afferent had much the same pattern of discharge under all the conditions: an abrupt increase in discharge frequency at the onset of movement, with a gradual lowering as the movement progresses. The pattern of discharge is very different from that of the muscle in which it is located, and very different from that of the reciprocal class of neurons in the motor cortex. The pattern is similar to that of the bidirectional class of neurons in the motor cortex, and similar to that of the majority of neurons in the interpositus and dentate. Furthermore, all five of the DRG cells thus identified as primary spindle afferents discharged in a similar bidirectional pattern.

What caused the bidirectional pattern in the spindle afferent discharge? Can it be explained by the two conventional means of activating spindle afferents –

passive stretch of muscle, and gamma motorneuron drive coactivated with alpha motor neurons [4, 34]? We concluded that it can not for three reasons: (a) the temporal profile of spindle afferent discharge, which abruptly increased at the start of all movements, was not matched by parallel EMG activity in the arm; (b) the varying combinations of passive stretch and gamma coactivation with alphas under such diverse constancy; and (c) in the extreme case illustrated in Fig. 6E, upper left graph, the discharging spindle receptor was located in a muscle that was both passively shortening and electrically silent (the opposite muscle was active under full load and slowly lengthening). The spindle afferent was therefore discharging in a situation quite without *either* of the two conventional means of activating spindles receptors. Neither can the spindle afferent discharge in Fig. 6E be explained as due to the threshold recruitment of the smaller gamma motorneurons before recruitment of any of the larger alpha motorneurons: if this were the case, one might have expected a much greater spindle afferent discharge when the conditions were optimal for driving the spindle afferents by the two conventional means. In Fig. 6E, lower right graph, the spindle was in a loaded muscle that was actively lengthening[1]; yet the pattern of spindle afferent discharge was qualitatively and quantitatively similar to that which was observed under the least conventionally favorable conditions in Fig. 6E, upper left graph. We must therefore assume that this pattern of constancy of spindle afferent discharge can only be brought about by changes in gamma drive that are sufficiently dissociated from alpha drive to keep the pattern constant.

But why should the pattern of spindle afferent discharge be kept constant? We surmise that in precise performances of this kind, the use of the primary spindle receptors is not to register the large lengthenings and shortenings that are planned and performed in the task, but rather to detect the small errors of muscle length (and joint position) that occur because of distraction of attention, friction of the device, and physiological tremor [15, 19]. These small errors can themselves be anticipated through the experience of the performance, and the spindle sensitivity optimally adjusted to detect them. We think it might be *only* through the long practice of such a difficult task, where small errors might be damaging but anticipatible, that alpha-gamma dissociation of this degree ever takes place. The facts that both (a) the gamma motor neuron and (b) the circuitry for its private control occur in an animal capable of making such movements (monkey), and not in animals that cannot (frog), seem to make some teleological sense.

How the information might be used to improve the performance of the movement is another question; we assume that it could be used at many levels, from the stiffening of the muscle through the segmental loop servo [20] to the automation of motor performance by longer loops, and even to the insertion of it into the consciousness of the monkey [9].

---

1 Before movement onset, the maintained discharge of the spindle is higher when the parent muscle is loaded (Fig. 6E lower graphs, left and right) than when unloaded (Fig. 6E upper graphs, left and right). This is presumably due to alpha-gamma coactivation

But whatever the cause and the effect of the alpha-gamma dissociation, we were impressed by the degree to which motor cortex, and especially the cerebellum, would appear to be involved in the operation.

References

1. Allen GI, Gilbert PFC, Marini R, Schultz W, Yin TCT (1977) Integration of cerebral and peripheral inputs by interpositus neurons in monkeys. Exp Brain Res 27:81–99
2. Allen GI, Gilbert PFC, Yin TCT (1978) Convergence of cerebral inputs onto dentate neurons in monkey. Exp Brain Res 32:151–170
3. Allen GI, Tsukahara N (1974) Cerebrocerebellar communication systems. Physiol Rev 54:957–1006
4. Burke D (1981) The activity of muscle spindle endings in normal motor behavior. In: Porter R (ed) International review of physiology, Neurophysiology IV. University Park Press, Baltimore pp 91–126
5. Chan-Palay V (1977) Cerebellar dentate nucleus. Springer, Berlin Heidelberg New York
6. Evarts EV (1968) Relation of pyramidal tract activity to force exerted during a voluntary movement. J Neurophysiol 31:14–27
7. Evarts EV (1969b) Methods for recording activity in individual neurons in moving animals. Methods Med Res:241–250
8. Gilbert PFC, Thach WT (1977) Purkinje cell activity during motor learning. Brain Res 128:309–328
9. Goodwin GM, McCloskey DI, Matthews PBC (1972) The contribution of muscle afferents to kinaesthesia shown by vibration induced illusions of movement and by the effects of paralysing joint afferents. Brain 95:705–748
10. Granit R, Holmgren B, Merton PA (1955) The two routes for excitation of muscles and their subservience to the cerebellum. J Physiol (Lond) 130:213–224
11. Kalil K (1977) Topographic organization of projections from dentate and interpositus nuclei in the Rhesus monkey: an autoradiographic study. Abstracts of the meeting of Society for Neuroscience 3:165
12. Koeze TH (1968) The independence of corticomotoneuronal and fusimotor pathways in the production of muscle contraction by motor cortex stimulation. J Physiol (Lond) 197:87–105
13. Goldberger ME, Growdon JH (1973) Patterns of recovery following cerebellar deep nuclear lesions in monkeys. Exp Neurol 39:307–322
14. Henneman E (1974) The cerebellum. In: Mountcastle VB (ed) Medical Physiology, 13th edn. Mosby, St. Louis, pp 722–746
15. Kuffler SW, Hunt CC, Quilliam JP (1951) Function of medulated small-nerve fibers in mammalian ventral roots: efferent muscle spindle innervation. J Neurophysiol 14:29–54
16. Loeb GE, Duysens J (1979) Activity patterns in individual hindlimb primary and secondary muscle spindle afferents during normal movements in unrestrained cats. J Neurophysiol 42:420–440
17. Mano N-I, Yamamoto J-I (1980) Simple spike activity of cerebellar Purkinje cells related to visually guided wrist tracking movement in the monkey. J Neurophysiol 43:713–728
18. Massion J, Rispal-Padel L (1972) Spatial organization of the cerebello-thalamo-cortical pathway. Brain Res 40:61–65
19. Matthews PBC (1981) Muscle spindles, their messages and their fusimotor supply with particular reference to the provision of information for motor control. In: Brooks VB (ed) Handbook on motor control. American Physiological Society, pp 189–228
20. Nichols TR, Houk JC (1976) Improvement in linearity and regulation of stiffness that results from action of stretch reflex. J Neurophysiol 39:119–142
21. Perry JG (1980) Somatotopy in deep cerebellar nuclei revealed by active movement of individual joints. Doctoral Dissertation. Washington University, Program in Neural Science
22. Sasaki K, Kawaguchi S, Oka H, Sasaki M, Mizuno N (1976) Electrophysiological studies on the cerebellocerebral projections in monkeys. Exp Brain Res 24:495–507

23. Schieber MH (1981) Muscle, motor cortex, cerebellar nucleus, and spindle afferent activity during slow hold ramp hold position tracking movements of the monkeys wrist. Doctoral Dissertation, Washington University, Program in Neural Science
24. Schultz W, Montgomery E, Marini R (1976) Stereotyped flexion of forelimb and hindlimb to microstimulation of dentate nucleus in Cebus monkeys. Brain Res 107:151–155
25. Stanton GB (1980) Topographical organization of ascending cerebellar projections from the dentate and interposed nuclei in Macaca mulatta. An anterograde degeneration study. J Comp Neurol 190:699–731
26. Thach WT (1968) Discharge of Purkinje cells and cerebellar nuclear neurons during rapidly alternating arm movements in the monkey. J Neurophysiol 31:785–797
27. Thach WT (1970a) Discharge of cerebellar neurons related to two maintained postures and two prompt movements. I. Nuclear cell output. J Neurophysiol 33:527–536
28. Thach WT (1970b) Discharge of cerebellar neurons related to two maintained postures and two prompt movements. II. Purkinje cell output and input. J Neurophysiol 33:537–547
29. Thach WT (1972) Cerebellar output: properties, synthesis and uses. Brain Res 40:89–97
30. Thach WT (1975) Timing of activity in the cerebellar dentate nucleus and cerebral motor cortex during prompt volitional movement. Brain Res 88:233–241
31. Thach WT (1978) Correlation of neural discharge with pattern and force of muscular activity, joint position, and direction of intended next movement in motor cortex and cerebellum. J Neurophysiol 41:654–676
32. Thach WT (1980) Complex spikes, the inferior olive and natural behavior. In: Courville J (ed) The inferior olivary nucleus. Raven, New York, pp 349–360
33. Thach WT, Jones EG (1979) The cerebellar dentatothalamic connection: terminal field, lamellae, rods and somatotopy. Brain Res 169:168–248
34. Vallbo AB (1971) Muscle spindle response at the onset of isometric voluntary contractions in man. Time differences between fusimotor and skeletomotor effects. J Physiol (Lond) 318:405–431

Discussion

Thach first noted that he did not intend to suggest that cerebellar function is only related to γ-motorneurons, since it is clear from phylogenetic considerations that the cerebellum has other functions. For example, the frog has a well-developed cerebellum, but no neurons that can give independent control of muscle spindles.

Evarts (Bethesda) congratulated Dr. Thach on providing clear evidence for independent control of α- and γ-motorneurons, a concept that has been considered likely for some time. He added that Dr. Taylor had also presented evidence for independent control at a recent conference in Montreal. Dr. Thach pointed out that the tracking test used in his own studies is a very difficult motor task, probably requiring optimal performance of spindles and sensory feedback, and is the kind of behavior that might be expected to engage such a control mechanism.

Ito referred to work by Madame Padel (Marseille) using microstimulation of cerebellar nuclei of the baboon. She finds movement at two or three joints evoked by stimulation of the dentate nucleus, but only at one joint with stimulation of the interpositus nuclei. Dr. Thach has not observed conspicuous differences between cerebellar nuclei of this kind, but has not looked at this question in detail.

Eccles commented that one might a priori expect rapid movements to be more closely related to the dentate nucleus and slower ones to the interpositus. Dr. Thach noted that in his studies there was no evidence for such a selective relationship.

Role of Cerebellar Purkinje Cells in Voluntary Limb Movement

N. Mano and K. Yamamoto *

"The disturbance of skill in voluntary limb movement" is one of the cardinal observations made in humans [6] and experimental animals [3] with injured or ablated cerebellum. In humans, the skill of the limb movement has often been analyzed quantitatively by the visually guided limb movement in the fields of control engineering, psychology, neurology, and so on [18]. In this article, we will present data showing that the monkey can also be trained to perform a skillful limb movement by a visual cue, and that we can analyze the neural discharges quantitatively in relation to the skilled limb movement in terms of movement parameters, such as holding position (P), velocity (dP/dt), force (F), rate of force change (dF/dt), and the direction of wrist movement (flexion or extension) [10, 14].

The second point which we will discuss is the complexity of the spatiotemporal pattern of muscle activity, even in a simple limb movement restricted to one joint and to one plane. This complexity has been one of the major obstacles in analyzing the neural correlate in relation to a specified limb movement [2]. To avoid this obstacle, many scientists have recently attempted to study the neural correlate of the cerebellum in relation to the eye movement [8, 9, 16, 17], in which the number of muscles involved and the pattern of these muscles' activities in the eye movement is well known. But, to elucidate the common and/or different features of the brain mechanisms of the eye and the limb movements, we should solve the complexity of limb muscle's activity. This obstacle could be overcome, at least in part, by analyzing the degree of temporal coupling of each muslce's activity and each cell's discharge-rate modulation with the beginning of the wrist movement, under the carefully adjusted forelimb posture [12, 14].

Based on these technical developments, we investigated the normal operations of the cerebellar cortex, by recording Purkinje-cell (P cell) discharges while the monkey performed visually guided, wrist tracking movements.

Visually Guided Wrist Tracking Movements in Monkeys

To instruct the monkeys (*Macaca mulatta*) to flex or extend the wrist with different velocities and to hold the wrist joint still at different angles, we displayed the target (Fig. 1, T) and the cursor line (Fig. 1, C) on a videoscope in front of

---

* The authors wish to thank Mrs. M. Sakai for typing the manuscript

Experimental Brain Research, Suppl. 6

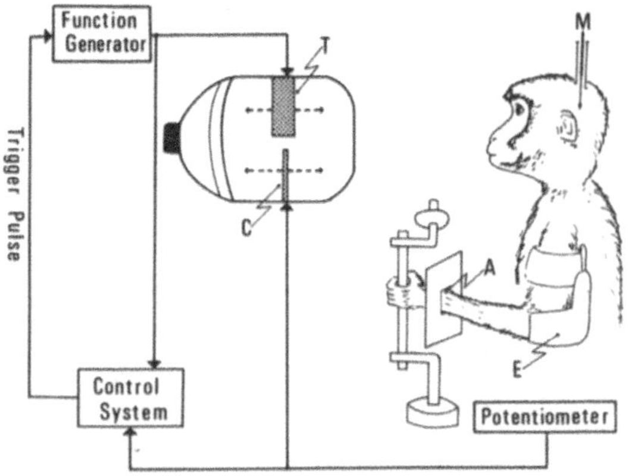

Fig. 1. Experimental arrangement for visually guided wrist-tracking movements. *T*, target strip; *C*, cursor line; *A*, narrow access hole to restrict the side-to-side movement of the wrist; *E*, elbow pad to restrict the push-pull and side-to-side movements of the forelimb; *M*, microelectrode. See text for explanation about the task. Mano and Yamamoto [14]

the monkey. The monkeys could move the cursor line by moving the handle to the left or right on a horizontal plane. The angular position of the handle was proportionally converted to the horizontal displacement of the line by a potentiometer coupled to the rotation axis of the handle. The target was initially still at the center of the scope. After the animal held the cursor line beneath the target for at least of 0.6 s, the target was triggered to move horizontally to the left or right by a step or ramp function voltage. The monkey had to track the target for at least 2.5 s within the allowance zone (the width of the target strip) by flexing or extending the wrist about 30° from a neutral position to receive a drop of fruit juice as a reward. When the monkey correctly performed the wrist tracking movement, the target returned to the center and the direction of the tracking movement was reversed.

By this visually guided movement, we could control the direction of the monkey's wrist movement: flexion and extension; the holding position at three different angles of the wrist joint – neutral, about 30° flexed and extended; and the velocity of the wrist movement in four ranges – (a) 10–30°/s (slow ramp, Fig. 2S), (b) 30–100°/s (ramp, Fig. 2R), (c) 100–300°/s (quick step, Fig. 2Q), and (d) 300–650°/s (ballistic, Fig. 2B).

The training procedures and the four kinds of tracking movements (Fig. 2S, R, Q, B) have been described in detail previously [14].

Muscles Involved in Task Performance

To reduce the complexity of the spatiotemporal pattern of the muscles' activities involved in the task performance, we restricted the side-to-side and push-pull movements of the forearm by restricting the wrist and elbow (Fig. 1A, E) and adjusted the distance of the grip rod from the rotation axis to coincide with the wrist-joint axis. Under these conditions, the muscles working as prime movers were confined to the wrist extensors and flexors, and the activities of upper arm, shoulder, and truncal muscles did not directly influence the handle movement, even if their activities incidentally accompanied the task performance. In other words, the wrist extensors (M. Ext. carpi radialis, M. Ext. carpi ulnaris) and flexors (M. Flex. carpi radialis, M. Flex. carpi ulnaris) contracted at fairly fixed times prior to the handle movement, while the other muscles (M. Pect. major, M. Infraspinatus, etc.) contracted at variable timings in reference to the beginning of the handle movement from trial to trial. Based on the dissociated timings of the muscle activities in between the prime movers and other muscles (see Fig. 2 in ref. [14]), we discriminated the P cells related directly to the wrist movement from other P cells that might be related to the activities of the muscles not working as prime wrist movers, as will be described in the following section.

Wrist-Related P Cells

The spike discharges of about 200 P cells were recorded in three monkeys by glass-coated Pt-Ir microelectrodes (Fig. 1, M) from the lobules IV–VII of the cerebellar hemispheres ipsilateral to the task-performing hand. Of these cells, 92 P cells significantly increased or decreased simple-spike discharge rate during task performance as compared to the tonic discharge rate while the monkeys were holding the handle at the neutral position, waiting for target displacement. For the analyses of the spike activities in relation to the movement parameters of the wrist flexion or extension, we further selected 45 P cells related to the wrist movement by analyzing the degree of temporal coupling of the discharge modulation with the wrist movement by a statistical method [12, 14]. In brief, the onset times of significant frequency modulation were determined in individual trials when the increase or decrease of instantaneous frequencies reached a significant level in the Kolmogorov-Smirnov one-sample test [12] and the temporal coupling of the discharge frequency modulation and electromyographic activities to the beginning of wrist movement was compared [14]. Based on the comparison of the degree in temporal coupling, we conjectured that 45 cells showing good timing of the frequency modulation with the wrist movement were related to wrist movement.

Discharge Patterns of Simple Spikes in Wrist-Related P Cells

In each of the four kinds of tracking movements (Fig. 2B, Q, S, R), the discharge pattern of simple spikes in wrist-related P cells was very similar to the velocity pattern of wrist movement (Fig. 2, V) but different from the angular position of the wrist joint (Fig. 2, P).

When following the step-function displacements of the target, the simple-spike frequency transiently increased (Fig. 2B, Q) or decreased (Fig. 5B) with transient velocity change, and recovered to the control level of the firing rate with the return of the velocity to zero. The maintained frequency differences of the simple spikes while holding still at the neutral position and at about 30°, flexed or extended, were mostly less than 10 spikes/s. For detailed quantitative ana-

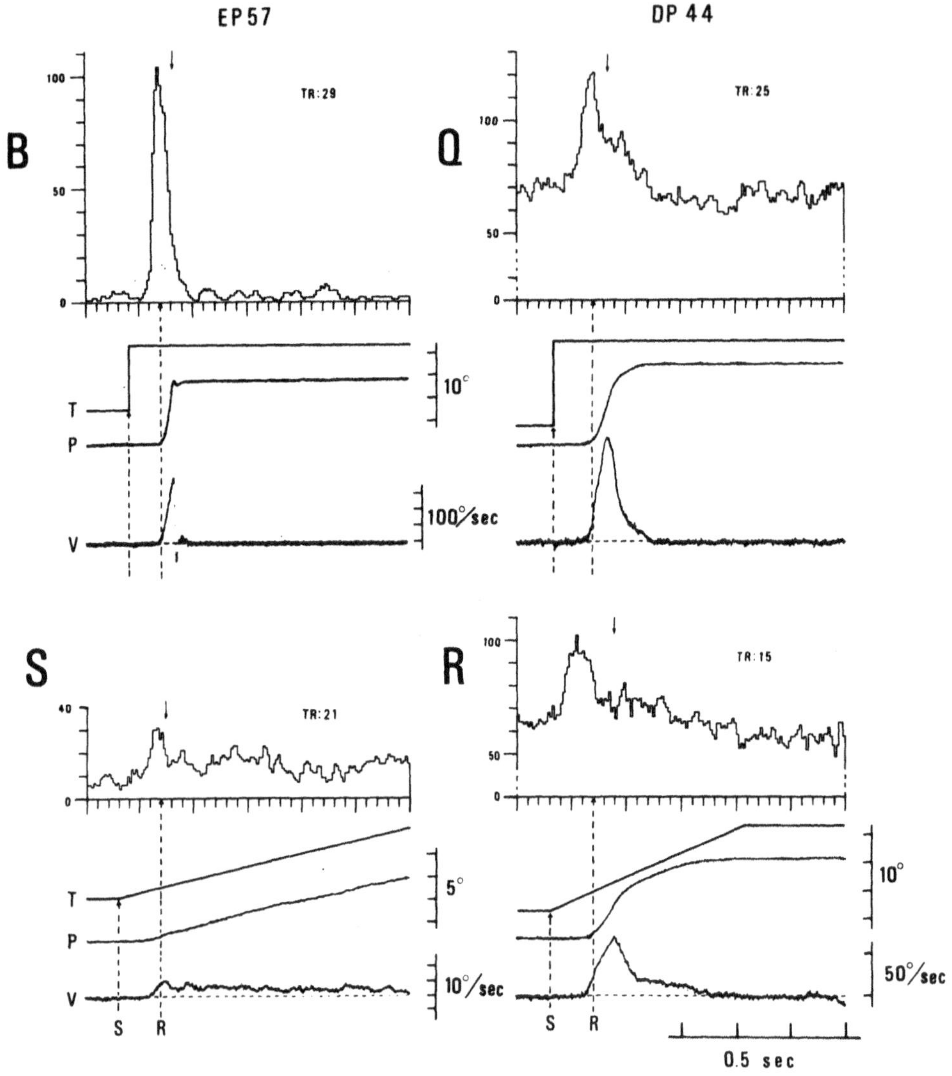

Fig. 2B, Q, R, S. Pattern of simple-spike discharges in wrist-related group I P cells with ballistic **B** and slow ramp **S** wrist movements (EP57), or quick **Q** and ramp **R** wrist movement (DP44). DP44 and EP57 identify the P cell numbers. The moving average histograms (window: 60 ms, bin: 20 ms) of spike frequencies (*ordinate*, simple spikes/s) were aligned at the beginning of wrist movement (event *R*). Positions (*P*) and velocities (*V*) of handle movements were averaged over ten successive trials, aligned at event *R*. Target displacement (*T*) is a single trial trace. *Downward arrows* on the histograms indicate the peak time of velocity. Note the precedence of spike activity to wrist movement in both onset and peak times. Mano and Yamamoto [14]

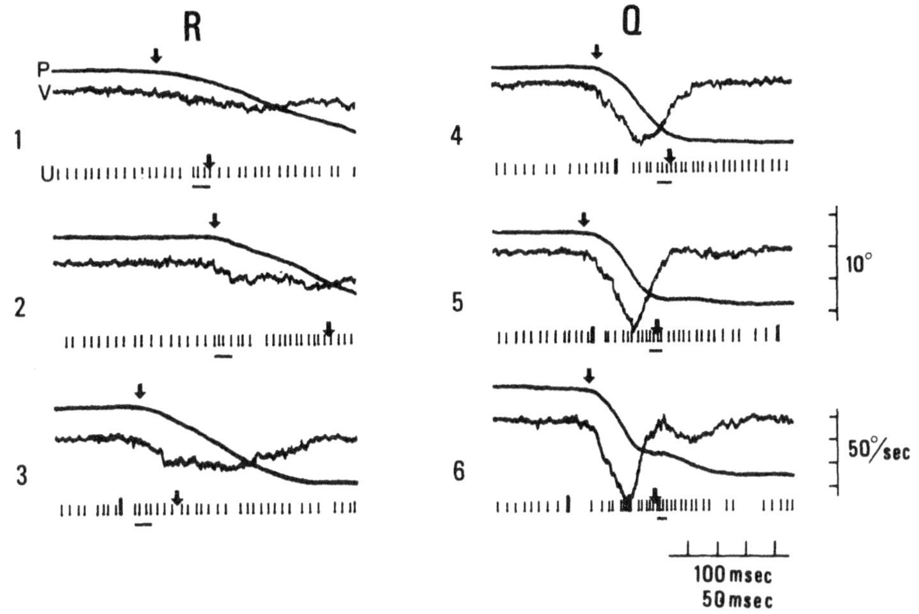

Fig. 3. Specimen trials of ramp **R** and quick **Q** wrist movements. In each trial set, the position (*P*) of the handle, the velocity (*V*) of the movement, and the unitary discharges (*U*) of the P cell (DP44) illustrated in Fig. 2 are shown from *top* to *bottom*. *Upper* two traces (*P* and *V*) were triggered to sweep (*time scale:* 100 ms) by the beginning of the target displacement (event *S*, *upward arrow S* in Fig. 2, not shown here), but the spike activities (*U*) were swept after a certain delay with expanded sweep speed (*time scale:* 50 ms). *Downward arrow* (event *R*) on the *P* trace corresponds in timing to the *arrow* on the *U* trace. A short *vertical bar* in the *U* trace represents a simple spike, and a longer *thick bar* a complex spike. *Underlining* in each *U* trace indicates the shortest inter-spike intervals of three successive intervals

lyses, refer to Figs. 5, 7 in ref. [10] and Figs. 5, 6B in ref. [14]. Thus, the firing rate of the simple spikes appeared to contain the information mainly about the velocity or some dynamic component of the wrist movement, and only poorly about the holding angular position of the wrist joint.

This suggestion was supported by the discharge patterns of simple spikes associated with the slow ramp and ramp movement of the wrist (Fig. 2S, R). The firing rate of the simple spikes maintained the slightly increased frequency as long as the wrist moved evenly with very slow velocity (Fig. 2S), and recovered to the control frequency when the velocity returned to zero (Fig. 2R).

The amount of firing-rate increase also appeared to be in proportion to the velocity of wrist movement. For example, the difference in maximum increase of simple-spike frequency between the ballistic and slow-ramp wrist movements (Fig. 2B, S) was much larger than the difference between the quick and ramp movements (Fig. 2Q, R), probably reflecting the much larger velocity difference in the former pair of movements than in the latter pair. This quantitative relation between the frequency and the velocity was observed even in individual trials.

As is illustrated in Fig. 3, the increase of simple-spike discharges (Fig. 3, U) became more and more prominent, as the peak velocity (Fig. 3, V) of wrist movement became faster, from trials 1 to 6. This positive correlation between the discharge frequency and the velocity is analyzed in more detail, in the next section.

Frequency-Velocity Relationship

To clarify the quantitative relation between the simple-spike activity and the velocity of wrist movement, the instantanous frequency change of simple spikes was analyzed in relation to the peak velocities in individual trials. The maximum instantaneous frequencies, defined as the reciprocal of the minimum moving average of three successive inter-spike intervals (underlined in Fig. 3, U), are plotted on the ordinate in relation to the peak velocities on the abscissa in Fig. 4, obtained in the P cell illustrated in Fig. 2Q, R and Fig. 3. Although there were large variations from trial to trial, the correlation between the two variables was highly significant, and the ratios of firing-rate increase to velocity, the slope of the regression line, was 0.39 spikes/s/degree/s. Thus, the linear gradations of the velocities were observed without a distinct gap in between the quick stepwise movement (white circles) and the ramp tracking movement (black circles). The lack of a distinct gap between the two tasks (white vs black circles) suggests that the discharge frequencies of the simple spikes were primarily correlated with the velocity of wrist movement, but were not correlated with the velocity of the target's displacement, nor with the error between the target and the cursor line (see Fig. 2Q, R-T).

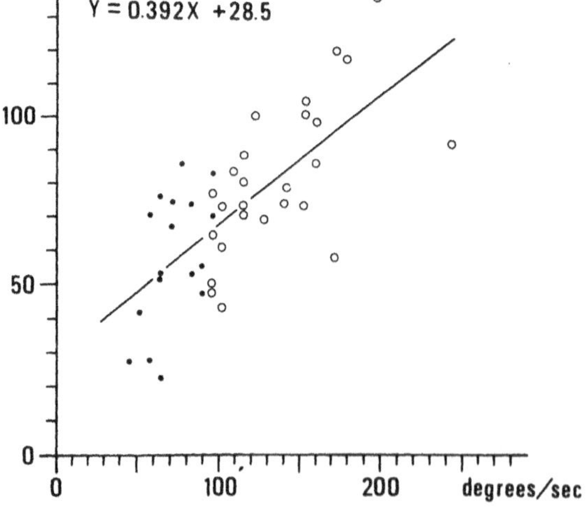

Fig. 4. Relationship between instantaneous frequency modulation (*ordinate*, Y) and the peak velocity of wrist movement (*abscissa*, X) in individual trials in the same P cell (DP 44) illustrated in Figs. 2, 3. A *black* or *white circle* indicates a single trial of ramp or quick wrist movement, respectively. The *regression line* was obtained by the least squares method from the combined 43 trials of ramp and quick movements. *r*, correlation coefficient of frequency increase on peak velocity; *P*, significance level to reject the null hypothesis; $r=0$. Mano and Yamamoto [14]

Discharge Patterns of Simple Spikes in Group II P Cells

In the preceding sections, we described a group of P cells (group I) whose discharge-rate modulation of simple spikes was best correlated with the velocity of wrist movement. Among the wrist-related P cells, another group of P cells (group II) was found [13]. They discharged essentially in a similar pattern to group I P cells, in the sense that the simple-spike frequency modulated in relation to the dynamic aspect of wrist movement, but not to the maintained posi-

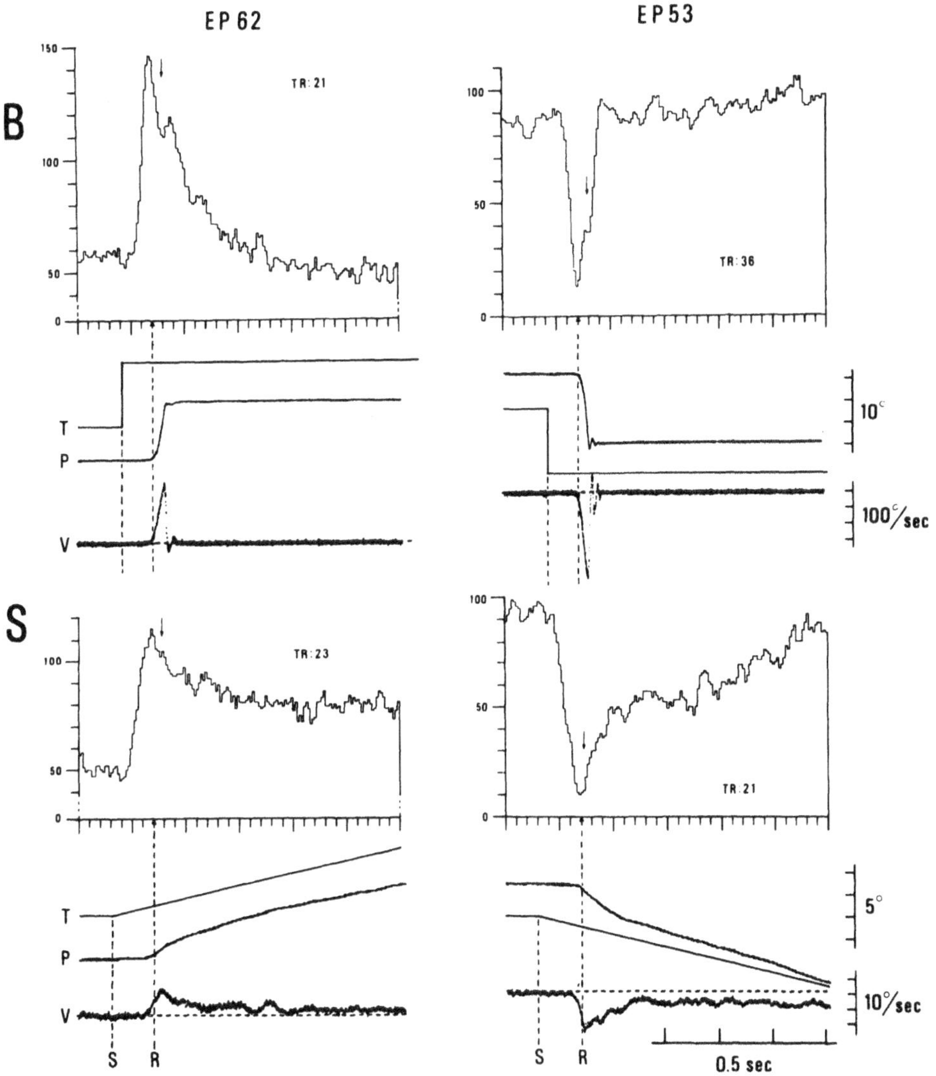

Fig. 5. Pattern of simple-spike discharges in group II P cells with ballistic **B** and slow-ramp **S** wrist movements. Conventions are same as in Fig. 2. Mano and Yamamoto [14]

tion (Fig. 5B). A prominent characteristic of the discharge pattern in group II P cells was the large amount of frequency modulation throughout the execution of slow wrist movement (Fig. 5S). The maximum increase or decrease of the discharge rate in the initial phase of slow-ramp movement was not so much different from that with ballistic movement, compared to the prominent difference between the amounts of frequency modulation in ballistic and slow-ramp movements (Fig. 2B vs Fig. 2S). Throughout the later phase of slow-ramp movement, the prominent frequency modulation was maintained (compare Fig. 5S and Fig. 2S).

The frequency-velocity analysis in individual trials in group II P cells reflected the discharge pattern characteristics. In group II P cells, the ratio of discharge rate modulation to the velocity was smaller than 0.11 spikes/s/degree/s, compared to the ratio larger than 0.19 in group I P cells, and the correlation between the frequency modulation and the velocity of wrist movement was not statistically significant ($r < 0.40$, $P > 0.05$).

Whether the two groups (I, II) of P cells suggest the presence of two distinct types bearing qualitatively different functions, or the difference between the two groups is a mere quantitative one, should be clarified in future.

Directionality of Simple-Spike Activity

The majority of P cells modulated their simple-spike discharge rate in a nonreciprocal fashion (see Fig. 5 in refs. [10, 14]): some P cells increased the discharge rate on either flexion and extension, and the other cells decreased on both directions of wrist movement. These nonreciprocal changes of spike activity cannot be attributed to cocontraction of wrist flexors and extensors because in our restricted limb positions these prime movers contracted in a reciprocal or unidirectional fashion (see Fig. 2 in ref. [14]). Another possible interpretation might be that these nonreciprocal activities of P cells are related to nonreciprocal activities of truncal muscles associated with wrist flexion and extension. This possibility was analyzed from the viewpoint of temporal coupling with the wrist movement.

The P cells showing a nonreciprocal change were 72.8% of the total 92 P cells that significantly modulated their discharge rate with the task performance. The percentage increased to 86.7 among the 45 P cells selected by good temporal coupling with the wrist movement. The percentage of the nonreciprocally changing P cells further increased to 94.7 among the 19 P cells further selected by their good temporal coupling with both rapid and slow wrist movement. Thus, among the P cells selected by this method, the nonreciprocal modulation in spike activity became a more common feature among the selected P cells [10]. Considering a poor temporal coupling of truncal muscles' activity with the wrist movement in the restricted experimental posture (Fig. 1), the second interpretation mentioned in the preceding paragraph appears to be implausible.

The nonreciprocal modulation of P-cell activities was also reported by Llinás and Wolfe [9] to be associated with the opposite direction of saccadic eye movement. Thus, the nonreciprocal change with either extension or flexion in the majority, if not all, of P cells appears to be one of the distinct features of the cerebellar cortex, contrasting with the predominantly reciprocal change of spike activities in the motor cortex [4].

Discharge Patterns of Complex Spikes

In about half of the P cells, whose simple-spike activities changed with the performance of the tracking task, the complex-spike activity also significantly changed with the wrist movement. In the cell illustrated (Fig. 3), the complex spike discharged more frequently with faster wrist movement (trial 6) than with slower movements (trials 1, 2). At present, this parallel increase of both simple and complex spike activities with faster velocities of wrist movements has not yet been quantitatively analyzed. But, it is quite clear that the complex spikes discharge in association with fairly slow limb movement [11], and the complex spike is not necessarily related specifically with fast limb movements [19].

Most commonly, a single complex spike appeared at the beginning of the simple-spike frequency modulation (Fig. 3, trials 3, 4, 5), or, rarely, at the quick recovery phase of the simple-spike frequency modulation (not shown). Significant frequency modulation of complex spikes was not observed when the simple-spike discharge rate was maintained at a constant level, as when the monkey held the handle still at a fixed position or when the monkey was tracking the target with fairly constant velocity.

Thus, the complex spike discharged in a phasic manner in close temporal coupling with the rapid modulation of the discharge rate of simple spikes. However, only one, or at most, a few complex spikes observed in one trial of wrist movement can hardly be considered to be conveying meaningful information to a target cell about a movement parameter of the wrist movement, as do the simple spikes. Some conjunctive interaction between the mossy- and climbing-fiber inputs at the level of cerebellar cortex might be a most probable functional role of the comodulation of simple- and complex-spike activities [1, 5, 7, 15].

Discussion and Conclusions

We briefly reviewed our recent studies on the Purkinje-cell (P cell) activity associated with voluntary limb movement. We offer a new paradigm which enables us to overcome the difficulties in studying the central mechanisms of voluntary limb movement. First, by the visually guided wrist tracking movement, we could dissociate the direction, position, and velocity of wrist movement as independent variables. By imposing different levels of load on the rotation axis of the handle by torque motors, we can add the force (F) and the rate of force change (dF/dt) to the dissociable movement parameters. We recently confirmed that a rhesus monkey can perform the skillful wrist tracking movement even under loaded condition (Mano and Kanazawa, unpublished observations). Thus, by the limb tracking movement, we are now able to analyze quantitatively the skilled limb movement in experimental animals, as in humans [18], in terms of those movement parameters. Second, we can select the central neurons that are related to a specified limb movement (in our study, wrist flexion and extension) by an objective criterion, the degree of temporal coupling between the neural activity and a specified movement [12]. This objective selection of movement-related cells not only qualifies us to analyze the neural activity in relation to the parameters of the specified limb movement, but also reduces the error due to the sampling bias when we compare the neural activities in different motor centers [10]. The temporal coupling of the neural activity with a specified limb movement is, however, only one of the necessary requirements in identifying the cells as related to a specified movement. In addition, the statistical criterion for the degree of temporal coupling is not an absolute but a relative criterion. To overcome these drawbacks of our present method in selecting the related cell we must seek another, better method in future.

Our study indicated that both simple- and complex-spike activities modulate with wide-range velocities of the wrist movements, suggesting the importance of the cerebellar cortex in controlling the slow limb movement as well as the rapid movement [11]. The P cells, selected as wrist-movement-related, also suggested that the discharge-rate modulation of simple spikes was closely related with the velocity, or some dynamic component coupled with the velocity, of the wrist movement, but was poorly related to the direction of the movement or to maintained wrist-joint position. These results roughly agree with the reports on the P cell activity in relation to eye movement [8, 9, 16, 17]. In some P cells, however, discharge rates of simple spikes during steady fixation of the eye were reported to be proportional to eye position [17]. So far, we have not found a P cell whose simple-spike-discharge rate was consistently correlated with the maintained wrist-joint angle. Whether this discrepancy suggests the essentially different involvement of the cerebellar cortex in controlling eye and limb movements or our failure to sample another subgroup of P cells related to maintained limb position, should be answered in future by sampling more P cells related to the wrist movement.

References

1. Albus JS (1971) A theory of cerebellar function. Math Biosci 10:25–61
2. DeLong MR, Strick PL (1971) Relation of basal ganglia, cerebellum, and motor cortex to ramp and ballistic movement. Brain Res 71:327–335
3. Dow RS, Moruzzi G (1958) The physiology and pathology of the cerebellum. University of Minnesota Press, Minneapolis
4. Fetz EE, Finocchio DV, Baker MA, Soso MJ (1980) Sensory and motor responses of precentral cortex cells during comparable passive and active joint movements. J Neurophysiol 43:1070–1089
5. Gilbert PFC, Thach WT (1977) Purkinje cell activity during motor learning. Brain Res 128:309–328
6. Holmes G (1917) The symptoms of acute cerebellar injuries due to gunshot injuries. Brain 40:461–535
7. Ito M (1970) Neurophysiological aspects of the cerebellar motor control system. Int J Neurol 7:162–176

8. Lisberger SG, Fuchs AF (1978) Role of primate flocculus during rapid behavioral modification of vestibular reflex. I. Purkinje cell activity during visually guided horizontal smooth-pursuit eye movements and passive head rotation. J Neurophysiol 41:733–763
9. Llinás R and Wolfe JW (1977) Functional linkage between the electrical activity in vermal cerebellar cortex and saccadic eye movements. Exp Brain Res 29:1–14
10. Mano N (1979) Analyses of cerebellar Purkinje cell activity in relation to the direction, position and velocity of wrist tracking movement. In: Massion J, Sasaki K (eds) Cerebro-cerebellar interactions. Elsevier North-Holland, New York Oxford Shannon, pp 163–183
11. Mano N, Yamamoto K (1975) Slow and rapid (quick or ballistic) tracking movements and a cerebellar Purkinje cell activity. J Physiol Soc Japan 37:383–384
12. Mano N, Yamamoto K (1979) Kolmogorov-Smirnov test applied to the onset time determination of the modulation in discharge rate. In: Ito M et al. (eds) Integrative control functions of the brain, vol II. Kodansha, Tokyo and Elsevier, Amsterdam, pp 146–148
13. Mano N, Yamamoto K (1979) Two groups of cerebellar Purkinje cells in relation to the velocity of wrist movement. Neurosci Lett [Suppl] 2:S 33
14. Mano N, Yamamoto K (1980) Simple-spike activity of cerebellar Purkinje cells related to visually guided wrist tracking movement in the monkey. J Neurophysiol 43:713–728
15. Marr D (1968) A theory of cerebellar cortex. J Physiol (Lond) 202:473–480
16. Noda H, Suzuki DA (1979) The role of the flocculus of the monkey in saccadic eye movements. J Physiol (Lond) 294:317–334
17. Noda H, Suzuki DA (1979) The role of the flocculus of the monkey in fixation and smooth pursuit eye movements. J Physiol (Lond) 294:335–348
18. Poulton EC (1966) Tracking behavior. In: Bilodeau EA (ed) Acquisition of skill. Academic Press, New York London, pp 361–410
19. Thach WT (1970) Discharge of cerebellar neurons related to two maintained postures and two prompt movements. II. Purkinje cell output and input. J Neurophysiol 33:537–547

Discussion

Thach commented that the observation by Dr. Mano that the Purkinje cells lack directional selectivity during slow tracking movements fits nicely with the results of his own work and perhaps indicates a different mechanism during such movements.

Responding to a question by Sir John Eccles, Dr. Mano identified the location of the recorded neurons as lobule V, in either the lateral or intermediate zone. To a question from Dr. Llinás, he replied that both the onset and peak time of simple-spike-frequency increase preceded the onset and peak time of movement velocity by between 50 and 200 ms. To a question by Dr. Altman, Dr. Mano said that he observed no correlation of cell activity and eye movements.

Chan-Palay asked about the consistency of responses in different Purkinje cells. Dr. Mano replied that he saw only a few wrist-movement-related cells of group I in each animal, but that the electrode penetrations had separations of 1 mm, so it is possible that correlated cells could be found in closer proximity.

Snider questioned whether both Dr. Thach and Dr. Mano disagreed with Kornhuber's suggestion that slower ramp movements are the domain of the basal ganglia whereas the cerebellum is more concerned with saccadic movements. Dr. Thach replied that they could not say whether cerebellar neurons cause the ramp movements, but the degree of activity of the cerebellar neurons during such movements suggests some kind of relationship.

Spinocerebellar Connections in the Cat with Particular Emphasis on Their Cellular Origin

G. Grant

Introduction

Of the many spinal pathways to the cerebellum [33] those projecting directly from the spinal cord without any intervening relay, i.e., the spinocerebellar tracts, have been the most accessible to anatomic studies. Still, our knowledge about the anatomic organization of these tracts has been rather restricted. It is only recently that considerable new information has been obtained, particularly with regard to the location of cells of origin. Much more detailed knowledge has been available about the functional organization of the spinocerebellar tracts [33]. This has been derived mainly from studies in the cat. The present paper will focus first generally on the anatomic organization of the spinocerebellar tracts in this species and then specifically on the recently obtained findings regarding cells of origin.

Anatomic Organization of the Spinocerebellar Tracts

The spinocerebellar tracts comprise the dorsal spinocerebellar tract (DSCT), the ventral spinocerebellar tract (VSCT), and the physiologically identified rostral spinocerebellar tract (RSCT) [21, 32, 34, 35].

The DSCT ist known to be an uncrossed tract originating from cells in the column of Clarke, which in the cat extends from the 2nd or 3rd thoracic segment to the 3rd or 4th lumbar segment [39]. Its axons run in the dorsal part of the lateral funiculus of the spinal cord. They enter the cerebellum via the inferior cerebellar peduncle. The DSCT terminates as mossy fibers, like the other spinocerebellar tracts [4, 13]. It has two main projection areas, one anteriorly, comprising anterior parts of the anterior lobe, and one posteriorly, comprising posterior parts of the pyramis and the paramedian lobule [13]. These areas have been shown in physiological studies to be influenced from hindlimb nerves (cf. [13]). This is in good agreement with the demonstration that the column of Clarke, regarded as the source of origin of the DSCT, receives dorsal spinal root afferents from levels caudal to the 1st thoracic segment [15]. Corresponding cerebellar areas influenced from forelimb nerves, including posterior parts of the anterior lobe and anterior parts of the pyramis and the paramedian lobule, receive mossy-fiber terminals from the external cuneate nucleus of the medulla oblongata [14]. This is supplied by dorsal root afferents from the upper parts of the body [26]. The rostral part of the main cuneate nucleus, which

Experimental Brain Research, Suppl. 6

has been demonstrated to project to the cerebellum [7, 40], has also been shown to contribute fibers to the posterior parts of the anterior lobe, in addition to fibers to the pyramis and the paramedian lobule [40, 42]. The connections both from the external and from the main cuneate nuclei are uncrossed. Together they form the cuneocerebellar tract, a forelimb equivalent of the DSCT [8, 14, 20]. The pathway via the external cuneate nucleus has been shown to forward proprioceptive information and the pathway via the main cuneate nucleus, exteroceptive information [8, 11, 20]. In physiological studies it has been demonstrated that these two pathways have a differential termination, the proprioceptive pathway influencing deep parts of the folia and the exteroceptive pathway superficial parts [11]. Anatomic studies have confirmed these findings [40].

The VSCT is known to be a mainly crossed tract in the spinal cord originating from groups of cells extending caudal to the level of the column of Clarke, running in the ventral part of the lateral funiculus and entering the cerebellum via the superior cerebellar peduncle (see [13]). The VSCT terminates bilaterally but with a predominance contralaterally in the cerebellar cortex. Most of its fibers terminate in the anterior, hindlimb part of the anterior lobe [13]. Fibers from the most caudal parts of the spinal cord terminate more anteriorly than fibers from more rostral spinal levels [13]. In the macaque the "border cells" of Cooper and Sherrington [9] were early shown to give rise to spinocerebellar fibers assumed to be VSCT fibers [25, 43, 44]. These border cells were described as large motoneuron-like cells located at the ventrolateral border of the spinal gray matter at the lowest thoracic and upper six lumbosacral segments being resistent to ventral root transection but showing chromatolytic changes following contralateral spinal cord hemisection at various levels from C3 to T11. The cells were found to be most numerous in the 4th and 5th lumbar segments. Similar cells in the cat did not show chromatolytic changes following cerebellar lesions [17, 44] or transections of the brachium conjunctivum [31]. Physiologic studies later demonstrated, however, that also in the cat spinal border cells give rise to VSCT fibers [5, 6]. Another group of VSCT cells has been described from physiologic studies in the cat to be located in the lateral parts of the intermediate zone and the base and neck of the dorsal horn at L4 and L5 [23, 24].

The RSCT, a functionally identified tract [21, 34], has been regarded as a forelimb equivalent of the VSCT [34, 35]. It is an uncrossed tract originating from cells located rostral to the column of Clarke. Its fibers run in the lateral funiculus, further ventrally than the DSCT. They enter the cerebellum via a dual route, partly via the inferior and partly via the superior cerebellar peduncle. The tract has been found to terminate bilaterally but with a predominance for an ipsilateral termination. Both hindlimb and forelimb areas are influenced from the tract.

Recent Findings Regarding Cells of Origin

Lower Lumbar and More Caudal Segments

Until recently no systematic anatomic studies covering large areas of the spinal cord had been made with regard to cells of origin of the spinocerebellar tracts.

The modified Gudden method of Brodal [3], which makes use of the strong retrograde reaction in very young animals exhibited by neurons subjected to axonal trauma, should have been a well-suited method. The principle of this method was used to begin with for a detailed investigation of the cells of origin of spinocerebellar tracts in the lower lumbar cord (L3–L7) of the kitten [1]. Following cerebellar lesions, chromatolytic nerve cells were found not only in the column of Clarke (L3–L4) but also laterally in the ventral horn (L3–L6), including the group of spinal border cells. The largest number of changed cells in the ventral horn was found in L4–L5. Furthermore, chromatolytic cells were found in laminae IV–VI of the dorsal horn. Since the material was taken from very young animals the location of cells in relation to different nerve cell groups and to spinal cord laminae was greatly facilitated (cf. [38]). It was found that most of the ventral horn cells were located in two separate nuclei, both of which are described in Rexed's cytoarchitectonic atlas of the cat's spinal cord [39]. In his description they are included in the lateral group of lamina IX, which is the motor-cell-group lamina. One of the nuclei is located dorsolaterally in the ventral horn, at the border towards the intermediate zone. This group is described by Rexed to extend from L3 to L6. The other nucleus is found in L4 and L5 just ventral to the dorsolateral nucleus. In addition to confirming the physiologic demonstration that spinal border cells project to the cerebellum also in the cat [5, 6], these findings confirmed that there are cerebellar projecting neurons in the dorsal horn at segmental levels caudal to the column of Clarke. This had been suggested from physiologic studies [2, 45]. They also confirmed physiologic findings regarding the presence of cerebellar projecting neurons in laminae IV–VI, i.e., outside the column of Clarke, at segmental levels L3 and L4 [37].

The introduction of the much more sensitive retrograde tracing method with the aid of horseradish peroxidase (HRP) made it more tempting to continue the investigations with that method. It was found that the number of HRP-labeled neurons in the lower lumbar cord after injections of HRP into the cerebellum of young kittens far exceeded the number of chromatolytic neurons found after cerebellar lesions [1, 16]. Furthermore, the use of tetramethylbenzidine (TMB) as a substrate [18, 30] instead of diaminobenzidine (DAB) [12], which was used originally, turned out to give details as to orientation of dendrites and the course taken by axons [16]. By combining the HRP injections into the cerebellum with unilateral spinal cord transections, information could also be obtained with regard to crossing-noncrossing of axons of the spinocerebellar neurons in the spinal cord [16].

In general, the findings to be discussed below regarding spinocerebellar cells of origin at lower lumbar and more caudal spinal cord levels are in agreement with those reported recently from two other HRP studies on spinocerebellar neurons in the cat [29, 41]. The differences between the three studies lie mainly in the way in which the location of the labeled neurons are described and in details regarding projection laterality or proportional density of certain groups of cells. The only more important difference regards labeled cells in lamina I. Such cells were reported in large numbers after cerebellar HRP injections in one of these studies [41], but not in the other [29], and the finding of labeled

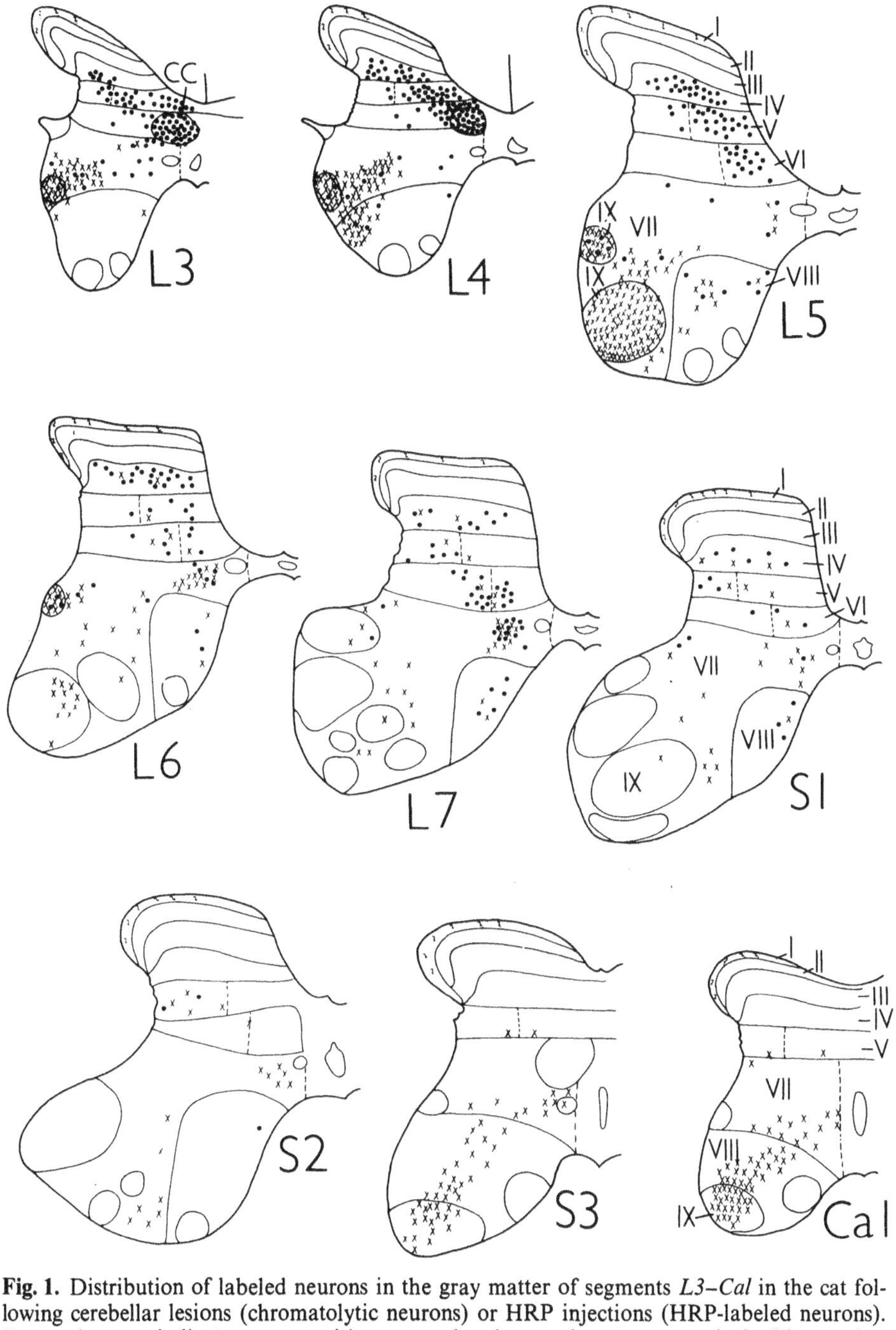

Fig. 1. Distribution of labeled neurons in the gray matter of segments *L3–Ca1* in the cat following cerebellar lesions (chromatolytic neurons) or HRP injections (HRP-labeled neurons). *Dots* and *crosses* indicate neurons with uncrossed and crossed axons, respectively. The number of *dots* and *crosses* indicates relative densities of labeled neurons. *Curved lines* in lamina I indicate neurons which were not consistently labeled. I–IX, laminae according to Rexed (1954)

lamina I cells in a few cases in our study could not be taken as an indication of a cerebellar connection from lamina I (see below).

Figure 1 is a diagram summarizing the location of HRP-labeled spinocerebellar neurons at different levels from L3 to Ca1 in the kitten, following injections of HRP into various cerebellar regions known to receive spinocerebellar fibers [13]. Filled circles and crosses represent neurons with uncrossed and crossed axons in the spinal cord, respectively. The density of the symbols indicates relative density of neurons. Labeled neurons were observed in the dorsal horn, the intermediate zone, and the ventral horn.

In the dorsal horn most labeled neurons were found in laminae IV–VI, as in the experiments with retrograde chromatolysis. The neurons were most numerous in the more rostral segments. In the caudal segments (S2–Ca1) only a few labeled neurons were observed in lamina V. The mediolateral distribution of the neurons in the dorsal horn laminae was rather even, except for lamina VI, where the neurons tended to accumulate medially. Labeled neurons were also seen in lamina I, the marginal layer of Waldeyer (Fig. 1, curved lines). This finding was not consistent, however. Labeled neurons were found only in TMB-treated material from cases where the cerebellar HRP injections also involved the area of the inferior colliculus.

In the intermediate zone, which corresponds approximately to lamina VII (except for the segments included in the spinal cord enlargements, where lamina VII also has a ventral extension into the ventral horn [39], labeled neurons were found both medially and laterally. The medially located neurons were found in the column of Clarke (L3–L4) and in a paracentral group caudal to this column (L6–S2). The neurons laterally were found close to, or rather close to, the dorsolateral nucleus of lamina IX (L3–L6).

In the ventral horn, labeled neurons were located in the two nuclei of the lateral nuclear group of lamina IX, where also chromatolytic neurons were found after cerebellar lesions, i.e., the dorsolateral and ventrolateral nuclei (Fig. 1). These two nuclei were found very close to each other in many sections and not separated as widely as they appear to be in the schematic drawing of Fig. 1. Furthermore, labeled neurons were observed in the ventromedial nucleus, which fills the apex of the ventral horn at S3 and Ca1. This nucleus is regarded by Rexed [39] as part of the medial group of nuclei of lamina IX. As can be seen in Fig. 1, labeled neurons were found also in areas outside lamina IX in the ventral horn, both in lamina VII (L5–S2) and in lamina VIII (L3–Ca1).

As regards crossing-noncrossing of spinocerebellar axons in the spinal cord it can be seen from Fig. 1 that ipsilaterally projecting neurons tended to be located more dorsally, particularly in the more rostral segments (L3–L5), than contralaterally projecting neurons, which had a tendency to be found more ventrally. In the intermediate zone neurons projected to either side.

The findings discussed clearly demonstrate a much more widespread origin of spinocerebellar neurons in the lower part of the spinal cord than hitherto assumed. The pattern that can be seen, e.g., with regard to crossing-noncrossing of axons at spinal level, indicates, however, that the traditional subdivision of the spinocerebellar tracts from these levels of the cord in a DSCT, being an uncrossed spinal tract, and the VSCT, being a crossed spinal tract, can be maintained.

Thoracic and Upper Lumbar Segments

Also in thoracic and upper lumbar segments spinocerebellar neurons have turned out to be more widely distributed than hitherto assumed. In the detailed study by Matsushita et al. [29], labeled neurons were found after cerebellar HRP injections not only in the column of Clarke but also in the dorsal horn (laminae IV–V), the intermediate zone outside the column of Clarke, and in the ventral horn. Both the column of Clarke and lamina V contained many labeled neurons, whereas the intermediate zone outside the column of Clarke and the ventral horn only had a small number of such neurons, at least rostral to T13. In segments T13–L3 labeled neurons laterally in laminae VII and VIII were identified as spinal border cells. Both the dorsal horn neurons and those of the column of Clarke were found to have their axons ascending on the ipsilateral side of the cord, whereas those of the group classified as spinal border cells were found to send their axons across the midline to ascend contralaterally.

Lower Cervical Segments

Earlier anatomic studies have given no evidence of spinocerebellar fibers originating from spinal levels rostral to the column of Clarke. In physiologic studies in the cat, a forelimb tract was revealed, however, originating from cells rostral to that column at, or slightly above, the level of the dorsal root entrance. This tract was called the RSCT and it was considered to be a forelimb homolog to the VSCT (see above). In the recent studies by Snyder et al. [41] and Matsushita et al. [29], labeled spinocerebellar cells were identified in the lower cervical cord after cerebellar HRP injections. Especially the paper by Matsushita et al. [29] gives a detailed account of the location of labeled cells in the cat. Such cells were found in all of the segments C5–C8 and among these should be the cells of origin of the RSCT. As in the lower parts of the spinal cord described above, labeled cells were found in the dorsal horn, the intermediate zone, and in the ventral horn. In the dorsal horn labeled neurons were particularly numerous medially in lamina VI and in the segments caudal to C6 also laterally in lamina V. Labeled neurons were found, however, also in other parts of laminae VI and V, as well as in the ventral part of lamina IV. In the intermediate zone one group of labeled neurons, which was well-developed in C8 and also in T1, was found medially, lateral to the central canal. In the ventral horn another group, which contained many labeled neurons, was found in C6–C8 and also in T1. This was located centrally in lamina VII, dorsomedial to the lateral group of motor nuclei of lamina IX. In experiments with spinal cord hemisections preceding cerebellar HRP injections it was shown that both the dorsal horn cells and those central in lamina VII had their axons ascending ipsilaterally in the spinal cord [29]. On the other hand, the medial cells in the intermediate zone were found to send their axons across the midline before they took their ascending course contralaterally. The RSCT is known to be an uncrossed tract. It should therefore take its origin from the neurons with uncrossed axons. For a further discussion of the cells of origin of this tract the reader is referred to the paper by Matsushita et al. [29].

Upper Cervical Segments

It is only recently that also the upper cervical cord was shown to have efferent connections with the cerebellum. This has been demonstrated not only in the cat [28, 46, 47] but also in the dog [10] and monkey [36]. In all these species the central cervical nucleus, which is present in C1–C4 and located lateral to the central canal, has been shown in HRP studies to project to the cerebellum. In experimental studies where anterograde transport of ^{3}H-leucine was used, it has been demonstrated, furthermore, that the central cervical nucleus projects bilaterally, mainly on lobule I, lingula, and adjoining parts of lobule II [48]. Nearly all the axons from the nucleus were found to cross in the spinal cord and to ascend contralaterally [47, 48]. The majority of them were found to enter the cerebellum via the superior cerebellar peduncle, but a few also via the inferior peduncle [48]. Earlier anatomic investigations have demonstrated afferents to the central cervical nucleus from dorsal spinal roots, mainly from upper cervical levels (see [46]). In accordance with this, recent physiologic studies have shown that central cervical neurons can be excited from upper cervical fibers, most probably innervating joints and adjacent ligaments of the upper cervical vertebrae [19]. Taken together it seems therefore that the central cervical nucleus is a spinocerebellar relay for impulses from joints and adjacent ligaments of the upper cervical vertebrae.

It is not only the central cervical nucleus, however, which shows labeled neurons in the upper cervical segments after cerebellar HRP injections. Although not in large numbers such neurons have been found also in the medial part of lamina VI, in lamina VII adjacent to the central cervical nucleus, and in the ventral horn [29, 47]. The medial neurons in lamina VI were found to have their axons uncrossed, ascending on the ipsilateral side of the spinal cord, whereas the other neurons were found to send their axons across the midline to ascend contralaterally [29, 47].

Concluding Remarks

From the above it appears that the recent studies of spinocerebellar connections with the aid of HRP have revealed a multitude of sources of origin for spinocerebellar fibers not previously known. In addition they have helped in confirming and extending previous knowledge with regard to certain groups of cells like that of the column of Clarke and the spinal border cells. Although in many ways these new findings make the pattern more complicated they help also to correlate findings from earlier physiologic studies. DSCT cells have been identified in physiologic studies at levels caudal to the column of Clarke, although this column was regarded as the only source of DSCT fibers [22, 45]. The HRP studies have now revealed ipsilaterally projecting spinocerebellar neurons at levels caudal to the column of Clarke (cf. [29]). Furthermore, certain types of cutaneous DSCT neurons have been found outside the column of Clarke in L3–L4, more precisely in laminae IV–VI of the dorsal horn [37]. The HRP studies have confirmed the presence of spinocerebellar neurons at these locations (cf. [41]). Physiologic studies have also demonstrated the presence of a forelimb spinocerebellar tract, the RSCT, originating from the level of the cervical enlargement, rostral to the column of Clarke [21, 27, 34]. The recent HRP studies have revealed spinocerebellar neurons located at this spinal cord level. Among these should be the cells of origin of the RSCT (cf. [29]). Future studies will hopefully reveal which of the many now known spinocerebellar groups of neurons form entities of their own and which specific cerebellar projections they may have.

References

1. Aldskogius H, Grant G, Wiksten B (1976) Cells of origin of spinocerebellar fibres from the lower lumbar spinal cord in the kitten. Anat Rec 184:342–343
2. Aoyama M, Hongo T, Kudo N (1973) An uncrossed ascending tract originating from below Clarke's column and conveying group I impulses from the hindlimb muscles in the cat. Brain Res 62:237–241
3. Brodal A (1940) Modification of Gudden method for study of cerebral localization. Arch Neurol 43:46–58
4. Brodal A, Grant G (1962) Morphology and temporal course of degeneration in cerebellar mossy fibers following transection of spinocerebellar tracts in the cat. Exp Neurol 5:67–87
5. Burke RE, Lundberg A, Weight F (1968) Gower's tract and "spinal border cells". Acta Physiol Scand 74:16A
6. Burke RE, Lundberg A, Weight F (1971) Spinal border cell origin of the ventral spinocerebellar tract. Exp Brain Res 12:283–294
7. Cheek MD, Rustioni A, Trevino DL (1975) Dorsal column nuclei projections to the cerebellar cortex in cats as revealed by the use of retrograde transport of horseradish peroxidase. J Comp Neurol 164:31–46
8. Cooke JD, Larson B, Oscarsson O, Sjölund B (1971) Origin and termination of cuneocerebellar tract. Exp Brain Res 13:339–358
9. Cooper S, Sherrington CS (1940) Gower's tract and spinal border cells. Brain 63:123–134
10. Cummings JF, Petras JM (1977) The origin of spinocerebellar pathways. I. The nucleus cervicalis centralis of the cranial cervical spinal cord. J Comp Neurol 173:655–692
11. Ekerot CF, Larson B (1972) Differential termination of the exteroceptive and proprioceptive components of the cuneocerebellar tract. Brain Res 36:420–424
12. Graham RC Jr, Karnovsky MJ (1966) The early stages of absorption of injected horseradish peroxidase in the proximal tubules of mouse kidney: Ultrastructural cytochemistry by a new technique. J Histochem Cytochem 14:291–302
13. Grant G (1962) Spinal course and somatotopically localized termination of the spinocerebellar tracts. An experimental study in the cat. Acta Physiol Scand 56 [Suppl 193]
14. Grant G (1962) Projection of the external cuneate nucleus onto the cerebellum in the cat. An experimental study using silver methods. Exp Neurol 5:179–195
15. Grant G, Rexed B (1958) Dorsal spinal root afferents to Clarke's column. Brain 81:567–576
16. Grant G, Wiksten B, Berkley KJ, Aldskogius H (1982) The location of cerebellar-projecting neurons within the lumbosacral spinal cord in the cat. An anatomical study using HRP and retrograde chromatolysis. J Comp Neurol 204:336–348
17. Ha H, Liu CN (1968) Cell origin of the ventral spinocerebellar tract. J Comp Neurol 133:185–206
18. Hardy H, Heimer L (1977) A safer and more sensitive substitute for diaminobenzidine in the light microscopic demonstration of retrograde and anterograde axonal transport of HRP. Neurosci Lett 5:235–240
19. Hirai N, Hongo T, Sasaki S (1978) Cerebellar projection and input organizations of the spinocerebellar tract arising from the central cervical nucleus in the cat. Brain Res 157:341–345

20. Holmqvist B, Oscarsson O, Rosén I (1963) Functional organization of the cuneocerebellar tract in the cat. Acta Physiol Scand 58:216–235
21. Holmqvist B, Oscarsson O, Uddenberg N (1963) Organization of ascending spinal tracts activated from forelimb afferents in the cat. Acta Physiol Scand 58:68–76
22. Hongo T, Okada Y, Sato M (1967) Corticofugal influences on transmission to the dorsal spinocerebellar tract from hindlimb primary afferents. Exp Brain Res 3:135–149
23. Hubbard JI, Oscarsson O (1961) Localization of the cells of origin of the ventral spinocerebellar tract. Nature 189:157–158
24. Hubbard JI, Oscarsson O (1962) Localization of the cell bodies of the ventral spinocerebellar tract in lumbar segments of the cat. J Comp Neurol 118:199–204
25. Lafleur J, DeLean J, Poirier LJ (1974) Physiopathology of the cerebellum in the monkey. Part I. Origin of cerebellar afferent nervous fibers from the spinal cord and brain stem. J Neurol Sci 22:471–490
26. Liu CN (1956) Afferent nerves to Clarke's and the lateral cuneate nuclei in the cat. Arch Neurol Psychiatry 75:67–77
27. MacKay WA, Murphy JI (1974) Responses of interpositus neurons to passive muscle stretch. J Neurophysiol 37:1410–1423
28. Matsushita M, Ikeda M (1975) The central cervical nucleus as cell origin of a spinocerebellar tract arising from the cervical cord: a study in the cat using horseradish peroxidase. Brain Res 100:412–417
29. Matsushita M, Hosoya Y, Ikeda M (1979) Anatomical organization of the spinocerebellar system in the the cat as studied by retrograde transport of horseradish peroxidase. J Comp Neurol 184:81–106
30. Mesulam MM (1978) Tetramethyl benzidine for horseradish peroxidase neurohistochemistry: a non-carcinogenic blue reaction product with superior sensitivity for visualizing neural afferents and efferents. J Histochem Cytochem 26:106–117
31. Morin F, Schwartz HG, O'Leary JL (1951) Experimental study of the spinothalamic and related tracts. Acta Psychiatr Scand 26:371–396
32. Oscarsson O (1965) Integrative organization of the rostral spinocerebellar tract in the cat. Acta Physiol Scand 64:154–166
33. Oscarsson O (1973) Functional organization of spinocerebellar paths. In: Iggo A (ed) Somatosensory system. Springer, Berlin Heidelberg New York (Handbook of Sensory Physiology, vol II, pp 338–380)
34. Oscarsson O, Uddenberg N (1964) Identification of a spinocerebellar tract activated from forelimb afferents in the cat. Acta Physiol Scand 62:125–136
35. Oscarsson O, Uddenberg N (1965) Properties of afferent connections to the rostral spinocerebellar tract in the cat. Acta Physiol Scand 64:143–153
36. Petras JM (1977) Spinocerebellar neurons in the rhesus monkey. Brain Res 130:146–151
37. Randić M, Myslinski NR, Gordon JH (1976) Spinal localization of neurons receiving inputs from cutaneous afferents in the cat hindlimb. Brain Res 105:573–577
38. Rexed B (1952) The cytoarchitectonic organization of the spinal cord in the cat. J Comp Neurol 96:415–496
39. Rexed B (1954) A cytoarchitectonic atlas of the spinal cord in the cat. J Comp Neurol 100: 297–379
40. Rinvik E, Walberg F (1975) Studies on the cerebellar projections from the main and external cuneate nuclei in the cat by means of retrograde axonal transport of horseradish peroxidase. Brain Res 95:371–381
41. Snyder RL, Faull RLM, Mehler WR (1978) A comparative study of the neurons of origin of the spinocerebellar afferents in the rat, cat and squirrel monkey based on the retrograde transport of horseradish peroxidase. J Comp Neurol 181:833–852
42. Somana R, Walberg F (1980) A reexamination of the cerebellar projections from the gracile, main and external cuneate nuclei in the cat. Brain Res 186:33–42
43. Sprague JM (1950) Cells of the ventral spinocerebellar tract. Anat Rec 106:289–290
44. Sprague JM (1953) Spinal "border cells" and their role in postural mechanism (Schiff-Sherrington phenomenon). J Neurophysiol 16:464–474
45. Tapper DN, Mann MD, Brown PB, Cogdell B (1975) Cells of origin of the cutaneous subdivision of the dorsal spinocerebellar tract. Brain Res 85:59–63

46. Wiksten B (1975) The central cervical nucleus – A source of spinocerebellar fibres, demonstrated by retrograde transport of horseradish peroxidase. Neurosci Lett 1:81–84
47. Wiksten B (1979) The central cervical nucleus in the cat. II. The cerebellar connections studied with retrograde transport of horseradish peroxidase. Exp Brain Res 36:155–173
48. Wiksten B (1979) The central cervical nucleus in the cat. III. The cerebellar connections studied with anterograde transport of ^{3}H-leucine. Exp Brain Res 36:175–189

Discussion

Eccles: Why don't we relabel the spinal border cells? As you showed, they're really not on the border as Cooper and Sherrington (1940) demonstrated, but are located more medially (see Hubbard & Oscarsson, 1962; Eccles et al., 1961). I just think why not simply call them VSCT cells and for the dorsal spinocerebellar tract, DSCT cells. The other thing is that those fibers outside of Clarke's column I think are relaying cutaneous impulses up the DSCT. They are not so sharply bunched as the ones bringing the motor input. Lundberg (1964) you know found some outside of Clarke's column and also they are more caudally located than the end of Clarke's column.
Grant: It is true that the cells that were described by Hubbard and Oscarsson (1962) were not found in the area of the Cooper and Sherrington cells, as they pointed out very precisely in their paper. But the cells we found are definitely also found in the border zone. So we have both types. For the sake of clarification Oscarsson (1973) has in his review described the neurons which he and Hubbard found as the Ib component of the VSCT, whereas the ones often activated by Ia afferents (Burke et al., 1971) Oscarsson described as the spinal border cell component of the VSCT. With regard to the dorsal horn cells I agree completely that there are several reports on cutaneous afferents coming to the cells located in the dorsal horn, laminae IV–VI and also caudal to the column of Clarke.
Marshall: I thought I noticed a curious pattern in the lamina-IX cell projection to the cerebellum within the lumbosacral spinal cord. The cells in the L2 to L5 region were labeled whereas those from L6 to S2, which should contain the heaviest innervation from the muscle fibers of the limb, weren't labeled. Is this pattern correct?
Grant: That is what also has been found for these cerebellar tracts by other investigators, but the reason is not clear.
Martin: Are there any data available as to whether or not any of these neurons that you show projecting to the cerebellum might also project to other areas of the neural axis like the thalamus and brainstem? Have double labeling techniques been applied to these neurons?
Grant: I do not know of any support for that so far, but naturally that is one kind of study which we are eager to do. Collaterals, for instance from the spinal border cells in the cat could come to, for example, the cervical enlargement area and that could be the reason why these cells do not react with chromatolytic changes following lesions of the cerebellum.

Haines: Are the labeled cells in the ventral horn large lower motoneurons?
Grant: They look like large motoneurons and their general appearance is such that one cannot distinguish them from motoneurons. I am aware of the description given by Romanes of the motor cell groups in which he described somewhat different Nissl patterns for some of the cells in these regions of the ventral horn. His description has been commented on in the literature and the suggestion has been made that the cells with a finer Nissl granular arrangement could be the VSCT cells.
Haines: Tolbert and his colleagues have shown that at least some of the projections of nucleocortical cells may be collaterals of cerebellar efferent fibers. Do you think that some of these ventral horn cells may be lower motoneurons which are projecting out to muscle and also sending collaterals to the cerebellar cortex?
Grant: One can only speculate about that, but it should be possible to use double labeling techniques to answer that question.
Palay: I want to call attention to the autoradiogram in which you showed mossy-fiber terminals ending in the granular layer with an injection in the central cervical nucleus. I noticed that the space in which this terminal ended was twice as large as the zone outlined by the grains. It's been thought that many glomeruli contain more than one mossy-fiber terminal ending, but I think this is the first time we have any real evidence. It would be extremely interesting if one could use differential labeling of different sources to see whether mossy fibers ending in the same glomerulus have different sources.
Grant: That's an interesting suggestion.
Chan-Palay: What do you suppose is so special about that vermian part of lobule I that makes its input so very different?
Grant: That's an interesting question. In the spider monkey lobule I is known to receive fibers from the most caudal part of the cord, but in the cat we know of only one projection from the spinal cord area. That's the one from the central cervical nucleus. It may be that this area is also influenced from the tail area in the cat, but not by a direct route. One observation which we are interested in following further experimentally is that the cells of the central cervical nucleus have dendrites oriented in three different directions. One group of dendrites is oriented dorsally or dorsolaterally and the incoming afferents from the upper cervical dorsal roots can be seen along these dorsally or dorsolaterally oriented dendrites. A second set of dendrites is oriented in the lateral direction and in preliminary studies we have found that these laterally oriented dendrites receive afferents from more caudal levels of the cord. It may be that these dendrites are influenced from the tail area. The third set of dendrites is probably the set of dendrites which receives the descending vestibular input found by Dr. Hirai and co-workers.

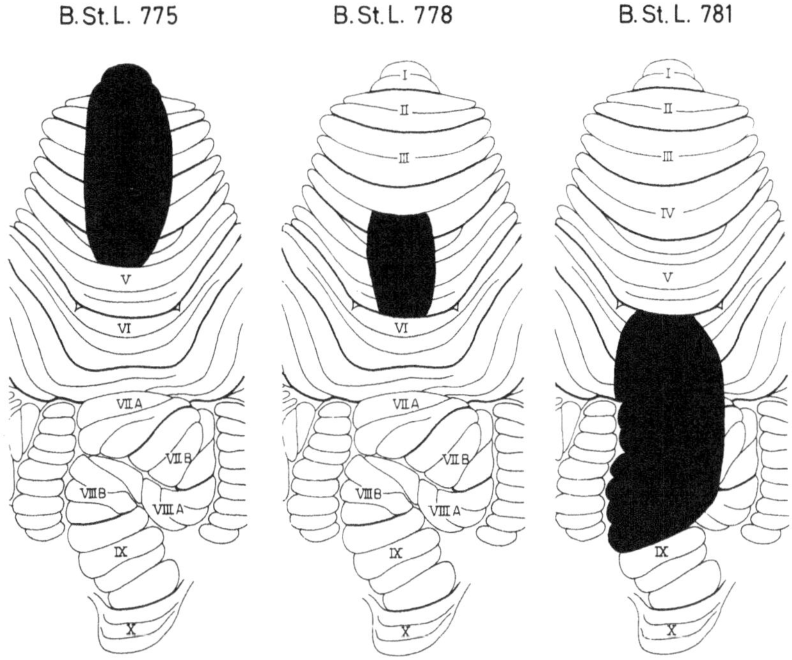

Fig. 1. Diagram of the injection sites in the cerebellar cortex in three cats where labeled cells are present bilaterally in the vestibular ganglion [29][1]

1 Abbreviations. *a*, accessory group of paramedian reticular nucleus; *B.c.*, superior cerebellar peduncle (brachium conjunctivum); *Br.c.*, brachium conjunctivum; *Br.p.*, brachium pontis; *C.i.*, inferior colliculus; *C.r.*, restiform body; *Cr.I*, *Cr.II*, crus I and II; *D*, descending (inferior) vestibular nucleus; *d*, dorsal group of paramedian reticular nucleus; *f*, cell group f in descending vestibular nucleus; *F.l.m.*, medial longitudinal fasciculus; *Flocc.*, flocculus; *g*, group rich in glia cells, caudal to the medial vestibular nucleus; *HII-HVI*, hemispheral lobules II–VI; *HVIIA (l. ans) Cr. Ia,p; Cr.IIa,p*, anterior and posterior folia of crus I and II of the ansiform lobule; *HVIIB, HVIIIA,B*, sublobules A and B of hemispheral lobules VII and VIII; *HIX*, hemispheral lobule IX; *i.c.*, nucleus intercalatus (Staderini); *L.*, *L*, left; lateral vestibular nucleus (Deiters); *l*, lateral small-celled part of lateral vestibular nucleus; *L.pm.*, paramedian lobule; *L.simpl.*, lobulus simplex; *M*, medial (triangular or dorsal) vestibular nucleus; *N.c.*, cuneate nucleus; *N.c.e.*, external cuneate nucleus; *N.c.t.*, nucleus of the trapezoid body; *N.cu.e.*, external cuneate nucleus; *N.f.*, *n.f.*, fastigial nucleus; *N.f.c.*, cuneate nucleus; *NIA*, *N.i.a.*, *n.i.a.*, nucleus interpositus anterior; *NIP*, *N.i.p.*, *n.i.p.*, nucleus interpositus posterior; *NL*, *N.l.*, *n.l.*, nucleus lateralis; *N.l.l.*, nucleus of the lateral lemniscus; *NM*, fastigial nucleus; *N.m.X*, dorsal motor vagal nucleus; *N.mes.*, *N.mes.V.*, mesencephalic nucleus of trigeminal nerve; *NRL*, *N.r.l.*, lateral reticular nucleus; *N.r.p.*, paramedian reticular nucleus; *N.r.t.*, nucleus reticularis tegmenti pontis of Bechterew; *N.tr.s.*, nucleus of the solitary tract; *N.V.*, trigeminal nerve; *N.VI*, abducent nerve; *N.VII*, facial nerve; *N.XII*, hypoglossal nerve, *Nucl.n.VII*, motor nucleus of facial nerve; *Ol.*, inferior olive; *Ol.s.*, superior olive; *Oliva inf.*, inferior olive; *Oliva sup.*, superior olive; *P.fl.d.*, *pfl.d.*, dorsal paraflocculus; *P.fl.v.*, *pfl.v.*, ventral paraflocculus; *P.h.*, *p.h.*, perihypoglossal nucleus; *p.t.l.*, processus tegmentosus lateralis of N.r.t.; *py.*, pyramis; *R.*, *R*, right; *r.f.XII*, hypoglossal nerve; *R.gc.*, nucleus reticularis gigantocellularis; *R.l.*, nucleus reticularis lateralis; *R.p.*, nucleus reticularis parvicellularis; *R.p.c.*, nucleus reticularis pontis caudalis; *R.p.o.*, nucleus reticularis pontis oralis; *R.v.*, nucleus reticularis ventralis; *S*, superior vestibular nucleus (Bechterew); *S.n.*, substantia nigra; *Sv.*, cell group probably representing the nucleus supravestibularis;

The Vestibulo- and Reticulocerebellar Projections in the Cat as Studied with Horseradish Peroxidase as a Retrograde Tracer

F. Walberg

Introduction

Experimental studies with tracer techniques have given evidence of a much more detailed pattern in cerebellar projections from the precerebellar relay nuclei than what has been revealed in previous anatomic studies where conventional methods were used. The new investigations, which have been performed during the last decade, have shown that not only is there a much more detailed and differentiated pattern in the projections already known, there are also cerebellar connections from brain stem nuclei and regions hitherto not thought to project to this part of the neuraxis.

In this review a survey will be given of the cerebellar projections of primary and secondary vestibular fibers and of the projections from the reticular formation when horseradish peroxidase (HRP) is used as a retrograde tracer in the cat.

The Cerebellar Projection from the Vestibular Nerve and from the Vestibular Nuclei

The Primary Vestibular Afferents

Primary vestibular afferents from the labyrinth have in experimental anatomic studies in mammals been shown to reach the flocculonodular lobe and the fastigial nucleus [1, 34, 35]. Actually, it was from this observation that the term "vestibulocerebellum" originated.

However, in later studies Brodal and Høivik [7] gave evidence that primary vestibular fibers were also distributed to the caudal folia of the uvula, the ventral and dorsal paraflocculus, the lingula, and the small-celled part of the ipsilateral dentate nucleus, and recent physiological observations have indicated a primary afferent projection also to the cerebellar vermis.

All these observations prompted a restudy of the primary vestibular afferent projection to the cerebellum by means of the method of retrograde transport of HRP [29]. Figure 1 shows some of the injections which resulted in labeled cells in the vestibular ganglion, and from these and other cases it could be concluded that primary vestibular fibers probably reach the entire cerebellar vermis. This part of the cortex, therefore, belongs to the "vestibulocerebellum," if this is defined as the area of the cerebellar cortex receiving projections from primary

Experimental Brain Research, Suppl. 6

vestibular fibers. In addition to illustrating that the HRP technique can be used for a demonstration of retrograde axonal transport from ganglion cells, our observations indicate that the entire vermis acts as a neuronal substrate for interactions between primary vestibular afferents and afferents from other sources of importance for the fine coordination of posture and movement.
Below, it will be shown that the new tracer studies have given evidence that the origin and distribution also of the secondary vestibulocerebellar fibers are larger than has hitherto been demonstrated.

The Secondary Vestibular Afferents

The first detailed account on the projection of the secondary vestibulocerebellar fibers was given by Brodal and Torvik [10], who based their conclusions on findings made with the modified Gudden method [2]. They found that most of the cerebellar afferents originated from the ventrolateral area of the caudal descending vestibular nucleus, including the cell group f. Some fibers originated from the cell group x of Brodal and Pompeiano [8] and a very few from the ventral part of the medial vestibular nucleus. However, since their conclusions were drawn from observations with only clear-cut retrograde cellular changes in the vestibular nuclei, they stressed that their findings represented a minimum of the projections from the nuclei to the cerebellum. Also, their cerebellar lesions were in most cases rather large.
An accurate mapping of the HRP-labeled cells requires a precise description of the cytoarchitectonic and topographic organization of the vestibular nuclear complex. This has been given in the cat [8], and our restudy of the distribution of the secondary vestibulocerebellar fibers [30] has been based on this description.
Figure 2 indicates the distribution of HRP-labeled cells in the vestibular complex in a case with a relatively large injection covering the cerebellar vermal lobules I–IV and the adjacent part of lobule V. The diagram shows that there are a large number of labeled cells in the superior vestibular nucleus (S), mostly localized in the most medial part at the medial and caudal level, approximately equally distributed on both sides. In addition, two medium-sized labeled cells[2] are present in the left lateral vestibular nucleus (L), and one smaller labeled cell in the nucleus on the right side. Furthermore, numerous labeled cells are present bilaterally in the medial (M) and descending (D) vestibular nuclei along

1 Continued: *T.*, trapezoid body; *Tr. s.*, solitary tract; *Tr. sp. V*, spinal tract of trigeminal nerve; *T.s.*, solitary tract; *v*, ventral group of paramedian reticular nucleus; *V.m.*, medial vestibular nucleus; *x*, small-celled group x, lateral to the descending vestibular nucleus; *y*, small-celled group y, lateral to the lateral vestibular nucleus (Deiters); *z*, cell group dorsal to the caudal part of the descending vestibular nucleus; *I-VI*, vermian lobules I-IV; *V*, motor nucleus of trigeminal nerve; *VIIA,B; VIIIA,B*, anterior and posterior sublobules of lobules VII and VIII; *IX*, uvula; *X*, nodulus; dorsal motor vagal nucleus; *XII*, nucleus of hypoglossal nerve

2 Small cells are less than 20 μm, medium cells between 20 and 50 μm, and large cells larger than 50 μm

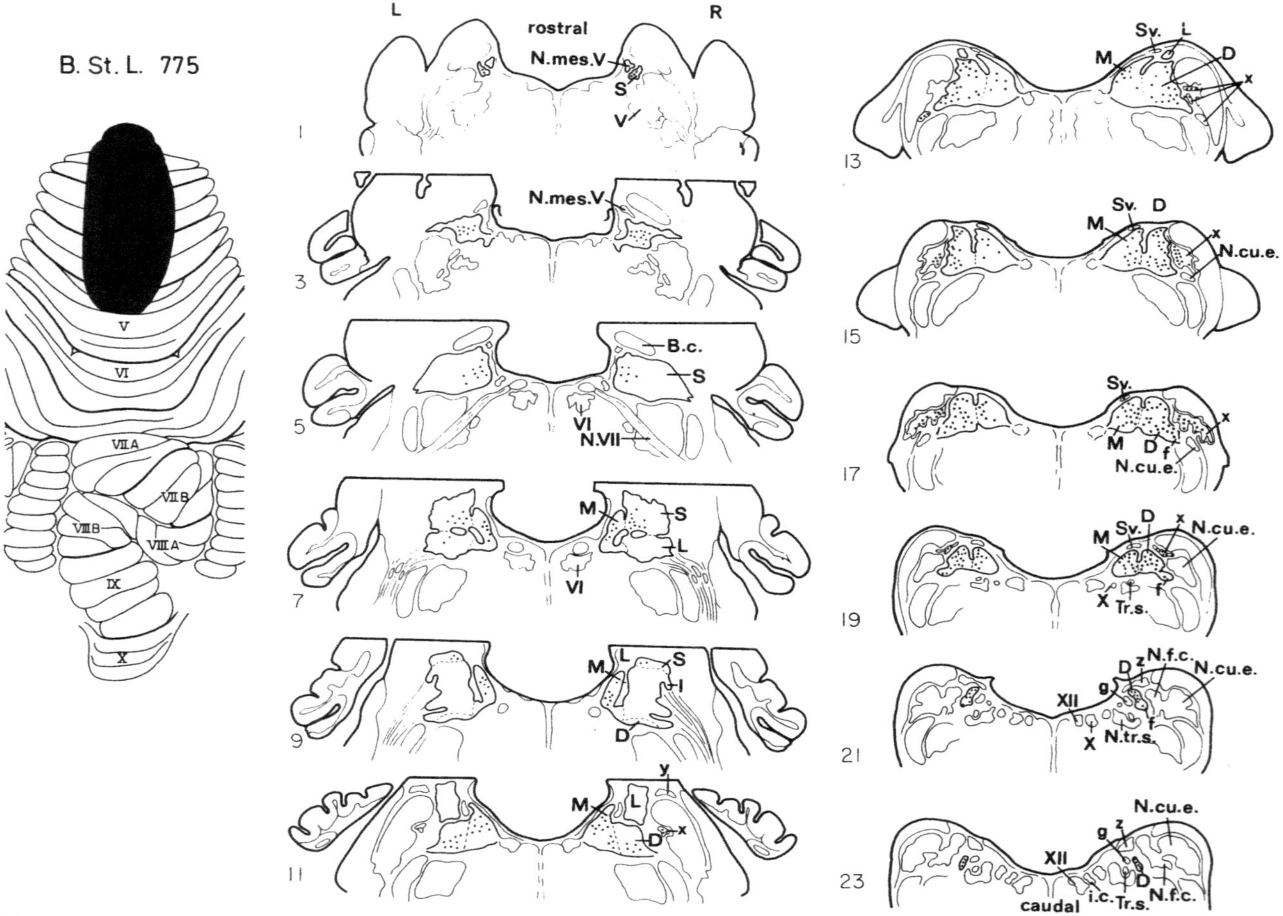

Fig. 2. Diagram illustrating the injection site and the distribution of labeled cells, indicated by *dots* (one *dot* represents one labeled cell) in the various subdivisions of the vestibular nuclear complex in a cat described in the text [30]. Abbreviations see p. 478–479

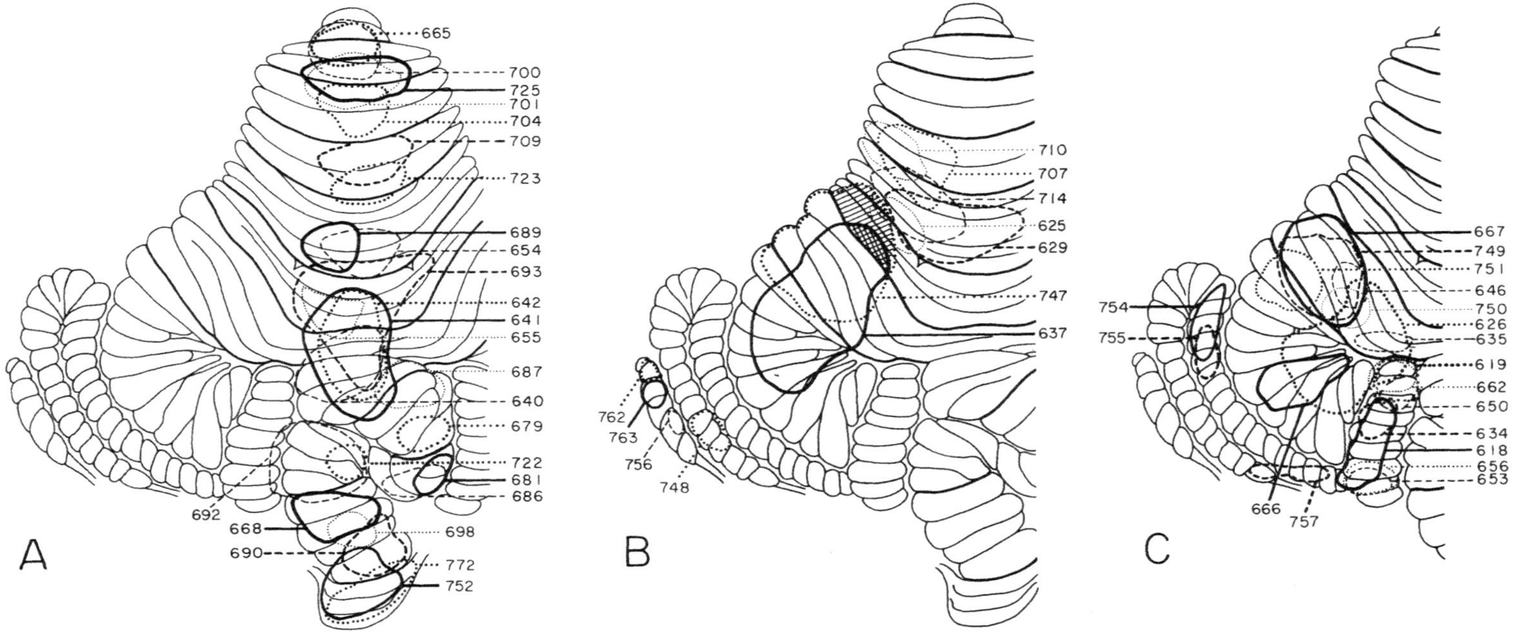

Fig. 3. Diagram of the cerebellar folia, visualized unfolded [26], showing the HRP injection sites in **A** vermis; **B** the intermediate-lateral part of the anterior lobe and the flocculus; and **C** the cerebellar hemisphere, paramedian lobule, and paraflocculus in the cats used for the description of the secondary vestibulocerebellar projection [30]

their entire rostrocaudal extent, and there is in addition a high density of labeled cells in group x and a few positive cells caudally in group f, but no labeled cells in other nuclear groups.

Large HRP injections in other parts of the cerebellar vermis (not illustrated) and the small localized injections shown in Fig. 3A made it possible for us to reach conclusions concerning details within the vestibular projection to the *cerebellar vermis*. Although labeled cells were present bilaterally in most parts of the nuclear complex also following the smaller injections, there was a projection from S only to the lingula and to the nodulus. On the other hand, consistent labeling was observed in M, D, and cell group x in all cases with vermal injections, but L projects only to lobules I–II, VI–VIIA, and to the nodulus. Finally, injections in the uvula resulted in a very high density of labeled cells bilaterally within cell group x.

The *intermediate-lateral part of the anterior lobe* receives afferents from the same vestibular nuclear groups as the vermis. Figure 3B shows our injections in this part of the cerebellum. In this figure are included two cases (B. St. L. 747 and 637) with injections in the transition zone between the lateral part of lobules V–VI and crus I–II. Since a large number of cases with injections in crus I and II did not show any evidence of labeling in the vestibular nuclear complex (see Fig. 3C and below), we concluded that the labeled cells in the vestibular nuclei in these two series occurred as a result of the injection of HRP into the lateral parts of lobules V and VI, i.e., the crosshatched area in Fig. 2B.

There is no vestibular projection to *crus I and II*, the *paramedian lobule*, and the *paraflocculus*. This is learnt from the cases illustrated in Fig. 3C (eight cases in crus I and II, seven cases in the paramedian lobule, four cases in the paraflocculus).

In contrast to this observation there was an ample distribution of labeled neurons in the vestibular complex following injections into the *flocculus*. Thus, in all cases illustrated in Fig. 3B there were a large number of labeled cells bilaterally in S and (at a lower density) in L, M, and D. In one of the cases, two labeled cells were observed in the left cellgroup y, otherwise the vestibular complex was free from labeled cells.

Our experimental material gives evidence that there also is a projection to the *fastigial* and to the *anterior and posterior interposite* nuclei. A comparison of the seven cases included in this group shows that the distribution of the labeled cells in the cases with HRP injections into these nuclei is similar to that described for most of the cases with injections in the cerebellar vermis. However, injections into the lateral cerebellar nucleus resulted in negative cases.

Figure 4 is a diagram of the total projection from the vestibular complex to the cerebellar cortex and nuclei.[1] As is seen, the fibers reach the greater part of the cerebellar cortex, but the flocculonodular lobe and the fastigial nucleus are most amply supplied with fibers. Only crus I and II, the paramedian lobule, and the paraflocculus lack afferents. The projection is bilateral with an ipsilateral preponderance.

---

1 Our observations are in good agreement with other recent HRP studies [16, 20, 21, 22, 41, 43, 45], but these do not include injections in all parts of the cerebellar cortex

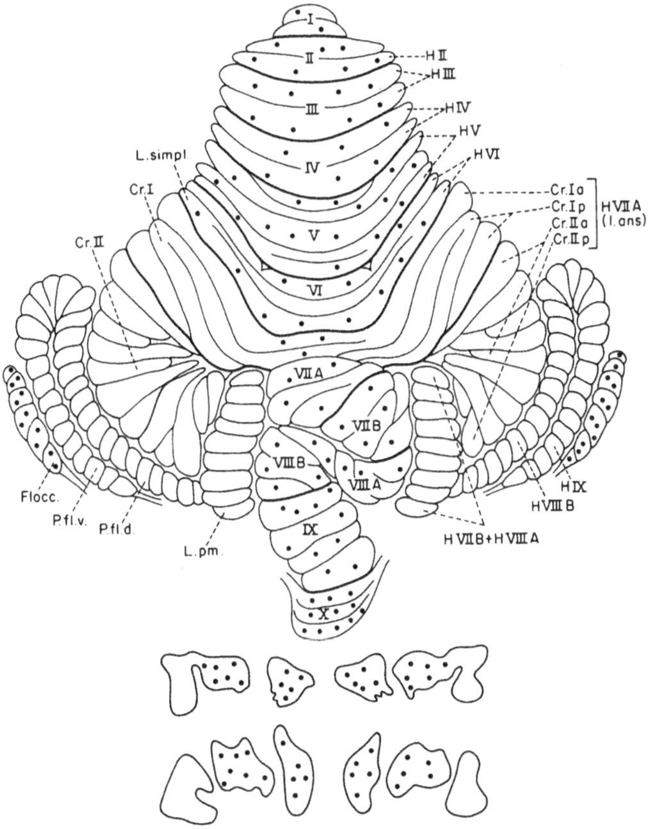

Fig. 4. Diagram showing the projection from the vestibular nuclear complex onto the various parts of the cerebellar cortex and nuclei. Variations in density of *symbols* indicate relative densities of the projections [30]. Abbreviations see p. 478–479

As mentioned above, with the modified Gudden method [2], Brodal and Torvik [10] found a projection to the cerebellum only from the caudoventral part of M, the ventrolateral part of D, and from cell groups f and x. These regions correspond to the projection zone of the spinal afferents to the vestibular complex [40], and they therefore concluded that the vestibular neurons projecting to the cerebellum probably mediated afferent information from spinal origin only. However, our observations give evidence that the cerebellum receives afferents also from the S, L, and cell group y. This observation, that positive cells are distributed almost to the entire territory of the nuclear complex and also to the part of this receiving primary afferents [55], indicates that afferent impulses, not only from the spinal cord but also from other regions including the eighth nerve, via the vestibular nuclei and their subgroups are mediated to larger areas in the cerebellum than previously known. In this context it should be recalled (see above) that we have recently given evidence that primary vestibular fibers project to the entire vermis [29]. The functional importance of this direct and indirect projection to the cerebellar cortex remains to be elucidated.

No conclusions can be made from negative findings when HRP is used as a tracer. We can not, therefore, definitely rule out the possibility that secondary vestibular afferents may reach the "negative" areas of the cerebellum (see Fig. 3). Actually, Saigal et al. [44], using HRP as a retrograde tracer, have recently shown that in ruminants there is a wider field of origin and termination of secondary vestibulocerebellar fibers than reported by us. This could, however, only mean that there are species differences in the terminal distribution of the cerebellar afferents from the vestibular nuclei.

The Cerebellar Projection from the Reticular Formation

In the cat the reticular formation (RF) can be divided into several nuclei. In the following account the subdivision given by Brodal is followed (Fig. 10). (See especially ref. [4].) On the basis of their efferent connections, he distinguishes between three separate nuclei and other nuclei, which constitute the greater part of the RF (here called the RF proper). The three separate nuclei are: the nucleus reticularis tegmenti pontis of Bechterew (N.r.t. in Fig. 10), the lateral reticular nucleus (N.r.l. in Fig. 10), and the paramedian reticular nucleus (N.r.p. in Fig. 10). The other RF nuclei (the RF proper) comprise seven areas whose delimitation can be given only arbitrarily. They are shown in Fig. 10. The nuclei are from caudal to rostral: the nucleus reticularis ventralis (R.v.), the nucleus reticularis lateralis[1] (R.l.), the nucleus reticularis parvicellularis (R.p.), the nucleus reticularis gigantocellularis (R.gc.), the nucleus reticularis pontis caudalis (R.p.c.), the nucleus reticularis pontis oralis (R.p.o.), and the reticular formation of the mesencephalon[2] (R.mes.). In the presentation given below, the three separate RF nuclei will be treated individually, and after this the cerebellar projection from the RF proper will be reviewed.

The Cerebellar Afferents from the N.r.t.

The N.r.t. is situated immediately dorsal to the pontine nuclei proper, but differs from these nuclei in many respects (for details, see ref. [6]). Earlier studies in our laboratory with the modified Gudden method [2] showed that the nucleus had a conspicuous connection with the cerebellum, but it was not until the tracer techniques were introduced that important details could be revealed. In this study [23] it was shown that virtually all parts of the cerebellar cortex are connected with the N.r.t. The diagram in Fig. 5 gives a summary of the projection. To simplify the presentation the areas of the N.r.t. containing labeled neurons following injections in lobules VI–VIII B and the flocculus are outlined by thick and broken lines, respectively. Furthermore, the same symbol is chosen for the cerebellar lobules in which injections of HRP give rise to a very similar distribution of labeled cells in the N.r.t.

1 Not to be confused with the lateral reticular nucleus (N.r.l.)

2 No labeled cells were found in Rmes in our experimental animal. The nucleus is therefore not indicated in Fig. 10

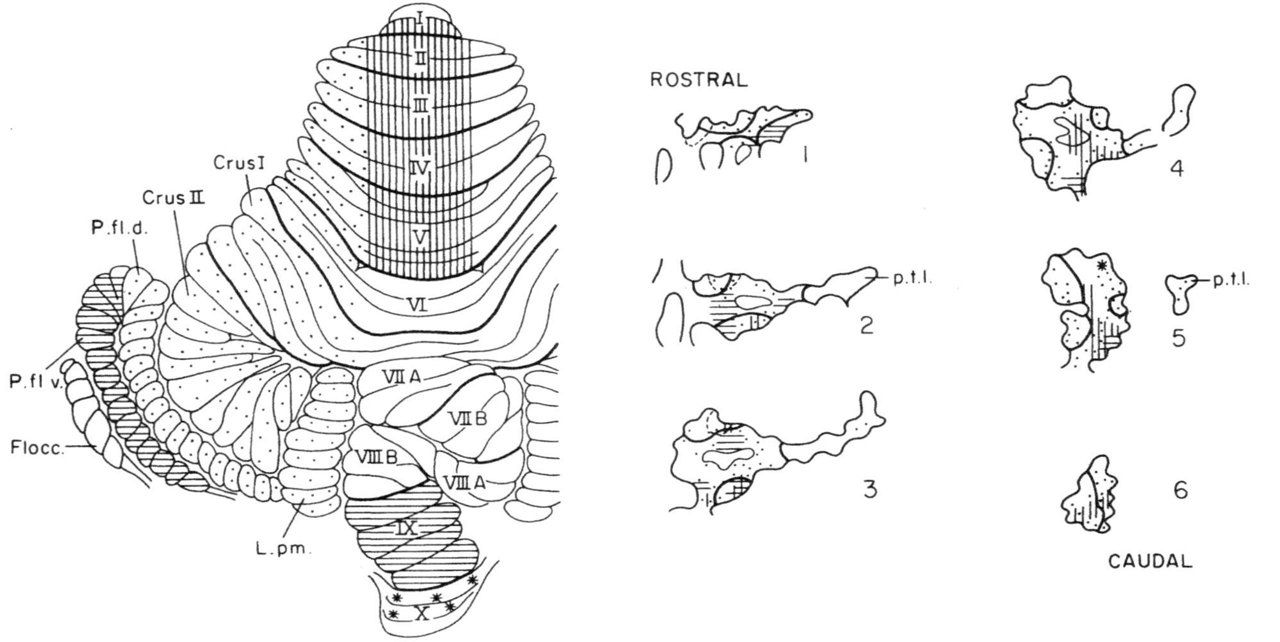

Fig. 5. Diagram summarizing the projections from the N.r.t. to the cerebellar cortex. To simplify presentation the areas of the nucleus containing labeled cells following injections in lobule VI–VIIIB and in the flocculus are outlined by *thick* and *broken lines*, respectively [23]. Abbreviations see p. 478–479

The pattern of projection from the N.r.t. onto the cerebellar cortex is rather precise and has many features in common with that from the pontine nuclei onto the cerebellum. Thus, the projection is bilateral with a contralateral preponderance, and the cells giving origin to axons to particular cerebellar lobules are arranged in groups which in the caudorostral direction constitute columns. The N.r.t. gives off fibers to all parts of the cerebellar cortex, and some cerebellar lobules receive fibers from the same areas of the N.r.t. Figure 5 shows that this is especially the case for vermal lobules VI–VIII B. Furthermore, the intermediate and lateral part of the anterior lobe, the hemispheres, the paramedian lobule, and the dorsal paraflocculus are connected with a common area of the N.r.t., but, as is evident from the figure, these regions overlap only partly with those projecting onto vermal lobules VI–VIII B. In addition, lobule IX and the ventral paraflocculus get fibers from areas of the N.r.t. partly different from those mentioned above. The diagram also shows that the fibers to the various lobules of the anterior lobe vermis take origin from common regions of the N.r.t., but these are to some extent different from those projecting onto the other cerebellar subdivisions. It should furthermore be noted that the small lateral extension of the N.r.t., the processus tegmentosus lateralis (p.t.l.), projects almost exclusively onto lobule VII A (not shown in Fig. 5). Thus, the total projection from the N.r.t. is very complex but it should be stressed that there is no separate projection from various parts of the nucleus onto the cerebellar longitudinal zones of Voogd.

The Cerebellar Afferents from the N.r.l.

The N.r.l. is a rather conspicuous nucleus. It is located laterally to the inferior olive and makes its appearance caudal to this. The nucleus can be divided into a main part, which is built up by a dorsal large-celled and a ventral small-celled portion, and a subtrigeminal part. Rostrally, the main part of the nucleus terminates somewhat caudal to the rostral pole of the inferior olive, the subtrigeminal part can be followed a little beyond the upper pole of the facial nucleus [53].

We have performed two HRP studies on the cerebellar projection from the N.r.l. [14, 19]. Like our other HRP studies they have given evidence of a much more detailed pattern in this reticulocerebellar projection than was revealed previously [19].

Figure 6 shows the distribution of the labeled cells within the N.r.l. following an injection into lobule VIII B of the posterior lobe vermis. Together with the anterior lobe, this lobule receives the majority of the cerebellar afferents from the nucleus. A greater number of labeled cells are present in the parvicellular and adjacent part of the magnocellular portion throughout the entire rostrocaudal extent of the nucleus. Many labeled cells are also present in the subtrigeminal part.

An analysis of our material shows that all cerebellar nuclei and all parts of the cerebellar cortex receive fibers from the N.r.l., and that there is a clear-cut topical pattern in the nuclear projection to the anterior lobe. There is a sequence in the projection to the lobules, so that lobule I is supplied from the most caudal area, lobule V from the rostromedial nuclear region, with the other lobules in between. The topical pattern is valid for the vermis as well as for the intermediate-lateral part, but there is considerable overlapping between the cerebellar projecting fields.

In addition to the anterior lobe and the posterior vermal lobule VIIIB, the paramedian lobule is the only cerebellar region which is amply supplied with fibers from the N.r.l. The other cortical areas are weakly connected with the nucleus and are supplied from the magnocellular portion and from the sub-

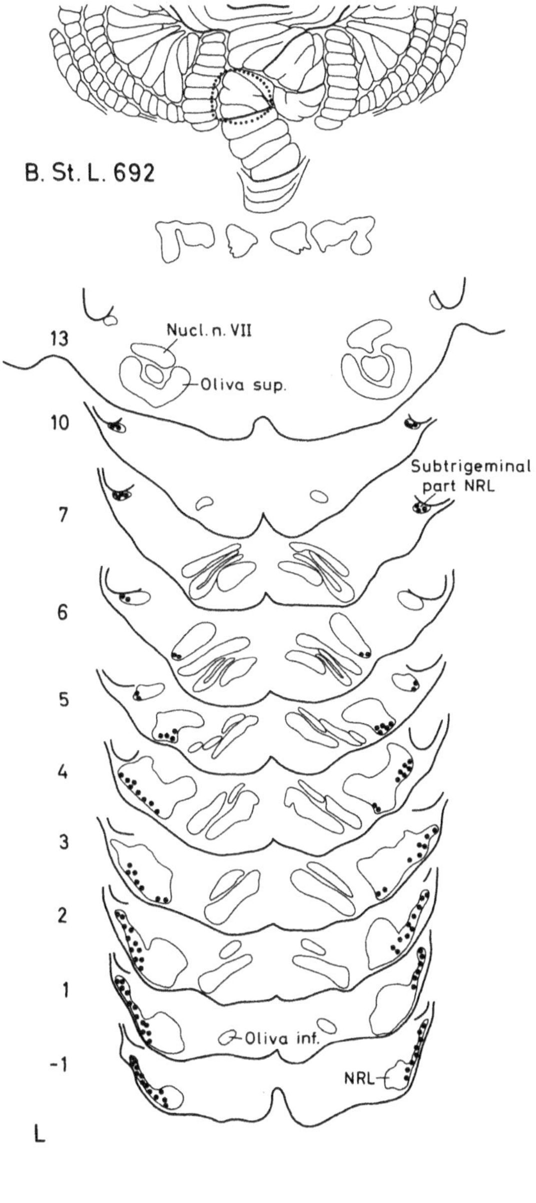

Fig. 6. Diagram illustrating the injection site and the distribution of labeled cells, indicated by dots (one dot does not represent one labeled cell) in the lateral reticular nucleus in one of the cats described in the text [19]. Abbreviations see p. 478–479

trigeminal part of the N.r.l. This is in contrast to the projection to lobule VIII B which has an especially heavy projection from the parvicellular portion of the nucleus. The cerebellar nuclei are supplied from the entire territory of the N.r.l., but receive the majority of their afferents from the magnocellular portion.

Figure 7 shows the total projection from the N.r.l. to the cerebellum. The cerebellar N.r.l. projection is bilateral, but there is a heavy ipsilateral preponderance. The filled triangles indicate the projection from the main part, the open circles the projection from the subtrigeminal part of the N.r.l. Variations in the density of symbols indicate relative densities in the projection to the different areas of the cerebellum. The diagram shows that the nuclear afferents reach the entire cerebellar cortex and all cerebellar nuclei, and that they are derived either from the parvicellular and magnocellular portion, or from the subtrigeminal part.

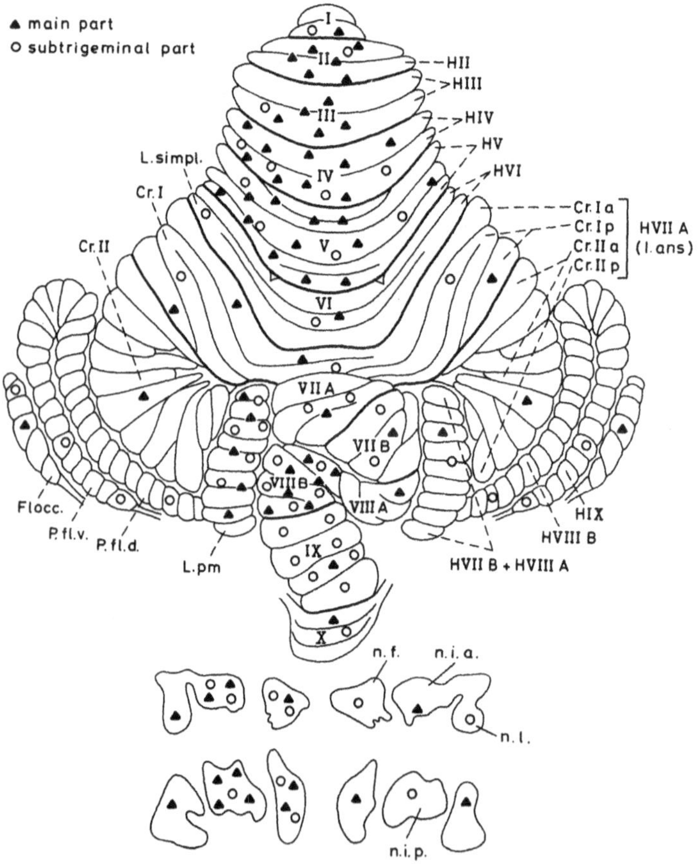

Fig. 7. Diagram of the projection from the main part (*filled triangles*) and from the subtrigeminal part (*open circles*) of the N.r.l. onto various parts of the cerebellar cortex and nuclei. Variations in density of *symbols* give relative densities in projections from the N.r.l. to different parts of the cerebellum [19]. Abbreviations see p. 478–479

The large majority of the labeled cells within the N.r.l. are of the small category, this is so also in the magnocellular portion. One explanation for this interesting observation is that there could be a difference in the terminal distribution within the cerebellar cortex of axons from small and large N.r.l. cells. More extensive terminal branching of an axon would make it less likely that its parent cell would be labeled following localized HRP injections. Further studies are needed for a clarification of this important point.

The Cerebellar Afferents from the N.r.p.

The N.r.p. is a separate nuclear entity with connections different from those of the cells of the main part of the RF. The cytoarchitecture of the nucleus in the cat was described by Brodal [3] and Brodal and Torvik [9]. The nucleus can be subdivided into an accessory (aPRN), a dorsal (dPRN), and a ventral (vPRN) group. The nucleus which is shown in Fig. 8 is laterally limited by the roots of the hypoglossal nerve, ventrally by the inferior olivary complex, and medially by the raphe nuclei. Large, medium-sized and small cells are present within the nucleus, partly interspersed, partly lying in groups.

The above mentioned studies by Brodal [3] and Brodal and Torvik [9] where the modified Gudden method [2] was used, showed that practically all cells of the N.r.p. project bilaterally onto the cerebellar cortex with the uncrossed connection being more abundant. All three nuclear subdivisions were found to send fibers to the anterior lobe, the pyramis, the uvula, with the adjacent part of lobule C_2, and probably to the fastigial nucleus. Our experimental HRP study [46] gave evidence of a more elaborate cerebellar projection from the N.r.p. Figure 8 gives the details in the distribution of the labeled cells in a typical case and Fig. 9 shows a diagram of the total cerebellar projection. Cells of all sizes were found to be labeled following the cerebellar HRP injections, and it is seen from the figure that the greater part of the cerebellar cortex receives afferents from the N.r.p. The majority of the fibers project to the anterior lobe and to the vermis of the posterior lobe (with the exception of lobules VII B and VIII A). There is a less conspicuous projection to the lobulus simplex, the crura, the flocculus, the cerebellar nuclei, and the paramedian lobule. The paraflocculus appears to be weakly connected with the N.r.p.

An interesting observation is that the three subgroups of N.r.p. are not equal in their projections (Fig. 9). Thus, while the dPRN is connected with the greater part of the cerebellar cortex and with all nuclei (the vermal lobules VII B, VIII A, the posterior parts of the flocculus and dorsal paraflocculus, and the entire ventral paraflocculus are free from connections), the vPRN lacks a connection with lobule IX, the flocculus, and the paraflocculus. The aPRN projects differently, and has its most substantial contribution to lobule I (lingula), the flocculus, and the vermal lobules VII–X.

We found no evidence for a topographic localization within the N.r.p. projection (cf. what is said above concerning the cerebellar projection from the N.r.l.), but we found that the variations in the relative density of labeled cells in the N.r.p. were not always related to the size of the HRP-stained cortical area.

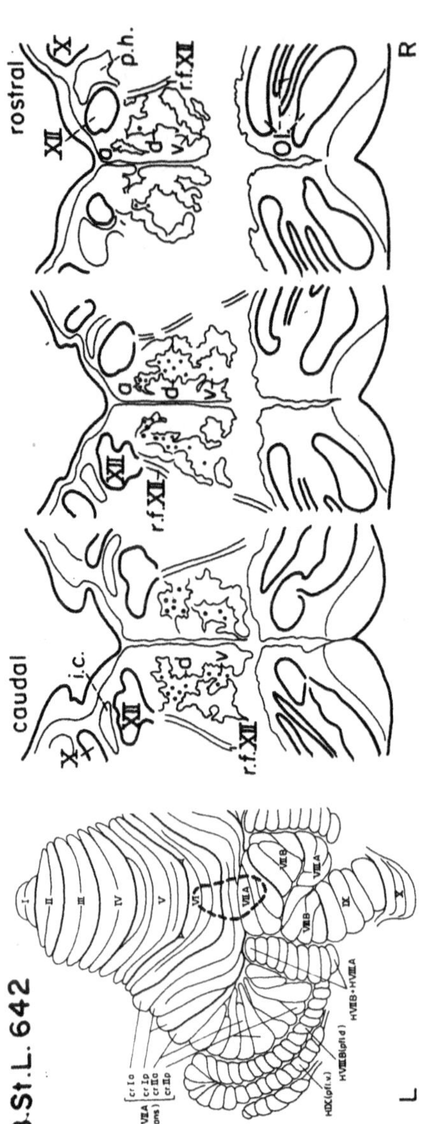

Fig. 8. Diagram of the injection site and the distribution of labeled cells, indicated by *dots* (one *dot* represents one labeled cell) in the N.r.p. in one of the cats described in the text [46]. Abbreviations see p. 478–479

This difference could of course only reflect biologic differences between the animals, but it cannot, in our opinion, be excluded that there might be local differences in the cerebellar cortical distribution of afferent fibers from a certain precerebellar relay nucleus. In this context two other findings should be mentioned. Rinvik and Walberg [42] in their study of the cerebellar projection from the main cuneate nucleus observed that HRP injections in the superficial parts of the cerebellar folia resulted in labeling of neurons in this nucleus, whereas injections into the deep parts of the cerebellar folia produced labeling of neurons in the external cuneate nucleus. Brodal and Walberg [12] made a similar observation; they found indications for a rostrocaudal pattern in the

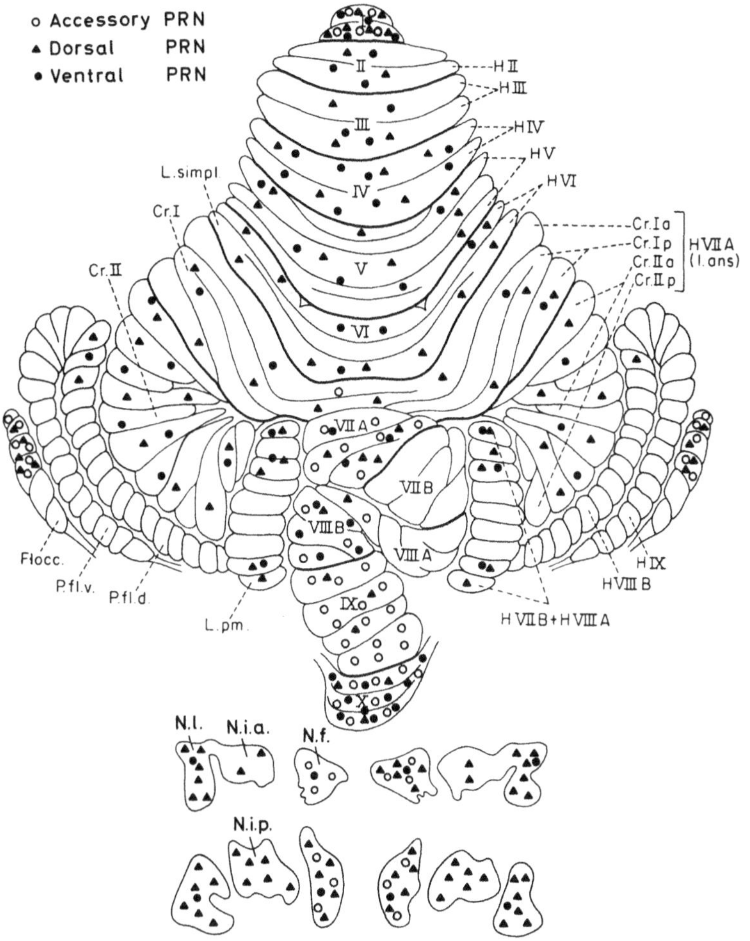

Fig. 9. Diagram of the projection from the three subdivisions of the N.r.p. onto the various parts of the cerebellar cortex and nuclei. Variations in density of *symbols* show relative densities in the projections from the three subdivisions [46]. Abbreviations see p. 478–479

projection from the dorsal accessory olive to deep versus superfical parts of the folia of the paramedian lobule. Our various findings clearly invite detailed investigations of the precerebellar relay nuclei concerning a possible variation in the density of distribution of mossy (and climbing) fibers within the various cerebellar lobules and folia.

The Cerebellar Afferents from the RF Proper

The experimental studies with the modified Gudden method [2] led Brodal and collaborators to conclude that of the reticular cell groups only the three well-

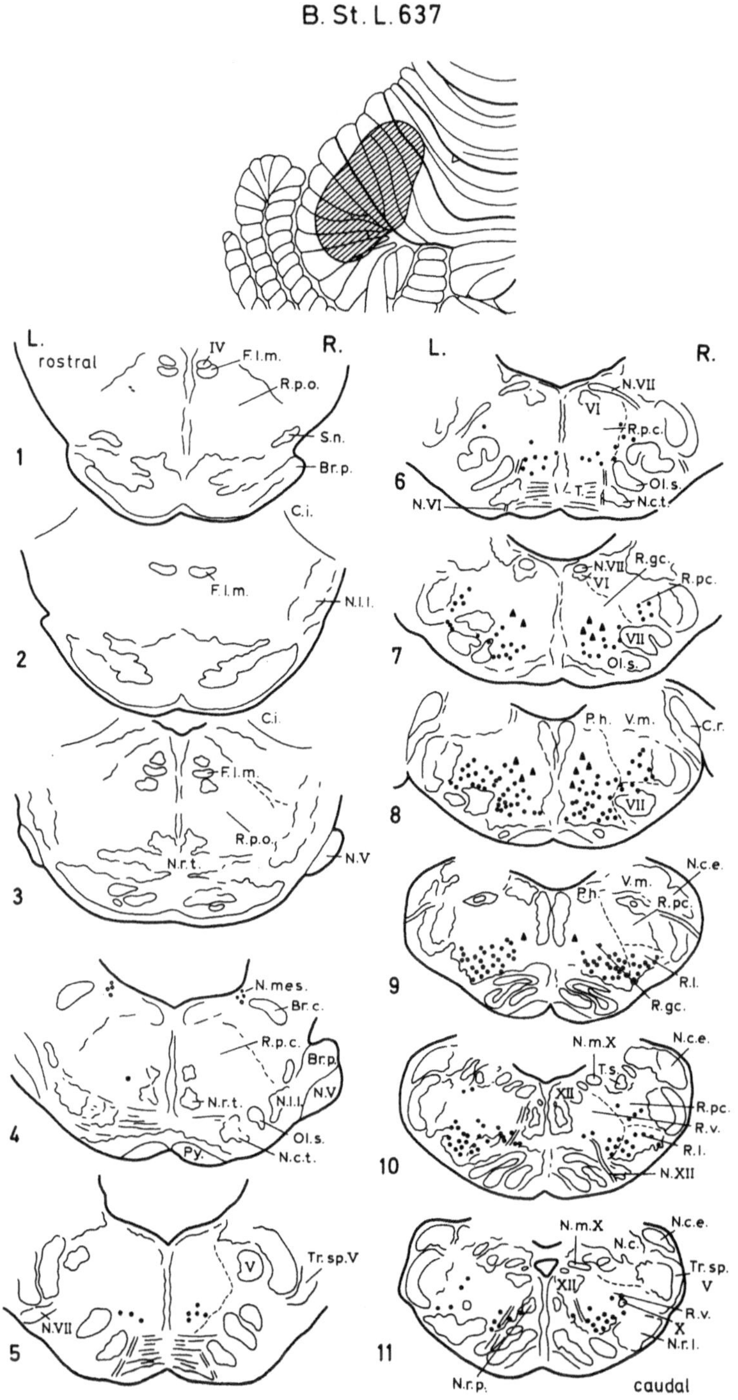

Fig. 10. Diagram showing the injection site and the distribution of labeled cells within the RF (one *dot* represents one labeled small and medium-sized cell, one *triangle* represents one labeled giant cell) in one of the cases described in the text [32]. Abbreviations see p. 478–479

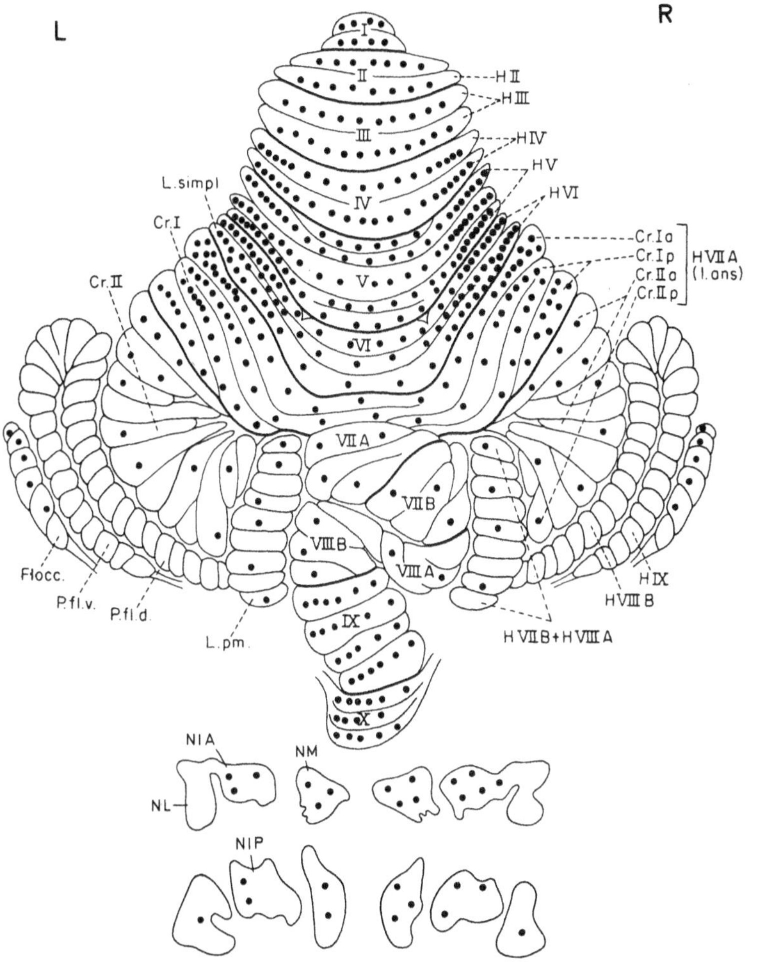

Fig. 11. Diagram showing the total projection from the RF to the cerebellum. The density of the *dots* indicates the relative densities in the projections [32]. Abbreviations see p. 478–479

circumscribed nuclei, the N.r.t., the N.r.l., and the N.r.p., send their fibers to the cerebellum. These experimental observations were taken to indicate that the three nuclei differed functionally from the remaining part of the RF and that they more or less constituted a separate entity. However, our recent HRP studies have shown that not only do the three above mentioned nuclei send their fibers to a much greater part of the cerebellum than was hitherto known, they also show that the cells in the RF proper are intimately connected with the cerebellum.

Our experimental findings [32] reveal that R.v., R.l., R.p., R.gc., R.p.c., and R.p.o. all show labeled cells after cerebellar HRP injections. The only negative observation was made as regards the R.mes., we had in none of our cases labeled cells within this part of the RF. The highest number of labeled neurons after cerebellar injections was found in the caudal area of the RF, especially within R.v., R.l., and R.gc. Another part of the RF with a conspicuous cerebellar projection is the rostral R.p.c. (at the level of N.r.t.). Figure 10 shows the distribution of labeled cells in a relevant case. In addition to showing the projection from the various RF nuclei, the diagram reveals that not only small and medium-sized cells, but also giant cells participate in the projection. This was always found to be the case in animals with large cortical injections. This finding, that large injections are required for a positive labeling of giant cells, is another finding indicating that there are differences in the terminal distribution of the mossy fibers from the various precerebellar relay nuclei (cf. what was mentioned above concerning the N.r.l.).

Figure 11 summarizes the cerebellar projection from the RF proper. Except for the paraflocculus, all cerebellar cortical areas and the nuclei receive afferents from one or more of the RF nuclei. By far the largest number of labeled neurons is observed in cases where the HRP injections include the intermediate-lateral part of the lobulus simplex with its adjacent anterior and posterior areas. However, it should be stressed that the projection is rather diffuse and that small cortical injections result in labeling of only a few RF cells. Likewise (because of this?), we have not been able to reveal a topical difference in the projection, but as mentioned above, it is clear that some of the reticular groups are more intimately connected with the cerebellum than are others.

Addendum

As stressed in the introduction, new techniques always make possible a more detailed mapping of well-known connections and a description of new projections. This has been shown to be the case for the cerebellar afferent fibers. In the list shown below, the upper part indicates the nuclei previously shown to be intimately connected with the cerebellum. Our HRP studies have added much new information concerning the details in these connections (in addition to the publications referred to above, the reader should consult ref. [5, 11, 13, 15, 24, 25, 26, 31, 33, 38, 51, 52, 54, 56, 57]). The fine last nuclei in the following list are brain stem nuclei hitherto not known to project to the cerebellum.

Pons
Nucleus reticularis tegmenti
Nucleus reticularis lateralis
Nucleus reticularis paramedianus
Inferior olive
Primary vestibular fibers
Vestibular nuclei
Trigeminal nuclei
Perihypoglossal nuclei
Raphe nuclei
Dorsal column nuclei
Locus coeruleus

Cranial nerve nuclei
Nucleus of solitary tract
Parabrachial nucleus
Paratrigeminal nucleus
Reticular formation

The RF efferents have been considered above; here brief reference will be made to the projections from the four other nuclei [28, 48, 49, 50].

The afferents from the neurons in the *motor nuclei of the cranial nerves* appear to reach only certain parts of the cerebellum [28]. Thus, positively labeled cells in the motor nuclei of the cranial nerves were found following HRP injections in the anterior lobe, the nodulus, the flocculus, and the fastigial nucleus. Most of the labeled cells were medium-sized or large and of an appearance similar to motoneurons. This observation concurs with the findings by Grant and coworkers, who have made similar observations in the spinal cord (this volume, p. 466).

The cerebellar afferents from the *nucleus of the solitary tract* [48] were traced to the cerebellar vermis and flocculus. The fibers to the anterior lobe vermis emanate from the caudal part of the nucleus, those to the posterior lobe vermis and the flocculus from the rostral part.

The *parabrachial nucleus* has recently been shown to be a relay station in the gustatory pathway from the nucleus of the solitary tract to the thalamus [36, 37]. Our experiments [49] reveal that it is the cerebellar vermis that receives the bulk of the fibers from the nucleus, but that in addition a few cells project to the anterior part of the paramedian lobule and to the ventral paraflocculus. The projection pattern is very similar to that found from the locus coeruleus [47] and it should be stressed that the parabrachial nucleus, like the locus coeruleus, displays a great number of catecholamine-containing cell bodies [27, 39].

The afferents from the *paratrigeminal nucleus* reach a larger part of the cerebellum than do the fibers from the two previously mentioned nuclei. The fibers reach the cerebellar lobules I, II, V (hemispheral part), VIII B, and IX, the paramedian lobule, and the fastigial nucleus [50]. Our observations are of particular interest since Chan-Palay [17, 18] recently has described details in the neuronal organization of the nucleus, and that substance P, catecholamine, and serotonin are present in terminal axons within the nucleus, and that some of the neurons contain substance P.

In the above review emphasis has been put on the description of cerebellar afferent fibers from certain precerebellar relay nuclei, as these appear when HRP is used as a retrograde tracer in the cat. The afferent connections to these nuclei have not been considered; the reader is referred to the original publications for details. Although our observations indicate that the cerebellum plays a much more active role in the integration of impulses than has hitherto been known, anatomic studies with more sensitive techniques will probably reveal further details in the mosaic of connections already described.

References

1. Alley K, Baker R, Simpson JI (1975) Afferents to the vestibulo-cerebellum and the origin of the visual climbing fibers in the rabbit. Brain Res 98:582–589
2. Brodal A (1940) Modification of Gudden method for study of cerebral localization. Arch Neurol 43:46–58
3. Brodal A (1953) Reticulo-cerebellar connections in the cat. J Comp Neurol 98:113–153
4. Brodal A (1957) The reticular formation of the brain stem. Anatomical aspects and functional correlations. Oliver and Boyd, Edingburgh London
5. Brodal A (1976) The olivocerebellar projection in the cat as studied with the method of retrograde axonal transport of horseradish peroxidase. II. The projection to the uvula. J Comp Neurol 166:417–426
6. Brodal A, Brodal P (1971) The organization of the nucleus reticularis tegmenti pontis in the cat in the light of experimental anatomical studies of its cerebral cortical afferents. Exp Brain Res 13:90–110
7. Brodal A, Høivik B (1964) Site and mode of termination of primary vestibulocerebellar fibres in the cat. An experimental study with silver impregnation methods. Arch Ital Biol 102:1–21
8. Brodal A, Pompeiano O (1957) Vestibular nuclei in the cat. J Anat 91:438–454
9. Brodal A, Torvik A (1954) Cerebellar projection of paramedian reticular nucleus of medulla oblongata in cat. J Neurophysiol 17:484–495
10. Brodal A, Torvik A (1957) Über den Ursprung der sekundären vestibulo-cerebellaren Fasern bei der Katze: Eine experimentell-anatomische Studie. Arch Psychiatr Nervenkr 195:550–567
11. Brodal A, Walberg F (1977) The olivocerebellar projection in the cat studied with the method of retrograde axonal transport of horseradish peroxidase. IV. The projection to the anterior lobe. J Comp Neurol 172:85–108
12. Brodal A, Walberg F (1977) The olivocerebellar projection in the cat studied with the method of retrograde axonal transport of horseradish peroxidase. VI. The projection onto longitudinal zones of the paramedian lobule. J Comp Neurol 176:281–294
13. Brodal A, Walberg F, Hoddevik GH (1975) The olivocerebellar projection in the cat studied with the method of retrograde axonal transport of horseradish peroxidase. I. The projection to the paramedian lobule. J Comp Neurol 164:449–470
14. Brodal P (1975) Demonstration of a somatotopically organized projection onto the paramedian lobule and the anterior lobe from the lateral reticular nucleus: An experimental study with the horseradish peroxidase method. Brain Res 95:221–239
15. Brodal P, Walberg F (1977) The pontine projection to the cerebellar anterior lobe. An experimental study in the cat with retrograde transport of horseradish peroxidase. Exp Brain Res 29:233–248
16. Chan-Palay V (1977) Cerebellar dentate nucleus: organization, cytology and transmitters. Springer, Berlin Heidelberg New York
17. Chan-Palay V (1978) The paratrigeminal nucleus. I. Neurons and synaptic organization. J Neurocytol 7:405–418
18. Chan-Palay V (1978) The paratrigeminal nucleus. II. Identification and interrelations of the catecholamine, indolamine axons and substance P immunoreactive cells in the neuropil. J Neurocytol 7:419–442
19. Dietrichs E, Walberg F (1979) The cerebellar projection from the lateral reticular nucleus as studied with retrograde transport of horseradish peroxidase. Anat Embryol 155: 273–290
20. Eller TW, Chan-Palay V (1976) Afferents to the cerebellar lateral nucleus. Evidence from retrograde transport of horseradish peroxidase after pressure injections through micropipettes. J. Comp Neurol 166:285–302
21. Frankfurter A, Weber JT, Harting JK (1977) Brain stem projections to lobule VII of the posterior vermis in the squirrel monkey: as demonstrated by the retrograde axonal transport of tritiated horseradish peroxidase. Brain Res 124:135–139
22. Gould BB, Graybiel AM (1976) Afferents to the cerebellar cortex in the cat: evidence for an intrinsic pathway leading from the deep nuclei to the cortex. Brain Res 110:601–611

23. Hoddevik GH (1978) The projection from nucleus reticularis tegmenti pontis onto the cerebellum in the cat. A study using the methods of anterograde degeneration and retrograde axonal transport of horseradish peroxidase. Anat Embryol 153:227–242
24. Hoddevik GH, Brodal A (1977) The olivocerebellar projection studied with the method of retrograde axonal transport of horseradish peroxidase. V. The projections to the flocculonodular lobe and the paraflocculus in the rabbit. J Comp Neurol 176:269–280
25. Hoddevik GH, Walberg F (1979) The pontine projection onto longitudinal zones of the paramedian lobule in the cat. Exp Brain Res 34:233–240
26. Hoddevik GH, Brodal A, Walberg F (1976) The olivocerebellar projection in the cat studied with the method of retrograde axonal transport of horseradish peroxidase. III. The projection to the vermal visual area. J Comp Neurol 169:155–170
27. Jones BE, Moore RY (1974) Catecholamine-containing neurons of the nucleus locus coeruleus in the cat. J Comp Neurol 157:43–52
28. Kotchabhakdi N, Walberg F (1977) Cerebellar afferents from neurons in motor nuclei of cranial nerves demonstrated by retrograde axonal transport of horseradish peroxidase. Brain Res 137:158–163
29. Kotchabhakdi N, Walberg F (1978) Primary vestibular afferent projections to the cerebellum as demonstrated by retrograde axonal transport of horseradish peroxidase. Brain Res 142:142–146
30. Kotchabhakdi N, Walberg F (1978) Cerebellar afferent projections from the vestibular nuclei in the cat: an experimental study with the method of retrograde axonal transport of horseradish peroxidase. Exp Brain Res 31:591–604
31. Kotchabhakdi N, Hoddevik GH, Walberg F (1978) Cerebellar afferent projections from the perihypoglossal nuclei: an experimental study with the method of retrograde axonal transport of horseradish peroxidase. Exp Brain Res 31:13–29
32. Kotchabhakdi N, Hoddevik GH, Walberg F (1980) The reticulocerebellar projection in the cat as studied with retrograde transport of horseradish peroxidase. Anat Embryol 160:341–359
33. Kotchabhakdi N, Walberg F, Brodal A (1978) The olivocerebellar projection in the cat studied with the method of retrograde axonal transport of horseradish peroxidase. VII. The projection to lobulus simplex, crus I and II. J Comp Neurol 182:293–314
34. Larsell O (1967) The comparative anatomy and histology of the cerebellum from myxinoids through birds. Jansen J (ed) University of Minnesota Press, Minneapolis
35. Larsell O (1970) The comparative anatomy and histology of the cerebellum from monotremes through apes. Jansen J (ed) University of Minnesota Press, Minneapolis
36. Norgren R (1978) Projections from the nucleus of the solitary tract in the rat. Neuroscience 3:207–218
37. Norgren R, Leonard CM (1971) Taste pathways in rat brainstem. Science 173:1136–1139
38. Pierce ET, Hoddevik GH, Walberg F (1977) The cerebellar projection from the raphe nuclei in the cat as studied with the method of retrograde transport of horseradish peroxidase. Anat Embryol 152:73–87
39. Poitras D, Parent A (1978) Atlas of the distribution of monoamine-containing nerve cell bodies in the brain stem of the cat. J Comp Neurol 179:699–718
40. Pompeiano O, Brodal A (1957) Spino-vestibular fibers in the cat. J Comp Neurol 108:353–382
41. Precht W, Volkind R, Blanks RHJ (1977) Functional organization of the vestibular input to the anterior and posterior cerebellar vermis of cat. Exp Brain Res 27:143–160
42. Rinvik E, Walberg F (1975) Studies on the cerebellar projection from the main and external cuneate nuclei in the cat by means of retrograde axonal transport of horseradish peroxidase. Brain Res 95:371–381
43. Ruggiero D, Batton III RR, Tayaraman A, Carpenter MB (1977) Brain stem afferents to the fastigial nucleus in the cat demonstrated by transport of horseradish peroxidase. J Comp Neurol 172:189–210
44. Saigal RP, Karamanlidis AN, Voogd J, Michaloudi H, Mangana O (in press) Cerebellar afferents from the vestibular and perihypoglossal nuclei in sheep studied with retrograde transport of horseradish peroxidase. J Hirnforsch

45. Shinnar S, Maciewicz RJ, Shofer RJ (1975) A raphe projection to cat cerebellar cortex. Brain Res 97:139–143
46. Somana R, Walberg F (1978) Cerebellar afferents from the paramedian reticular nucleus studied with retrograde transport of horseradish peroxidase. Anat Embryol 154:353–368
47. Somana R, Walberg F (1978) The cerebellar projection from locus coeruleus as studied with retrograde transport of horseradish peroxidase in the cat. Anat Embryol 155:87–94
48. Somana R, Walberg F (1979) Cerebellar afferents from the nucleus of the solitary tract. Neurosci Lett 11:41–47
49. Somana R, Walberg F (1979) The cerebellar projection from the paratrigeminal nucleus in the cat. Neurosci Lett 15:49–54
50. Somana R, Walberg F (1979) The cerebellar projection from the parabrachial nucleus in the cat. Brain Res 172:144–149
51. Somana R, Walberg F (1980) A reexamination of the cerebellar projections from the gracile, main and cuneate nuclei in the cat. Brain Res 186:33–42
52. Somana R, Kotchabhakdi N, Walberg F (1980) Cerebellar afferents from the trigeminal sensory nuclei in the cat. Exp Brain Res 38:57–64
53. Walberg F (1952) The lateral reticular nucleus of the medulla oblongata in mammals. A comparative anatomical study. J Comp Neurol 96:283–343
54. Walberg F, Brodal A (1979) The longitudinal zonal pattern in the paramedian lobule of the cat's cerebellum: an analysis based on a correlation of recent HRP data with results of studies with other methods. J Comp Neurol 187:581–588
55. Walberg F, Bowsher D, Brodal A (1958) The termination of primary vestibular fibers in the vestibular nuclei in the cat. An experimental study with silver methods. J Comp Neurol 110:391–419
56. Walberg F, Brodal A, Hoddevik GH (1976) A note on the method of retrograde transport of horseradish peroxidase as a tool in studies of afferent cerebellar connections, particularly those from the inferior olive; with comments on the orthograde transport in Purkinje cell axons. Exp Brain Res 24:383–401
57. Walberg F, Kotchabhakdi N, Hoddevik GH (1979) The olivocerebellar projections to the flocculus and paraflocculus in the cat, compared to those in the rabbit. A study using horseradish peroxidase as a tracer. Brain Res 161:389–398

Discussion

Voogd: I would like to make some comments on the parasagittal termination pattern and on the central nuclear terminations of spinal and reticular mossy fiber pathways. On the basis of degeneration and autoradiographic experiments it is clear that the dorsal spinocerebellar tract and the external cuneate nucleus terminate mainly in different parts of the anterior lobe, but in both cases there is a zonal system in the termination. The fibers terminate in parasagittal concentrations. It is very spectacular to see how the fibers of the external cuneate projection, both in the white matter and in the overlying granular layer, are arranged in parasagittal bands which actually reach up to the Purkinje cell layer. So when someone tells you that spinocerebellar fibers terminate in the depths of the granular layer that is certainly not true – they terminate all through the thickness of the granular layer, but they terminate in bands. The tegmental reticular nucleus projections show some indication of parasagittal banding, but it is not as clear as for the spinocerebellar tracts. It is especially clear in the bottom of the fissures, but on the rest of the surface it is not that distinct. The projections from the basal pontine nuclei show a kind of organization, a kind of banding, you could say, but it is mainly restricted to the fact that the lateral part of the anterior lobe, approximately corresponding to the C zones and D zones, receives an extremely large projection. Now when we looked at the central cerebellar nuclei we did not find any real evidence of termination from spinocerebellar, cuneocerebellar, or basal pontine nuclei pathways. But after injections into the reticular formation or into the reticular nucleus of the pons we found clear projections to the central nuclei. After injection into the reticular nucleus of the pons, we found the following distribution of terminals bilaterally in the three central nuclei: in the dentate laterally and ventrally and mainly caudally, in the posterior interposed nucleus laterally and ventrally, in the tail of the fastigial nucleus, but not in the anterior interposed nucleus. After large injections into the lateral reticular nucleus or the paramedian reticular nucleus, the distribution of terminals in the central nuclei is exactly to the other parts of the central nuclei; the lateral and ventral parts of the dentate nucleus are free of terminals, but now the dorsomedial part of the dentate nucleus, the anterior interposed nucleus, and the ventral portion of the fastigial nucleus show terminals. These investigations, of course, are very crude as to the origin of the system, but as far as the termination of the system is concerned, there is a parasagittal banding in "phylogenetically" old systems; it is much less clear in the neocerebellar (pontocerebellar) system. Evidence for nuclear terminations, as far as I know, is only really there for reticulocerebellar systems. It doesn't mean that spinocerebellar systems do not terminate in the central nuclei at all, only that we do not have real evidence.

Llinás: When Dr. Berthoz and I investigated inputs to the vermis (lobules 5–6) we found, very much to our surprise, a vestibular mossy fiber input (Berthoz and Llinás, 1974). Do you know if Dr. Walberg has any idea how large this vestibular projection is and whether it is a well-defined or, rather, a diffuse projection?

Grant: I don't know, maybe Dr. Brodal knows about it.

Brodal: I think it's hard to find out because you have to use large injections to get labeled cells, but I don't think there is a very special small group projecting to the anterior lobe.

Llinás: Are you saying that it is a diffuse projection?

Brodal: I could not be definite.

Voogd: When you make injections of leucine into the vestibular nuclei and look in the vermis you see that there is an important projection to lobule 1 of the anterior lobe and then only a few fibers until near the primary fissure, where there is a concentration that goes rather far laterally, then in lobule 7 it's again almost nothing. In lobule 8 it increases a little bit more while in the ventral parts of lobule 9 and in lobule 10, it's extremely hot. Of course, there could be more because we do not have injections of the superior vestibular nucleus nor of the extreme caudal part of the vestibular complex, but that is what we saw with large injections in the central part of the vestibular nucleus.

Mugnaini: A student of mine, Dr. Korte, and I looked at primary vestibular projections to the cerebellum and the vestibular nuclei using be Fink-Heimer method. The reason we did this was that previous studies were done with the Nauta method, which is known not to show everything, and its is recognized that the Fink-Heimer method is going to reveal more. We ended up finding more projections in the vestibular nuclei, but fewer in the cerebellum. Now using HRP, Dr. Walberg finds the reverse. I have tried to put my comment to rhyme.

> The method that shows you too little here
> May show you too much there,
> HRP, which we did not have before
> Will always show you that there is more.
> It may then take another touch
> To help decide what is too little and what is too much.

Martin: Does my memory serve me correctly that there has been some controversy concerning the collaterals of the lateral reticular nucleus (N.r.l.) to the deep nuclei. We saw them in the opossum, and as I remember in the cat there was some question about whether Dr. Voogd saw them.

Voogd: Künzle (1975) didn't see them. And we didn't see them in older experiments with injections in the N.r.l. I don't know why.

Martin: On the question of a direct spinal input to the cerebellar nuclei, I think the literature is fairly clear that they are present in the fastigius. There may be a question about which parts of the interpositus, but I don't think there is too much question about the status of the interpositus.

Voogd: But I think there is. When you inject the external cuneate nucleus, you see some fibers passing through the central nuclei. But when you inject the reticular formation the whole nucleus is covered by a massive number of dots so it looks quite different. I am not quite convinced that what you see in autoradiograms after external cuneate injections really signifies termination. We should do EM autoradiography to determine if it really terminates there or not.

Martin: I was talking about what you can see after midthoracic transection as far as direct spinocerebellar collaterals to the deep nuclei.

Voogd: You see some fibers in the central nuclei corresponding in distribution to what I showed for the reticular formation. Whether these fibers really terminate there is open to doubt because there is a difference in intensity of labeling in the autoradiograms after external cuneate and reticular formation injections. In the latter case, it is very intense, but after external cuneate injections you have difficulty in seeing whether there is something in the nuclei or not.

The Signal Processing and Function of the Flocculus During Smooth Eye Movement in the Monkey

S. G. Lisberger *

Introduction

It has long been known that the flocculus, as part of the vestibulo-cerebellum, receives mossy-fiber inputs directly from the vestibular nerve [5] and projects to the vestibular nuclei in the brainstem [7]. A decade ago, several groups discovered in the rabbit and cat that these projections are quite specific; Purkinje cells in the flocculus inhibit brainstem neurons responsible for transmitting vestibular information to the oculomotor system [2, 10, 12]. Since the function of the brainstem vestibulo-oculomotor pathways was already well understood, the discovery that interneurons within them were the targets of output from the flocculus raised the hope that it might be possible to understand the role of the flocculus in eye movements. At least in the monkey this hope has been fulfilled; however, our initial expectation that the flocculus would be important for the eye movements produced by vestibular inputs has proved to be inaccurate, and available data indicate that the monkey flocculus is much more important for the smooth eye movements used to track a small, slowly moving object.

Before reviewing the evidence on which our current understanding of the monkey flocculus is based, we will briefly discuss the smooth eye movements evoked by visual and vestibular stimuli. Next, we will present physiologic data on the flocculus, paying special attention to recording experiments in which the signal processing of single Purkinje cells has been documented in behaving animals. Finally, we will attempt to fit the signal processing of the flocculus into a general description of the smooth oculomotor control system and suggest how the function of the flocculus might be generalized to the rest of the cerebellum.

Smooth Eye Movement

The smooth oculomotor control system can be divided into two subsystems having distinctly different functions: *smooth pursuit*, which attempts to track the motion of small visual targets, and the *vestibulo-ocular reflex* (VOR), which operates in light and dark and responds to head movement with an oppositely

* I am grateful to A. Fuchs, who contributed extensively to the design, execution, and interpretation of the experiments reviewed here. In addition, I want to thank F. Miles for many useful discussions and for commenting on an earlier draft of this paper. This work was supported by Grants RR00166, GM00260, and EY00745 from the National Institutes of Health

directed, "compensatory" eye movement. Figure 1 shows a schematic representation of these two subsystems; for simplicity, all variables are shown as velocities, the flow of neural signals is shown by solid lines, and physical variables are represented by dashed lines. In the VOR pathway, head velocity with respect to the world ($\dot{H}_W$) is (a) sensed by the semicircular canals of the vestibular apparatus (SCC), (b) inverted (by the −1), and (c) transmitted to the eyeball where it causes oppositely directed eye velocity with respect to the head ($\dot{E}_H$). In the pursuit pathway, target velocity with respect to the world ($\dot{T}_W$) produces retinal image slip which, ultimately, causes eye velocity appropriate to reduce and almost eliminate that slip. It should be pointed out that the smooth eye movements of pursuit and the VOR are interrupted at times by rapid, saccadic eye movements; these serve quite a different function from pursuit and the VOR and will not be treated here.

To evaluate the functions of the VOR and pursuit, it is best to consider their effect on the final output of the smooth oculomotor control system, eye velocity with respect to the world ($\dot{E}_W$). Although $\dot{E}_W$ is seldom measured in the laboratory, it can be reconstructed [6] from $\dot{E}_H$ and $\dot{H}_W$ (which are generally measured) using the equation:

$$\dot{E}_W = \dot{E}_H + \dot{H}_W \qquad \text{(Eq. 1)}$$

In monkeys, the VOR responds to head movement by producing eye velocity ($\dot{E}_H$) equal in amplitude and opposite in direction to head velocity [17]. As a result, eye velocity with respect to the world ($\dot{E}_W$) is little affected by head movement; this is clearly advantageous when the monkey attempts to fixate objects that are stationary in the world. If the monkey elects to track an object that is moving with respect to the world, the pursuit system is activated and

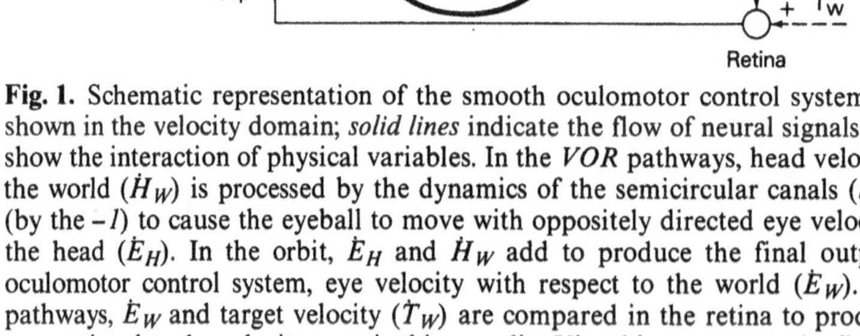

Fig. 1. Schematic representation of the smooth oculomotor control system. All variables are shown in the velocity domain; *solid lines* indicate the flow of neural signals, while *dashed lines* show the interaction of physical variables. In the *VOR* pathways, head velocity with respect to the world ($\dot{H}_W$) is processed by the dynamics of the semicircular canals (*SCC*) and inverted (by the *−1*) to cause the eyeball to move with oppositely directed eye velocity with respect to the head ($\dot{E}_H$). In the orbit, $\dot{E}_H$ and $\dot{H}_W$ add to produce the final output of the smooth oculomotor control system, eye velocity with respect to the world ($\dot{E}_W$). In the *PURSUIT* pathways, $\dot{E}_W$ and target velocity ($\dot{T}_W$) are compared in the retina to produce a visual input proportional to the velocity to retinal image slip. Visual inputs access the final motor pathways at summing junction *b*, and cause an eye velocity ($\dot{E}_W$) appropriate to reduce retinal image slip. Note that this representation of the smooth eye-movement system produces an appropriate $\dot{E}_W$ regardless of whether smooth tracking is accomplished with $\dot{E}_H$, $\dot{H}_W$, or any combination of the two

generates nonzero eye velocity with respect to the world. Equation 1 emphasizes that the required $\dot{E}_W$ could be generated by any combination of $\dot{E}_H$ and $\dot{H}_W$ – and a number of groups have shown that the quality of tracking does not depend on what combination is chosen [4, 16].

If monkeys are allowed to turn their heads freely, they track a slowly moving object by turning the head smoothly and keeping the eyes roughly fixed with respect to the head [13]; the required $\dot{E}_W$ is provided mainly by $\dot{H}_W$. To accomplish this, both pursuit and the VOR remain active: the pursuit system responds to the target moving with respect to the world, while the vestibular system responds to the head movement component of the tracking maneuver. As would be anticipated from the addition of signals shown occurring at summing junction b in Fig. 1, the visual and vestibular inputs counterbalance each other, thereby preventing either input from causing the eyes to move with respect to the head. This "natural" tracking condition emphasizes the different functions of pursuit and the VOR. Pursuit produces nonzero values of $\dot{E}_W$ when objects of interest are moving with respect to the world. The VOR insures that any perturbations of head movement always induce a compensatory eye movement (with respect to the head); since the compensatory eye movement is equal in amplitude and opposite in direction to any head movement, $\dot{E}_W$ is unaffected by such perturbations, regardless of whether the objects the monkey is attempting to track are moving or stationary with respect to the world.

Output of the Flocculus During Smooth Eye Movement

To evaluate the role of the flocculus in the VOR and pursuit, several laboratories [14, 18, 19] have made unit recordings from monkeys trained to track a small, movable target spot either with the head stationary or during vestibular stimulation produced by sinusoidal oscillation of the entire animal. Such stimuli make it possible to evaluate the responses of Purkinje cells and mossy fibers during repeated, controlled sensory stimuli and motor output, yet can be related to the tracking conditions normally encountered in the real world. For example, oscillating the monkey while it tracks a target that moves exactly with the monkey produces vestibular inputs and eye-movement outputs comparable to those occurring during free-head tracking of a moving target. Since the responses of Purkine cells and mossy fibers in the flocculus have already been published in some detail (cf. [14, 15, 18]), only general results will be repeated here.

When a monkey is oscillated in complete darkness (Fig. 2A), Purkinje cells show little modulation of either simple spike (SS) or complex spike (CS) activity. However, when the monkey tracks a single, small light that moves exactly with its oscillating chair, the same Purkinje cells show deep modulation of SS activity, with increases in firing during ipsilateral head movement (Fig. 2B). This observation, which was true in all Purkinje cells that could be driven by vestibular stimulation at all, suggests that the flocculus is relatively unimportant for the VOR. Since the tracking conditions in which SS activity is modulated require that the pursuit system generate eye velocity with respect to the

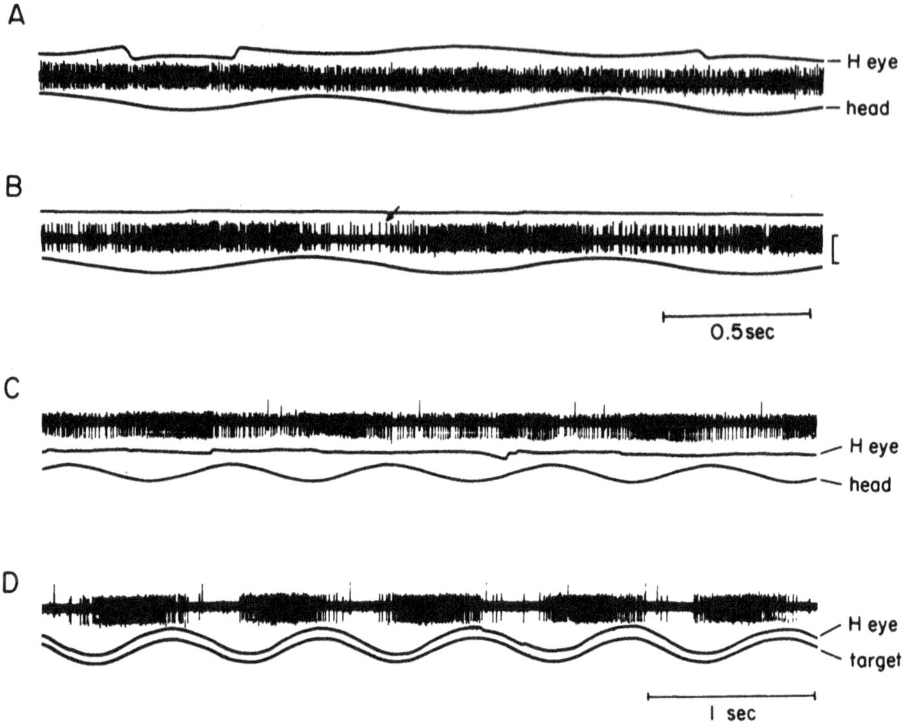

Fig. 2A–D. Activity of two Purkinje cells recorded in the flocculus during smooth eye movement. One cell was studied during sinusoidal head oscillation in darkness **A** and while the monkey fixated a target that moved exactly with the oscillating chair **B**. Although complex spikes were difficult to discriminate for this cell, one example is shown by the *diagonal arrow* in **B.** The second cell shown was studied in two conditions of pursuit: in **C** the monkey tracked a target that moved exactly with its oscillating chair, while in **D** its head was held stationary and the monkey tracked a sinusoidal target movement of ±70°/s. Traces shown are horizontal eye position (*H eye*), horizontal head position (*head*) and horizontal target position (*target*). Note that the *time calibrations* are different for the two cells; in all four panels, sinusoidal target and head movements were at 0.9 Hz. The amplitude of head oscillation was always ±10°. The amplitude calibration is 40° in **A** and **B,** and 25° in **C** and **D.** For all traces, *upward* deflections represent movement toward the side on which the recording was made (ipsilateral)

world, it seems likely that the flocculus is instead important for pursuit. Lesion experiments have supported this suggestion; bilateral flocculectomy has a minor and idiosyncratic effect on the VOR evoked by head oscillation in darkness, but severely disrupts pursuit with the head stationary or moving [24].

More detailed analysis of Purkinje-cell firing showed that SS activity is related to eye velocity with respect to the world whenever the animal pursues a target moving with respect to the world. For example, the Purkinje cell shown in the bottom two traces of Fig. 2 displayed SS modulation when the monkey tracked a target spot that oscillated exactly with it (Fig. 2C) and when the monkey tracked sinusoidal target motion with the head held stationary (Fig. 2D). In these and all other tracking conditions, most Purkinje cells show increased SS firing when eye velocity with respect to the world is towards the side on which the recording was made. This is consistent with electrophysiologic experiments on the cat and rabbit (Purkinje cells inhibit interneurons that cause contralateral eye movement, refs. [2, 10, 12]), and with the results of stimulating the flocculus of awake monkey (ipsilateral smooth eye movement, ref. [21]), and suggests that increases in SS output from the flocculus are important for the generation of ipsilateral pursuit eye velocity.

The Purkinje cell shown in Fig. 2C, D is somewhat atypical in that there was a profound modulation of CS as well as SS firing. Modulation of CS firing, when apparent, was always 180° out of phase with SS firing, i.e., CS activity increased in relation to contralateral pursuit eye velocity. Modulation of CS activity occurs only in relation to large values of eye velocity; it was often observed by Lisberger and Fuchs [14], who routinely used eye velocities of 60–70°/s, but was seldom seen by Miles et al. [18], who used eye velocities of 25°/s or less. In contrast, SS firing is modulated in relation to both high and low eye velocities.

Signal Processing in the Flocculus

The machinelike nature of the oculomotor system has made it possible to go beyond simply recording the output of the flocculus during eye movement. Some information has also been gained about the inputs entering the flocculus and how they are combined to form Purkinje-cell SS output. This has been done by (a) assessing the quantitative relationships between SS firing rate and head, eye, or target velocity, and (b) analyzing recordings made in the flocculus from elements believed to be mossy-fiber afferents. Both laboratories that have studied this problem [14, 18] agree that SS firing is due largely to the linear addition of two separate components related to head and eye velocity and transmitted to the flocculus over separate mossy-fiber pathways.

The head-velocity component of SS firing can be studied by requiring the monkey to generate eye velocity with respect to the world while keeping its eyes fixed in the head, i.e., by requiring the monkey to track a target that moves exactly with the oscillating chair. The resulting SS activity shows features already documented in the discharge of neurons known to be responding to vestibular stimulation (e.g., refs. [8, 9]): sinusoidal chair oscillation produces sinusoidal modulation of SS firing with peak firing rate occurring just prior to peak ipsilateral head velocity; increases in the peak-to-peak velocity of the vestibular stimulus produce increases in the peak- to-peak modulation of SS firing. The existence of quantitative relationships between SS firing and vestibular stimulation make it likely that the head-velocity component of SS firing represents inputs provided by the well-documented vestibular inputs to the flocculus; in agreement with this possibility, one of two major groups of mossy fibers encountered in the flocculus show discharge patterns like those found in cells of the vestibular nuclei of alert monkeys [9]. All such mossy fibers discharge in relation to vestibular stimulation, few discharge in relation to pursuit and, like the example appearing in Fig. 3A, all show modulation of firing rate during the VOR evoked by head oscillation in total darkness.

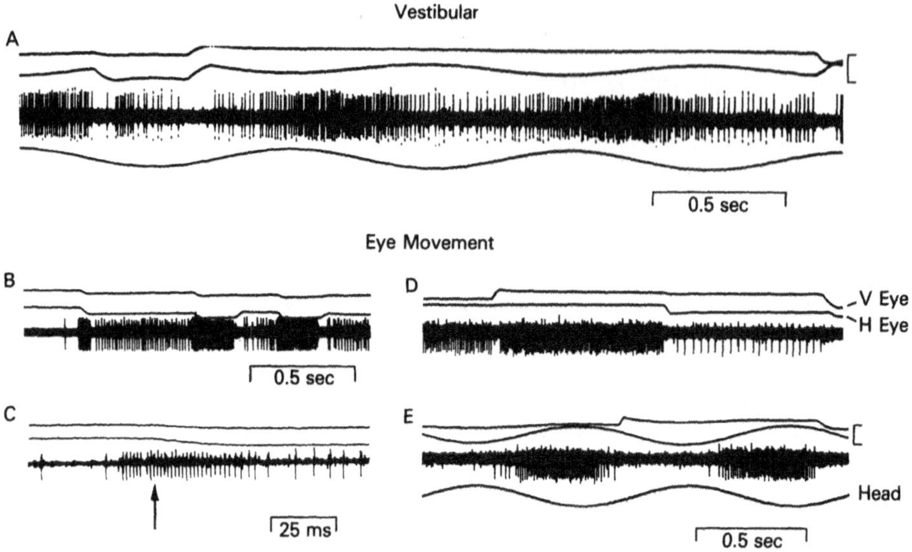

Fig. 3. Activity of mossy-fiber afferents transmitting information about vestibular stimulation **A** or eye movement **B–E** to the flocculus. **A** Vestibular fiber studied during head oscillation in darkness. Note that this fiber also shows a complete cessation of activity during saccadic eye movements. **B** "Burst-tonic" eye-movement fiber showing increased activity during contralateral positions of fixation, burst of activity during contralateral saccades, and a cessation of activity during ipsilateral saccades. **C** High-sweep-speed record of a single contralateral saccade from **B**, showing that the onset of the burst in activity precedes the onset of the saccade (indicated by the *arrow*). **D** Activity of a "tonic" mossy fiber that showed increased firing in relation to ipsilateral positions of steady fixation and a cessation of activity during all saccades. **E** Activity of the fiber in **D** during sinusoidal head oscillation in darkness. From *top* to *bottom* in each panel, the traces are vertical eye position (*V Eye*), horizontal eye position (*H Eye*), fiber activity, and (where applicable) horizontal head position (*Head*). The *time calibration* in **E** also applies to **D**. The amplitude calibration in **A** represents 40°. That in panel **E** represents 40° in **B, C,** and **D,** and 20° in **E.** *Upward* deflections represent upward or ipsilateral eye and head movement

The eye-velocity component of SS firing, which can be studied alone during pursuit with the head held stationary, appears to be related to ongoing smooth eye velocity. During tracking of sinusoidal target movement, Purkinje-cell SS firing shows sinusoidal modulation, with peak firing rate occurring in phase with peak ipsilateral eye velocity. Careful analysis of eye velocity, firing rate, and the velocity at which retinal images were slipping revealed a strong correlation between SS firing and eye velocity and no correlation between SS firing and visual inputs. Recordings from mossy-fiber afferents revealed few that discharged in relation to visual stimuli, but many that discharged in relation to eye movement (with respect to the head). Two eye-movement mossy fibers are documented in Fig. 3: during steady fixation, they show firing related to eye position (Fig. 3B, D); preceding saccadic eye movements, many emit a high-frequency burst of spikes (Fig. 3C); during head oscillation in darkness (Fig. 3E) and sinusoidal pursuit (not shown) they show a relationship to both eye position and eye velocity; during fixation of a target oscillating exactly with the monkey, they show no modulation of firing rate. Similar cells have been recorded in the feline nucleus prepositus hypoglossi [3], which is known to project to the flocculus [1].

Based on the large number of eye-movement mossy fibers and the strong correlation between Purkinje-cell SS firing and eye velocity, we believe that the eye-velocity component of SS firing is transmitted to the flocculus over the eye-movement mossy fibers. This raises the problem that the input fibers discharge with equal sensitivity to eye position and eye velocity, whereas Purkinje cells are much more sensitive to eye velocity and often show no firing in relation to eye position. Although our data do not suggest any specific mechanism for solving this problem, we presume that the inhibitory interneurons of the cerebellar cortex are connected in a way that removes all but the velocity component of the eye-movement inputs to the flocculus. Since the vestibular inputs do not require this kind of signal processing, and since the addition of eye- and head-velocity inputs to a given Purkinje cell is extraordinarily linear, it seems likely that the eye movement and vestibular inputs to the flocculus terminate on two separate groups of granule cells and converge only at the level of the Purkinje cell.

Functional Consequences of Purkinje-Cell Output

The addition of neural signals in the flocculus is summarized in the schematic diagram of Fig. 4. Here, some neural signals have been labeled using the prime (′) to distinguish them from the physical variables of which they are correlates. In keeping with the known electrophysiology, the output of the flocculus is shown inhibiting summing junction b, which is part of the direct VOR pathways. Purkinje-cell SS activity is formed at summing junction f by adding two signals: one is transmitted directly from the vestibular system and provides a neural correlate of head velocity with respect to the world ($\dot{H}'_W$); the other is transmitted from the oculomotor system and, by the time it affects Purkinje-cell firing, has been transformed into a neural correlate of eye velocity with respect to the head ($\dot{E}'_H$). The resulting output of the flocculus is a neural correlate of eye velocity with respect to the world ($\dot{E}'_W = \dot{E}'_H + \dot{H}'_W$).

The absence of modulation of SS firing during head oscillation in the dark can now be accounted for by a counterbalancing of the two major inputs to the flocculus when $\dot{E}_W$ is zero (i.e., $\dot{E}_H$ is equal and opposite to $\dot{H}_W$). In effect, an afferent signal related to the head-velocity input for the VOR and a corollary of the eye-velocity output of the entire smooth oculomotor system are continuously compared in the flocculus. When eye velocity is exactly that of the VOR (i.e., when the VOR alone is sufficient to track the object of interest) Purkinje-cell SS activity shows no modulation – the flocculus does not affect the brainstem VOR pathways if they are already producing the required eye movement. If the comparison of afferent inputs with corollaries of motor output is a general property of signal processing in the cerebellum, failure in the alert animal to drive Purkinje-cell SS activity with a given afferent input cannot necessarily be taken as evidence that the particular input is not important. Rather, it may be

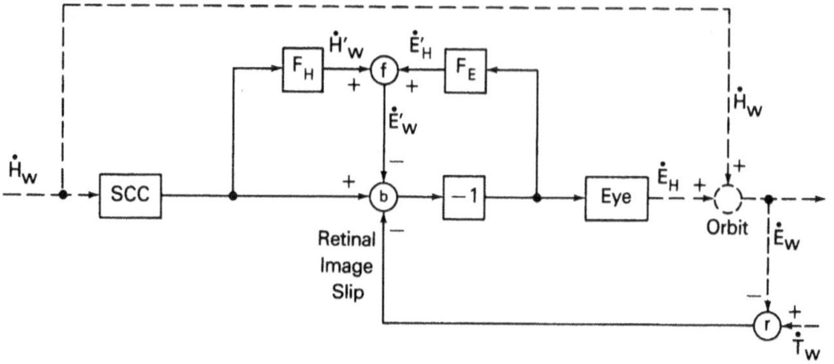

Fig. 4. Schematic representation of the smooth oculomotor control system, incorporating the head and eye velocity pathways through the flocculus. Extra-floccular pathways and the *abbreviations* labeling them are just as in Fig. 1, except that the retina is indicated here as summing junction *r*. In this and the subsequent diagram, neural signals are distinguished from physical variables by the use of the prime (′) and *solid signal flow lines.* The flocculus (summing junction *f*) is shown receiving a vestibular signal proportional to head velocity ($\dot{H}'_W$) and an eye-movement signal proportional to eye velocity with respect to the head ($\dot{E}'_H$). Recording experiments indicate that the sensitivity of Purkinje cells to head and eye velocity is equal (i.e., $F_H = F_E$) and that these two inputs add to form the output of the flocculus, which is a neural signal proportional to eye velocity with respect to the world ($\dot{E}'_W$). In keeping with its known connections to the brainstem, the flocculus is shown inhibiting summing junction *b.* Note the parallels between the addition of neural signals in the flocculus and the addition of physical variables in the orbit

that the afferent input is causing the correct motor output via other pathways and would affect Purkinje-cell activity in a different behavioral condition.

The modulation of SS firing whenever the monkey generates nonzero eye velocity with respect to the world has been taken as evidence that the flocculus is involved specifically in pursuit. This involvement is emphasized by the striking analogy between the addition of signals producing the output of the flocculus and the addition of $\dot{E}_H$ and $\dot{H}_W$ in the orbit to produce the final output of the smooth oculomotor control system, eye velocity with respect to the world. Regardless of what combination of smooth eye and head movement is used to accomplish pursuit, the output of the flocculus is always related to eye velocity with respect to the world. Since $\dot{E}_W$ is in fact the eye velocity of pursuit, the output from the flocculus can be viewed as a neural correlate of pursuit eye velocity, regardless of how pursuit is ultimately accomplished.

Role of Positive Feedback Through the Flocculus in Sustaining Pursuit

One important aspect of the diagram in Fig. 4 is that the eye-velocity pathway through the flocculus is shown as part of a positive-feedback loop. Such an arrangement is based on observations indicating that the discharge of the flocculus is both an output from and an input to the pursuit system. That *inputs* to the flocculus originate from the *output* of the pursuit system is suggested by the fact that eye-movement mossy fibers signal the final output of the oculomotor system during all eye movements, including pursuit; it seems unlikely that proprioceptive inputs play a role here, since many such mossy fibers show bursts prior to saccadic eye movements. That the *outputs* from the flocculus provide an important *input* to the pursuit system is shown by the severe disruptive effects of bilateral flocculectomy on pursuit with the head held stationary. It should be point out the existence of eye-velocity positive feedback in the pursuit system is not a new idea; it has been suggested a number of times based on both theoretical [20, 23] and experimental [11, 22] considerations.

The functional implications of eye-velocity positive feedback can be most easily appreciated by considering pursuit with the head held stationary. This makes it possible to work with the simpler schematic diagram shown in Fig. 5, where all vestibular pathways have been deleted. In this representation, $\dot{E}'_p(t)$ represents the neural command for pursuit eye velocity, and the visual inputs for pursuit are a neural correlate of the rate at which the target is moving with respect to the retina ($\dot{T}'_E$), produced by comparing target and eye velocity at summing junction r. The role of the positive-feedback pathway representing the flocculus can be seen by considering the equation:

$$\dot{E}'_p(t) = F \cdot \dot{E}'_p(t - \Delta t) + \dot{T}'_E \qquad \text{(Eq. 2)}$$

which describes the pursuit command in Fig. 5. If F is close to 1 (lesion studies [24] indicate it is 0.8 or 0.9), this equation would become $\dot{E}'_p(t) = \dot{E}'_p(t - \Delta t) + \dot{T}'_E$. Even in the absence of visual inputs ($\dot{T}'_E = 0$), the pursuit eye velocity command at any given time [$\dot{E}'_p(t)$] would be equal to that of an instant before [$\dot{E}'_p(t - \Delta t)$]; thus, the positive feedback representing the flocculus insures that ongoing pursuit is sustained.

If the function of the head- and eye-velocity components of Purkinje-cell SS firing is to sustain pursuit eye velocity, visual inputs would be expected to change

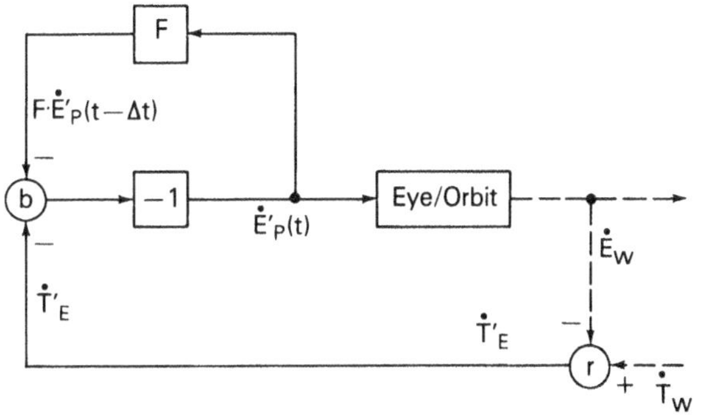

Fig. 5. Schematic representation of the pursuit system showing the use of positive feedback to sustain ongoing pursuit eye velocity. The neural command for pursuit [$\dot{E}'_p(t)$] is formed at summing junction *b* by adding two signals: one represents positive feedback of the pursuit command from the previous instant [$F \cdot \dot{E}'_p(t - \Delta t)$]; the other is a visual signal originating at the retina (*r*) and proportional to the rate at which the target is moving with respect to the (moving) eye ($\dot{T}'_E = \dot{T}_W - \dot{E}_W$). *F* represents the gain of the eye-velocity positive-feedback pathway and, based on lesion experiments [24], is assumed to be just less than 1. As before, $\dot{T}_W$ and $\dot{E}_W$ represent target and eye velocity with respect to the world

eye velocity. Specifically, nonzero values of $\dot{T}'_E$ would be expected to add or subtract from the old pursuit command [$\dot{E}'_p(T-\Delta t)$] to produce a new pursuit command [$\dot{E}'_p(t)$] that is changed by an amount related to the magnitude and direction of retinal image slip. The changed pursuit command should cause changes in pursuit eye velocity, e.g., eye acceleration. Recent experiments in primates have provided some support for this idea [16]; detailed analysis of the smooth eye movements used to track a wide range of frequencies and amplitudes of sinusoidal and nonperiodic target movements revealed that eye *acceleration* was uniquely related to the velocity of retinal image motion. In contrast, eye velocity was essentially unrelated to the velocity of retinal image motion. This lead to the suggestion that visual inputs provide an eye acceleration command to a positive-feedback network (the flocculus) that is already sustaining the previously programmed pursuit eye velocity.

Thus, the pursuit system, in which external inputs (retinal image motion) lead to *changes* in motor output (eye acceleration), behaves in the way expected of a simple physical system, in which the application of forces leads to acceleration of a mass ($F = ma$). One property of such systems is inertia – a body at rest tends to remain at rest, a body in motion tends to remain in motion. The smooth oculomotor control system also exhibits this property – eye velocity with respect to the world tends to be sustained, whether zero or nonzero. Whereas in physical systems inertia is a property of mass, in the smooth oculomotor system it is provided by the underlying neural pathways. One such pathway is the VOR, which insures that eye velocity with respect to the world is sustained despite expected or unexpected head movements. The other such pathway includes the inputs and outputs of the flocculus, which insure that nonzero values of $\dot{E}_W$ are sustained.

It is possible in this context to view the flocculus as a mechanism that compensates for the shortcomings of the eyeball and restores the physical properties of inertia to the smooth oculomotor system. This raises the possibility that other parts of the cerebellum might serve a similar function for other parts of the body. The obvious advantage of such an arrangement is that it then becomes possible for afferent inputs to access the final motor pathways without regard for the physical limitations of the effector organ – inputs can be regarded as error signals indicating the need to change motor output.

References

1. Alley K, Baker R, Simpson JI (1975) Afferents to the vestibulo-cerebellum and the origin of the visual climbing fibers in the rabbit. Brain Res 98:582–589
2. Baker R, Precht W, Llinás R (1972) Cerebellar modulatory action on the vestibulo-trochlear pathway in the cat. Exp Brain Res 15:364–385
3. Baker R, Gresty M, Berthoz A (1975) Neuronal activity in the prepositus hypoglossi nucleus correlated with vertical and horizontal eye movement in the cat. Brain Res 101:366–371
4. Benson AJ, Barnes GR (1978) Vision during angular acceleration: the dynamic interaction of visual and vestibular mechanisms. Aviat Space Environ Med 49:340–345
5. Brodal A, Hoivik B (1964) Site and mode of termination of primary vestibulo-cerebellar fibres in the cat: an experimental study with silver impregnation methods. Arch Ital Biol 102:1–21

6. Dichgans J, Bizzi E, Morasso P, Tagliasco V (1973) Mechanisms underlying recovery of eye-head coordination following bilateral labyrinthectomy in monkeys. Exp Brain Res 18:555–562
7. Dow RS (1938) Efferent connections of the flocculo-nodular lobe in Macaca Mulatta. J Comp Neurol 68:297–305
8. Fernandez, C, Goldberg JM (1971) Physiology of peripheral neurons innervating semicircular canals of the squirrel monkey. II. Response to sinusoidal stimulation and dynamics of peripheral vestibular system. J Neurophysiol 34:661–675
9. Fuchs AF, Kimm J (1975) Unit activity in vestibular nucleus of the alert monkey during horizontal angular acceleration and eye movement. J Neurophysiol 38:1140–1161
10. Fukuda J, Highstein SM, Ito M (1972) Cerebellar inhibitory control of the vestibulo-ocular reflex investigated in rabbit IIIrd nucleus. Exp Brain Res 14:511–526
11. Heywood S, Churcher J (1971) Eye movements and the afterimage I. Tracking the afterimage. Vision Res 11:1163–1168
12. Highstein SM (1973) Synaptic linkage in the vestibulo-ocular and cerebello-vestibular pathways to the VIth nucleus in the rabbit. Exp Brain Res 17:301–314
13. Lanman J, Bizzi E, Allum J (1978) The coordination of eye and head movement during smooth pursuit. Brain Res 153:39–53
14. Lisberger SG, Fuchs AF (1978) Role of primate flocculus during rapid behavioral modification of vestibuloocular reflex I. Purkinje cell activity during visually guided horizontal smooth pursuit eye movements and passive head rotation. J Neurophysiol 41:733–763
15. Lisberger SG, Fuchs AF (1978) Role of primate flocculus during rapid behavioral modification of vestibuloocular reflex II. Mossy fiber firing patterns during horizontal head rotation and eye movement. J Neurophysiol 41:764–777
16. Lisberger SG, Evinger C, Johanson GW, Fuchs AF (to be published) Relationship between eye acceleration and retinal image velocity during foveal smooth pursuit in man and monkey
17. Miles FA, Eighmy BB (1980) Long-term adaptive changes in primate vestibuloocular reflex. I. Behavioral observations. J Neurophysiol 43:1406–1425
18. Miles FA, Fuller JH, Braitman DJ, Dow BM (1980) Long-term adaptive changes in primate vestibuloocular reflex. III. Electrophysiological observations in flocculus of normal monkeys. J Neurophysiol 43:1437–1476
19. Noda H, Suzuki DA (1979) The role of the flocculus of the monkey in fixation and smooth pursuit eye movements. J Physiol 294:335–348
20. Robinson DA (1971) Models of oculomotor neural organization. In: Bach-y-Rita, Collins (eds) The control of eye movements. Academic Press, New York, p 519
21. Ron S, Robinson DA (1973) Eye movements evoked by cerebellar stimulation in the alert monkey. J Neurophysiol 36:1004–1022
22. Yasui S, Young LR (1975) Perceived visual motion as effective stimulus to pursuit eye movement system. Science 190:906–908
23. Young LR, Forster JD, van Houtte N (1968) A revised stochastic sampled data model for eye tracking movements. Ann. NASA – University Conf. on Manual Control, 4th, University of Michigan, Ann Arbor
24. Zee DS, Yamazuki A, Gucer G (1978) Ocular motor abnormalities in trained monkeys with floccular lesions. Soc Neurosci 4:168

Discussion

Llinás: Regarding the absence of vestibular modulation of floccular Purkinje cells in nonsuppressing animals, there are many ways in which this lack of responsiveness can occur. One of them is that the vestibular input is simply not reaching the cerebellum. Another is that something is happening in the granular layer or at basket and stellate cells. Do you have any ideas regarding the mechanism for this lack of response?
Lisberger: No, but my initial reaction is that it is actually occurring at the Purkinje cell because the addition is so remarkedly linear. The other mechanisms (e.g., the basket cells, the feedback mechanisms) are probably involved in processes like removing the position component of the eye-movement input and sorting out the eye velocity component of it.
Llinás: In that regard, it is significant that direct stimulation of Purkinje cells in the range below calcium spike threshold yields a rather linear relation between current and frequency.
Lisberger: That fits with the suggestion that it is occurring at the Purkinje cell.
Voogd: You were talking about the function of the flocculus. Would you tell me exactly what part of the flocculus?
Lisberger: That's a very good question, for the monkey flocculus is very large. It contains 11 folia and we have been dealing primarily with folia 6 through 11.
Voogd: What parts of these folia? Because there are at least three partitioning zones in this part of the flocculus.
Lisberger: Unfortunately we really cannot say. The cells we encounter are in patches to a certain extent, but when your are inserting a microelectrode into the flocculus of an alert monkey, traversing some 25–30 mm of tissue before even arriving there, you have very little idea exactly where in the flocculus you were when you do the histology 2 months later.
Voogd: What is the significance then of the Purkinje cells which are not modulated? Is it possible that they are outside the region?
Lisberger: Very possible. The significance of no modulation when the animal is oscillated in the dark becomes important only when you show that the same cell, in fact, responds in other conditions. Roughly 50% of the cells in the flocculus fall into this category.
Voogd: That means that your conclusions concern about one-third of the flocculus and in that region you do not know which part you hit.
Lisberger: That's correct. We can add that many of the cells that are not modulated by horizontal eye movement and vestibular stimulation are in fact related to the vertical, and we also know that there are other Purkinje cells in other parts of the flocculus that are related to eye movement in a somewhat different way.
Ito: As far as I understand it, in smooth pursuit an animal makes an effort to match the eye velocity with the target velocity. To get information about the target velocity, an animal has to process three kinds of information – visual, vestibular, and oculomotor. I could not see any visual information story in your talk. Therefore, I wonder how an animal achieves smooth pursuit without that.
Lisberger: In fact, very few of the Purkinje cells in the monkey flocculus studied

by Miles, Fuchs, and myself show any visual responsiveness. It seems that the visual input to the pursuit system occurs at the brainstem level and that by the time the eye-movement signals have reached the flocculus they are in fact related to eye movement. The relationship between the eye movements and the visual inputs has, by then, been obscured. The flocculus is providing two of the three components required for tracking: the head velocity in the world and the eye velocity in the head. The target velocity across the eye has to access the pathway somewhere else.

Ito: In a recent paper, Noda (Kase et al., 1979) emphasized that in your experimental paradigm, oculomotor and visual information are not completely dissociated. What is your comment on this point?

Lisberger: First of all, the data I have shown today was obtained from animals tracking a foveal target spot in otherwise dark surroundings. Thus, there was no influence from the surround. It is correct that Noda has shown that some Purkinje cells do respond, in addition, to the surround. It seems, however, that those are different Purkinje cells, located in the posterior part of the flocculus and they must subserve quite a different function. Unfortunately, he has not tested his cells during vestibular stimulation so that makes it more difficult to compare our samples.

Thach: Do you suggest an extrapolation of your proposal on floccular function to other parts of the cerebellum? I wonder if you could speculate a bit in terms easy to understand how that might work, say with regard to two or more joints in the limb. Now the joints in the limb have similarities with the relation of the eye to the head, in that movement of one will cause movement of the other. They have to be internally compensated to produce a particular trajectory. The signals from two joints must be combined so as to give a desired trajectory, say of a finger along a straight line. In addition, the positive feedback to the system could help program the trajectory.

Lisberger: I think you've said it very well.

Marshall: Other signals that change with head movement are those from muscle afferents and neck sensory afferents. Can these contribute to Purkinje-cell activity?

Lisberger: There certainly is a projection to the flocculus from neck afferents. In our experiments the whole body was oscillated with the head fixed to the chair and the neck afferents were not stimulated.

Collewijn: Do I understand correctly that you have a positive-feedback loop in your diagram in the smooth pursuit system?

Lisberger: Yes.

Collewijn: What kind of effect would you predict then on the dynamic properties of smooth pursuit? I am wondering whether this would introduce all kinds of aftereffects, difficulties in changing direction and so on. What are the dynamic properties of this loop?

Lisberger: It has a relatively short time constant in the order of several hundred milliseconds, so that it would be really a very short-term sustaining effect.

Chan-Palay: Is there something you could do in future experiments to try and localize anatomically where you have been and also to determine where you're going to go?

Lisberger: I think it is very difficult in the alert primate and that it is more readily done in the acute animal. It would be best I think to try and deal with this problem by first determining the location of the cells that project to these Purkinje cells so that one can identify the Purkinje cells in an acute preparation by their anatomic inputs, say stimulating the various sites in the brain. But in the monkey, where you have to go so far to reach the flocculus, mapping experiments are very difficult. I personally do not particularly trust microstimulation in a structure that's known to receive afferents that are related to movements. The possibility of axon reflex effects makes interpretation difficult.

Eye Movements and the Cerebellum

M. Ito

Eye Movements for Studies of Cerebellar Functions

An eye embedded in the orbit occupies a unique position in the motor system, often expressed as a limb afforded with a single joint. This simplicity allows accurate, quantitative assessments of movement dynamics. Eye movements therefore provide a sensitive preparation for evaluating even the most subtle aspects of cerebellar control of motor activity. Recent advances in studies of eye movements have facilitated investigation of neuronal mechanisms of the cerebellum related to eye-movement control.

However, detailed studies of cerebellar control of eye movements are complicated both by the multiplicity of planes and axes for eye rotation and by the apparent diversity of neuronal control mechanisms. Contraction and relaxation of six extraocular muscles permit horizontal, vertical, and rotatory eye movements. These movements can be either *reflexive* or *voluntary*. Two well-known examples of reflexive eye movements are the vestibulo-ocular reflex (VOR) and the optokinetic response (OKR). The VOR is driven by labyrinthine signals and compensates for head movements, while the OKR is a reflexive movement which follows movements of the entire visual surround. Since movement of the full-field visual surround occurs during head movement under natural conditions, it is likely that both the VOR and the OKR provide visual stability during head movement. The interrelationship of the VOR and OKR is further indicated by the fact that perceived motion during the OKR is indistinguishable from that induced by head rotation [11]. Other examples of reflexive eye movements are the cervico-ocular reflex [79], trunk-ocular reflex [80], and a possible stretch reflex in extraocular muscles [60, 62].

Voluntary eye movements may be classified as either saccades or smooth-pursuit movements. A saccade is a jerky, quick eye movement which positions a visual target on a region of the retina specialized for high acuity. By contrast, smooth-pursuit eye movements continuously follow a moving target with a high-acuity retinal region. Unlike the OKR, a small dot is an effective target for smooth-pursuit movements.

In dealing with eye movements, it is also important to recognize species differences in predominant eye-movement types. Rabbits display reasonably good VOR and OKR, but hardly any saccade or smooth-pursuit movements. Hence, rabbits are suitable for studying reflexive eye movements, but not for voluntary ones. On the other hand, well-developed saccades in cats, and both saccades and smooth-pursuit movements in monkeys and human subjects tend to mask

Experimental Brain Research, Suppl. 6

pure reflexive effects of the OKR. It is also important to be aware of the possibility that different types of eye movements utilize the same neuronal mechanisms. For example, there have been arguments as to the identity of the saccade with the quick set-back movement of an eye which takes place during excessive VOR or OKR, forming quick phases of the vestibular or optokinetic nystagmus [15]. The fact that an animal such as a rabbit exhibits quick phases of the VOR or OKR but not saccades is taken as evidence that they are different types of movements. Nevertheless, these seemingly analogous eye movements may share common neural control mechanisms.

With precautions for these complexities, eye movements provide excellent material for studying motor control mechanisms in the cerebellum. Two major classic methods for investigating brain functions, electric stimulation and lesion experiments, have been applied by numerous workers in order to reveal functional involvement of the cerebellum in eye movements [17, 18]. These analyses have recently been supplemented by dissection of neuronal connections with morphological and electrophysiologic techniques and also by recording from cerebellar Purkinje cells in alert, behaving animals, which provide new insight into cerebellar contributions to the control of eye movements. This article reviews recent data correlating eye movements to cerebellar functions, and then introduces new data from the author's laboratory concerning possible neuronal mechanisms in the cerebellar flocculus involved with the VOR of rabbits.

Vestibulo-Ocular Reflex

The flocculus projects Purkinje-cell axons to vestibular nuclei [4, 16]. Electrophysiologic studies in rabbits [23, 37] and cats [7] further demonstrated that flocculus Purkinje cells supply inhibitory synapses specifically to relay cells of the VOR. From a viewpoint of control theory, the VOR is a feedforward control system (a class of open-loop control systems) equipped with no direct feedback loop. Such a system cannot perform any precision work without extrinsic signals substituting a feedback. This attaches a cybernetic meaning to involvement of the flocculus in the VOR [32, 33, 34].

Dissection of neuronal circuitry is best advanced in the flocculus-VOR system as compared with other eye-movement systems (Fig. 1). One interesting feature is that the flocculus has a mosaic structure composed of at least five microzones having different input and output connections. Purkinje cells in zone II of the rabbit flocculus project to the rostral portion of the ipsilateral medial vestibular nucleus [85] and establish inhibitory connections with relay cells of two components of the VOR, arising from the ipsilateral horizontal canal and ending at the ipsilateral medial and lateral rectus muscles [42]. Zone II thus is involved specifically in control of the horizontal VOR to the ipsilateral eye. Zones I and III, on the other hand, project to the superior vestibular nucleus [85] and inhibit relay cells for the vertical and rotatory components of the VOR [42]. Functional implications of the projections from zone IV to the caudal part of the lateral cerebellar nucleus and from zone V to the perihypoglossal nucleus [83] are not clear at present.

The flocculus receives vestibular afferents bilaterally as a mossy-fiber input. These afferents involve collaterals of primary vestibular axons passing into the medulla and polysynaptic projections relayed by vestibular nuclei [13, 69, 76]. Activity of Purkinje cells in rabbits is modulated very effectively either by horizontal head rotation [21, 25] or by electric stimulation of vestibular nerves [45]. Therefore, it has been suggested that the flocculus contributes to dynamic characteristics of the VOR as a sidepath to the VOR arc [33].

Ablation of the cat vestibulocerebellum including the flocculus causes an abnormally high VOR gain [74]. However, ablation of the rabbit flocculus results

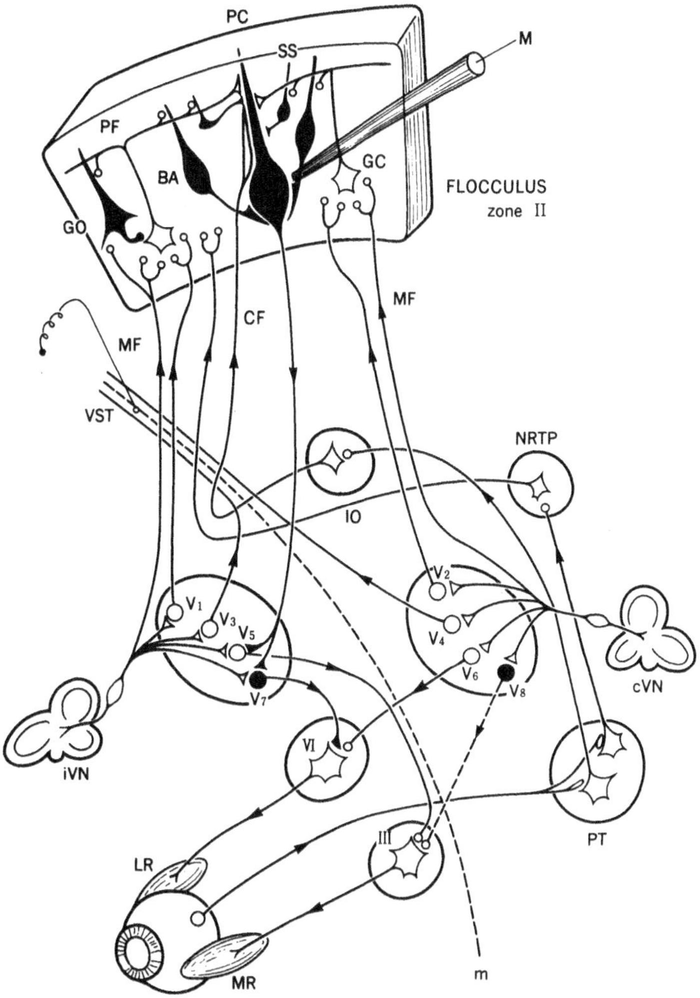

Fig. 1. Structure of the rabbit flocculus-VOR system for horizontal eye movements. *III, VI,* 3rd and 6th cranial nuclei; *MR, LR,* medial and lateral rectus muscles; *PT,* pretectal area; *IO,* inferior olive; *MF,* mossy fiber; *CF,* climbing fiber; *PC,* Purkinje cell; *PF,* parallel fiber; *GO,* Golgi cell; *BA,* basket cell; *GC,* granule cell; *SS,* superficial stellate cell; *iVN, cVN,* ipsi- and contralateral vestibular nerve; $V_1 - V_8$, vestibular nuclei cells; *VST,* vestibulospinal tract; *m,* midline. Inhibitory neurons are filled in black

in a moderate reduction of the VOR gain specifically in the ipsilateral eye and preferentially for a relatively small head rotation [39]. Ablation of the nodulus and uvula or lobules VI and VII does not cause such an effect. Direction and amount of contribution of the flocculus to the VOR gain under usual circumstances may vary among different animal species. Cerebellectomy also causes an advancement in the phase shift of the VOR [14, 73]. In rabbits, this was demonstrated to arise specifically after ablation of the nodulus and uvula, but not from flocculectomy which causes only a slight delay in the VOR phase [39].

Existence of climbing-fiber afferents conveying visual signals [3, 52, 54] is also an interesting aspect of the flocculus. At least three different visual climing-fiber pathways to the flocculus have been identified. One pathway arising from the ipsilateral eye passes to the contralateral pretectum and then runs down to the caudal part of the dorsal cap of the contralateral inferior olive [55]. This climbing-fiber pathway projects preferentially to zone II of the flocculus and activates Purkinje cells controlling the horizontal VOR of the ipsilateral eye [41, 42]. A second visual climbing-fiber pathway arising from the contralateral eye passes to the ipsilateral pretectal area [54]. Thereafter, it crosses back to the contralateral side through the posterior commissure and is relayed by cell groups located ventrolateral to the red nucleus and descends to the rostral portion of the dorsal cap [55]. This second pathway projects to zones I and III of the flocculus and activates Purkinje cells controlling the rotatory VOR of the contralateral eye [41, 42]. The third pathway takes a course similar to the second, although the linkage from the retina to the pretectum has not yet been demonstrated [42]. It reaches zones I and III, and activates Purkinje cells involved in the vertical VOR of the ipsilateral eye [41, 42].

Dorsal-cap neurons in rabbits are excited by large, contrast-rich stimuli moving forward in front of the contralateral eye at a velocity of 1–2°/s, and are depressed by stimuli moving in the opposite direction [9]. Similar responses are observed in *complex*-spike activity of flocculus Purkinje cells during optokinetic stimulation [25].

These basic neuronal arrangements found in the flocculus have lead to a suggestion that the flocculus adaptively modifies dynamic characteristics of the VOR according to climbing-fiber information about visual stability during reflex movements [32, 33, 34]. Occurrence of an adaptive depression and even reversal in polarity of the VOR was demonstrated in human subjects wearing dove prism goggles [27, 28]. Similar adaptation in the cat VOR can be removed by ablation of the vestibulocerebellum including the flocculus [74]. The rabbit VOR also undergoes an adaptive modification during sustained imposition of compined head rotation and optokinetic stimulation [47]; the VOR-gain either increases or decreases depending on the stimulus conditions. These adaptive changes in eye movements are abolished after ablation of the ipsilateral flocculus. The complication that surgical ablation of the flocculus causes retrograde degeneration in the interferior olive can be avoided by using local application of kainic acid, which spares axons while destroying Purkinje cells [31]. This chemical flocculectomy also abolishes the adaptive gain change in the VOR [39].

Interruption of the visual climbing-fiber pathway to the flocculus also abolishes the adaptability of the VOR [29, 40]. Such lesion experiments must be interpreted with caution, because destruction of the dorsal-cap neurons not only deprives the flocculus of climbing-fiber afferents but also reduces or even nullifies the inhibitory action of Purkinje cells upon relay cells of the VOR. After destruction of the dorsal cap, stimulation of flocculus Purkinje cells no longer inhibits relay cells of the VOR [19]. Similarly, the inhibitory action of Purkinje cells on Deiters neurons in rats was reduced without recovery after destruction of the inferior olive by poisoning with 3-Acetyl-pyridine [44]. In rabbit Deiters neurons, it was further shown that the depression in Purkinje-cell inhibition progresses rapidly; the effect is substantiated within 5 h [43]. This complication can be avoided by placing lesions rostral to the dorsal cap to interrupt preolivary fibers mediating visual signals. Such preolivary lesions still abolish the adaptability of the VOR [40].

There now seems to be a firm basis for the initial hypothesis [32, 33 34] that the flocculus adaptively modifies dynamic characteristics of the VOR to improve visual stability under circumstances of vestibular-visual interaction. Further support from studies of Purkinje-cell responses in the flocculus will be dealt with separately in the last section.

Optokinetic Response

The OKR is essentially a closed-loop control system, with a direct negative feedback from an eye-movement output to a visual input. Therefore, if the OKR system is equipped with a sufficiently high internal gain (open-loop gain) cerebellar assistance is unnecessary. This may account for a relatively minor contribution of the cerebellum to the cat OKR, which performs effectively even after total cerebellectomy [49]. However, if the OKR system has a relatively low internal gain, there may be a need for the cerebellum to intervene to improve its performance. Since the OKR is velocity-dependent, with a smaller gain for higher velocities of optokinetic stimuli [6, 10], contribution of the cerebellum to the OKR may be particularly important in the range of relatively fast optokinetic stimuli. In albino rabbits, this situation occurs in the range around 1 °/s, where after flocculectomy the OKR is nearly abolished. Even in a slower range (0.2–0.4 °/s), where the OKR gain is relatively unaffected, flocculectomy causes an unusually wide deviation of the OKR phase shift removing stimuli [39].

The existence of a major brain-stem pathway for the OKR is suggested by the fact that cerebellectomy does not abolish the OKR [39, 49]. In cats, it has been postulated that the brain-stem OKR pathway involves vestibular nuclei neurons in common with the major VOR pathway and that relay cells for this brain-stem OKR pathway are located in the nucleus reticularis tegmentis pontis (NRTP [70]). In rabbits, a connection from the NRTP to vestibular nuclei has not yet been shown. Instead, the supraparafascicular region of the midbrain has been proposed as a relay site for the rabbit OKR pathway [8].

A mossy-fiber pathway conveying visual signals to the flocculus [53, 54] appears to contribute to control of the OKR. The relay site for this visual mossy-fiber pathway is located in the medial terminal nucleus in chinchillas [82], and in the NRTP in rabbits [56, 58]. Unilateral lesions in the rabbit NRTP cause a depression in the OKR to the contralateral eye in a degree similar to flocculectomy. Lesions of the NRTP do not impair the adaptability of the VOR [63]. On the other hand, although interruption of the visual climbing-fiber pathway abolishes the adaptability of the VOR, it has no effect upon the OKR [40].

These observations suggest that the visual mossy-fiber afferents from the flocculus in rabbits form a sidepath to the brain-stem OKR pathway, just as the vestibular mossy-fiber afferents to the flocculus form a sidepath to the VOR arc. These arrangements match the current hypothesis that mossy-fiber inputs produce cerebellar outputs which subserve control of ongoing bodily movements, while climbing-fiber inputs play a key role in adaptive or learning processes in the cerebellar cortex.

Purkinje cells in the rabbit flocculus exhibit modulation of activity during optokinetic stimulation [36]. This modulation occurs such that Purkinje-cell activity normally facilitates the OKR, in agreement with the fact that either flocculectomy or interruption of the visual mossy-fiber pathway to the flocculus reduces the OKR gain [39, 63]. Since Purkinje-cell discharges in the monkey flocculus during smooth-pursuit eye movements are correlated predominantly with eye velocity, significance of visual input to the flocculus has been questioned [50]. In the rabbit flocculus, however, Purkinje cells are frequently modulated during the OKR, but rather rarely during the reversed postoptokinetic eye movements (13 of 76 cells tested, ref. [64]). This indicates that eye velocity is not a dominant input to the rabbit flocculus.

Optokinetic stimulation instantaneously modifies eye movements induced by head rotation. In rabbits, this rapid visual-vestibular interaction is due to a linear summation of the VOR and OKR [6, 10]. Impairment of rapid visual-vestibular interaction of rabbits after flocculectomy may thus be due to reduction of the OKR gain [39]. The rapid action of the flocculus to improve eye movements by referring to visual information, as proposed earlier [46], is now understood to be effected through a contribution of the flocculus to the OKR [39].

Visual suppression of the VOR in monkeys [77, 78] may involve more than a simple interaction of the VOR and OKR, as monkeys have a well-developed, smooth-pursuit eye-movement mechanism. The loss of visual suppression of the VOR in flocculectomized monkeys [78] should be considered from this point of view (see below).

Saccade

Quick saccadic eye movements do not allow the oculomotor system to utilize visual feedback for accurately locating a visual target in the central retinal region. In this sense, a saccade must be guided by a mechanism predicting its goal on the basis of information available before initiation of an eye movement. This predictive control for a saccade is of the same nature as feedforward control of the VOR in the sense that both have to operate without feedback. Here again, a cybernetic reason is found for involvement of the cerebellum in saccades.

Saccade-like, rapid eye movements can be evoked by electric stimulation in restricted areas of the monkey cerebellum: lobules V–VII of the vermis, and crus I and II and the lobulus simplex of the hemisphere [75]. Direction of eye movements is highly dependent on the site of stimulation. When represented on the dorsal aspect of lobules V–VII, it diverges radially from the intercept of the primary fissure and the mid sagittal line [75]. Damage to vermal cortices of lobules VI and VII results in dysmetric saccadic eye movements [5, 72]. Similarly, dysymetric saccades induced by partial tenotomy of extraocular muscles no longer recover after ablation of lobules VI and VII [68].

In cat lobules VI and VII, Purkinje cells fire 11–24 ms before the beginning of saccades [51], with peak activity falling at the time of onset of eye movements. Intensity of neuronal activity is inversely proportional to the amplitude of eye movement, suggesting that Purkinje cells in these areas are involved in initiation of saccades.

Purkinje cells in lobules VI andVII project to fastigial and interpositus nuclei. Since electric stimulation in monkeys produces saccade-like eye movements from all of the cerebellar nuclei including the dentate nucleus [75], it has not been possible to identify neuronal pathways underlying cerebellar control of saccades. Purkinje cells in lobule VII were found to establish inhibitory connections with those fastigial neurons which receive horizontal canal signals [24]. Functional implications of this connection, though, are not clear at present.

Electric stimulation of the monkey flocculus does not evoke saccades [75]. However, the majority of Purkinje cells in the monkey flocculus respond to saccadic eye movements by pausing spontaneous firing or by firing a burst [65]. The pause precedes the eye movement by an average of 9.6 ms and the burst by 3.8 ms.

As mentioned above, lesion experiments indicate that the cerebellum is not directly responsible for initiation and execution of saccades, but it contributes to the precision with which a saccade locates a visual target with a high-acuity retinal region. Such contribution may be effected by adding cerebellar signals to central command signals executing a saccade, so that an algebraic sum of the two types of signals determines the amount of eye movement in a saccade. By analogy with the model of the VOR-flocculus system, one may suppose that a cerebellar area forms a modifiable sidepath to the major brain-stem pathway for saccades. The modifiability is assumed to be under control of visual calibration to secure the accuracy of saccades. Purkinje-cell activity during saccades may have such a meaning. However, since a saccade is a voluntary motor function, another interpretation is also probable; Purkinje-cell activity represents corollary discharges accompanying central command signals for saccades that remove any conflict between execution of a saccade and other motor control activities going on at the same time. Unfortunately, there is little basis to determine which of these possibilities is correct.

Smooth-Pursuit Eye Movement

Effectiveness of a smooth-pursuit eye movement depends on prediction of a future position of a moving target. To perform this predictive control, an animal attempts to match the eye-movement velocity to the instantaneous velocity of the target [71]. This predictive control problem indicates a functional requirement for a cerebellar contribution to smooth-pursuit eye movements.

The cerebellar areas where electric stimulation evokes a smooth eye movement overlap those inducing saccades: Crus I and II and lobulus simplex of the hemisphere, and lobules VI and VII of the vermis [75]. Impairment of smooth pursuit and inability to maintain eccentric gaze occurs after hemicerebellectomy of monkeys, with or without removal of the vermis [81]. The deficit is unilateral; the animal is unable to track with smooth-pursuit movements a target moving away from the midline toward the side of the lesion.

Purkinje-cell activities during smooth-pursuit eye movements have been related to postulated neural processes extracting information about target velocity in space from a mixture of (a) visual, (b) oculomotor, and (c) vestibular signals [48, 50, 61, 66, 67]. These signals convey information of (a) target velocity relative to eye velocity, (b) eye velocity relative to head velocity, and (c) head velocity in space. Although Purkinje-cell activity reflecting target velocity (exclusive of head velocity and eye-movement velocity) was claimed to exist in the monkey flocculus [61], the visual component was not sufficiently dissociated from vestibular and oculomotor components in the experiments [48]. Subsequently, predominance of eye-velocity input over target-velocity signals to the monkey flocculus has been claimed [50]. Vestibular and oculomotor components can be eliminated under conditions where a monkey fixates a stationary point, while a target oscillates sinusoidally [48]. Acitivity so induced in Purkinje cells of lobules VI and VII is almost identical with that obtained during smooth-pursuit eye movement following the oscillating target [48]. Similar responses were recorded from mossy-fiber afferents, indicating that target-velocity information is extracted from a mixture of visual and oculomotor components already in the brain stem and/or cerebrum before reaching lobules VI and VII.

Smooth-pursuit eye movements, like saccades, are a voluntary motor function and therefore provide an interesting experimental material for studying neuronal mechanisms of voluntary motor control. Unfortunately, there is little knowledge about the neuronal circuitry responsible for smooth-pursuit eye movements. It is also important to note that studies on the monkey flocculus have been performed without consideration of microzonal structure. Thus, the relationship between observed Purkinje-cell activity and execution of horizontal eye movements is not certain. In rabbits, Purkinje cells involved in horizontal eye movements are restricted to zone II, which occupies only one-fifth of the total floccular area. Purkinje cells outside of zone II frequently exhibit modulation of impulse discharges in response to head rotation or optokinetic stimuli on the horizontal plane [21]. This situation, then, leaves the following questions still open: (a) Does the monkey flocculus contain a microzone equivalent to zone II in rabbits which is specifically involved in an adaptive control of the

VOR? (b) If so, is there another microzone specifically involved in smooth-pursuit eye movements? (c) If such a microzone exists, does it project to relay cells of the VOR, or does it join the cerebrocerebellar communication loop via a caudal part of the lateral cerebellar nucleus? Caudal areas of the flocculus project to the caudal part of the lateral cerebellar nucleus instead of vestibular nuclei [83]. (d) Is visual suppression of the VOR in monkeys [77, 78] primarily due to an interaction of the VOR with smooth-pursuit eye movement? This raises the possibility that visual suppression of the VOR is impaired by flocculectomy simply through depression of smooth-pursuit eye movements, just as is the case with the interaction of the VOR with the OKR in rabbits. (e) Is adaptive control of the VOR related to a neuronal mechanism equivalent to the model proposed for zone II of the rabbit flocculus, or is there another mechanism specific to the primate flocculus?

Neuronal Mechanisms in the Rabbit Flocculus for Adaptive Control of the Vestibulo-Ocular Reflex

A remarkable feature of the flocculus-VOR system is that its neuronal layout is extremely consistent with the learning-machine hypothesis of the cerebellum proposed by Marr [60]. This hypothesis assumes that signal transfer from mossy-fiber pathways, through granule cells and their axons (parallel fibers) to Purkinje cells, can be reorganized according to instruction signals from climbing-fiber afferents. Two basic assumptions adopted in the hypothesis are: (a) efficacy of synaptic transmission from parallel fibers to Purkinje cells is modifiable, and (b) this modifiability is effected when parallel-fiber and climbing-fiber impulses arrive simultaneously at the same Purkinje-cell dendrites. In this model, as later pointed out by Albus [1], the climbing-fiber afferents play a role as a teacher in a man-made learning machine, the *Simple Perceptron.* Different directions of modification of parallel-fiber–Purkinje-cell synapses have been assumed in two models. Marr [60] assumed an enhancement and Albus [1] a depression of synaptic transmission following conjunctive activation of a parallel fiber and a climbing fiber.

The fact that the flocculus receives visual climbing-fiber afferents may mean that the climbing-fiber system acts as a "teacher" by detecting retinal slip signals arising from an erroneous performance of the VOR, and "instructing" the vestibular mossy-fiber–Purkinje-cell circuitry of the flocculus to improve performance of the VOR. Since retinal slip is essentially an error signal, visual climbing-fiber afferents to the flocculus are likely to depress cerebellar synapses involved in an erroneous performance during the VOR. In this sense, Albus's assumption seems more reasonable than Marr's. This speculation has been tested and supported by recording from Purkinje cells of the rabbit flocculus under two experimental conditions.

First, flocculus Purkinje cells were sampled from alert rabbits rotated on a turntable with or without optokinetic stimulation (a vertical slit light). *Simple*-spike discharges of Purkinje cells, representing an integrated effect of bombardment through parallel fibers and intracortical inhibitory neurons, are modulated effectively by head rotation in darkness [21, 25]. These cells are probably driven by vestibular mossy-fiber inputs. The modulation was either inphase or 180° outphase with instantaneous head velocity during ipsilateral rotation. Zone II of the rabbit flocculus can be identified by microstimulation through a recording microelectrode, which evokes a horizontal abduction of the ipsilateral eye. When only Purkinje cells in zone II were examined, dominant responses to head rotation were of the outphase type [21]. Outphase modulation in zone II Purkinje cells should facilitate the VOR, as inhibitory signals from such Purkinje cells wane and wax oppositely to the excitatory signals of primary vestibular neurons on relay cells of the VOR. This is consistent with the fact that flocculectomy in rabbits causes a moderate reduction of the VOR gain.

Complex spikes representing climbing-fiber inputs to Purkinje cells are modulated effectively in phase with forward (temporonasal) movements of the slit light relative to the head. Thus, during rotation with the slit light fixed in space, complex spikes are modulated in phase with the ipsilateral head rotation, that is in conjunction with activity in the ipsilateral vestibular nerve. By contrast, rotation with the slit light moving in phase with the turntable, at an angular amplitude twice as large as that of the turntable, modulates complex spikes outphase with the ipsilateral head rotation; that is, in conjunction with activity in the contralateral vestibular nerve.

During sustained rotation with either a fixed or a moving slit light, the VOR-gain adaptively increases or decreases, respectively. The adaptation attains a plateau within 1 h [38, 39]. Concomitantly, outphase responses to rotation in darkness of flocculus Purkinje cells exhibit larger or smaller amplitudes, respectively [20]. This suggests that the flocculus controls the VOR-gain through outphase modulation of zone II Purkinje cells. Larger modulation yields an enhanced VOR and smaller modulation, a depressed VOR. The outphase modulation in flocculus Purkinje cells may result from an interaction of the following four factors: it is driven by (a) facilitation from the contralateral vestibular nerve or (b) inhibition from the ipsilateral vestibular nerve, and is antagonized by (c) facilitation from the ipsilateral nerve or (d) inhibition from the contralateral nerve. Provided that modification occurs only in facilitatory connections from mossy fibers to Purkinje cells via granule cells [1, 60], factors (a) and (c) should be involved in modification of Purkinje-cell responses. The increase of outphase modulation, induced by rotation with the fixed slit light, should therefore be effected through either enhancement of factor (a) or depression of factor (c). Since climbing-fiber afferents are activated during rotation with the fixed slit light in conjunction with activity of the ipsilateral vestibular nerve (see above), depression of factor (c) is likely to account for the observed enhancement of outphase modulation. The decrease of outphase modulation during rotation with the moving slit light may be induced by either depression of factor (a) or enhancement of factor (c). Since activation of climbing-fiber afferents occurs in conjunction with activity in the contralateral vestibular nerve (see above), depression of factor (a) is likely to be involved in the decrease of outphase modulation. This situation is consistent with Albus's assumption about modifiability of transmission [1]. Reciprocal behavior of simple- and complex-spike activity was also observed in the monkey cerebellum during

adaptation of hand movements to a suddenly imposed load change, and has been interpreted as supporting Albus's assumption [26].
A more direct test of the hypothesis has been performed by substituting electric pulse stimulation of a vestibular nerve and the inferior olive in decerebrate rabbits for natural vestibular and visual stimulation in alert rabbits [45]. These experiments demonstrate that olivary stimulation in conjunction with stimulation of either the ipsilateral or contralateral vestibular nerve produces a drastic depression in facilitatory responses of flocculus Purkinje cells to vestibular mossy-fiber inputs from that vestibular nerve. Although vestibular nerve stimulation also produced inhibitory responses in flocculus Purkinje cells, these inhibitory responses were not affected consistently by conjunctive-vestibular-nerve and inferior-olive stimulation. In those Purkinje cells receiving facilitation from both vestibular nerves, it was confirmed that depression occurs specifically in responses to the vestibular nerve involved in conjunctive stimulation with the inferior olive.

Comment

Studies of the VOR and OKR have been fruitful in giving concrete shape to concepts of cerebellar motor control of reflexive movements and provide favorable preparations for investigating intrinsic mechanisms of cerebellar neuronal networks. Investigation of saccades and smooth-pursuit eye movements will provide a new insight into the cerebellar mechanisms for voluntary motor control. Highly attractive problems of central motor programming may be expected to be approached from these eye movements. In conducting such investigations, it is important to employ a comprehensive approach utilizing all of the studies of neuronal circuitry, overall system performance, and recording neuronal signals in a dynamic behaving state of the cerebellum. This approach has been successful in studies of the flocculus-VOR system, and provides an excellent model of the cerebellar adaptive control system.

References

1. Albus JS (1971) A theory of cerebellar function. Math Biosci 10:25–61
2. Alley KA (1974) Anatomical basis for interaction between cerebellar flocculus and brainstem. In: Baker R, Berthoz A (eds) Control of Gaze by Brain Stem Neurons. Elsevier, Amsterdam (Developments in Neuroscience, vol 1, pp 109–117)
3. Alley K, Baker R, Simpson JI (1975) Afferents to the vestibulocerebellum and the origin of the visual climbing fibers in the rabbit. Brain Res 98:585–589
4. Angaut P, Brodal A (1967) The projection of the vestibulocerebellum onto the vestibular nuclei in the cat. Arch Ital Biol 105:441–479
5. Aschoff JC, Cohen B (1972) Cerebellar ablations and spontaneous eye movements in monkey. Bibl Ophthalmol 82:169–177
6. Baarsma EA, Collewijn H (1974) Vestibulo-ocular and optokinetic reactions to rotation and their interaction in the rabbit. J Physiol (Lond) 238:603–625
7. Baker RG, Precht W, Llinás R (1972) Cerebellar modulatory action on the vestibulo-trochlear pathway in the cat. Exp Brain Res 15:364–385

8. Barmack NH, Henkel CK, Pettorossi VE (1979) A subparafascicular projection to the medial vestibular nucleus of the rabbits. Brain Res 172:339–343
9. Barmack NH, Hess DT (1980) Multiple-unit activity evoked in dorsal cap of inferior olive of the rabbit by visual stimulation. J Neurophysiol 43:151–164
10. Batini C, Ito M, Kado RT, Jastreboff PJ, Miyashita Y (1979) Interaction between the horizontal vestibuloocular reflex and optokinetic response in rabbits. Exp Brain Res 37:1–15
11. Brandt TH, Dichgans J, Koenig E (1973) Differential effects of central versus peripheral vision on egocentric and exocentric motion perception. Exp Brain Res 16:476–491
12. Brodal A, Høivik B (1964) Site and mode of termination of primary vestibulocerebellar fibres in the cat. Arch Ital Biol 102:1–21
13. Brodal A, Torvik A (1957) Über den Ursprung der sekundären vestibulocerebellären Fasern bei der Katze, eine experimental-anatomische Studie. Arch Psychiatr Nervenkr 195:550–567
14. Carpenter RHS (1972) Cerebellectomy and the transfer function of the vestibulo-ocular reflex in the decerebrate cat. Proc R Soc Lond [Biol] 181:353–374
15. Carpenter RHS (1977) Movements of the eye. Pion, London pp 420
16. Dow RS (1938) Efferent connections of the flocculo-nodular lobe in Macaca mulatta. J Comp Neurol 68:297–305
17. Dow RS, Manni E (1964) The relationship of the cerebellum to extraocular movements. In: Bender MB (ed) The oculomotor system. Harper and Row, New York Evanston London, pp 280–292
18. Dow RS, Moruzzi G (1958) The Physiology and Pathology of the Cerebellum. University of Minnesota Press, Minneapolis
19. Dufossé M, Ito M, Miyashita Y (1978) Diminution and reversal of eye movements induced by local stimulation of rabbit cerebellar flocculus after partial destruction of the inferior olive. Exp Brain Res 33:139–141
20. Dufossé M, Ito M, Miyashita Y (1977) Functional localization in the rabbit's cerebellar flocculus determined in relationship with eye movements. Neurosci Lett 5:273–277
21. Dufossé M, Ito M, Jastreboff PJ, Miyashita Y (1978) A neuronal correlate in rabbit's cerebellum to adaptive modification of the vestibulo-ocular reflex. Brain Res 150:511–616
22. Fernandez C, Goldberg JM (1971) Physiology of peripheral neurons innervating semicircular canals of the squirrel monkey. II. Response to sinusoidal stimulation and dynamics of peripheral vestibular system. J Neurophysiol 34:661–675
23. Fukuda J, Highstein SM, Ito M (1972) Cerebellar inhibitory control of the vestibulo-ocular reflex investigated in rabbit IIIrd nucleus. Exp Brain Res 14:511–526
24. Furuya N, Kawano K, Shimazu H (1976) Transcerebellar inhibitory interaction between the bilateral vestibular nuclei and its modulation by cerebellocortical activity. Exp Brain Res 25:447–463
25. Ghelarducci B, Ito M, Yagi N (1975) Impulse discharges from flocculus Purkinje cells of alert rabbits during visual stimulation combined with horizontal head rotation. Brain Res 87:66–72
26. Gilbert PFC, Thach WT (1977) Purkinje cell activity during motor learning. Brain Res 128:309–328
27. Gonshor A, Melvill-Jones G (1976a) Short-term adaptive changes in the human vestibulo-ocular reflex arc. J Physiol (Lond) 256:361–379
28. Gonshor A, Melvill-Jones G (1976b) Extreme vestibulo-ocular adaptation induced by prolonged optical reversal of vision. J Physiol (Lond) 256:381–414
29. Haddad GM, Demer JL, Robinson DA (1980) The effect of lesions of the dorsal cap of the inferior olive on the vestibulo-ocular and optokinetic systems of the cats. Brain Res 185:265–275
30. Hassul M, Daniels PD, Kimm J (1976) Effects of bilateral flocculectomy on the vestibulo-ocular reflex in the chinchilla. Brain Res 118:339–343
31. Herndon RM, Coyle JT (1977) Selective destruction of neurons by a transmitter agonist. Science 198:71–72
32. Ito M (1970) Neurophysiological aspects of the cerebellar motor control system. Int J Neurol 7:162–176
33. Ito M (1972) Neural design of the cerebellar motor control system. Brain Res 40:81–84

34. Ito M (1974) The control mechanisms of cerebellar motor system. In: Schmitt FO, Worden FG (eds) The neurosciences, third study program. MIT Press, Boston. pp 293–303
35. Ito M (1976) Cerebellar learning control of vestibuloocular mechanisms. In: Desiraju T (ed) Mechanisms in transmission of signals for conscious behavior. Elsevier, Amsterdam. pp 1–22
36. Ito M (1977) Neuronal events in the cerebellar flocculus associated with an adaptive modification of the vestibuloocular reflex of the rabbit. In: Baker B, Berthoz A (eds) Control of gaze by brain stem neurons. Developments in Neuroscience, vol 1. Elservier, Amsterdam. pp 391–398
37. Ito M, Highstein SM, Fukuda J (1970) Cerebellar inhibition of the vestibulo-ocular reflex in rabbit and cat and its blockage by picrotoxin. Brain Res 17:524–526
38. Ito M, Jastreboff PJ, Miyashita Y (1979) Adaptive modification of the rabbit's horizontal vestibulo-ocular reflex during sustained vestibular and optokinetic stimulation. Exp Brain Res 37:17–30
39. Ito M, Jastreboff PJ, Miyashita Y (1982) Specific effects of unilateral lesions in the flocculus upon eye movements of albino rabbits. Exp Brain Res 45:233–242
40. Ito M, Miyashita Y (1975) The effects of chronic destruction of inferior olive upon visual modification of the horizontal vestibulo-ocular reflex of rabbits. Proc Jpn Acad 51:716–720
41. Ito M, Miyashita Y, Ueki A (1978) Functional localization in the rabbit's inferior olive determined in connection with the vestibulo-ocular reflex. Neurosci Lett 8:283–287
42. Ito M, Nisimaru N, Yamamoto M (1977) Specific patterns of neuronal connections involved in the control of the rabbit's vestibulo-ocular reflexes by the cerebellar flocculus. J Physiol (Lond) 265:833–854
43. Ito M, Nisimaru N, Shibuki K (1979) Destruction of inferior olive induces rapid depression in synaptic action of cerebellar Purkinje cells. Nature 277:568–569
44. Ito M, Orlov I, Shimoyama I (1978) Reduction of the cerebellar stimulus effect on rat Deiters neurons after chemical destruction of the inferior olive. Exp Brain Res 33:143–145
45. Ito M, Sakurai M, Tongroach P (1982) Climbing fibre induced depression of both mossy fibre responsiveness and glutamate sensitivity of cerebellar Purkinje cells. J Physiol (Lond) 324:113–134
46. Ito M, Shiida T, Yagi N, Yamamoto M (1974) Visual influence on rabbit horizontal vestibulo-ocular reflex presumably effected via the cerebellar flocculus. Brain Res 65:170–174
47. Ito M, Shiida T, Yagi N, Yamamoto M (1974) The cerebellar modification of rabbit's horizontal vestibulo-ocular reflex induced by sustained head rotation combined with visual stimulation. Proc Jpn Acad 50:85–89
48. Kase M, Noda H, Suzuki DA, Miller DC (1979) Target velocity signals of visual tracking in vermal Purkinje cells of the monkey. Science 205:717–720
49. Keller EL, Precht W (1979) Visual-vestibular responses in vestibular nuclear neurons in the intact and cerebellectomized, alert cat. Neuroscience 4:1599–1613
50. Lisberger SG, Fuchs AF (1978) Role of primate flocculus during rapid behavioral modification of vestibulo-occular reflex. I. Purkinje cell activity during visually guided horizontal smooth-pursuit eye movements and passive head rotation. J Neurophysiol 41:733–763
51. Llinás R, Wolfe JW (1977) Functional linkage between the electrical activity in the vermal cerebellar cortex and saccadic eye movements. Exp Brain Res 29:1–14
52. Maekawa K, Simpson JI (1973) Climbing fiber responses evoked in vestibulocerebellum of rabbit from visual system. J Neurophysiol 36:649–666
53. Maekawa K, Takeda T (1975) Mossy fiber responses evoked in the cerebellar flocculus of rabbits by stimulation of the optic pathway. Brain Res 98:590–595
54. Maekawa K, Takeda T (1976) Electrophysiological identification of the climbing and mossy fiber pathways from the rabbit's retina to the contralateral cerebellar flocculus. Brain Res 109:169–174
55. Maekawa K, Takeda T (1977) Afferent pathways from the visual system to the cerebellar flocculus of the rabbit. In: Control of gaze by brain stem neurons. Elsevier, Amsterdam. pp 187–195

56. Maekawa K, Takeda T (1978) Origin of the mossy fiber projection to the cerebellar flocculus from optic nerves in rabbits. In: Ito M, Tsukahara N, Kubota K, Yagi K (eds) The integrative control functions of the brain, vol 1. Kodansha, Tokyo, Elsevier, Amsterdam. pp 93–95
57. Maekawa K, Kimura M (1980) Mossy fiber projections to the cerebellar flocculus from extraocular muscle afferents. Brain Res 191:313–325
58. Maekawa K, Kimura M (1980) Electrophysiological study of the nucleus of the optic tract that transfers optic signals to the nucleus reticularis tegmenti pontis – the visual mossy fiber pathway to the cerebellar flocculus. Brain Res 211:456–462
59. Manni DE (1950) Localizzazioni cerebellari corticali nella cavia nota 29: effectti de lesioni delle "parti vestibolari" del cervelletto. Arch Fisiol 50:110–123
60. Marr D (1969) A theory of cerebellar cortex. J Physiol (Lond) 202:437–470
61. Miles F, Fuller JH (1975) Visual tracking and the primate flocculus. Science 189:1000–1002
62. Mitsui Y, Hirai K, Akazawa K, Masuda K (1979) The sensorimotor reflex and strabismus. Jpn J Ophthal 23:227–256
63. Miyashita Y, Ito M, Jastreboff PJ, Maekawa K, Nagao S (1980) Effect upon eye movements of rabbits induced by severance of mossy fiber visual pathway to the cerebellar flocculus. Brain Res 198:210–215
64. Neverov VP, Sterc J, Bures J (1980) Electrophysiological correlates of the reversed postoptokinetic nystagmus in the rabbit: activity of vestibular and floccular neurons. Brain Res 189:355–367
65. Noda H, Suzuki DA (1979) The role of the flocculus of the monkey in saccadic eye movements. J Physiol (Lond) 294:317–334
66. Noda H, Suzuki DA (1979) The role of the flocculus of the monkey in fixation and smooth pursuit eye movements. J Physiol (Lond) 294:335–348
67. Noda H, Suzuki DA (1979) Processing of eye movement signals in the flocculus of the monkey. J Physiol (Lond) 294:349–364
68. Optican LM, Robinson DA (1980) Cerebellar-dependent adaptive control of primate saccadic system. J Neurophysiol 44:1058–1076
69. Precht W, Llinás R (1969) Functional organization of the vestibular afferents to the cerebellar cortex of vestibular afferents to the cerebellar cortex of frog and cat. Exp Brain Res 9:30–52
70. Precht W, Strata P (1980) On the pathway mediating optokinetic responses in vestibular nuclear neurons. Neuroscience 5:777–787
71. Rashbass C (1961) The relationship between saccadic and smooth tracking eye movements. J Physiol (Lond) 159:326–338
72. Ritchie L (1976) Effects of cerebellar lesions on saccadic eye movements. J Neurophysiol 39:1246–1256
73. Robinson DA (1974) The effect of cerebellectomy on the cat's vestibulo-ocular integrator. Brain Res 71:195–207
74. Robinson DA (1976) Adaptive gain control of vestibulo-ocular reflex by the cerebellum. J Neurophysiol 39:954–969
75. Ron S, Robinson DA (1973) Eye movements evoked by cerebellar stimulation in the alert monkey. J Neurophysiol 36:1004–1022
76. Shinoda Y, Yoshida K (1975) Neural pathways from the vestibular labyrinths to the flocculus in the cat. Exp Brain Res 22:97–111
77. Takemori S, Cohen B (1974) Visual suppression of vestibular nystagmus in rhesus monkey. Brain Res 72:203–212
78. Takemori S, Cohen B (1974) Loss of visual suppression of vestibular nystagmus after flocculus lesion. Brain Res 72:213–224
79. Takemori S, Suzuki J (1971) Eye deviations from neck torsion in humans. Ann Oto Rhino Laryngol 80:439–444
80. Warabi T, Matsushima J (1979) Trunk-ocular reflex in the rabbit. Neurosci Lett 13:117–120
81. Westheimer G, Blair SM (1974) Functional organization of primate oculomotor system revealed by cerebellectomy. Exp Brain Res 21:463–472

82. Winfield JA, Hendrickson A, Kimm J (1978) Anatomical evidence that the medial terminal nucleus of the accessory optic tract in mammals provides a visual mossy fiber input to the flocculus. Brain Res 151:175–182
83. Yamamoto M (1978) Localization of rabbit's flocculus Purkinje cells projecting to the cerebellar lateral nucleus and the nucleus propositus hypoglossi, investigated by means of the horseradish peroxidase retrograde axonal transport. Neurosci Lett 7:197–202
84. Yamamoto M (1979) Topographical representation in rabbit cerebellar flocculus for various inputs from the brainstem investigated by means of retrograde axonal transport of horseradish peroxidase. Neurosci Lett 12:29–34
85. Yamamoto M, Shimoyama I (1977) Differential localization of rabbit's flocculus Purkinje cells projecting to the medial and superior vestibular nuclei, investigated by means of the horseradish peroxidase retrograde axonal transport. Neurosci Lett 5:279–283

Discussion

Llinás: Are you saying that the climbing fiber rather than reinforcing the parallel-fiber–Purkinje-cell synapse is actually doing the opposite?
Ito: Our result is consistent with Gilbert and Thach's (1977) results and supports Albus's (1971) assumption that conjunction between parallel-fiber and climbing-fiber impulses will cause depression of the parallel-fiber–Purkinje-cell synapses.
Llinás: Also you said that the contralateral input, which was not paired with the inferior-olivary stimulus, could activate the same Purkinje cell which was depressed by joining the ipsilateral stimulus with climbing-fiber activation.
Ito: Exactly. I neglected to make an important point. Conjunction never influences inhibitory action. It influences only facilitatory action of the vestibular mossy-fiber impulses, which argues against the possibility that plasticity happens at the mossy-fiber–granule-cell junction or somewhere else in the cerebellar cortex.
Llinás: How long does this effect last?
Ito: This is difficult to say since we have not followed the process to complete recovery. However, probably from observations which I showed we can make a guess. Recovery may have two time courses. A very fast one followed by a slow one. The slow one has a time scale of 1–2 h.
Simpson: If you stimulated just the olive over a period of 100 min in the same fashion as you described but without pairing with stimulation of the vestibular nerve is there any effect on subsequent vestibular activity?
Ito: No effect. And there is no need for exact conjunction. We use 4/s stimulation of the olive and 20/s stimulation of the mossy fibers and that's enough.
Collewijn: In relation to the question of Dr. Simpson, I want to comment that I have been able to modify the VOR, as you know, by only visual input, so there was no conjunction at all and yet I found modification. I don't know whether you can explain that.
Ito: Even when no vestibular stimuli were applied, there may be spontaneous vestibular mossy fiber impulses which would collide with visual climbing fiber impulses.

Collewijn: I have another question. You assume that there is a specific interaction of visual and vestibular information in this long-term adaptation of the VOR. Now, you did not say anything about changes in optokinetic reflexes when you make a lesion in the flocculus. Did you check the optokinetic reflexes? Were they decreased and, if so, can you show that there is really a specific effect of the interaction of the vestibular and visual input or is it merely the absence of the visual effects?

Ito: With lesion in the NRTP the OKR gain goes down and the results of the flocculectomy are essentially the same. There is a significant reduction in the OKR.

Collewijn: In other words, isn't this reduction in itself sufficient to explain the changes that you see?

Ito: It explains the impairment of the rapid interaction between OKR and VOR but doesn't explain anything about the adaptation.

Collewijn: If you have no short-term effect how would you get a long-term effect?

Ito: They are two separate processes.

Collewijn: Yes.

Ito: After lesions of the flocculus there is no adaptation. Still, there is a bit of OKR with a reduced gain and there is a rapid sort of interaction with a much reduced efficacy.

Collewijn: I just wonder if you can dissociate the loss of the optokinetic reflex and the loss of adaptation or whether they are just the same?

Ito: They can be removed separately from each other by interrupting the visual mossy fiber pathway at NRTP or the visual climbing fiber pathway [63].

Lisberger: You have shown that stimulating the vestibular nerve and the olive simultaneously changes the sensitivity of the mossy-fiber pathways to vestibular inputs. The extrapolation you want to make is that it is that change which causes the change in VOR-gain, but perhaps the change that is really causing the VOR-gain change is somewhere completely different, secondary to the stimulation that you're doing. Do your stimulation conditions produce a convergence of visual and vestibular information at other synapses?

Ito: We are stimulating the dorsal-cap area and I don't know where such convergence happens.

Lisberger: When you stimulate the dorsal cap does that cause simple-spike activity in the Purkinje cell or some change in it that is consistently related to the climbing fiber? Because if it does, what you may be producing is a consistent relationship between the output of the flocculus and the input from the vestibular nerve at the site where those two pathways converge (where the Purkinje-cell axons converge with the vestibular nerve), and it may be the consistent relationship between these activities that produces the VOR-gain changes.

Ito: I see, you mean if we were to stimulate Purkinje cells in combination with vestibular impulses would something happen or not? We don't know. We are observing Purkinje-cell responses and assuming that they account for the VOR adaptation.

Lisberger: It's that assumption I don't agree with.

Thach: Could you say how critical the pattern of electric stimulation is?

Ito: I think the stimulus frequency to the inferior olive is very crucial. Initially, we used very high frequencies – 200, 100, 500/s. Then most Purkinje cells showed a very peculiar behavior. They were activated and then completely silenced. We thought that they were lost, but after waiting many minutes they suddenly came back. Therefore, we really don't like to use high-frequency stimulation of the inferior olive. Four pulses/s is nearly what we get for the natural rotation condition.

Sotelo: Just a short comment on the use of kainic acid. If you look at the *nervous* mutant mouse where 90% of the Purkinje cells are degenerating in the hemispheres and look at the olive, the principal olive is gone.

Ito: There may be some other reason for this. Not simply removal of Purkinje cells.

Krnjevic: Exactly how do you do your stimulation of the vestibular nerve and to what extent does the rabbit have an efferent projection from the olive to the inner ear? Could you possibly have interactions from the olive affecting your vestibular input?

Ito: We adjusted the vestibular nerve stimulation just to maximum by observing the descending vestibulospinal volley.

Llinás: Following inferior-olive stimulation at 4/s, do you see increased activity in the olive beyond the time of stimulation?

Ito: Yes, very often, for a few seconds.

Llinás: We also know that the inferior olive is modified by the stimulus itself and that modification should be taken into account.

Ito: Yes, I agree. They can be activated and the activation will outlast the stimulus, but sometimes they are inhibited and the inhibition persists. Nevertheless, these phenomena finish in about a minute and then the normal response pattern comes back.

Llinás: And the normal response pattern does not require that the climbing fiber be activated during this period?

Ito: As far as Purkinje cells are concerned, I don't think so. Inputs are important. Purkinje-cell-output signals are not really important during conjunction.

Llinás: But, if you happened to have left an inferior olive that was slightly hyperexcitable one wonders whether the reduction of Purkinje-cell activity was not related more to biased activation of the inferior olive by the ipsilateral vestibular stimulation. We know that climbing fibers can inhibit the Purkinje cells indirectly.

Ito: But in those Purkinje cells which are initially excited by both ipsilateral and contralateral vestibular nerve stimulation modification is found only for that vestibular input which was conjugated with olivary stimulation. The nonconjugated vestibular input is not affected. It is fair to assume that only the synapses involved in the conjunctive stimulation are altered.

Thach: Dr. Llinás, can you conceive of any kind of simultaneous activity produced by the climbing-fiber input and the mossy-fiber input which would provide a mechanism whereby temporal correlation of two different kinds of electric activity would induce a more or less long-term change in one or the other heterosynaptically?

Llinás: The fact that you apparently don't need a precise conjunction of the two inputs means obviously that it is not really the EPSP but probably something else that is controlling this modulation. Calcium could of course be such a modulator. The question to be posed is whether this is a presynaptic or a postsynaptic change. If this modulation does happen at the Purkinje-cell level, it is probably going to be a postsynaptic change at the subsynaptic region.

GABA and Other Transmitters in the Cerebellum

K. Krnjević

Introduction

GABA and Glutamate as Neurotransmitters

Over the last 20 years, a large amount of information has been accumulated about gamma aminobutyric acid (GABA) and its probable function as perhaps the most important inhibitory transmitter in the vertebrate central nervous system. It has been extensively reviewed in recent years [65, 77]. Therefore only the main points of general interest will be summarized here before considering in greater detail the role(s) of GABA in cerebellar function.

The first aspect of GABA that is of importance is its very close relationship to glutamic acid; GABA is simply obtained from glutamate by α-decarboxylation. The change from an acidic amino acid to a neutral omega amino acid results in a startling reversal in physiologic activity: from a powerful excitant action, exerted on a wide variety of cells throughout the brain, to a powerful inhibitory action, which is perhaps even more widespread. Since glutamate is readily available from glucose and pyruvate via the tricarboxylic acid cycle, the supply of glutamate is unlikely to run out under normal conditions. The conversion of glutamate is promoted by glutamate decarboxylase (GAD), an enzyme with a specific distribution; indeed a high level of GAD activity is sufficiently unusual to be a useful mark of inhibitory synaptic function (as demonstrated particularly clearly with GAD-specific antibodies [61, 76]).

Mechanism of Postsynaptic Inhibition

The best established inhibitory actions of GABA result from its ability to increase the neuron's membrane permeability to Cl^- (P_{Cl}). There is every reason to believe that in most central neurons, the internal Cl^- concentration is well below the concentration that would be in equilibrium at the resting potential – presumably because Cl^- is actively transported out of central neurons, by a "pump" that has not yet been fully characterized. Hence, usually there is a net electrochemical outward gradient for Cl^-, and any increase in Cl^- permeability leads to an efflux of Cl^-, and consequently, hyperpolarization.

This action readily explains the widespread postsynaptic type of inhibition seen in many parts of the brain and often ascribable to GABA [24, 42].

Experimental Brain Research, Suppl. 6

Presynaptic Inhibition

Presynaptic inhibition is also widely believed to be mediated by GABA [59]. Its mechanism is less clear, but a plausible hypothesis runs as follows. Presynaptic inhibition, which is seen most characteristically at primary afferent synapses in the spinal cord and brain stem, is closely associated with depolarization of afferent terminals. This depolarization can be explained by a P_{Cl}-augmenting action of GABA if the Cl^- gradient is in the outward direction because primary afferent neurons contain an excess of Cl^-. Since this indeed appears to be the case, it is supposed that because of such a depolarization, nerve-terminal action potentials are diminished in amplitude and therefore become less effective in triggering transmitter release at the synapse. The precise mechanism of this is not established; it may be due to voltage-dependent inactivation of the Ca^{2+} inward current that presumably initiates transmitter release. At any rate there is significant evidence that at a variety of synapses, presynaptic depolarization (or the increase in terminal excitability, which is more often measured) reduces the efficacy of synaptic transmission [23, 52, 85].

Another Presynaptic Receptor for GABA?

A very different, more direct presynaptic mechanism of GABA action has been proposed recently by Dunlap and Fischbach [21]. Having identified what appears to be a Ca^{2+}-mediated, slow component of the action potential of dorsal-root ganglion cells, they found somewhat unexpectedly that this was blocked selectively by GABA (as well as by other postulated presynaptic inhibitory transmitters) in the absence of any significant depolarization. Thus GABA seems to interfere directly with the Ca^{2+} inward current. This action is insensitive to bicuculline and other GABA antagonists, and therefore is not mediated by the GABA receptors that are involved in post-synaptic inhibition. Dunlap and Fischbach's finding is supported by Bowery et al.'s [9] observations on frog dorsal-root fibers, where a presynaptic inhibitory action of GABA can be demonstrated after its depolarizing effect has been eliminated by bicuculline (or picrotoxin). A particularly attractive feature of this mechanism is that it does not require an outward gradient of Cl^- for its operation. Most investigations have indicated a relative *deficiency* of Cl^- in central neurons, which would preclude the possibility of GABA-evoked, Cl^--mediated presynaptic inhibition in the CNS. A relatively direct inhibition of Ca^{2+} influx would be of wide relevance and could account, for example, for the presynaptic inhibition believed to be exerted by cerebellar Golgi cells [25].

Time Course of Action of GABA

Another significant characteristic of GABA is a comparatively prolonged duration of action. This was first emphasized by Diamond and Roper [18] who compared the effects of glycine and GABA on goldfish Mauthner cells. It could be explained by either a particularly prolonged interaction between GABA and its receptors, or a longer duration of opening of Cl^--channels. The latter would evidently have to be a specific property of Cl^- channels controlled by GABA, since glycine, which activates comparable Cl^- channels, does not have such a prolonged action. The second possibility is supported by the results of an analysis of membrane "noise" generated, respectively, by GABA or glycine in spinal cells from fetal mice. According to Barker and McBurney [2] the elementary conductance change evoked by GABA consistently has a longer duration. But very recent measurements of the "noise" produced in Mauthner cells by GABA and glycine showed no such difference [30]. Therefore it is not yet clear whether the longer action of GABA will prove to be a peculiarity of the relevant membrane receptors or of some Cl^- channels.

Fading or Desensitization

A further characteristic of the action of GABA in vertebrates is that it tends to "fade" during a maintained application [1, 4, 18, 20, 54]. The falloff in GABA action is fully evident when measuring the membrane resistance change produced by GABA, and therefore reflects a true loss of effectiveness and not simply a change in Cl^- equilibrium potential consequent on the large Cl^- fluxes evoked by GABA. This characteristic, which again is not shown by glycine, could be explained by: (a) rapid GABA uptake [27, 50, 54], (b) true desensitization of GABA receptors, or (c) inactivation of Cl^- channels. Although some evidence is in keeping with the first hypothesis (accelerated uptake), "fading" can be such a striking phenomenon [4] that some further mechanism such as (b) or (c) is likely to be at least as important.

GABA Antagonists

The action of GABA can often be blocked quite effectively by a number of agents [46]; the best known are picrotoxin and bicuculline (both plant alkaloids). These antagonists can be applied directly (e.g., by iontophoresis) or systemically. The blocking action is quite quickly reversible, especially after local applications. Although such antagonist drugs can also block quite strongly synaptic inhibition (especially where mediated by GABA or GABA-like agents), their value as agents for identifying GABAergic synapses is limited, because they are at best only partly specific for some GABA receptors. For example, the action of GABA on cerebral cortical neurons grown in culture is blocked almost as readily by strychnine as by bicuculline [19]. The variability in the action of the antagonists has led Nistri and Constanti [65] to postulate the existence of two kinds of GABA receptors, which differ systematically in their susceptibility to block by bicuculline (etc.). As already mentioned, a new population of presynaptic GABA receptors has recently been described that is quite insensitive to bicuculline or picrotoxin [9, 21].

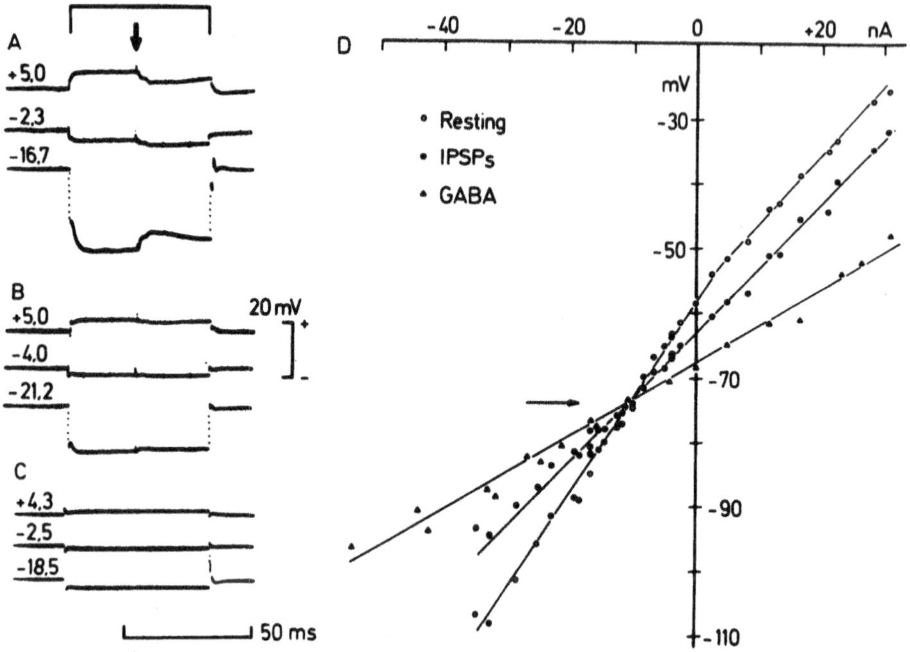

Fig. 1A–D. Identification GABA as inhibitory transmitter responsible for IPSPs evoked in Deiters neurons of the cat by cerebellar stimulation. **A–C** Examples of experimental data. In **A** reversal potential for IPSP (evoked at *arrow*) is demonstrated by applying depolarizing or hyperpolarizing current, indicated in nA; **B** similar series during iontophoretic administration of GABA (270 nA); **C** control runs performed extracellularly; **D** graph of the voltage current data showing fall in resistance during IPSP (*full circles*), and GABA application (*open triangles*), and common reversal level, at *horizontal arrow*. From Fig. 5 in Obata et al. [69]

GABA in the Cerebellum

With the single exception of granule cells, all types of intrinsic cerebellar neurons appear to be predominantly GABAergic.

Purkinje Cells

These cells have the distinction of being the first inhibitory neurons to be clearly identified as such in vertebrates [25, 44], as well as being the first to be recognized as GABAergic [66, 69]. Intracellular studies of Deiters neurons demonstrated an excellent agreement between the properties of inhibitory postsynaptic potentials (IPSPs) evoked in the Deiters nucleus by Purkinje-cell activation and the effects of GABA applied directly by iontophoresis [the parallel extended to the direction of potential and conductance changes, as well as the reversal potentials (Fig. 1)]. Strong supporting evidence came from the demonstration by Obata and Takeda [68] that stimulation of the cerebellar cortex leads to the release of GABA into the 4th ventricle (near Deiters and other deep nuclei). Obata, Otsuka, and Tanaka [67] further showed that Purkinje cells probably contain GABA, though the amount of GABA in the cell bodies is relatively small and therefore the absence of Purkinje cells (in *nervous* mutants) makes no significant difference to the total GABA content of the cerebellar cortex [79, 80]. Similarly, although it is generally expected that GABA-releasing terminals would be manifested by a high rate of GABA uptake, this does not seem to be the case in the Deiters nucleus [40, 84]. On the other hand, GABA is present in high concentration in inhibitory terminals on Deiters neurons [70]; curiously enough, according to the same authors significant amounts of GABA are found in the cytoplasm of Deiters neurons, probably indicating an appreciable postsynaptic uptake of GABA (Fig. 2). Strong GAD activity has been demonstrated in Purkinje-cell nerve terminals on Deiters and other deep nuclei [this volume, Chap. 26, 33, 61]. GAD activity is also present in the Purkinje cell bodies, but this is clearly demonstrable only after treatment with colchicine (Fig. 6), presumably because GAD manufactured in the soma is normally rapidly removed to the terminals by axoplasmic transport; by blocking such transport, colchicine causes GAD to accumulate in the cell bodies.

The results of experiments with convulsant agents in general support the other evidence that GABA is the main transmitter released by Purkinje cell terminals in deep cerebellar nuclei. Thus picrotoxin and bicuculline given intravenously or directly are usually better antagonists of GABA than of glycine (Fig. 3), and they suppress synaptic inhibition quite effectively [16, 69, 86]. As the latter authors point out, however, strychnine is also quite potent, sometimes more so

	cell dissection	dissected area	GABA mmoles/kg ± S.E.M.
A	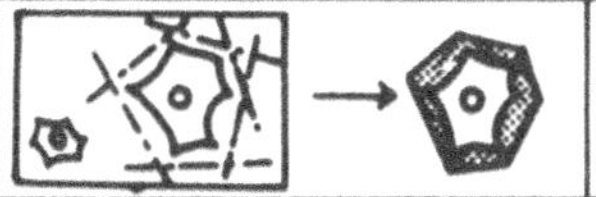	cell + surrounding tissue	28.8 ± 2.9. (11)
B	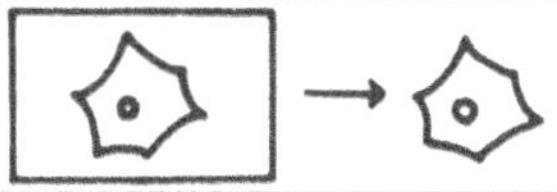	tapped out cell	26.3 ± 3.7 (23)
C	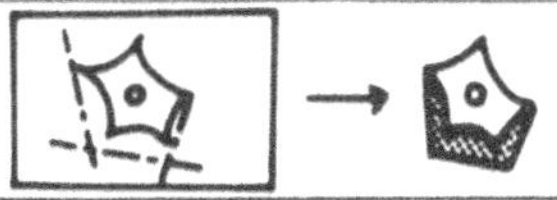	cell together with area surrounding half membrane	21.2 ± 1.6 (20)
D	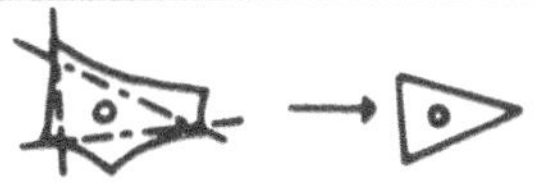	cell without membrane fragments	16.4 ± 1.6 (12)
E	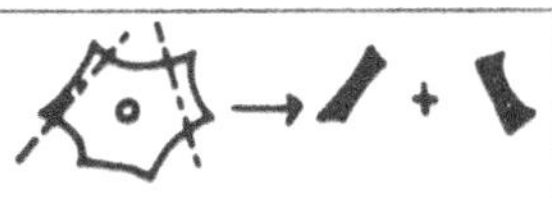	membrane fragments	32.2 ± 2.1 (5)

Fig. 2. Diagram demonstrating technique for measuring GABA content inside Deiters neurons and in their immediate surroundings, in thin sections of frozen tissue. Table 1 from Okada and Shimada [70]

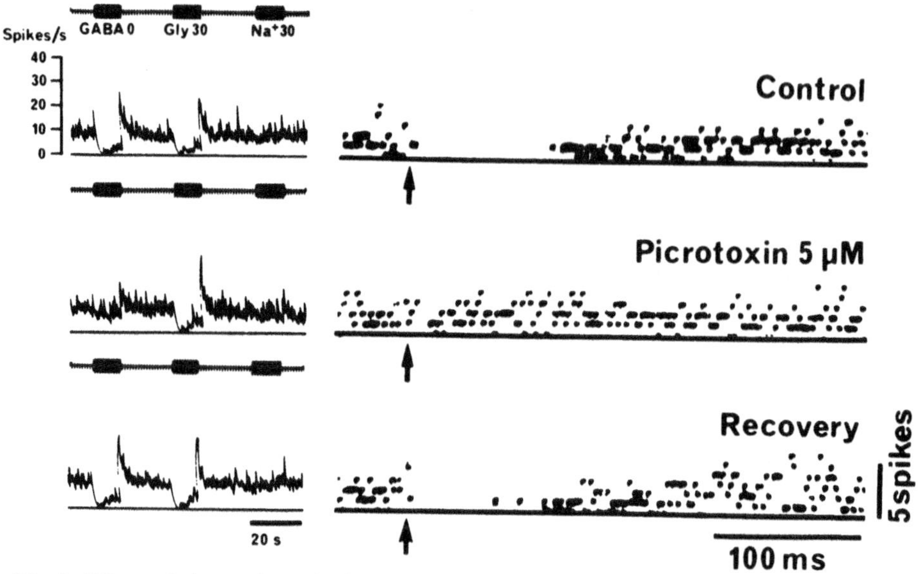

Fig. 3. Effects of picrotoxin on inhibitory responses in a deep cerebellar nucleus neuron. *Left column,* polygraph records showing the effects of a 5 μM solution of picrotoxin on iontophoretic applications of GABA and glycine. *Black bars* above each record show 10-s periods when retaining current (10 nA) was switched off and indicated positive ejected currents were switched on. GABA, 0 nA; glycine, 30 nA; and Na^+, 30 nA. *Right column,* peristimulus histograms showing effects of picrotoxin on evoked inhibition of same neuron (bin width, 2 ms, 70 sweeps). Figure 8 from Wojtowicz et al. [86]

than GABA. Whether this indicates the release of some other inhibitory amino acid (such as glycine, β-alanine, or taurine) from certain Purkinje-cell terminals, or is simply another example of the relatively low specificity of the antagonists [19, 71] remains to be established.

Cerebellar Inhibitory Interneurons

It is well known that Purkinje cells are themselves subject to an important inhibitory regulation ([25]; this volume, p. 412). This is exerted by three kinds of cells. Basket cells and stellate cells directly inhibit Purkinje cells. Basket-cell terminals are situated mainly on or near the Purkinje-cell somata, and therefore exert a particularly powerful control on their firing (on theoretical grounds, the operation performed can be expected to be a *division* of ongoing discharge, [7]). By contrast, stellate-cell axons terminate on the dendrites of Purkinje cells, and therefore control in a more discrete manner the excitatory influence of various parallel-fiber inputs (presumably by a subtractive operation [7]). The terminals of Golgi cells are said to act both postsynaptically on dendrites of granule cells and presynaptically on mossy-fiber terminals; so they influence Purkinje cells firing only indirectly. It appears that all three types of inhibitory interneurons operate mainly by releasing GABA.

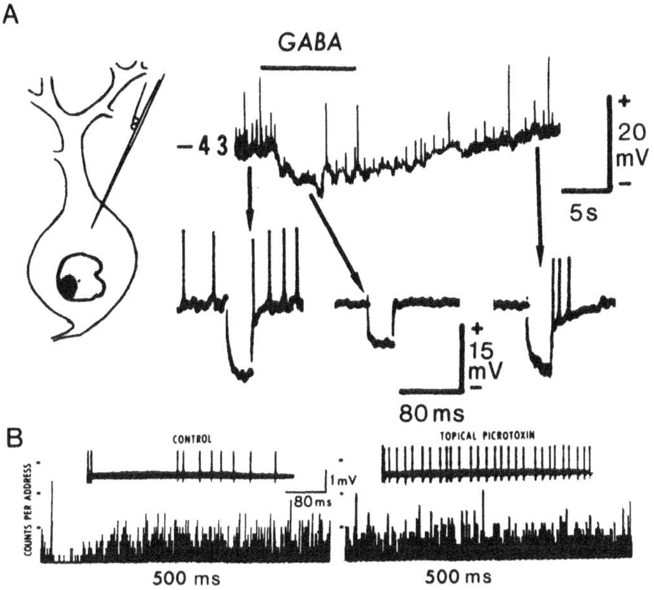

Fig. 4A, B. GABA and inhibition of frog cerebellar Purkinje cells. **A** Iontophoretic application of GABA causes hyperpolarization (*upper trace*) and marked reduction in resistance as shown by diminution of resistance-testing pulses (*below*). *Calibrations* indicate 5 s and 20 mV (*top*) and 80 ms and 50 mV (*bottom*). **B** Synaptic inhibitory action evoked by local stimulation of parallel fibers is blocked by topical application of picrotoxin (5×10^{-5} M). At *left*, controls show inhibitory pause in extracellularly recorded unit firing (*above*) and corresponding poststimulus time histogram (*below*). Traces at *right* illustrate disappearance of inhibition during application of picrotoxin. From Figs. 1, 2 in Woodward et al. [87]

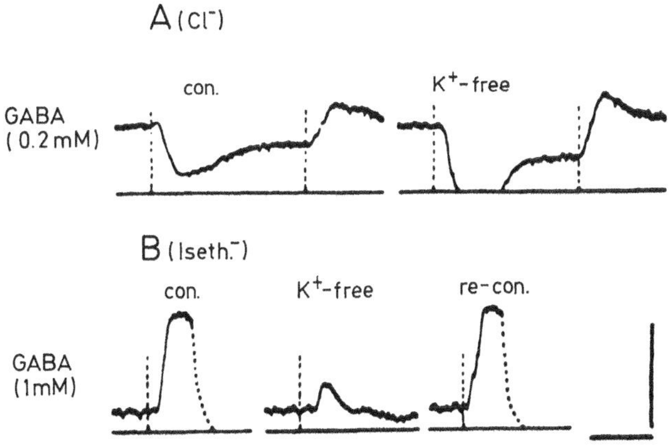

Fig. 5A, B. Effects of GABA in low-Cl⁻ and K⁺-free media. **A** Neuronal firing in slice of guinea-pig cerebellar cortex in 136 mM Cl⁻, and **B**, in 4 mM Cl⁻ and 125 mM isethionate. GABA was applied at times indicated by *vertical interrupted lines* or for periods between two *vertical interrupted lines*. Each transfer to K⁺-free medium was approximately 1 min before application of GABA. *Calibrations, vertical:* 60 spikes/s **(A)**, and 200 spikes/s **(B)**, *horizontal:* 10 s. Figure 6 from Okamoto et al. [71]

Basket and Stellate Cells

Action of GABA on Purkinje Cells. The first indication that Purkinje cells might be a target for GABAergic inhibition was their exquisite sensitivity to the inhibitory action of GABA [53], subsequently confirmed by numerous authors. Intracellular studies in cats and frogs have shown a marked similarity of this action with that observed in the cerebral cortex or Deiters nucleus: as illustrated in Fig. 4, there is a hyperpolarization and marked conductance increase [81, 87], generated principally by an increase in Cl^- conductance; but some evidence from a study of guinea-pig cerebellar slices in vitro indicates a possibly significant increase in K^+ conductance as well [71] (Fig. 5).

Selective inactivation of the inhibitory effects of basket and stellate cells by picrotoxin and bicuculline (but not strychnine) was demonstrated by Bisti et al. [6], Curtis and Felix [17], and Woodward et al. [87], and there is now excellent

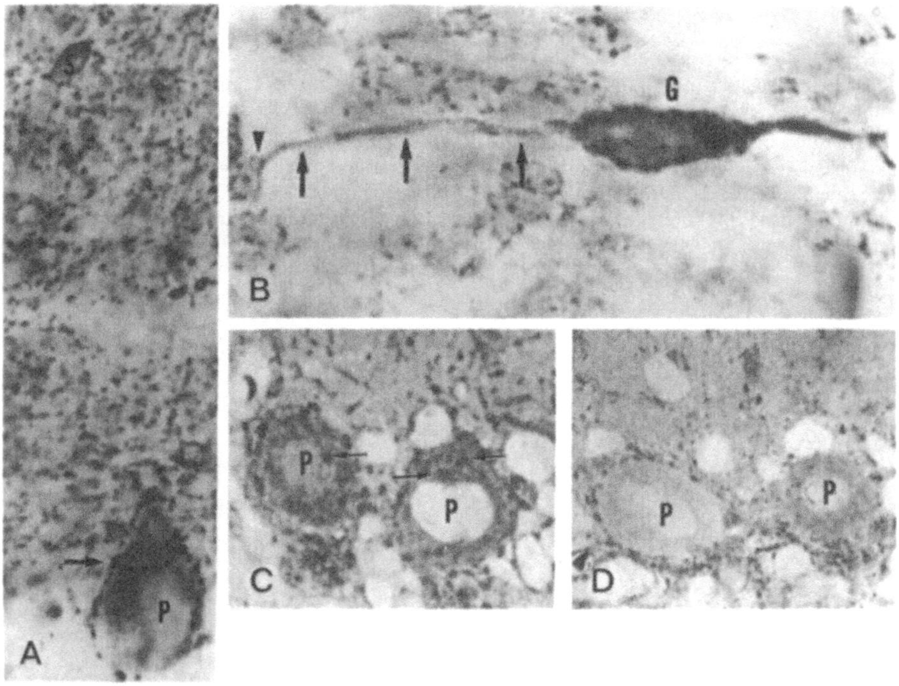

Fig. 6A–D. GAD activity in neuronal elements of cerebellar cortex. **A–C** frozen sections of colchicine-injected rat cerebellum incubated in anti-GAD serum. **A** Purkinje (*P*) and stellate (*S*) neurons show GAD-positive reaction within soma. Perimeter of P soma is also studded with GAD-positive axon terminals, e.g., *arrow*. ×1350. **B** Golgi neuron (*G*) within granule layer, with dense GAD-positive reaction within soma and proximal processes. Note thin axon-like process (*arrows*) terminating in glomerulus (*arrowhead*). ×1300. **C, D** Indistinct clumps of GAD-positive reaction (*arrows*) in somata of Purkinje neurons (*P*) may correspond to Golgi complex. ×1100. Comparable section of cerebellum *not* treated with colchicine: Purkinje somata (*P*) lack GAD-positive reaction. ×1100. From part of Fig. 1 and Figs. 4, 5, 6 of Ribak et al. [76]

immunohistochemical evidence that basket and stellate cells (and especially their terminals on Purkinje cells) are rich in GAD activity [this volume, Chap. 26, 62, 76]. This GAD activity can be seen in Fig. 6, both in numerous perineuronal boutons on Purkinje cells, as well as in a stellate-cell body (after treatment with colchicine).

However, GABA may not be the only transmitter released by stellate cells: selective destruction of these cells by x-irradiation is followed by a substantial reduction of the usually high concentration of taurine in the molecular layer [64]. This would be consistent with the possibility that taurine is a (the) transmitter released by at least some stellate cells, especially as Purkinje cells are quite sensitive to taurine [71], particularly when this is applied to their dendrites [34].

Golgi Cells

The main evidence favoring GABA as the transmitter released by Golgi cells is that they take up GABA [40] [not a very strong argument because GABA may be taken up by glia, as well as noninhibitory cells (Fig. 2)]; they are rich in GAD (Fig. 6) [this volume, Chap. 26, 61, 76]; and their inhibitory effects on granule cells are suppressed by relatively large doses of picrotoxin and bicuculline, but resistant to strychnine [6].

On the basis of more limited evidence some other transmitters have been proposed as transmitters released by Golgi cells: notably acetylcholine [because Golgi cells have a high content of "cholinergic" enzymes [48]) and glycine [because Golgi cells take up glycine (this volume, Chap. 16)].

Excitatory Transmitters in the Cerebellum

The most likely excitatory transmitter released by intrinsic cerebellar neurons is glutamate, at the synapse between parallel fibers and Purkinje cells. Glutamate was first proposed as ae widespread central excitatory transmitter some 15 years ago [51], and much evidence has now accumulated in support (for an up to date review, see ref. [45]). There is still much uncertainty about its precise mode of action [29], but the recent studies of Bürhle et al. [10] on spinal motoneurons provide strong evidence that it is associated with a substantial influx of Ca^{2+}. Another unusual feature is that after release, glutamate is probably taken up by glia, and returned to nerve terminals only after its transformation to the synaptically inactive form glutamine [5].

Parallel-Fiber Pathway

Several kinds of evidence point to glutamate as the excitatory transmitter released by the granule cell and parallel-fiber terminals on Purkinje-cell dendrites. In the first place, Purkinje cells are highly sensitive to glutamate [36, 49,

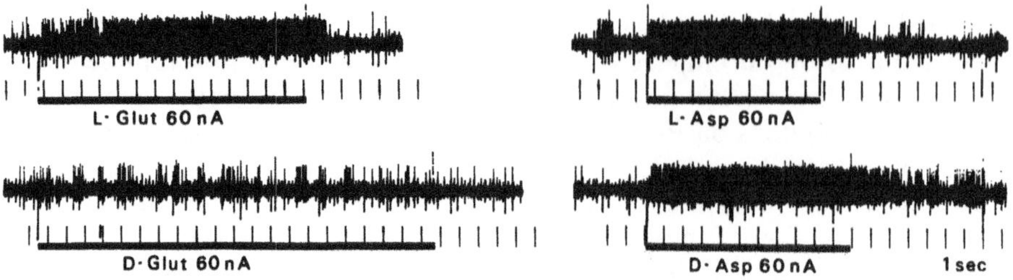

Fig. 7. Excitation of presumed Purkinje cell in cerebellar cortex of the cat by microiontophoretic applications of L-glutamate, L-aspartate, D-glutamate, and D-aspartate, in equal iontophoretic doses. Krnjević K and Phillis JW, unpublished observations

53] particularly in the region of the dendrites [12]. The strong firing readily evoked by L-glutamate (but not D-glutamate) is illustrated in Fig. 7. This figure shows that cerebellar cells can also be strongly excited by aspartate, but neurochemical evidence makes it unlikely that aspartate is released by parallel fibers, though it may be relevant in another context (cf. subsection "Climbing Fibers" below). A more recent study by Hackett et al. [37] has confirmed that glutamate excites Purkinje cells directly, since its action is not prevented by Mn^{2+}, applied in a concentration sufficient to block indirect (synaptic) responses. By intracellular recording (Fig. 8), Hackett et al. [37] were further able to demonstrate a good correspondence between the reversal potential of EPSPs evoked by stimulating parallel fibers and the reversal potential for the action of glutamate, applied by iontophoresis (in both cases near −30 mV). Stone [83] has attempted to distinguish between excitation by glutamate and aspartate through the use of a pharmacologic antagonist, but this proved unselective in its action on Purkinje cells.

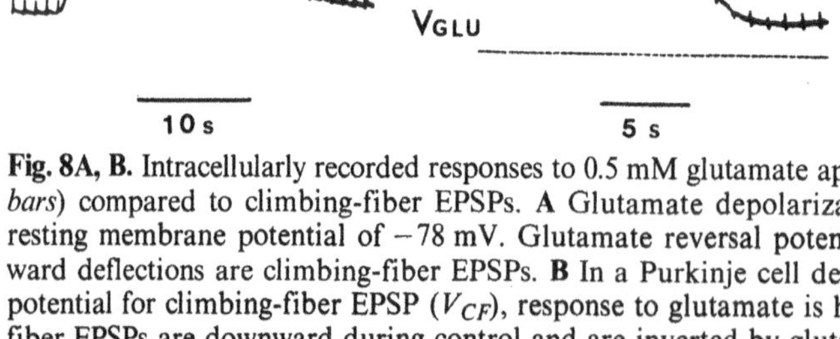

Fig. 8A, B. Intracellularly recorded responses to 0.5 mM glutamate applications (marked by *solid bars*) compared to climbing-fiber EPSPs. **A** Glutamate depolarization in Purkinje cell with resting membrane potential of −78 mV. Glutamate reversal potential is −26 mV. Small upward deflections are climbing-fiber EPSPs. **B** In a Purkinje cell depolarized past the reversal potential for climbing-fiber EPSP (V_{CF}), response to glutamate is hyperpolarizing. Climbing-fiber EPSPs are downward during control and are inverted by glutamate (*solid bar*). Figure 2 from Hackett et al. [37]

There is a high concentration of glutamate in the cerebellar [31], especially in the molecular and the granule-cell layers [64]. Even more direct evidence that this is located in parallel fibers is the selective reduction in tissue (or synaptosomal) glutamate content in animals that lack granule cells and their axons owing to a genetic defect [78, 79], as a consequence of a viral infection [90], or after selective x-irradiation [80].

Extrinsic Inputs

The only clearly defined pathways with a well-established action are the excitatory climbing fibers and mossy fibers. Curiously enough, in neither case is the identity of the main transmitter known with any certainty.

Climbing Fibers

In spite of the very characteristic excitatory action of the terminals of olivary cells, including EPSPs that are unusually easily reversed by depolarization [22, 26, 37], it has not yet been possible to identify the corresponding transmitter. Most of the evidence available is based on negative results that tend to exclude certain agents. Thus, though the presence of large, dense-core granules [58] might seem to point to a monoamine transmitter, various catecholamines and serotonin have predominantly depressant actions on most Purkinje cells [49, 81, 89] (Fig. 9). The reversal potential of the climbing-fiber-evoked EPSP is close to zero, and therefore more positive than the reversal potential for EPSPs evoked in the dendrites of the same cell by parallel fibers (Fig. 8) [37]. The transmitter is therefore unlikely to be glutamate. (The possibility that parallel fibers also release GABA, thus making the reversal potential more negative, seems to have been excluded by the lack of any effect of bicuculline or picrotoxin [22].)

Other authors have tackled the problem by looking for changes in the tissue content of amino acids when climbing fibers are destroyed selectively either by disease in humans [73] or by the action of 3-acetyl-pyridine in rats [63, 75]. Apart from some loss of taurine (probably irrelevant in view of its predominant inhibitory action on Purkinje cells), the most significant observation is a consistent reduction in aspartic acid. Hence aspartate must be considered the only serious contender for this neurotransmitter role. It is evident from Fig. 7 that aspartate is at least as effective an excitant as glutamate, but more searching tests, including an intracellular comparison of climbing-fiber EPSPs and the effects of aspartate, are very much needed to confirm this hypothesis.

A more complex interaction between climbing fibers and Purkinje-cell activity, possibly including some chemical modulation, is indicated by certain other observations, such as the rapid loss of synaptic efficacy of Purkinje-cell terminals in deep nuclei following inactivation of climbing fibers [43], as well as the prolonged depression of parallel-fiber synapses induced by concurrent climbing-fiber activation [described very recently by M. Ito (this volume, p. 523)].

Mossy Fibers

On the basis of a relatively high content of choline acetyltransferase in the middle cerebellar peduncle, the afferent cerebellar pathway was suggested to be cholinergic by Feldberg and Vogt [32] as early as 1948. This observation was later confirmed by Hebb and Silver [38], Kasa and Silver [48], and Kan et al. [47], and supported by the presence of acetylcholinesterase in the granule-cell layer [74, 82], and acetylcholine (ACh) itself in mossy-fiber terminals [41]. Iontophoretic applications of ACh, however, have yielded conflicting results: strong excitation of granule cells in the hands of McCance and Phillis [60], but only a slow excitation of Purkinje cells according to Crawford et al. [13]. (Some mossy fibers contain serotonin (5HT) [11] and there is evidence that certain granule cells may be excited by serotonin [18].) On the whole, the evidence does not strongly favour ACh, serotonin (5HT), or indeed any other particular agent as the main transmitter released by mossy fibers.

One should perhaps keep in mind some earlier reports that cerebellar extracts contain a special excitatory factor that is not found in the cerebral hemispheres [14]. This material was later identified as ergothioneine [15], which, however, did not seem to live up to its promise when tested iontophoretically in the cerebellum [56]. On the other hand, it is likely that most of the cells tested in these experiments were *not* granule cells, and it may be necessary to reexamine the effects of ergothioneine (or possible some related sulphur-containing agents) to exclude a significant role at mossy-fiber synapses.

Modulatory Agents

There is no hard and fast rule by which neuroactive agents can be definitively classed as either transmitters or modulators. The same agent (e.g., ACh) may operate as a transmitter at peripheral junctions (and on Renshaw cells) and probably as a modulator at excitatory muscarinic receptors in the CNS; there its action leads to increased responsiveness to other inputs rather than simple excitation [55]. The disinhibitory action of ACh seen in the thalamus [3] and the hippocampus [57] is also more easily categorized as modulation of activity. To what extent comparable modulations are mediated by cholinergic pathways extrinsic or intrinsic to the cerebellum is largely a matter of speculation (cf. section on mossy fibers above).

Monoamine-containing pathways have also been studied in some detail [8, 11, 35 39, 72]. In most regions of the cerebellum, monoamines tend to depress neuronal firing [49, 81, 89], though, in the cat particularly, noradrenaline has an excitatory effect on archicerebellar neurons. The depressant action was considered for some years to indicate an inhibitory function for noradrenaline; but later tests have revealed a curious potentiation by noradrenaline of various transmitter actions, most notably that of GABA [62, 88]. Noradrenergic pathways, which originate from the locus coeruleus especially, may thus operate principally by modulating other synaptic responses.

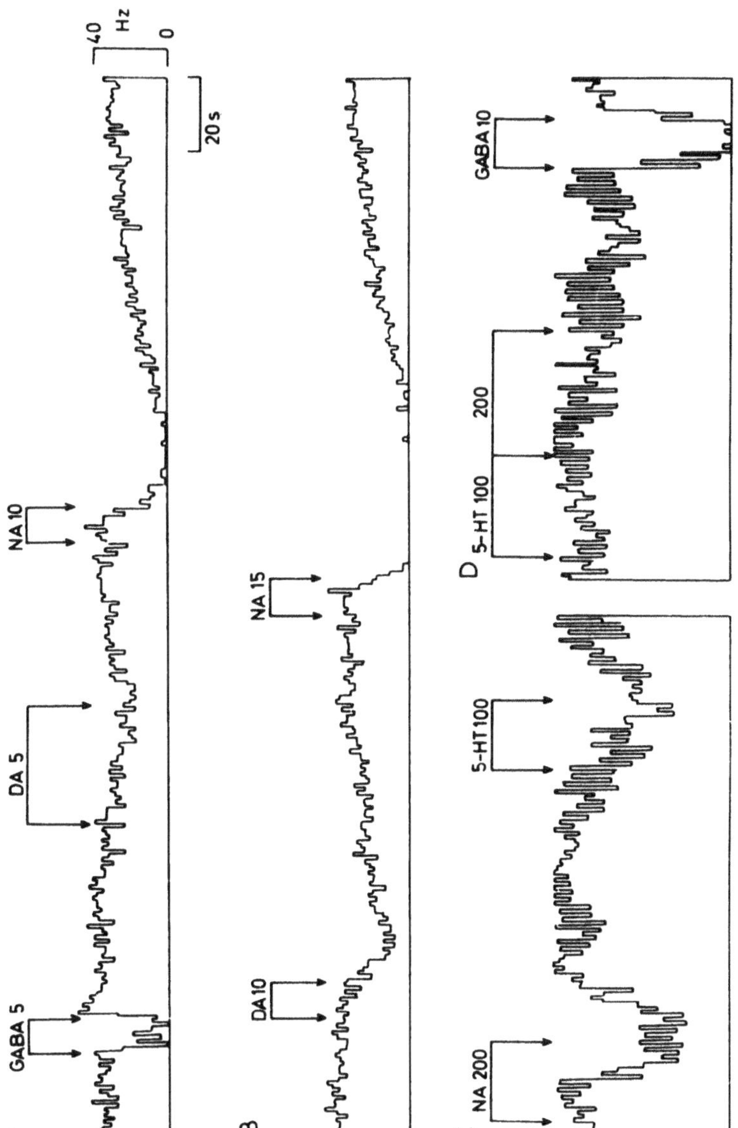

Fig. 9A–D. Purkinje-cell firing affected by monoamines. Firing rate of the Purkinje cell illustrated in **A** and **B** has an unusual sensitivity to administration of small amounts of noradrenaline (*NA*) and dopamine (*DA*). Slow time course of catecholamine action contrasts with quick effect of GABA. Cells illustrated in **C** and **D** were depressed only with strong currents of noradrenaline or serotonin (*5HT*), both of which had a relatively quick action. Record **D** was taken a few minutes after **C** when cell was becoming desensitized to *5HT*. Figure 4 from Kawamura and Provini [49]

Unlike many other parts of the brain, the cerebellum is deficient in neuroactive peptides (substance P, opioids, cholecystokinin, etc.) [28]. This is perhaps in keeping with the lack of prominence of other likely modulators such as ACh and the monoamines, and therefore supports the notion that the cerebellum is a relatively hard-wired organ, where a great deal of learning may not take place continuously, in contrast to structures like the cerebral cortex and hippocampus.

References

1. Adams PR, Brown DA (1975) Actions of γ-aminobutyric acid on sympathetic ganglion cells. J Physiol 250:85–120
2. Barker JL, McBurney RN (1979) GABA and glycine may share the same conductance channel on cultured mammalian neurones. Nature 277:234–236
3. Ben-Ari Y, Dingledine R, Kanazawa I, Kelly JS (1976) Inhibitory effects of acetylcholine on neurones in the feline nucleus reticularis thalami. J Physiol 261:647–671
4. Ben-Ari Y, Krnjević K, Reinhardt W (1979) Hippocampal seizures and failure of inhibition. Can J Physiol Pharmacol 57:1462–1466
5. Benjamin AM, Quastel JH (1975) Metabolism of amino acids and ammonia in rat brain cortex slices in vitro: a possible role of ammonia in brain function. J Neurochem 25:197–206
6. Bisti S, Iosif G, Strata P (1971) Suppression of inhibition in the cerebellar cortex by picrotoxin and bicuculline. Brain Res 28:591–593
7. Blomfield S (1974) Arithmetical operations performed by nerve cells. Brain Res 69:115–124
8. Bloom FE, Hoffer BJ, Siggins GR, Barker JL, Nicoll RA (1972) Effects of serotonin on central neurons: microiontophoretic administration. Fed Proc 31:97–106
9. Bowery NG, Hill DL, Hudson AL, Dogle A, Middlemiss DN, Shaw J, Turnball M (1980) (–) Baclofen decreases transmitter release in the mammalian CNS by an action at a novel GABA receptor. Nature 283:92–94
10. Bührle Ch Ph, Richter DW, Sonnhof U (1978) The action of glutamate upon the motoneurone membrane investigated by measuring extra- and intracellular ion activities. J Physiol 294:44–45P
11. Chan-Palay V (1975) Fine structure of labelled axons in the cerebellar cortex and nuclei of rodents and primates after intraventricular infusions with tritiated serotonin. Anat Embryol 148:235–265
12. Chujo T, Yamada Y, Yamamoto C (1975) Sensitivity of Purkinje cell dendrites to glutamic acid. Exp Brain Res 23:293–300
13. Crawford JM, Curtis DR, Voorhoeve PE, Wilson VJ (1966) Acetylcholine sensitivity of cerebellar neurones in the cat. J Physiol 186:139–165
14. Crossland J, Mitchell JF (1956) The effect on the electrical activity of the cerebellum of a substance present in cerebellar extracts. J Physiol 132:391–405
15. Crossland J, Woodruff GN, Mitchell JF (1964) Identity of the cerebellar factor. Nature 203:1388–1389
16. Curtis DR, Duggan AW, Felix D (1970) GABA and inhibition of Deiters' neurones. Brain Res 23:117–120
17. Curtis DR, Felix D (1971) The effect of bicuculline upon synaptic inhibition in the cerebral and cerebellar cortices of the cat. Brain Res 34:301–321
18. Diamond J, Roper S (1973) Analysis of Mauthner cell responses to iontophoretically delivered pulses of GABA, glycine and L-glutamate. J Physiol 232:113–128
19. Dichter MA (1980) Physiological identification of GABA as the inhibitory transmitter for mammalian cortical neurons in cell culture. Brain Res 190:111–121
20. Dreifuss JJ, Kelly JS, Krnjević K (1969) Cortical inhibition and γ-aminobutyric acid. Exp Brain Res 9:137–154
21. Dunlap K, Fischbach GD (1978) Neurotransmitters decrease the calcium component of sensory nerve action potentials. Nature 276:837–839
22. Dupont JL, Crepel F, Delhaye-Bouchaud N (1979) Influence of bicuculline and picrotoxin on reversal properties of excitatory synaptic potentials in cerebellar Purkinje cells of the rat. Brain Res 173:577–580
23. Eccles JC (1964) The physiology of synapses. Springer, Berlin Heidelberg New York
24. Eccles JC (1969) The inhibitory pathways of the central nervous system. Charles C Thomas, Springfield
25. Eccles JC, Ito M, Szentagothai J (1967) The cerebellum as a neuronal machine. Springer, Berlin Heidelberg New York

26. Eccles JC, Llinás R and Sasaki K (1966) The excitatory synaptic action of climbing fibres on the Purkinje cells of the cerebellum. J Physiol 182:268–296
27. Edwards C, Kuffler SW (1959) The blocking effect of γ-aminobutyric acid (GABA) and the action of related compounds on single nerve cells. J Neurochem 4:19–30
28. Emson PC (1979) Peptides as neurotransmitter candidates in the mammalian CNS. Progr Neurobiol 13:61–116
29. Engberg I, Flatman JA, Lambert JDC (1979) The actions of excitatory amino acids on motoneurones in the feline spinal cord. J Physiol 288:227–261
30. Faber DS, Korn H (1980) Single-shot channel activation accounts for duration of inhibitory postsynaptic potentials in a central neuron. Science 208:612–614
31. Fahn S (1976) Regional distribution studies on GABA and other putative neurotransmitters and their enzymes. In: Roberts E, Chase TN, Tower DB (eds) GABA in nervous system function. Raven, New York, pp 169–186
32. Feldberg W, Vogt M (1948) Acetylcholine synthesis in different regions of the central nervous system. J Physiol 107:372–381
33. Fonnum F, Storm-Mathisen J, Walberg F (1979) Glutamate decarboxylase in inhibitory neurons. A study of the enzyme in Purkinje cell axons and boutons in the cat. Brain Res 20:259–275
34. Frederickson RCA, Neuss M, Morzorati SL, McBride WJ (1978) A comparison of the inhibitory effects of taurine and GABA on identified Purkinje cells and other neurons in the cerebellar cortex of the rat. Brain Res 145:117–126
35. Fuxe K, Hökfelt T, Ungerstedt U (1970) Morphological and functional aspects of central monoamine neurons. Int Rev Neurobiol 13:93–126
36. Geller HM, Woodward DJ (1974) Responses of cultured cerebellar neurons to iontophoretically applied aminoacids. Brain Res 74:67–80
37. Hackett JT, Hou SM, Cochran SL (1979) Glutamate and synaptic depolarization of Purkinje cells evoked by parallel fibers and by climbing fibers. Brain Res 170:377–380
38. Hebb CO, Silver A (1956) Choline acetylase in the central nervous system of man and some other animals. J Physiol 134:718–728
39. Hökfelt T, Fuxe K (1969) Cerebellar monoamine nerve terminals, a new type of afferent fibers to the cortex cerebelli. Exp Brain Res 9:63–72
40. Hökfelt T, Ljungdahl A (1972) Autoradiographic identification of cerebral and cerebellar cortical neurons accumulating labelled gamma-aminobutyric acid (^{3}H-GABA). Exp Brain Res 14:354–362
41. Israel M, Whittaker VP (1965) The isolation of mossy fibre endings from the granular layer of the cerebellar cortex. Experientia 21:325–327
42. Ito M (1976) Roles of GABA neurons in integrated functions of the vertebrate CNS. In: Roberts E, Chase TN, Tower DB (eds) GABA in nervous system function. Raven, New York, pp 427–448
43. Ito M, Nisimaru N, Shibuki K (1979) Destruction of inferior olive induces rapid depression in synaptic action of cerebellar Purkinje cells. Nature 277:568–569
44. Ito M, Yoshida M (1966) The origin of cerebellar-induced inhibition of Deiters' neurones. I. Monosynaptic initiation of the inhibitory postsynaptic potentials. Exp Brain Res 2:330–349
45. Johnson JL (1978) The excitant aminoacids glutamic and aspartic acid as transmitter candidates in the vertebrate central nervous system. Progr Neurobiol 10:155–202
46. Johnston GAR (1978) Amino acid receptors. In: Smythies JR, Bradley RJ (eds) Receptors in pharmacology. Dekker, New York, pp 295–333
47. Kan KSK, Chao LP, Eng LF (1978) Immunohistochemical localization of choline acetyltransferase in rabbit spinal cord and cerebellum. Brain Res 146:221–229
48. Kasa P, Silver A (1965) The correlation between choline acetyltransferase and acetylcholinesterase activity in different areas of the cerebellum of rat and guinea pig. J Neurochem 16:389–396
49. Kawamura H, Provini L (1970) Depression of cerebellar Purkinje cells by microiontophoretic application of GABA and related amino acids. Brain Res 24:293–304
50. Kehoe J (1975) Electrogenic effects of neutral amino acids on neurons of *Aplysia Californica.* Cold Spring Harbor Symp Quant Biol 40:145–155

51. Krnjević K (1965) Transmitters in the cerebral cortex. Proc 23rd Int Congr Physiol Sci, Tokyo. Lectures and Symposia, pp 435–443. Int Congress Series 87. Excerpta Medica Foundation, Amsterdam, New York
52. Krnjević K, Morris ME (1976) Input-output relation of transmission through cuneate nucleus. J Physiol 257:791–815
53. Krnjević K, Phillis JW (1963) Iontophoretic studies of neurones in the mammalian cerebral cortex. J Physiol 165:274–304
54. Krnjević K, Puil E, Werman R (1977) GABA and glycine actions on spinal motoneurons. Can J Physiol Pharmacol 55:658–669
55. Krnjević K, Pumain R, Renaud L (1971) The mechanism of excitation by acetylcholine in the cerebral cortex. J Physiol 215:247–268
56. Krnjević K, Randic M, Straughan DW (1965) Ergothioneine and central neurones. Nature 205:603–604
57. Krnjević K, Reiffenstein RJ, Ropert N (1981) Disinhibitory action of acetylcholine in the hippocampus. Neuroscience 6:2465–2474
58. Larramendi LMH, Victor T (1967) Synapses on the Purkinje cell spines in the mouse. An electron microscopic study. Brain Res 5:15–30
59. Levy RA (1977) The role of GABA in primary afferent depolarization. Progr Neurobiol 9:211–267
60. McCance I, Phillis JW (1968) Cholinergic mechanisms in the cerebellar cortex. Int J Neuropharmacol 7:447–462
61. McLaughlin BJ, Wood JG, Saito K, Barber R, Vaughn JE, Roberts E, Wu JW (1974) The fine structural localization of glutamate decarboxylase in synaptic terminals of rodent cerebellum. Brain Res 76:377–391
62. Moises HC, Woodward DJ (1980) Potentiation of GABA inhibitory action in cerebellum by locus coeruleus stimulation. Brain Res 182:327–344
63. Nadi NS, Kanter D, McBride WJ, Aprison MH (1977) Effects of 3-acetylpyridine on several putative neurotransmitter amino acids in the cerebellum and medulla of the rat. J Neurochem 28:661–662
64. Nadi NS, McBride WJ, Aprison MH (1977) Distribution of several amino acids in regions of the cerebellum of the rat. J Neurochem 28:453–455
65. Nistri A, Constanti A (1979) Pharmacological characterization of different types of GABA and glutamate receptors in vertebrates and invertebrates. Prog in Neurobiol 13:117–235
66. Obata K, Ito M, Ochi R, Sato N (1967) Pharmacological properties of the postsynaptic inhibition by Purkinje cell axons and the action of γ-aminobutyric acid on Deiters' neurones. Exp Brain Res 4:43–57
67. Obata K, Otsuka M, Tanaka Y (1970) Determination of γ-aminobutyric acid in single nerve cells of cat central nervous system. J Neurochem 17:697–698
68. Obata K, Takeda K (1969) Release of γ-aminobutyric acid into the fourth ventricle induced by stimulation of the cat's cerebellum. J Neurochem 16:1043–1047
69. Obata K, Takeda K, Shinozaki H (1970) Further study on pharmacological properties of the cerebellar-induced inhibition of Deiters' neurones. Exp Brain Res 11:237–342
70. Okada Y, Shimada C (1976) Gamma-aminobutyric acid (GABA) concentration in a single neuron – localization in Deiters' neuron. Brain Res 107:658–662
71. Okamoto K, Quastel DMJ, Quastel JH (1976) Action of amino acids and convulsants on cerebellar spontaneous action potentials *in vitro:* effects of deprivation of Cl^-, K^+ or Na^+. Brain Res 113:147–158
72. Olsen L, Fuxe K (1971) On the projections from the locus coerulus noradrenaline neurons: the cerebellar innervation. Brain Res 28:165–171
73. Perry TL, Currier RD, Hansen S, MacLean J (1977) Aspartate-taurine imbalance in dominantly inherited olivoponto cerebellar atrophy. Neurology 27:257–261
74. Phillis JW (1968) Acetylcholinesterase in the feline cerebellum. J Neurochem 15:691–698
75. Rea, MA, McBride WJ, Rohde BH (1980) Regional and synaptosomal levels of amino acid neurotransmitters in the 3-acetylpyridine deafferentated cat cerebellum. J Neurochem 34:1106–1108

76. Ribak CE, Vaughn JE, Saito K (1978) Immunocytochemical localization of glutamic acid decarboxylase in neuronal somata following colchicine inhibition of axonal transport. Brain Res 140:315–332
77. Roberts E, Chase TN, Tower DB (eds) (1976) GABA in nervous system function, vol 5. Raven, New York
78. Roffler-Tarlov S, Beart PM, O'Gorman S, Sidman RL (1979) Neurochemical and morphological consequences of axon terminal degeneration in cerebellar deep nuclei of mice with inherited Purkinje cell degeneration. Brain Res 168:75–95
79. Roffler-Tarlov S, Sidman RL (1978) Concentrations of glutamic acid in cerebellar cortex and deep nuclei of normal mice and weaver, staggerer and nervous mutants. Brain Res 142:269–283
80. Rohde BH, Rea MA, Simon JR, McBride WJ (1979) Effects of X-irradiation induced loss of cerebellar granule cells on the synaptosomal levels and the high affinity uptake of amino acids. J Neurochem 32:1431–1435
81. Siggins GR, Oliver AP, Hoffer BJ, Bloom FE (1971) Cyclic adenosine monophosphate and norepinephrine: effects on trans-membrane properties of cerebellar Purkinje cells. Science 171:192–194
82. Silver A (1967) Cholinesterases of the central nervous system with special reference to the cerebellum. Int Rev Neurobiol 10:57–109
83. Stone TW (1979) Selective antagonism of amino acids by α-aminoadipate on pyramidal tract neurones but not Purkinje cells. Brain Res 166:217–220
84. Storm-Mathisen J (1975) High affinity uptake of GABA in presumed GABAergic nerve endings in rat brain. Brain Res 84:409–427
85. Takeuchi A, Takeuchi N (1962) Electrical changes in pre- and post-synaptic axons of the giant synapse of *Loligo*. J Gen Physiol 45:1181–1193
86. Wojtowicz JM, Marshall KC, Hendelman WJ (1980) Electrophysiological and pharmacological studies of the inhibitory projection from the cerebellar cortex to the deep cerebellar nuclei in tissue culture. Neuroscience 3:607–618
87. Woodward DJ, Hoffer BJ, Siggins GR, Oliver AP (1971) Inhibition of Purkinje cells in the frog cerebellum. II. Evidence for GABA as the inhibitory transmitter. Brain Res 33:91–100
88. Woodward DJ, Moises HC, Waterhouse BD, Hoffer BJ, Freedman R (1979) Modulatory actions of norepinephrine in the central nervous system. Fed Proc 38:2109–2116
89. Yamamoto C (1967) Pharmacologic studies of norepinephrine, acetylcholine and related compounds on neurons in Deiters nucleus and the cerebellum. J Pharmacol Exp Ther 156:39–47
90. Young AB, Oster-Granite ML, Herndon RM, Snyder SH (1974) Glutamaic acid: selective depletion by viral induced granule cell loss in hamster cerebellum. Brain Res 73:1–13

Discussion

Marshall: In our culture system we studied one pathway, particularly in relation to GABA transmission, the projection of Purkinje cells to the deep cerebellar nuclei. In reference to the question of selectivity of the blockers brought about by Dr. Krnjević. Here is one slide showing with extracellular recording the correlates of the intracellular recordings I presented on Thursday. If you record from a deep cerebellar nuclear cell and obtain the rate of firing, when you apply GABA you get a strong depression of the activity of the cell. You see the rebound that Dr. Krnjević mentioned also. Application of glycine, always in higher doses, will give a similar depression. If we stimulate the cortical region electrically, a depression of the rate of glycine ensues with return to the control or higher values later. With bicuculline usually at 5–10 μM, one gets a selective depression of the GABA inhibition but not of the glycine inhibition. One obtains a block of the electrical inhibition as well, at least the negative inhibition. This selectivity of bicuculline with respect to the GABA versus glycine inhibition holds true only for concentrations up to 10 μM. Above this concentration the glycine inhibition will also be affected. The same is true for picrotoxin in doses of up the 10 μM or slightly more. One should also remember that with iontophoretic applications in situ it is very difficult to titrate the dose. We had the blocking solution in the culture bath so we had an absolute knowledge of the concentration of the blocker. With this sensitivity to dosage and selectivity, it is hazardous to draw conclusions from the iontophoretic experiments. I wish also to point out that this is one of the few cases where this pathway has been studied directly. Most previous studies were done on the projection of the cerebellar cortex to the lateral vestibular nucleus where the target cells are larger. So another advantage of the cerebellar explant culture is that you can test directly intracerebellar connections.

In a small number of cells strychnine would block both the inhibition and selectively the glycine action without affecting the GABA effect. This could be related to the effects of bath application or could indicate some peculiarities of some of the receptors of these neurons.

Krnjevic: Was the inhibition blocked by both bicuculline and strychnine?

Marshall: Yes!

Korn: Do you imply that the same receptors could be involved?

Marshall: I am not sure. It is possible. If taurine or β-alanine receptors were involved they can be blocked by either GABA-blockers or glycine-blockers. We do not have the definitive explanation.

Eccles: In 1956 Grundfest and Purpura were trying the effect of strychnine on the cerebellum because we had shown that it blocks inhibition. In finding no effect of strychnine, they concluded that there is no inhibition in the cerebellum. So we had to come back and use picrotoxin showing that there are other kinds of inhibition. Obviously, there are traps in the pharmacology! Another point to remember is that it has been shown that there are depolarizing IPSPs in the dendrites of the hippocampus, which probably are due to excess chloride in the dendrites compared to the reduced chloride in the cell bodies.

Krnjevic: Per Andersen also had similar findings in the hippocampal slice. He could not be completely sure whether this was due only to excess chloride in the dendrites or to a small sodium component which was being activated as well.

Balazs: Turning to the evidence of glutamate as the parallel fiber transmitter, I think that the biochemistry in this respect is still quite inconclusive. There have been conflicting reports on the effects of applied glutamate. The best evidence remains that release of endogenous glutamate is diminished in the agranular cerebellum.

With respect to the cholinergic system, at least in rat, during ontogenesis there is an enormous amount of CAT-activity and muscarinic cholinergic receptors that subsequently subside. I think that the possibility that ACh activity is concentrated in certain parts of the cerebellum is very much open.

Krnjevic: Cholinergic functions are very hard to pin down. As you know, AchE pattern in the cerebellum of different animals varies considerably and it is very difficult to make sense of it. In kittens the staining seems to accompany the migrating granule cells. The functions of this enzyme remain uncertain.
Balazs: I think it is more interesting to concentrate on what happens to CAT, as with this enzyme one obtains more meaningful results.

Neurotransmitters and Receptors in the Cerebellum: Immunocytochemical Localization of Glutamic Acid Decarboxylase, GABA-Transaminase, and Cyclic GMP and Autoradiography with ^{3}H-Muscimol

V. Chan-Palay

GABA Pathways in the Cerebellum Studied by Retrograde and Anterograde Transport of GAD Antibody After In Vivo Injections

Gamma aminobutyric acid (GABA) is an inhibitory neurotransmitter in the mammalian central nervous system, and deficits of GABA have been implicated in certain neurologic and psychiatric disorders, such as Huntington's chorea, Parkinson's disease, and schizophrenia. Considerable interest attaches to the identification of GABA-containing neurons and receptor sites for GABA. Although cells and processes with GABA-synthesizing enzymes and with GABA-uptake systems have been identified morphologically [9, 35, 42, 47], the receptor binding sites for GABA have been visualized only recently in various parts of the central nervous system at the light- and electron-microscope level and also in cultures of the mammalian spinal cord ([10, 11, 12, 16, 18] see Figs. 1 a, b).

The present investigations extend the applications of a new technique for the retrograde and anterograde tracing of chemically specific pathways by the injection of specific, characterized antibodies directly into the central or peripheral nervous system ([12, 13], see Fig. 1 c). A specific antibody can be used to localize and to identify neurons known to contain the antigen in the live animal by in vivo injections directly into nervous tissue. The method allows localization of a putative transmitter molecule in the central and peripheral nervous system without the use of agents such as colchicine, which are necessary in most experiments that apply the primary antibody onto fixed tissue. The antigen-antibody complex is largely associated with lysosomal or prelysosomal particles in the somatic cytoplasm, and such complexes mark the dendritic and axonal processes of Substance P (SP) immunoreactive cells. Further, the antigen-antibody complexes are carried by axoplasmic flow in retrograde or anterograde directions and therefore the method can be adapted for use in tracing chemically specific pathways.

Glutamic acid decarboxylase (GAD) is the enzyme that converts glutamic acid to GABA; GAD has been isolated and purified from mouse brain and its properties extensively characterized [41, 61, 62, 63]. Antibodies specific to GAD have been obtained for immunocytochemical studies [48, 59, 61]. These antibodies have been applied to fixed tissue sections in order to detect GAD in the brain. In the mammalian cerebellum, GAD immunoreactivity has already been localized to stellate, basket, and Golgi cells and their processes [1, 42, 60] and to Purkinje-cell somata after treatment with colchicine [47]. Other his-

Experimental Brain Research, Suppl. 6

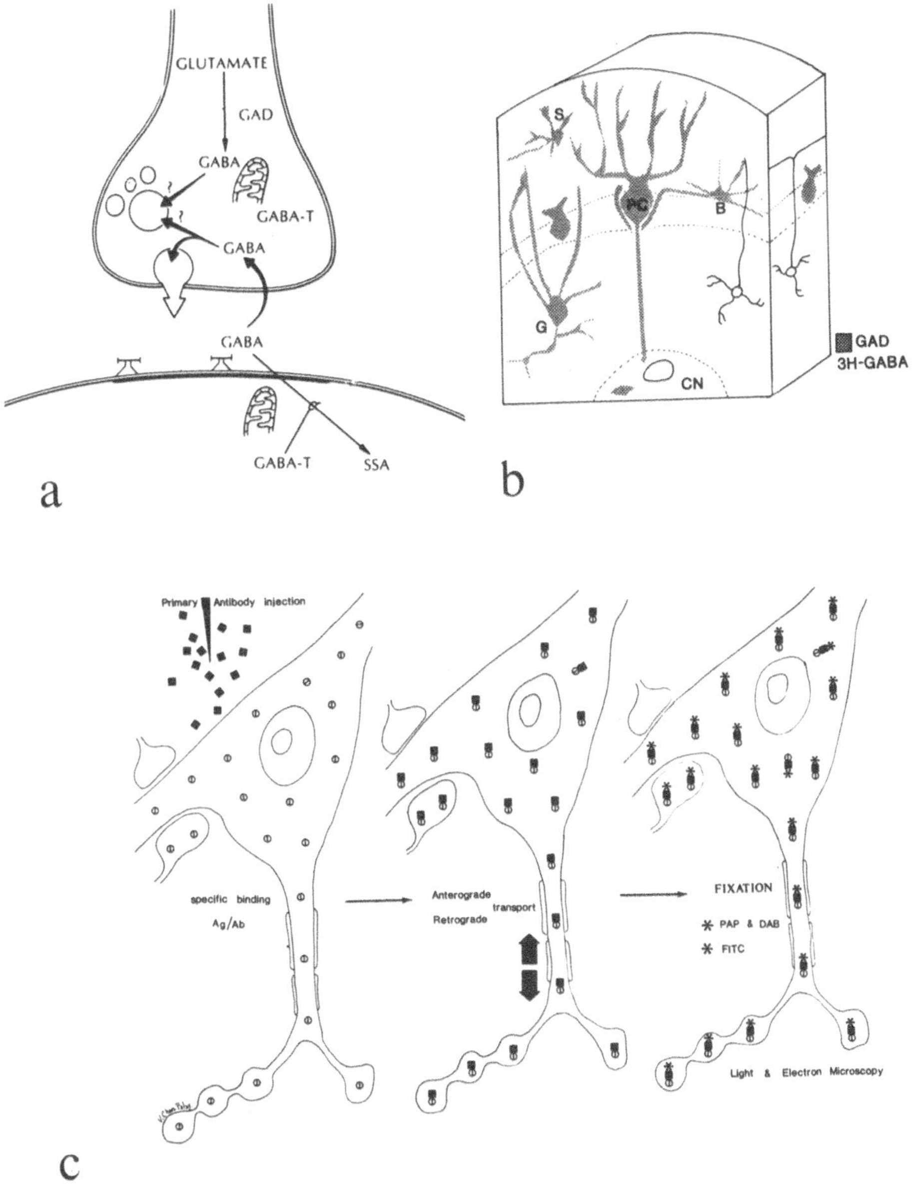

Fig. 1. **a** Schematic diagram to show the synthesis and metabolism of GABA. **b** The cerebellar cortical and nuclear neurons with GAD immunoreactivity and uptake capacities for ^{3}H-GABA are indicated by *stippling*. These are the stellate (*S*), basket (*B*), Purkinje (*PC*), Golgi (*G*) cells of the cortex, and some small neurons in the deep cerebellar nuclei (*CN*). **c** Schematic diagram to summarize the steps involved in chemically specific labeling by in vivo injection of the primary antibody. Primbary antibody molecules are indicated by *black squares;* antigen molecules (or precursor molecules) are indicated by *circles;* subsequent immunocytochemical labels are indicated by *asterisks*

tochemical studies with ^{3}H-GABA uptake [40], GABA-transaminase immunoreactivity [1, 18], and ^{3}H-muscimol have strengthened the evidence for GABA as a transmitter in most of the intracortical cerebellar neurons (except for granule cells and Lugaro cells) and some neurons of the deep cerebellar nuclei [1, 9, 10, 11, 18].

Up to the present time GAD immunoreactivity has been found to be confined to neuronal sites and is not apparently found in neuroglia. In a series of recent experiments, a characterized antibody against GAD was used to study the reciprocal pathways in the cerebellum [18]. These studies validated the known corticonuclear projections from Purkinje cells to the deep cerebellar nuclei and vestibular nuclei by utilizing chemically specific transport of GAD antigen-antibody complexes in the anterograde and retrograde directions, and investigated the chemical nature of the nucleo-cortical pathways recently demonstrated to run between the deep cerebellar nuclei and the cortex [9, 33, 56].

Experiments were designed to label GAD-containing neurons, particularly the Purkinje cells, and to study the transport of GAD antigen-antibody complexes in anterograde transport from the cerebellar cortex to the corresponding underlying deep cerebellar nucleus, as well as retrograde transport of the tracer from cerebellar cortical terminals to the deep nuclei. Multiple doses of 0.025 μl of undiluted antibody were ejected by pressure from a glass micropipette [9, 12, 13] into the cerebellar cortical surface less than 0.1–0.5 mm deep into the brains of rats. Single amounts of 0.01 μl were injected into the dentate nucleus and care was taken to avoid leakage of the label into the overlying cortex and to secure as small an injection site as possible, confined within the boundaries of the dentate nucleus. A dorsal posterior approach through the occipital cortex was used to avoid damaging the cerebellar cortex as much as possible. These injections were intended to label dentate neurons by means of immunoreactivity to GAD and to examine the transport of GAD antigen-antibody complexes from the dentate nucleus to Purkinje cells in the cortex.

Controls were carried out by injecting undiluted preimmune sera in equal volumes (0.025 μl) unilaterally into the vermis, simple lobule, and lateral hemispheres of the cerebellar cortex. In other control animals, colchicine, a drug that inhibits fast axonal transport [23], was given as a single intracisternal injection into the fourth ventricle (3 μg/μl; 10 μl/100 g body weight) 24 h prior to injections of GAD antibody into the cerebellum. These controls were intended (a) to alter the rate of retrograde and anterograde transport of GAD antigen-antibody complexes, and (b) to enhance the visualization of GAD immunoreactivity.

GAD was isolated and purified from mouse brain [60]. The purity of GAD preparations was established from the following experiments: (a) polyacrylamide gel electrophoresis, (b) high-speed sedimentation equilibrium in dilute buffer solution, in D_2O solution, and in guanidine HCl solution, and (c) sodium dodecyl sulfate polyacrylamide gel electrophoresis. Antiserum to GAD purified from mouse brain was produced in rabbits by biweekly injections of 50 μg of the decarboxylase in complete Freund's adjuvant into the infrascapular muscles. The rabbits were bled 1 week after the fourth injections, and the GAD antiserum was characterized by enzyme inhibition test, immunodiffusion test, microcomplement fixation test, and immunoelectrophoresis as previously described [48, 59, 60]. Preimmune and/or normal rabbit sera served as controls. Antibody against GAD was used undiluted throughout these studies. Three separate batches of antibody against GAD were tested; each produced equivalent results. Pilot studies with sera diluted at 1 : 10, 1 : 50, and 1 : 100 showed less intense and less reliable results. On the basis of previous experience with in vivo injections of SP antibodies into the rat medulla, the technique for tissue preparation was standardized and used as described previously [12, 13].

After survival times of 1, 2, 4, 24, and 48 h, tissues from the separate groups of animals were examined in order to evaluate (a) the initial size of the injection, (b) the rate of regression of the injection site, and (c) the GAD immunoreactivity obtained in cells and terminals at various times after injection. Optimal results as judged by the number and intensity of cells and terminals labeled at the injection site, after anterograde and retrograde transport of GAD, were obtained from animals with postinjection survival times of 2–4 h.

The animals were fixed by perfusion through the heart [9, 45]. The animals were anesthetized with ether for the perfusion and maintained under artificial respiration through a tracheotomy tube with a mixture of 95% oxygen and 5% carbon dioxide. The blood was washed out with cold Ca^{2+}-free Tyrode's buffer (50 ml at 4 °C), followed immediately with cold 4% formaldehyde in 0.2 M phosphate buffer, pH 7.4 (500 ml at 4 °C) for 20 min. Throughout, the animal was immersed in ice. Following perfusion the brain was dissected from the skull and soaked in fresh fixative. The optimum duration of this postperfusion fixation was 2 h; then the entire cerebellum was sectioned on a freezing microtome or in a cryostat. Through the region of the injection site and the deep cerebellar nuclei and vestibular nuclei, all sections were saved and mounted in series.

Two light-microscopic immunocytochemical techniques were performed; the indirect immunofluorescence method of Coons [20] and the peroxidase-antiperoxidase (PAP) method of Sternberger [55]. Immunofluorescence studies were conducted on coronal serial sections through the cerebellum and brainstem on a cryostat (Dittes, −20 °C), 10 μm thick, or on a freezing microtome, 30 μm thick. The sections were mounted on chrome alum-gelatin-coated slides, treated directly with goat anti-rabbit immunoglobulin (IgG) conjugated to fluorescein isothiocyanate (FITC), and the coverslips were mounted in buffer-glycerol (3:1 v/v). No other application of primary antibody was used [12, 13]. Sections were examined with a Zeiss fluorescence microscope fitted with epi-illumination.

More permanent preparations were obtained by using the PAP technique. Coronal sections through the injection sites in the cerebellar cortex and the deep cerebellar nuclei were cut serially, 20–25 μm thick, on a Vibratome. The sections were treated with goat anti-rabbit IgG (1:10 in 0.05 M Tris buffer, Triton X 100 0.5%, room temperature, 30 min), then with rabbit PAP followed by a reaction with 0.022% diaminobenzidine (DAB) in the presence of 0.03% H_2O_2. No further application of primary antibody was introduced [12, 13]. The sections were mounted on chrome alum-gelatin-coated slides, counterstained lightly with 0.5% cresyl violet, and the coverslips were mounted in Permount for examination by light- or darkfield microscopy.

The injection sites of GAD antibody were readily located in the cerebellum by either immunofluorescence or the PAP method. In cerebellar cortical folia injected discretely with 0.025 µl of undiluted GAD antibody, only neuronal elements were found to be immunoreactive. The neurons most intensely reactive were Purkinje cells (Fig. 1 a, b) with intense label in their perikarya and less label in their dendrites. Sections parallel to the Purkinje-cell layer (Fig. 1 a) showed that even within the injection site all Purkinje cells did not exhibit the same level of immunoreactivity to GAD antibody. Some cells were intensely labeled (arrows) and others less so (crossed arrows), and still others in between these were not GAD immunoreactive at all. This observation brings up several questions: (a) Does this patchy labeling of Purkinje cells reflect deficiencies in the sensitivity of the GAD antibody or in the method of displaying it? Similar results were obtained with three different samples of GAD antibodies. (b) Does the patchy labeling reflect the biology of the Purkinje cells? Is it possible that not all Purkinje cells contain GABA and GAD immunoreactivity? (c) Does the GABA content of Purkinje cells undergo cycles so that GAD and therefore GAD immunoreactivity is present in low and barely detectable levels at certain phases in the cell's life? This question is made more pointed by the fact that blockers of fast axonal transport effectively raised intensities of GAD immunoreactivity in material obtained after in vivo injections (Chan-Palay, unpublished data) as well as in material prepared according to the more conventional postfixation immunocytochemical methods [47], but do not increase the numbers of labeled cells.

The other cerebellar cortical elements labeled by GAD antibody at the injection site included many stellate and basket cells of the molecular layer, Golgi cells in the granular layer, and the dendrites and axons belonging to these

Fig. 2 a–f. Comparison of the injection sites in cerebellar cortex 4 h after injections with 0.025 µl undiluted GAD antibody **(a, c)** and preimmune control sera **(b, d).** Immunofluorescence, 10-µm sections. **a** Photomicrograph of a section through the Purkinje-cell layer showing neuronal somata, excluding nuclei, intensely labeled by GAD immunoreactivity (*arrows*), others lightly GAD labeled (*crossed arrows*) and still others not reactive at all in between. ×200. **b** Photomicrograph through the Purkinje-cell layer (*PC*) and granular layers (*gr l*) of the cerebellar cortex showing unlabeled Purkinje-cell somata (*arrows*) surrounded by intense nonspecific fluorescence with control preimmune sera in Golgi epithelial neuroglial cells (*double arrows*). Nonspecifically labeled protoplasmic and velate astrocytes of the granular layer surround unlabeled granule cells (*crossed arrows*). ×200. **c** Coronal section through the molecular (*mol*), Purkinje-cell (*PC*), and granule cell layers (*gr l*) of the cerebellar cortex showing intense GAD immunoreactivity in *PC* somata (*arrows*) and Golgi-cell somata, and light specific labeling in the neuropil of the granular and molecular layers. ×100. **d** Coronal section through the molecular layer (*mol*), Purkinje-cell layer (*PC*), and granule-cell layer (*gr l*) of the cerebellar cortex showing no label within the cerebellar neurons of Purkinje cells (*arrow*). Intense nonspecific staining is seen in two Golgi epithelial neuroglial cells and their processes (*crossed arrows*). ×100. **e** A group of GAD immunoreactive mossy-fiber rosettes (*crossed arrows*) and intervaricose segments (*arrows*) near the location of a GAD antibody injection into the cerebellar cortex. Immunofluorescence with FITC, 4 h postinjection survival. ×150. **f** Cerebellar dentate neurons after retrograde labeling by GAD immunoreactivity due to an injection of GAD antibody into the cortical lateral hemisphere. Intensely labeled neurons (*crossed arrows*) and moderately labeled neurons (*arrow*) intermingle with completely nonreactive ones. Vibratome section, 20 µm thick, immunofluorescence method, 4 h postinjection survival. ×60

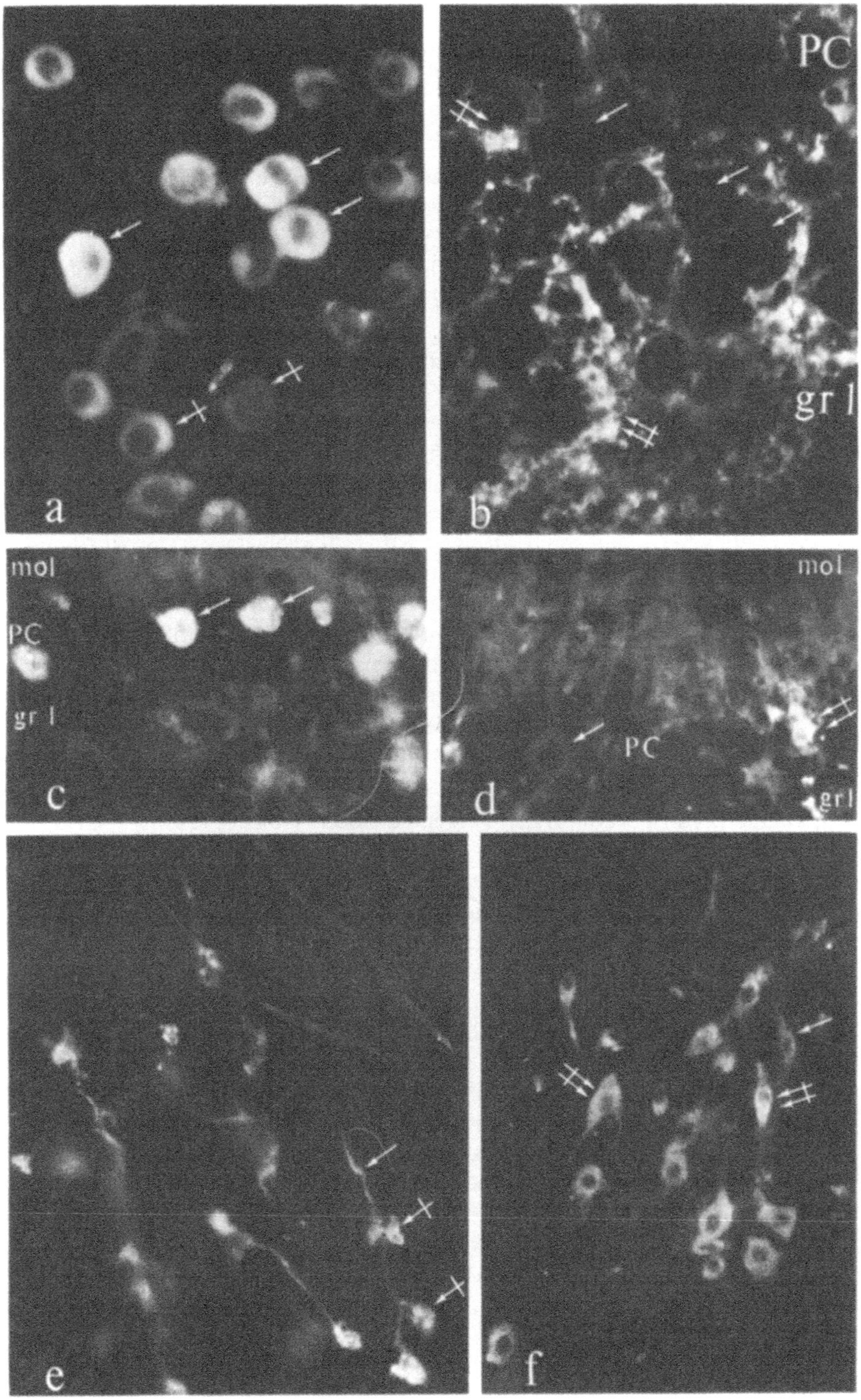
PC
gr l
a
b
mol
PC
gr l
c
mol
PC
d
grl
e
f

neurons throughout the cortex. Golgi axons surrounding glomeruli were also labeled, but not granule cells. A significant observation is that neuroglial cells were not GAD immunoreactive (see Fig. 2a, c; compare with Fig. 2b, d).
Control injections with preimmune sera provided different results (Fig. 2b, d). Within the injection sites no Purkinje, stellate, basket, Golgi, or granule cells were immunoreactive. Instead, intense nonspecific staining was found in neuroglial cells and their processes throughout the cortex (Fig. 2b, d). The cell bodies of the Golgi epithelial neuroglial cells (double arrows) between unstained Purkinje-cell somata (arrows) were intensely stained, as were their processes, the Bergmann fibers, in the molecular layer. Protoplasmic and velate astrocytes and their processes were also well stained and their veil-like sheets (Fig. 2b), crossed arrows) defined the spaces occupied by unreactive granule cells in the granule cell layer. Occasionally, entire single neuroglial cells were delineated by the uptake of injected preimmune sera (Fig. 2d, crossed arrows). A comparison of Fig. 2a, c with Fig. 2b, d shows the difference between GAD-specific immunoreactivity and nonspecific staining at the injection sites after in vivo injection of GAD antibody and preimmune sera, respectively.
Injections of GAD antibody into the dentate nucleus resulted in the labeling of approximately 5–10% of the neurons, mostly multipolar or fusiform cell bodies ranging between 8 μm and 14 μm in diameter. In the neuropil numerous boutons and fibers were also GAD immunoreactive and these were probably the processes of intrinsic dentate cells as well as terminals of Purkinje-cell axons from the cortex. Control injections with preimmune sera into the dentate nucleus did not label neurons; only neuroglial elements were stained, providing data corresponding to that already presented above for the cortex.

Anterograde Transport of GAD Antigen-Antibody Complexes (Fig. 3a)

Injections of GAD antibody into the cerebellar cortex produced two distinct forms of specific labeling in the deep cerebellar and vestibular nuclei. There was an anterograde corticonuclear transport of label from GAD-immunoreactive neurons. Since a vast literature shows that the major cortical projection GABA neuron is the Purkinje cell, the following description of the observations will presume that the GAD-immunoreactive anterograde transport path is the Purkinje-cell corticonuclear projection. A second, retrograde transport in the nucleocortical system also exists. Microinjections of GAD antibody unilaterally into the vermis on one side of the midline allowed anterograde transport into axons en route to the ipsilateral fastigial nucleus and consequent labeling of axons and terminal projectional fields of GAD-immunoreactive Purkinje cells. Corresponding injections into the paravermal cortex and simple lobule allowed specific immunoreactive labeling of projection axons and terminal fields in the anterior and posterior interpositus complex and a small lateral portion of the fastigius nucleus. Injections into the folia of the lateral hemisphere (e.g., in Cruss II) produced specific GAD-immunoreactive labeling of axons en route to their terminal projections in the dentate nucleus and neighboring lateral portions of the interpositus nucleus. The GAD-immunoreactive axons were individually and discretely labeled so that each could be followed separately, and in fascicles, on their corticonuclear trajectory among unlabeled axons in the white matter. The arrangement of the projections of GAD-immunoreactive axons from Purkinje cells to deep cerebellar and vestibular nuclei conformed to the traditional topographic distribution patterns as described in detail for the cerebellum of many experimental species [6, 58]. These results are summarized schematically in Fig. 3 a. An example of a GAD-labeled injection site in the cortex (lobulus simplex), the axonal trajectory, and the terminal projection fields in the fastigius and interpositus nucleus are illustrated in Fig. 3 c.

The GAD-immunoreactive terminals of Purkinje cells labeled by in vivo injections in the cortex were observed in the ipsilateral cerebellar and lateral vestibular nuclei. The GAD-immunoreactive boutons and terminals, 1–4 μm in diameter, were found in the neuropil in large numbers directly applied to the somatic and dendritic surfaces (Fig. 3 d, arrows) of large and medium-sized neurons. The boutons were intensely labeled with dense grains that could be resolved with the oil-immersion lens in the light microscope. The GAD-immunoreactive boutons not directly applied against neuronal surfaces were found in groups (crossed arrow, Fig. 3 d) in the neuropil participating in nucleocortical connections. Conversely, injections of GAD antibody into the dentate nucleus also resulted in anterograde labeling which was detectable in approximately 25% of the cases studied. Small groups of mossy-fiber rosettes, intensely GAD immunoreactive, with labeled intervaricose segments were seen in the cerebellar cortex of the lateral hemispheres. These regions were not near or within the track of the injecting micropipette and were not likely artifacts of the injection itself. These GAD-immunoreactive mossy-fiber rosettes may be part of the projections of the dentatocortical mossy-fiber system (see Fig. 2 e). Nucleocortical axons that terminate as mossy fibers in a topographic manner have been described in a number of species [9, 56]. In addition, other investigators have contributed to establishing the presence and organization of nucleocortical projections by means of horseradish peroxidase (HRP) and amino acid autoradiography, without specifically defining the terminal formations [33, 34]. The present evidence suggests that some dentatocortical mossy fibers are GAD-containing and GABA-synthesizing as well.

Retrograde Transport of GAD Antigen-Antibody Complexes (Fig. 3 a)

Injections of GAD antibody into small, discrete zones of the cerebellar cortex produced GAD immunoreactive labeling of Purkinje, stellate, basket, and Golgi cells and their processes (see above), as well as intense GAD immunoreactivity in small groups of mossy-fiber rosettes and their intervaricose segments (Fig. 2 e). GAD immunoreactive mossy-fiber rosettes were not found in control tissues from animals injected with preimmune sera.

In the cases in which injections into the vermis or paravermal cortex resulted in GAD-immunoreactive mossy fibers, groups of diffusely labeled GAD-immunoreactive cells were found in the fastigius and interpositus nuclei, most

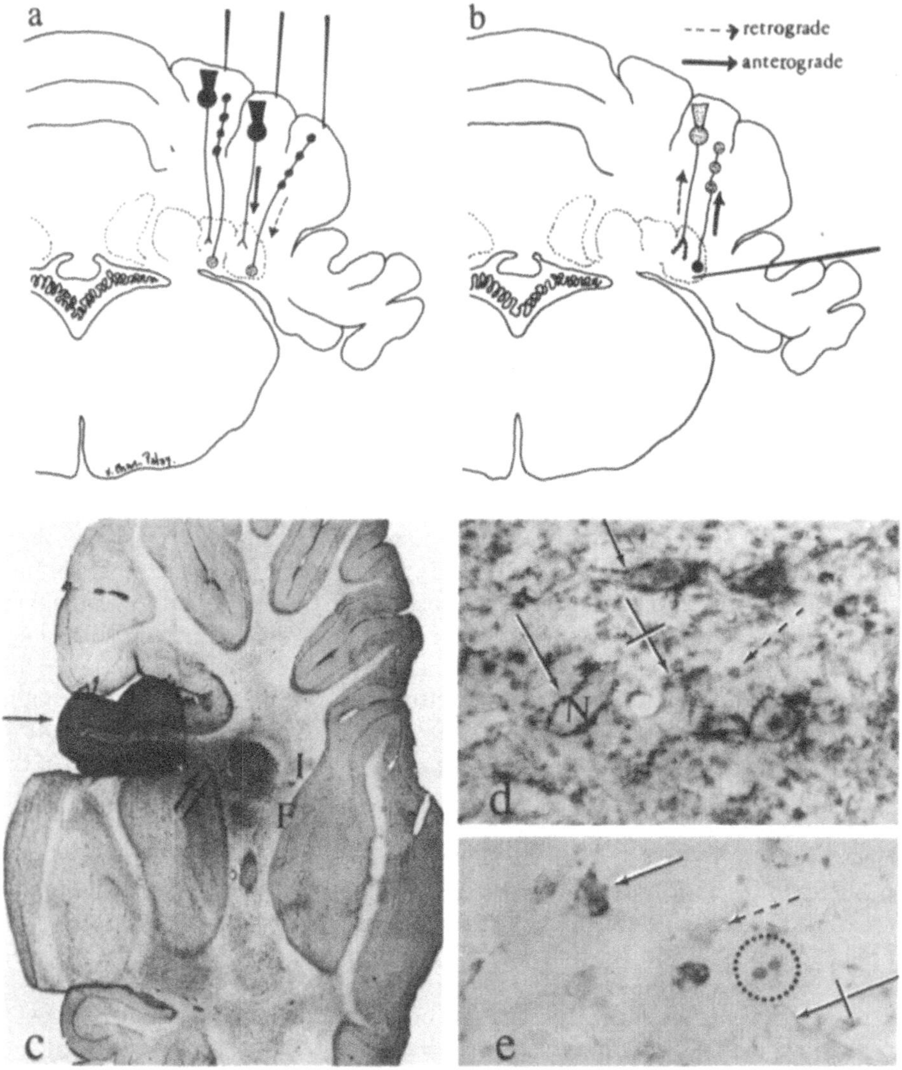

Fig. 3a–e. The results of anterograde and retrograde transport of GAD antigen-antibody complexes after in vivo injections of GAD antibody into the cerebellar cortex. The concepts of reciprocity and topographic GABA projections are illustrated in these tracings of corticonuclear and nucleocortical projections. **a** Unilateral injections of GAD antibody into the cerebellar cortex produce GAD-immunoreactive Purkinje cells (black), which project anterogradely and topographically to the ipsilateral dentate nucleus, indicated by numerous GAD-immunoreactive boutons. The GAD-immunoreactive mossy-fiber rosettes cause a diffuse labeling in smaller cerebellar nuclear neurons (stipple circles) via retrograde transport. **b** Unilateral injections of GAD antibody into the dentate nucleus produces a number of diffusely labeled Purkinje cells ipsilaterally (stipple) by retrograde transport. In the dentate nucleus, GAD-immunoreactive neurons (*black circles*) can effect labeling of small groups of mossy fibers in the overlying cerebellar cortex through anterograde axonal transport. Anterograde and retrograde transport in these systems does not appear to be inhibited by short-term application of colchicine. **c** Low-magnification photomicrograph to show injection sites of GAD antibody into the simple lobule on the right side (*arrow*) and the resulting labeled axonal tracts

commonly in the ventral posterior interpositus nucleus, in a thin band arranged above the roof of the fourth ventricle. These cells (Figs. 3e, 2f, arrows) were neuronal and not neuroglial. They measured 9–18 µm in diameter and were either multipolar or fusiform with labeled perikarya and dendrites (arrow). Compared with the remaining unlabeled neurons (crossed arrow) these GAD-labeled cells were small.

Injections of GAD antibody into the lateral hemisphere induced labeling in a small number of mossy fibers which transport GAD-immunoreactive material to cells in the dentate nucleus in accordance with its expected topography [9, 56]. These neurons were found in groups of 2 or 3 to 18. They were usually diffusely labeled in their perikaryal cytoplasm and denrites. The intensity of GAD immunoreactivity ranged from great (Fig. 2f, crossed arrows) to moderate (arrow) and they were surrounded by numerous unlabeled cells. These GAD-immunoreactive nucleocortical neurons ranged from 8 µm to 16 µm in diameter and were multipolar or fusiform. In some cases, these neurons occurred at the boundaries of the dentate nucleus, particularly within the rostral trabeculae [7]. Thus GAD-immunoreactive mossy-fiber rosettes and preterminal segments apparently transport the GAD antigen-antibody complexes retrogradely and in an ipsilateral and topographic order to their neurons of origin in the deep cerebellar nuclei.

Corticonuclear Projections (Fig. 3b)

Injections of GAD antibody into the dentate nucleus retrogradely labeled a small number of Purkinje cells in the overlying cerebellar cortex. The cells were identifiable as Purkinje cells because of their location in the cortex and the size of their somata. The GAD immunoreactivity was generally of low intensity and the cells were widely dispersed over the folium. This disposition may be due to (a) the small amounts of GAD antigen-antibody complexed accumulated in the

Fig. 3a–e (Continued). From cortex through the white matter (*double arrows*) to terminal projection fields in the ipsilateral fastigial nucleus (*F*) and interpositus nuclei (*I*) following a typical corticonuclear topographic distribution. Frozen section 30 µm, treated with the PAP technique and counterstained with thionin; 4 h postinjection survival. Coronal section. Control injections with preimmune sera show injection sites (see Fig. 2a, c) without transport or terminal field labeling. ×80. **d** Anterograde transport of GAD antigen-antibody complexes after a GAD antibody cortical injection. Photomicrograph of unreactive neurons (*N*) in the cerebellar dentate nucleus showing numerous dark GAD-immunoreactive terminals and boutons upon the dendritic and somatic surfaces (*arrows*). Other GAD-immunoreactive terminals are found in the neuropil (*crossed arrows*). Vibratome section, 20 µm thick, PAP technique, 4-h postinjection survival. The tissue has been lightly counterstained with cresyl violet to show non-GAD-reactive neurons and neuroglial cells (*broken arrow*) ×120. **e** Photomicrograph of neurons in the ventral posterior interpositus nucleus of the cerebellum labeled retrogradely after injection of GAD antibody into the cerebellar cortex. The labeled cells and dendrites (*arrow*) are usually smaller than the larger unlabeled ones (*crossed arrow*) and are readily differentiated from neuroglia (*circle*). Vibratome section 20 µm, 4 h postinjection survival, PAP method, lightly counterstained with cresyl violet to show non-GAD-immunoreactive neurons and neuroglia (*broken arrow*) ×200

Purkinje-cell body, (b) the fact that not all neighboring Purkinje cells project to the same cerebellar nuclear area [8], (c) the fact that the Purkinje cells in general are difficult to demonstrate reliably by morphological techniques for the localization of GABA mechanisms. Studies of ^{3}H-GABA uptake do not consistently reveal labeling of Purkinje cells in adult animals [40, 53]; GAD immunocytochemistry reveals Purkinje-cell somata irregularly [1] and more consistently if colchicine is applied. Similar observations have been made with studies using antibodies with GABA transaminase [18].

Colchicine

In experiments in which GAD antibody was injected into animals pretreated with colchicine, there was an apparent increase in the detectability of GAD immunoreactivity at injection sites and in terminal projection areas after retrograde and anterograde transport, with both immunofluorescence and the PAP method. Except for the enhanced levels of immunoreactivity, there was no difference in the localization or distribution of labeled cells and fibers. The increased intensity of immunoreactivity obtained indicates that colchicine treatment increased the accumulation of GAD antigen-antibody complexes in neurons and their processes, but it did not block fast axonal transport to the point of preventing the phenomena of retrograde and anterograde labeling. In general we suggest that experiments with antibody injections for afferent- and efferent-pathway tracing are best done without colchicine pretreatment. However, colchicine-pretreated controls, as used here, are necessary in order to determine whether any negative results obtained are due (a) to low sensitivity of the immunocytochemical detection method used and therefore reflect a technical inadequacy, or (b) to a genuine absence of afferent or efferent projections in the chemically specific system studied.

Specificity

Throughout these studies it has been accepted that detectable staining in neural structures by the purified, characterized GAD antibody indicates the presence of specific GAD-immunoreactive sites. Control studies with preimmune sera substantiate this by indicating no staining in the same neural structures in the absence of GAD-specific antibodies.

The control studies with preimmune sera injections into the cerebellum compared with injections of GAD antisera indicate that whereas anti-GAD sera bind specifically to neurons with previously demonstrated GAD and GABA-transaminase immunoreactivity, ^{3}H-GABA uptake, and ^{3}H-muscimol-GABA receptor binding properties, preimmune sera bind nonspecifically to non-neuronal sites. Small localized injections with the GAD antisera showed that immunoreactive neurons can bind and transport the antigen-antibody complex from cortex to nuclei or vice versa, but injections with preimmune control sera showed no comparable results. The present experiments indicate that when neurons in a specified location in the cerebellum are injected with GAD antiserum, the antigen-antibody complex can be detected in their projection targets or in cell bodies at more distant sites from the injection points. It is presumed that these complexes are transported to these sites in anterograde or retrograde fashion. No indication can be gained from these studies as to whether this process is one of active transport or of passive diffusion.

In conclusion, the present investigations utilized in vivo injections of antibody against GAD to demonstrate reciprocal projections within the cerebellum between cortex and nuclei. Based upon the retrograde and anterograde transport of GAD antigen-antibody complexes taken up from the injection site, these studies indicate that known corticonuclear and nucleocortical projections within the cerebellum can be confirmed. In addition, this technique imparts important information on the chemical specificity of these pathways and suggests that some of the nucleocortical projections are GABA-containing. The method promises to be a significant means for investigation of chemically specific connections in the central and peripheral nervous systems.

Immunocytochemical Localization of GABA Transaminase at Cellular and Ultrastructural Levels

There is considerable interest in the identification of cellular sites of the biosynthesis [42, 43] and metabolism of GABA. Localization of GABA transaminase (GABA-Tase; 4-aminobutyrate: 2-oxoglutarate aminotransferase), an enzyme involved in GABA degradation, has been attempted by histochemical stains [36, 57], by light-microscope and by electron-microscope immunocytochemistry [1, 13]. In our experiments we employed the indirect immunofluorescence method [20], and the PAP method [55] for light and electron microscopy. The GABA-Tase was purified from mouse brain and its purity was established by gel electrophoresis, high-speed sedimentation equilibrium in dilute buffer, deuterium oxide, and guanidine hydrochloride solution, and polyacrylamide gel electrophoresis as described by others [50, 51, 61]. Antisera to GABA-Tase were produced in rabbits by weekly infrascapular injections of 30 μg of enzyme in complete Freund's adjuvant; serum was collected after the fourth injection. The GABA-Tase antisera were characterized by immunodiffusion microcomplement fixation and immunoelectrophoresis as described [48, 51, 59, 61]. The GABA-Tase antisera were used at dilutions of 1:100 or 1:200, and normal rabbit preimmune sera served as the controls for cytochemical specificity in light- and electron-microscope studies.

In the molecular layer, numerous stellate- and basket-cell somata (greater than 80%) were immunoreactive. The neuroglial somata surrounding Purkinje cells and their radial fibers [45] displayed the most intense reaction. Purkinje-cell somata were unreactive when glutaraldehyde was present in the fixative, but appeared as single immunoreactive cells or as groups of up to 10 or 12 immunoreactive cells when formaldehyde was used alone or after colchicine treatment, respectively (Fig. 4a, b). These results indicate that the content of

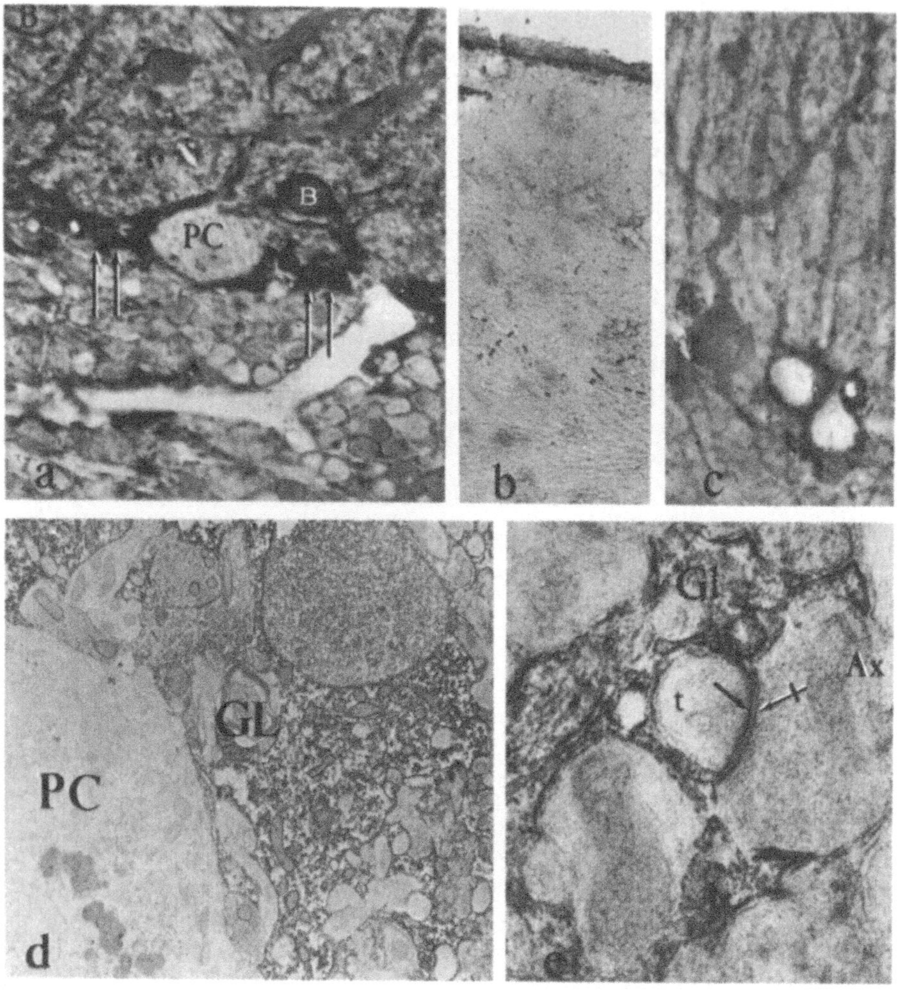

Fig. 4a–e. Light micrographs (**a, b**) of cerebellar cortex with immunoreactive neuronal and neuroglial elements visualized by GABA-Tase antisera using the PAP method. **a** Unlabeled Purkinje cell (*PC*) and primary dendrites surrounded by intensely immunoreactive neuroglial cells (*arrows*) and their processes. Labeled basket cells (*B*) are also present. ×480. **b** Control tissue treated with normal rabbit preimmune sera. ×120. **c** Normal, untreated, ether-anesthetized animal treated with cAMP antisera. ×100. **d, e** Electron micrographs of GABA-Tase immunoreactive cells in the cerebellar cortex from normal untreated animals anesthetized with ether and visualized by the PAP method without counterstains. **d** A neuroglial cell (*GL*) with immunoreactive surface membranes, organelles, and cytoplasmic matrix surround an unlabeled Purkinje-cell soma (*PC*) and other unlabeled neuronal elements. ×6000. **e** GABA-Tase labeled glial (*GL*) process. ×25,000

GABA-Tase may differ from one Purkinje cell to another. In the granular layer, Golgi neurons were always intensely reactive, as were neuroglial cells, but granule cells and axons were not. In the deep nuclei, some large neurons and neuroglial cells were reactive and this reactivity was most intense in large and small neurons after harmaline treatment. The total amount of immunoreactivity was considerably lower in the deep nuclei than in the cortex. Labeled structures were randomly scattered in the cerebellum, and no sagittal microzonation [18] in GABA-Tase distribution was seen. Changes in the intensity of GABA-Tase immunoreactivity were detectable on administration of various drugs. Increased reactivity was obtained by treatment with colchicine, GABA and oxamic acid, GABA, harmaline, norepinephrine and glutamate, or diazepam, in order of decreasing effectiveness. Serotonin produced no detectable increase in GABA-Tase reactivity above normal, and apomorphine and muscimol decreased it. No specific staining was obtained in control tisues treated with preimmune rabbit serum.

Electron microscopy confirmed the light-microscope results. Labeled neurons included Golgi cells, basket and stellate cells, and Purkinje-cell somata and their dendrites. Neuroglial cells between Purkinje cells were also labeled, as were their processes surrounding neural elements in the molecular layer, other cells in the granular layer, and blood vessels. In the labeled neuron or neuroglial cell, two components were recognized – membranous and cytoplasmic. The reactive material was detectable on the plasma membranes, on outer nuclear membranes, on outer mitochondrial membranes, on membranes of the granular and smooth endoplasmic reticulum, and on microtubules and neurofilaments. The cytoplasmic matrix appeared as a dark, reactive, flocculent material between the cellular organelles. Where the label occurred only in neuroglial cells, the unlabeled neuronal elements were encircled by reactive glial processes around Purkinje cells (Fig. 4d), stellate cells, Purkinje-cell dendrites, and mossy fibers. At the synaptic interface, the presynaptic and postsynaptic membranes alone could be specifically labeled (Fig. 4e).

Evidence is provided for the presence of GABA-Tase in the neuronal and neuroglial compartments of the cerebellum. In the neuronal pool, cells that have been observed with GABA-Tase immunoreactivity in their cytoplasm and membranes are cerebellar GABA neurons previously shown to have GAD immunoreactivity [1] and ^{3}H-GABA uptake [9, 40]. GABA-Tase immunoreactivity was also observed on postsynaptic membranes alone, opposite terminals of axons belonging to non-GABA-containing neurons, such as granule cells. This indicates that GABA-Tase is a major cytoplasmic and membrane-related degradative enzyme in GABA-synthesizing neurons but is, in addition, selectively bound to the postsynaptic membrane at synapses formed by non-GABA-containing axons on GABA-containing neurons. Neuroglial cells, particularly those enveloping GABA-containing neurons, have significant amounts of cytoplasmic and membrane-bound GABA-Tase. Although many Purkinje cells have GABA-Tase immunoreactivity, some have none. All Purkinje cells and their dendrites, however, are ensheathed by GABA-Tase immunoreactive neuroglial processes. The presence of GABA-Tase in GABA neurons, neuroglia, and non-GABA neurons associated with GABA synapses indicates the partici-

pation of these cells in important mechanisms for terminating transmitter action – the uptake and degradation of GABA.
The GABA-Tase immunoreactivity was greater: (a) in cerebella from animals anesthetized with ether than with barbiturates; (b) in tissues treated by the PAP method than by the immunofluorescence method; (c) in tissues fixed in formaldehyde without glutaraldehyde than in unfixed frozen material (the presence of glutaraldehyde in the primary fixative enhanced morphological preservation for electron microscopy but decreased immunoreactivity); and (d) in tissues obtained after colchicine administration. An increase in GABA-Tase immunoreactivity can be induced by application of GABA and intensified with the use of oxamic acid and glutamate. These effects may be explained by increases in enzyme substrate (GABA), in coenzyme-ligand interactions (oxamic acid) and in enzyme-product interactions (glutamate). Colchicine, a drug that blocks axoplasmic transport of proteins, also increase demonstrable GABA-Tase. The finding that muscimol, a potent GABA agonist, does not increase GABA-Tase levels suggests that binding sites for GABA-Tase and transmitter receptor sites are separate. With the exception of muscimol and apomorphine, the selective changes elicited in levels of GABA-Tase reactivity by pharmacologic treatments indicate that drugs and neurotransmitter substances that increase the activity of cerebellar GABA neurons directly (GABA, norepinephrine, glutamate), or indirectly (diazepam, harmaline) increase immunologically detectable levels of the enzyme. These studies indicate that the ability to localize the precise sites of a degradative enzyme such as GABA-Tase provides a powerful means for investigation of neurotransmitter mechanisms at cellular and subcellular levels.

Immunocytochemical Localization of Cyclic GMP

The mammalian cerebellum contains unusually high concentrations of endogenous guanosine 3′,5′-cyclic monophosphate (cGMP) [29, 30]. Experiments on brain slices, cultures, and in vitro preparations suggest that cGMP may be associated with a variety of possible neurotransmitter substances in mechanisms that are not understood. Selective changes of cerebellar cGMP independent of adenosine 3′,5′-cyclic monophosphate (cAMP) can be produced by a number of agents and conditions such as alcohol, excitatory and inhibitory transmitter substances, decapitation, and benzodiazepines. Considerable speculation marks the interpretation of the correlations among cGMP levels, putative transmitter substances, and their possible localization in cerebellar neurons, particularly Purkinje cells. Although the presence of cGMP in Purkinje cells has not been demonstrated [21], the cellular and subcellular location of cGMP in some cerebellar neurons and particularly in neuroglial cells has [17].
Adult 200–300-g Sprague-Dawley rats, the indirect immunofluorescence method [20], and the PAP method [55] for light and electron microscopy were used. Rabbit antisera were raised against the 2′-O-succinyl derivative of cGMP or cAMP conjugated to limpet hemocyanin [54]. More than 50% of 2′-O-succinyl-cGMP ^{125}I-iodotyrosine methyl ester derivative (<0.01 pmol) was bound

at a serum dilution of 1:2000. Specificity was determined by radioimmunoassay. The antisera raised against cGMP gave 20–30% displacement of bound ^{125}I-labeled cGMP with 5 fmol of acetylated cGMP. Acetylated cAMP did not produce significant displacement up to 1000 fmol. Corresponding experiments with antisera raised against cAMP produced the equivalent appropriate result, indicating its specificity. The IgG fractions of these antisera were used. The basic cytochemical methods have been described [9]. Cryostat sections (10 μm thick) of cerebella from formaldehyde-perfused brains and unfixed cerebella frozen in liquid nitrogen 1–2 min after decapitation were treated with the IgG and stained by the immunofluorescence method, using a fluorescein isothiocyanate-conjugated goat IgG. Vibratome sections (20–30 μm thick, cut in cold 0.05 M Tris-HCl buffer, pH 7.6) of cerebella from perfused brains were treated sequentially with cGMP IgG, PAP antiserum, and diaminobenzidine with hydrogen peroxide prior to postfixation in 2% osmium tetroxide, dehydration with methanol, and embedding in epoxy resin. These sections were then examined with the light microscope and subsequently thin- sectioned in serial order for electron microscopy. No counterstains were used for electron microscopy. Two forms of anesthesia were employed and their results were compared: 2% sodium pentobarbital (0.1 ml/100 g of body weight) injected intraperitoneally, and diethyl ether by inhalation. Two fixatives were used in the perfusions, either 4% (wt./vol.) formaldehyde in Na phosphate buffer, pH 7.4, or 4% formaldehyde and 0.25% glutaraldehyde in phosphate buffer, pH 7.4 both at 4 °C; each was preceded by a wash with cold Ca^{2+}-free Tyrode's buffer. The cGMP immunoreactivity was greater (a) in the cerebella from animals anesthetized with ether than in those from animals anesthetized with sodium pentobarbital; (b) with the more sensitive PAP method than with immunofluorescence; (c) in tissues fixed in formaldehyde without glutaraldehyde than in unfixed frozen material. The presence of glutaraldehyde in the primary fixative enhanced morphological preservation for electron microscopy but reduced immunoreactivity. Colchicine treatment did not enhance cGMP immunoreactivity. In the molecular layer, some stellate and basket somata (approximately 30%) were cGMP immunoreactive. The Golgi epithelial neuroglial somata surrounding Purkinje cells and their radial fibers displayed the most intense immunoreactivity. Purkinje-cell somata remained unreactive with all modes of fixation and drug manipulations attempted, except for superfusion with norepinephrine and glutamate. Neuroglial cells in the granular layer and their processes [15, 45] were immunoreactive, whereas Golgi neurons and granule cells somata were not. In the white matter, some oligodendroglial cells and some axons were immunoreactive. In the cerebellar nuclei, neuroglial cells were generally reactive, whereas the neurons were not, and the total amount of cGMP immunoreactivity was considerably lower in the cerebellar nuclei than in the cortex. Intracerebellar injections of GABA, with or without aminooxyacetic acid, induced cGMP immunoreactivity in some large neurons. Labeled cells and their processes were randomly scattered in the cerebellum and no indication of sagittal microzonation was observed in cGMP distribution (17; see Fig. 5a, b). No specific staining was obtained when normal rabbit serum and cGMP IgG adsorbed with cGMP were used (Fig. 5c, d); cGMP IgG adsorbed

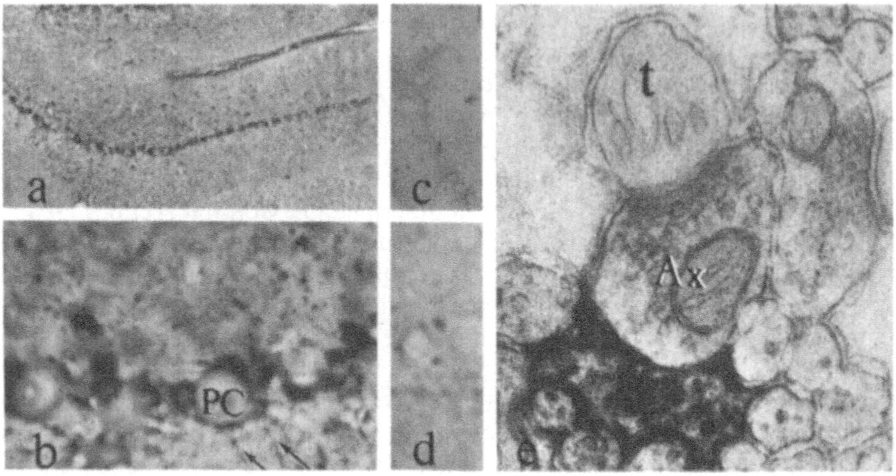

Fig. 5a–d. Light micrographs of immunoreactive neuroglial and neuronal elements of the cerebellar cortex visualized by cGMP IgG by using the PAP method. **a, b** Tissue from normal, untreated, ether-anesthetized animal showing cGMP immunoreactivity in glial cells surrounding Purkinje cells (*PC*) and in the granular layer (*arrows*). **a** ×120; **b** ×480; **c, d** Control tissues reacted with cGMP IgG preadsorbed with 1 mM cGMP. **c** ×120; **d** ×480. **e** Electron micrograph of cerebellar cortex from normal, untreated, ether-anesthetized animals, treated with cGMP IgG, and visualized after the PAP reaction; no counterstains. Examples of unreactive synapses of thorns (*t*) with axons (*Ax*) surrounded by reactive neuroglial processes. ×35,000

with cAMP showed a labeling pattern no different from that obtained with unadsorbed cGMP IgG. Comparative studies with cAMP antibody repeatedly indicated immunoreactivity in Purkinje cells (Fig. 4c), granule cells [4], stellate and basket cells, Golgi cells, numerous Golgi epithelial neuroglial cells and their processes, and some large and small neurons in the deep cerebellar nuclei. Because these results differ significantly from the sites of cGMP immunoreactivity, the data indicate that the cytochemical activities of cGMP and cAMP antisera are distinguishable.

Electron microscopy confirmed the findings of light microscopy that the majority of labeled cells and processes were neuroglial: Golgi epithelial cells in between Purkinje cells, their processes (the Bergmann fibers) in the molecular layer, and other neuroglial cells in the granular layer and around blood vessels. Rarely were labeled stellate or basket cells observed. There were two components of immunoreactivity in labeled cells – membranous and cytoplasmic. The membranous reactive material is detectable on the plasma membranes, on outer nuclear membranes but not in the nucleus itself, on outer mitochondrial membranes but not within mitochondria or on the cristae, on the membranes of the granular and smooth endoplasmic reticulum but not within the lumen, and on microtubules and neurofilaments. The cytoplasmic matrix appears as a dark, reactive, flocculent material between the cellular organelles. Where the label occurs in glial cells, the unlabeled neuronal elements are encircled by reactive processes, for example, around Purkinje cells, around synapses between Purkinje-cell thorns and axonal boutons (Fig. 5e), around mossy-fiber rosettes and granule cells, and surrounding a blood capillary. No specifically labeled glial or neuronal elements were found in control tissue treated with cGMP IgG adsorbed with cGMP.

Immunocytochemical methods can be used to demonstrate the cellular and subcellular locations of cGMP immunoreactivity. These are to a large extent in neuroglial cells throughout the cerebellum but, in particular, those adjacent to and surrounding Purkinje cells. The intensity and distribution of cGMP immunoreactivity are affected by pharmacologic manipulation, and the cellular locations and levels of such changes can be studied. Substances that increase cerebellar activity increase cGMP immunoreactivity, and substances that decrease cerebellar activity decrease cGMP immunoreactivity. Because the majority of cGMP is in neuroglial cells, it would be expected that their activity would fluctuate in response to activity of adjacent or related neurons. Although the data indicate that these substances can alter levels of cGMP detectable by immunocytochemical methods, their mechanisms of action remain obscure. Interpretation of the pharmacologic data is impeded by the reduction in cerebellar activity imposed by the necessary anesthesia of the experimental animals. It is not clear, for example, whether the increase in cGMP immunoreactivity after drug treatment is the direct result of drug action or selective neuronal activity, or is secondary to other effects, such as interference with calcium influx or GABA release and uptake. The present study provides evidence for the presence of membranous (particulate) and cytoplasmic (soluble) cGMP, particularly in neuroglial cells, and indicates that cGMP is in a position to interact with externally applied substances, including putative neurotransmitters, as well as to participate in the regulation of intracellular processes. This focuses our attention on the possible nonneuronal, nonsynaptic functions of cGMP and forces us to recognize the importance of the neuroglia in neurotransmitter-related neuronal events.

Localization of GABA Receptors in the Cerebellum by Means of ^{3}H-Muscimol Autoradiography

In the mammalian cerebellum, the cortical neurons that have been demonstrated to have immunoreactivity for antibody against GAD, the GABA-synthesizing enzyme, are stellate cells, basket cells, Golgi cells, and Purkinje cells and their various dendritic and axonal processes. These neurons and some small neurons in the deep cerebellar nuclei have also been demonstrated by autoradiography to have uptake capacity for ^{3}H-GABA [9]. Figure 1 a indicates schematically the GABA-containing neurons (stipple) of the cerebellum. Granule cells, Lugaro cells, the large cerebellar nuclear neurons, and other small nuclear neurons have not been demonstrated to contain GABA; GABA-receptor sites have been localized by only one method so far. This approach is to manipulate the GABA system pharmacologically by using molecules structurally related to it that can specifically simulate the action of the transmitter. Muscimol (3-hydroxy-5-aminomethyl-isoxazole) is one of a group of compounds that have been reported to be GABA-receptor agonists in the central nervous system [26,

37, 38, 39]. It is a psychotomimetic compound isolated from the mushroom *Amanita muscaria* [28] and is structurally analogous to GABA according to X-ray crystallography [5]; it appears to be a powerful GABA agonist at bicuculline-sensitive postsynaptic receptors [22], weakly inhibits high-affinity uptake of GABA in brain slices, is not a substrate for GABA: 2-oxoglutarate aminotransferase [2], and has a dissociation constant of approximately 2 nM.

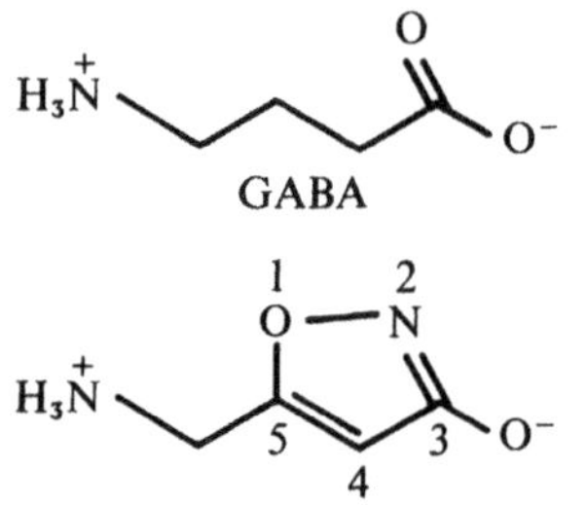

GABA

MUSCIMOL

Studies comparing the binding of ^{3}H-muscimol (^{3}H-M) with that of ^{3}H-GABA in rat-brain homogenates indicate that the high-affinity binding characteristics of both substances are similar, although not identical. The regional distributions of ^{3}H-M receptor binding and ^{3}H-GABA uptake are comparable: cerebellum > cerebral cortex > hippocampus > corpus striatum > midbrain and hypothalamus > medulla and spinal cord [27]. Furthermore, it has been indicated [3] that ^{3}H-M is displaced stereospecifically only by drugs or related amino acids known to interact with the synaptic GABA receptor and is unaffected by other agents that activate or inhibit other neurotransmitter receptors.

In the present situation, ring-labeled, ^{3}H-M was used as a histochemical marker for GABA receptor sites; ^{3}H-M has a free amino group that enables the substance, when it is bound to receptor sites in tissue constituents, to be covalently

Fig. 6a–d. Sites of GABA receptors in the cerebellar cortex demonstrated by ^{3}H-M autoradiography. **a** After exposure to ^{3}H-M. Low-magnification, dark-field microscopy of several cortical folia in the sagittal plane of the cerebellum (1 µm epoxy section). Silver grains are generally distributed over the neuropil of the molecular layer (*ml*), and over the granular layer (*grl*), and the white matter (*wm*) is virtually label-free. Intracortical neurons of the molecular layer are heaviley labeled (*horizontal arrows*). The highest amount of silver-grain deposition is over the basket-axon formation around the Purkinje-cell body and the axonal initial segment (*vertical arrows*). ×100. **b** Systemic injection of unlabeled muscimol 1 h prior to administration of ^{3}H-M causes a significant loss of ^{3}H-M binding and autoradiographic label throughout the cerebellar cortical layers, particularly over intracortical neurons and the basket-axon formations over Purkinje-cell somata and axonal initial segments (*arrows*). Sagittal plane of rat cerebellum, 1 µm epoxy section, ×100 **c** Purkinje-cell layer and basket-axonal formations around the cell somata heavily labeled (*triangles*) after ^{3}H-M binding. One µm expoxy section, ×600 **d** Diagram of distribution of GABA receptors, indicated in actual numbers of autoradiographic silver grains after ^{3}H-M binding within 20-µm^2 squares of a grid placed over the basket formation of two Purkinje-cell somata. The Purkinje-cell somata have minimal grains per unit area (0–5), the region surrounding the basket formation has 5–10, and within the basket itself the grain-counts rise considerably from 10 to 35

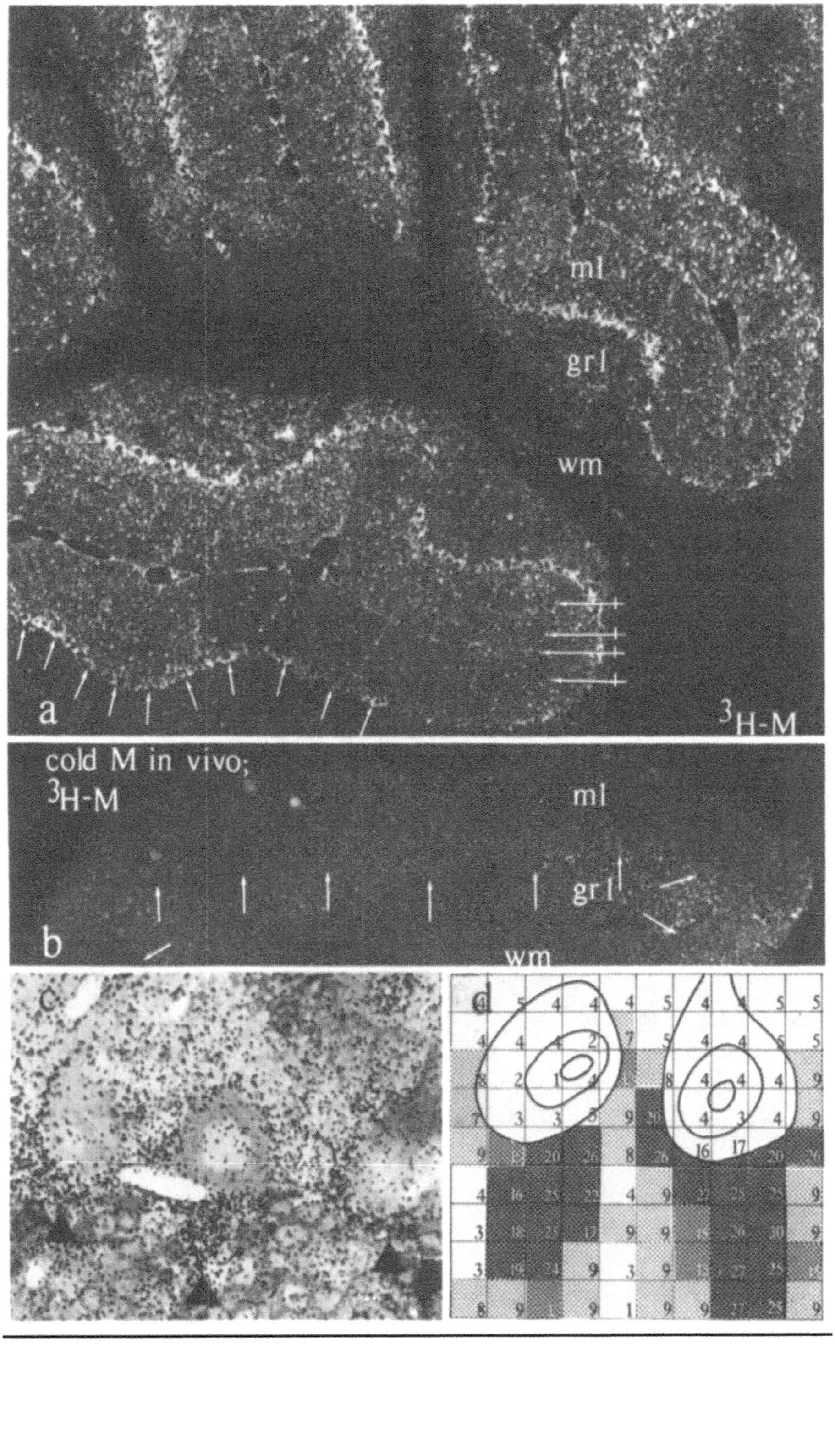
ml
gr l
wm
a
^{3}H-M
cold M in vivo;
^{3}H-M
ml
gr l
b
wm
c
d

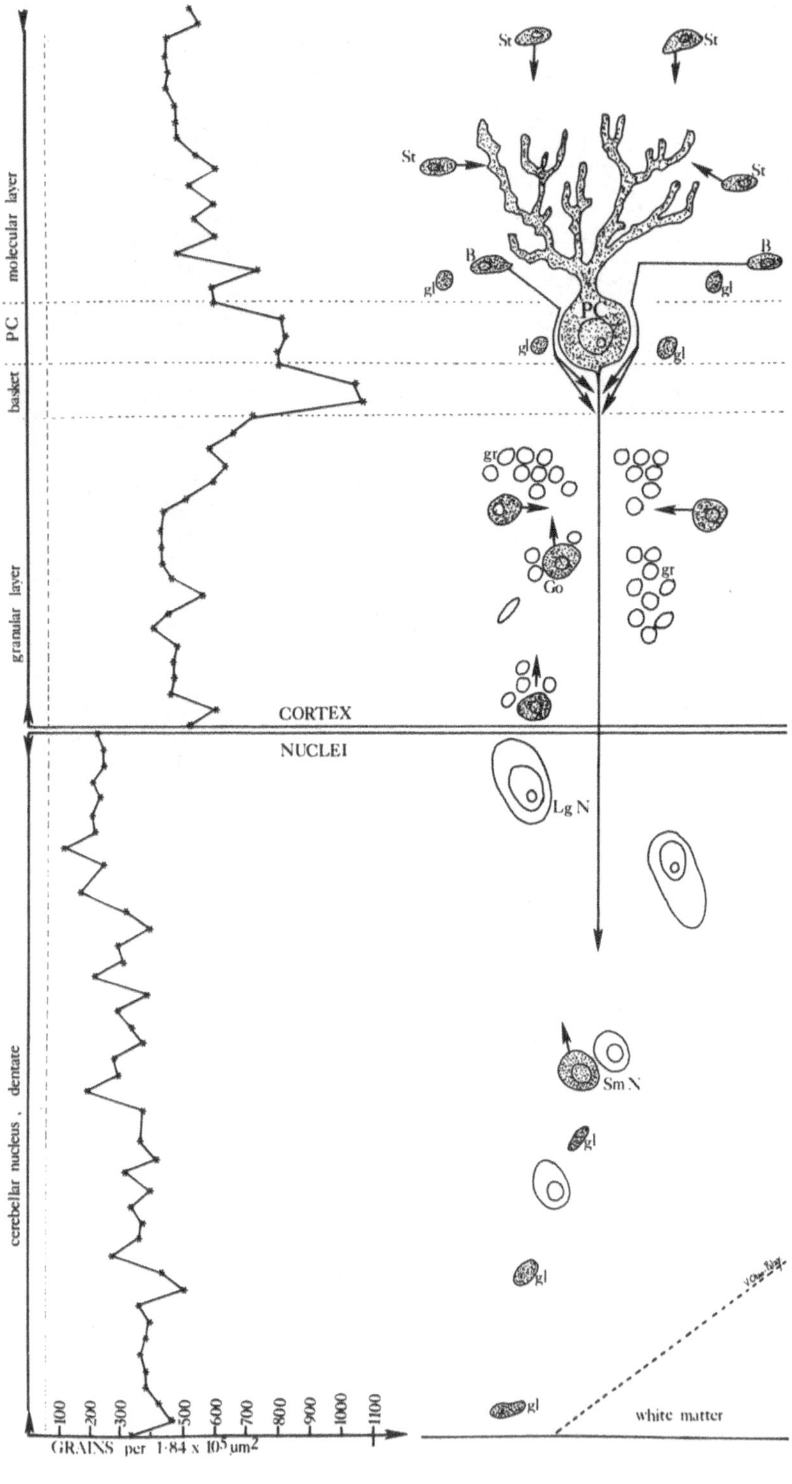

molecular layer
PC
basket
granular layer
cerebellar nucleus, dentate
St
B
gl
PC
gr
Go
CORTEX
NUCLEI
Lg N
Sm N
white matter
100
200
300
500
600
700
800
900
1000
1100
GRAINS per 1·84 x 10⁵ μm²

linked by aldehyde fixation. Subsequent manipulations are then possible for autoradiographic visualization of the bound ^{3}H-M. At the light-microscope level the quantitative analysis of resulting autoradiograms provides data on the distribution of ^{3}H-M binding sites in the cerebellum both in a laminar display across the layers of the cerebellar cortex and nuclei, and in a cellular manner. It is also imperative to know the subcellular locations of these ^{3}H-M binding sites and this ultrastructural definition can be provided by electron-microscopic autoradiography. The major questions to be addressed include whether or not GABA receptors are associated with (a) membranes of neuronal or neuroglial elements, (b) synaptic sites, (c) specific cellular types, or (d) unusual non-synaptic relationships.

A differential distribution of ^{3}H-M binding was displayed in the cerebellar cortex and nuclei (Fig. 6a–d) – a laminar distribution with the highest density of autoradiographic signal around, but not including, the Purkinje-cell somata and in basket and stellate neurons of the molecular layer. There was binding of ^{3}H-M throughout the cerebellar neuropil, highest in the molecular layer and in the granular layer, low in the cerebellar nuclei, and insignificant over the white matter.

Examination of the autoradiograms in stained sections readily revealed the identity of the various structures labeled (Fig. 7). Counts of the silver grains over selected fields that sample the molecular, Purkinje-cell, and granular layers of the cortex, dentate nucleus, and white matter provided a quantitative display of the laminar distribution of the autoradiographic signal generated by ^{3}H-M binding. The highest binding of ^{3}H-M occurred on the Purkinje-cell somatic surface and in the basket axon formation surrounding the Purkinje-cell body and its axon initial segment. Neuroglial cells of the cortex have no ^{3}H-M binding capacity, some glial cells in the cerebellar nuclei do. The role of these glial cells in GABA-receptor-mediated mechanisms remains to be clarified. Table 1 compares the relative distribution of autoradiographic grains over identified cells within the cerebellar cortex and nuclei. In the cortex, almost all basket and stellate cells were heavily labeled; Purkinje-cell dendritic surfaces and the somatic surface surrounded by basket axons were well labeled, but the cell body itself was not. The highest density of label was found in the region of the Purkinje-cell initial axonal segment.

Specificity of ^{3}H-M binding was indicated by control experiments summarized in Fig. 6. In order to examine whether ^{3}H-M binding could be attributable in part to the GABA-uptake and -transport system, it was necessary to pretreat

Fig. 7. The quantitative distribution (*left side*) of silver grains in autoradiograms after ^{3}H-M binding in laminase of the cerebellar cortex, in the dentate nucleus, and in white matter. The estimated background level is indicated by the *vertical dotted line*. Each point on the chart was obtained by counting the grains overlying 1.84×10^5 μm^2 of tissue. The cerebellar neurons and neuroglial cells present in each layer are indicated on the *right*. Cells with previously reported ^{3}H-GABA uptake or containing GABA-synthesizing or degradative enzymes are indicated by *stippling*. *B*, basket cell; *gl*, neuroglial cell; *Go*, Golgi cell; *gr*, granule cell; *LgN*, lage neuron in dentate nucleus; *PC*, Purkinje cell; *SmN*, small neuron in dentate nucleus; *St*, stellate cell

Table 1. Relative distributions of autoradiographic grains over the cells and neuropil of the cerebellar cortex and nuclei

Cell type	Grains per unit area
Cortex	
Basket/stellate cells	25
Purkinje cell	
Primary and secondary dendrites	12
Somata	5
Initial segment/basket	35
Neuroglial cells	0–3
Granule cells	5
Golgi cells	5–10
Neuropil of molecular and granular layers	5
Nuclei	
Large neurons	3
Small neurons	3
Neuroglial cells	15
Neuropil	5
White matter	0–3

brain slices with inhibitors of GABA uptake before incubation with ^{3}H-M. (−)Nipecotic acid, and guvacine, a psychoactive agent found in betel nuts, are potent inhibitors of GABA uptake and combine with the carrier. When cerebellar slices were incubated with either of these substances for 10 min prior to incubation with ^{3}H-M, there was no detectable change in the pattern of distribution or quantity of silver grains in the autoradiograms. These results indicate that the ^{3}H-M binding to GABA receptors is not interfered with by GABA-transport or − uptake inhibitors and thus that the binding of ^{3}H-M is selective for receptors.

The GABA-receptor antagonists, bicuculline and picrotoxin, were equally effective in preventing subsequent binding with ^{3}H-M and no autoradiographic labeling occurred. Pretreatment with nonradioactive GABA also effectively prevents further binding with ^{3}H-M and no labeling occurred in the autoradiograms. Systemic administration of muscimol can cause a number of behavioral changes, including lethargy and hallucinations, an observation that suggests that the substance penetrates the blood/brain barrier. However, the possibility exists that the effects elicited may be the result of the action of metabolites of muscimol. In the present study, unlabeled muscimol administered intravenously 1 h prior to exposure of cerebellar slices to ^{3}H-M produced a significant decrease in autoradiographic silver grains. In the cerebellum, the sites most severely affected were the basket and stellate cells of the molecular layer and the basket axon formation around Purkinje cells, which are the sites with the highest binding of ^{3}H-M (Fig. 6e, d). These results show that muscimol administered parenterally can enter the brain and bind to available receptor sites, blocking most of these sites from subsequently binding ^{3}H-M. Thus, unlabeled muscimol or its metabolites are effective competitors in vivo for receptors of ^{3}H-M subsequently introduced in vivo or in vitro into brain tissue. On the other hand, pretreatment of brain slices in vitro with nonradioactive muscimol prior to incubation with ^{3}H-M only partially inhibits binding with the radioactive ^{3}H-M, presumably because some exchange between bound and unbound muscimol (M) and ^{3}H-M occurs. Pretreatment of cerebellar slices with cold GABA in the presence or absence of amino-oxyacetic acid (AOAA) inhibits binding with ^{3}H-M and no labeling occurs in autoradiograms. The same result occurs with pretreatment with two GABA agonists THIP (isoxazole 16) and isoguvacine. These pharmacologic/morphological tests for specificity of binding suggest that ^{3}H-M binding indicates binding at GABA-receptor sites.

Several interesting observations deserve comment at this point: (a) The failure to obtain significant autoradiographic labeling in the brain after systemic intravenous injections of ^{3}H-M suggests that the majority of the injected material may be metabolized in blood plasma with only minute quantities possibly binding in the brain sites examined; (b) ^{3}H-M binding on certain neuroglial cells in the deep cerebellar nuclei needs to be further examined for possible GABA-receptor-mediated mechanisms; (c) the discrepancy in the relative distribution between the M-binding GABA-receptor sites and the distribution of GAD- and ^{3}H-GABA-uptake sites needs further examination. For instance, although the terminals of Purkinje cells have considerable GAD content and capacity to take up ^{3}H-GABA, the amount of ^{3}H-M binding in the deep cerebellar nuclei is low. Several possible explanations can be entertained. First, that these regions were less accessible to autoradiographic labeling because of their distance from the injection sites. Repeated injections into the cerebellar nuclei have not changed this result, suggesting that the technical explanation is unlikely. Second, it can be proposed that there may be more than one class of GABA receptors, one that can be demonstrated by M and others that cannot, under the present experimental conditions. Third, the conditions for the visualization procedures used here may have favored the demonstration of only a portion of the GABA-receptor binding sites; perhaps others are masked by the presence of endogenous GABA; or can only be demonstrated by the use of ^{3}H-M in concentrations other than the 2-nM range.

Thus it appears reasonable at this time to conclude that ^{3}H-M autoradiography is useful for the morphological demonstration of GABA receptors. Nevertheless, a possibility remains that the receptors detected by M may be only one set of possible GABA receptors. The characteristics and locations of others may be discovered by the application of similar procedures with different GABA mimetics. The fundamental aim of all these studies is to define and visualize the sites at which GABA acts in order to discover safe pharmacological tools for the treatment of those nervous and mental disorders in which GABA may be deficient.

Ultrastructural Localization of GABA Receptors: Cellular Localization

The deposition of phenidone-developed silver grains was selectively localized to the plasma membranes of several neuronal types and their processes. Back-

ground label was low. Serial section autoradiograms exposed for 3 weeks exhibited half the number of silver grains encountered in those exposed for 5 weeks; however, the grains were on comparable structures in adjacent serial sections exposed for either period. Silver grains in the cerebellar cortex were associated with plasma membranes of the following structures: (a) somata and primary denrites of basket and stellate cells in the molecular layers; (b) somata and primary and secondary dendritic shafts of Purkinje cells; (c) axons and axon terminals of basket cells in the pinceau region; (d) initial axonal segments and myelinated axons of Purkinje cells; (e) the dendrites of granule cells and Golgi cells in the granular layer; (f) somata and dendritic shafts of large and small neurons in the cerebellar nuclei.
These data correspond well to the distribution and density of GABA receptors on cells in the cerebellar cortex and nuclei in light microscopic autoradiograms [10]. In almost all cases the label was associated with neuronal plasma membranes and not with the neuroglial investment. However, one example was found of label on the membranes of an opposing axon and a neuroglial cell in the dentate nucleus. Furthermore, the label occurred in relation to the cellular surface membranes and not to internal cytoplasmic membranes.

Synaptic Terminal Localization

One hundred and thirty-five electron microscopic autoradiograms were obtained in which silver grains were deposited on membranes belonging to axonal varicosities and to postsynaptic elements bearing visible snyaptic junctions. In 88.9% of these examples, the label was associated with axodendritic synapses on Purkinje cells and in 11.1% the label was associated with axosomatic synapses on Purkinje, stellate, and basket cells.

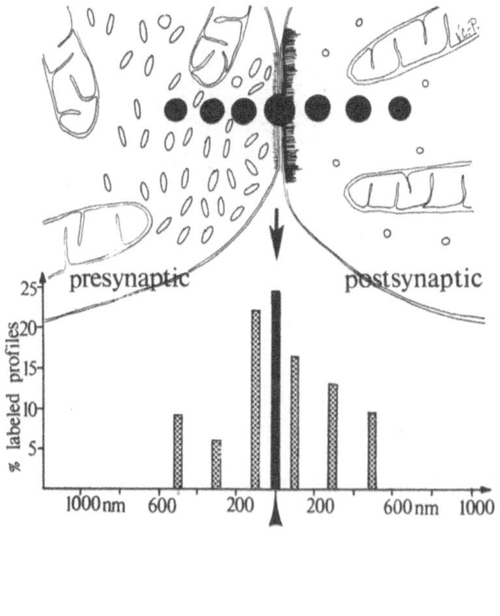

Fig. 8. The distribution of phenidone-developed autoradiographic silver grains produced by bound ^{3}H-M on the membranes of profiles bearing synaptic junctions. The sample includes 135 profiles, 24% of which have grains on the synaptic interfaces; the remaining 37.5% and 38.5% were disposed on pre- and postsynaptic sides, respectively, within 500 nm of the synaptic interfaces. This scatter of grains is within the limits of resolution of the autoradiographic method for tritium source and the Ilford L4 emulsion

Of the 135 examples of labeled synaptic terminals, 24% had the silver grain directly upon the opposing pre- or postsynaptic membrane at or near the synaptic junction. The remaining examples had silver grains scattered on either the pre- or postsynaptic side, close to the synaptic membranes: 37.5% had label on the presynaptic side – 22.2% contained silver grains within the first 100 nm of the synaptic junction and the remaining 15.3% had silver grains within 450 nm of the synaptic junction; 38.5% had silver grains on the postsynaptic side, all of which lay within the first 500 nm of the synaptic membranes. These results are summarized diagrammatically in Fig. 8. The data show that the silver grains were clearly localized upon and near synaptic junctions. The spread of grains reported here reflects the scatter of β-particles from the bound ^{3}H-M. The 500-nm maximal spread is well within the limits of resolution of this technique utilizing tritium and Ilford L4 emulsion [31].

The diameters of silver grains ranged from 110 to 150 nm. The neuronal plasma membrane was approximately 8 nm wide and the extracellular space between neuronal appositions was 20–25 nm wide. At symmetric synapses the synaptic cleft was 20–25 nm wide, whereas at asymmetric synapses the cleft was usually widened to 30 nm [46]. Therefore, the diameter of one silver grain is three to four times the combined widths of pre- and postsynaptic membranes and the synaptic cleft. Thus, although the elctron-microscope autoradiographic technique indicates that labeling occurs directly in conjunction with membranes at or near synapses, it is not possible to decide whether or not the source for the label, i.e., ^{3}H-M bound to GABA receptors, is associated with either the pre- or postsynaptic membrane (Fig. 8).

Nonsynaptic Locations

Sixty-four examples of neuronal profiles were obtained with silver grains located on plasma membranes of structures without visible synaptic contacts. Of these, 66% were on plasma membranes between axons and 34% were on dendrites. The basket region around the Purkinje-cell body and initial axon segment presented the most examples of silver grains over axonal plasma membranes. Here, the axons belonging to the GABA-containing basket cells of the molecular layer are complexly intertwined with one another, with some neuroglial processes between them [45]. Few, if any, true axo-axonal synapses exist, although specialized, septate junction-like formations have been described [32, 44, 45, 52]. The label over the pinceau was found on the membranes between apposed basket axons that were bare of neuroglia and not at any specialized junction. These observations confirm the earlier report from light-microscopic autoradiograms that the basket region around Purkinje cells was most densely labeled with ^{3}H-M binding GABA-receptor sites [10].

The presence of GABA receptors on the membranes of GABA-containing axons raises the obvious question of their function. Do the basket-axon terminals within this region release GABA at nonsynaptic locations? If so, does binding of GABA to the receptors in the basket produce self-inhibition of the basket and consequently a self-regulated inhibition of discharges from the Purkinje-cell axon that it surrounds, or does it produce a presynaptic facilitation? Because the basket formation around each Purkinje cell consists of axon collaterals from a number of different basket cells [25, 45], the effect of activation of any one basket-cell axon is difficult to predict. It could result in inhibition of the other members of the basket and thus a reduction of the effect. Alternatively, is it conceivable that the membrane events in the terminals could lead to synchronized activation of the whole formation and to reinforcement of the effect of exciting a single basket cell? Moreover, is it possible that presynaptic suppression of the inhibitory action of basket cells on the Purkinje cell could result? The inhibitory effect of basket-cell activation on the Purkinje-cell discharge builds up and decays relatively slowly [24, 25]. Some aspects of these electric properties may be explainable by the general distribution of GABA receptors throughout the axons of the basket formation. The present findings suggest that reexamination of the physiology of the complicated synapse between basket and Purkinje cells would be useful.

Several issues will be brought up at this point for discussion. The present studies demonstrate that ^{3}H-M or a labeled metabolite can be utilized to demonstrate the location and distribution of a GABA receptor which will be termed the M receptor of GABA. This receptor appears to be most heavily distributed over the molecular layer interneurons, basket and stellate cells, and especially over the basket-cell axon membrane relations with the Purkinje cell. Although the M GABA receptor can also be found in the granular layer neuropil within and around glomeruli and in the cerebellar nuclear neuropil, it is not as numerous as in the previously mentioned layers of the cortex.

GABA Autoreceptors

Although GABA-synthesizing enzymes and ^{3}H-GABA uptake have been consistently demonstrated in basket and stellate cells, the demonstration of these mechanisms in the Purkinje-cell body has been less consistent. For example, ^{3}H-GABA uptake has been shown only in immature Purkinje cells in culture [53], in intraocular transplants [40], and inconsistently in the mature cerebellar cortex in vivo [9]; GAD immunoreactivity is more readily demonstrable after the application of colchicine [47]. In the light of the M GABA receptor distribution demonstrated here, it appears that many GABA-containing cerebellar neurons, in particular the basket, stellate, and Purkinje cells, have receptors for the same transmitter on their various membrane surfaces. These may be regarded as examples of identified GABA autoreceptors.

Data to support this interpretation were obtained when the cerebella were prepared for autoradiography after recording experiments [14]; ^{3}H-M binding was detectable over all cortical surfaces exposed to a superfusate of ^{3}H-M and intense labeling was found over the basket-axon–Purkinje-cell-axon initial segment area and less intensely over the molecular layer. Further studies are needed to clarify the details of the functional interaction of M on cerebellar neurons.

Conclusions

The conclusions are summarized in Fig. 9. In vivo injections of characterized antibody against GAD, the enzyme responsible for the synthesis of GABA, into cerebellar cortex produced labeled stellate, basket, Purkinje, and Golgi cells and their processes at the injection site. Anterograde transport of GAD antigen-antibody complexes in Purkinje-cell axons caused intense labeling of terminals in deep cerebellar and several vestibular nuclei. Small groups of mossy-fiber rosettes labeled and produced retrograde labeling and GAD immunoreactivity in a small number of pleomorphic neurons in the deep cerebellar nuclei. Injections

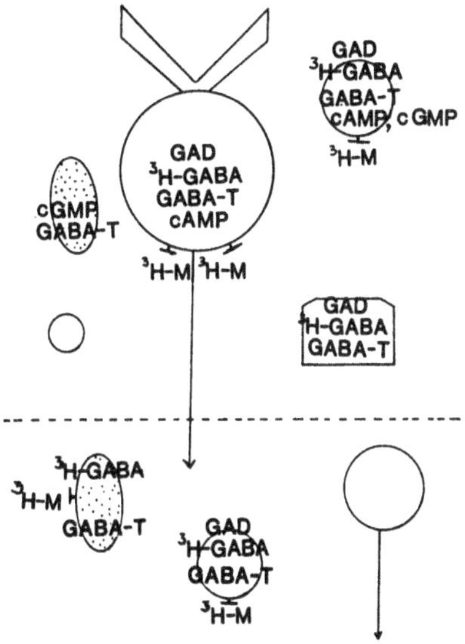

Fig. 9. Schematic diagram to summarize the distribution of ^{3}H-GABA uptake; GAD, GABA-T, cAMp, cGMP immunoreactivity; and ^{3}H-M binding in Purkinje cells, stellate and basket neurons (*round*), Golgi cells (*rectangle*) and neuroglia (*oval*) of the cerebellar cortex and nuclei

into the dentate nucleus produced retrograde labeling in Purkinje-cell bodies and anterograde labeling in a small number of mossy-fiber rosettes. All projections conformed to previously reported topographic distributions of corticonuclear and nucleocortical cerebellar pathways. These findings confirm the GABA content of most Purkinje-cell–deep-nuclei connections and provide new evidence for a GABA component in part of the nucleocortical pathway in the cerebellum. Immunocytochemical controls for specificity were conducted by injections of preimmune rabbit serum as a substitute for GAD antibody which produced only nonspecific labeling. Colchicine caused a cumulative enhancement of GAD immunoreactivity in all cases.

In the rat cerebellum, GABA-Tase immunoreactivity was studied by light and electron microscopy with indirect immunofluorescence and PAP methods. Evidence is presented for neuronal and neuroglial compartments of GABA-Tase. Labeled neurons included stellate, basket, Purkinje, and Golgi cells of the cortex and a few large neurons in the deep nuclei. Labeled neuroglia included those surrounding Purkinje cells, their radial fibers in the molecular layer, and astrocytes in the granular layer and deep nuclei. No evidence for sagittal microzonation was found. At the ultrastructural level, GABA-Tase immunoreactive sites were localized to cell-surface membranes, intracellular organelles, and the cytoplasmic matrix. The GABA-Tase immunoreactivity at synapses could be localized precisely to pre- and postsynaptic membranes in GABA-containing as well as non-GABA-containing neurons. Specific label was absent from tissues treated with normal rabbit preimmune sera.

The cGMP immunoreactivity in the rat's cerebellum was studied with light and electron microscopy by the indirect fluorescence method and the PAP method. Labeled cells included neuroglial cells in the cerebellar cortex, white matter, and deep nuclei, some stellate and basket cells in the cortex, and some large neurons in the deep nuclei. No evidence was found for sagittal microzonation in the cGMP distribution. In the labeled cells, cGMP immunoreactive sites were localized to surface membranes, organelles, and the cytoplasmic matrix. Specificity was indicated by the same pattern of labeling after treatment with cGMP IgG that had been adsorbed with cAMP and by the failure to label after treatment with normal rabbit sera or with cGMP IgG that had been adsorbed with 1 mM cGMP. Cerebella treated with cAMP antisera, however, showed immunoreactivity in Purkinje cells, granule cells, and Golgi cells, in addition to neuroglia in cortex and deep nuclei. These studies suggest that some neurons and many neuroglial cells are the major sites of cGMP in the cerebellum.

Muscimol, a structural analog and potent agonist of GABA was used in its tritiated form for the autoradiographic localization of GABA receptors in the rat cerebellum; ^{3}H-M was incubated with brain slices or was injected intracortically or into intraocular brain transplants. As indicated by ^{3}H-M binding and autoradiographic silver grains, GABA receptors display a laminar distribution over the cerebellar cortex. Quantitative analysis of the distribution of autoradiographic silver grains in the cerebellar cortex and dentate nucleus showed a general distribution of GABA receptors in the neuropil: molecular layer $>$ granular layer $>$ cerebellar nuclei $>$ white matter. The highest binding of ^{3}H-M occurred on the Purkinje-cell somatic surface, in the basket-axon formation surrounding the cell body and its axon initial segment, and somewhat less on basket and stellate cell somata. Neuroglial cells of the cortex have no ^{3}H-M binding capacity; some glial cells in the cerebellar nuclei do bind ^{3}H-M. The role of glial cells in GABA uptake, metabolism, and GABA-receptor-mediated mechanisms remains to be clarified. The distribution of GABA receptors as indicated by ^{3}H-M binding differs from the distribution of ^{3}H-GABA uptake and GABA-synthesizing and degradative sites.

Tritiated muscimol binding and electron microscope autoradiography localized GABA-receptor sites in the cerebellum of the rat. In the cerebellar cortex, silver grains were associated with somata and dendrites of basket and stellate cells in the molecular layer, with somata and primary and secondary dendritic shafts of Purkinje cells, with axons and terminals of basket cells in the pinceau or basket, initial axonal segments and myelinated axons of Purkinje cells, with dendrites of granule and Golgi cells in the granular layer, and with somata and dendritic shafts of large and small cells in the cerebellar nuclei. Label over GABA-receptor sites can be localized to the plasma membranes between pre- and postsynaptic elements at synaptic junctions, of which 88.9% of the samples are axodendritic and the remaining 11.1% are axosomatic. GABA-receptor sites are also found along axonal membranes of the GABA-containing basket cell, within the basket surrounding Purkinje cells, where true axo-axonal synapses are rare. It is speculated that GABA receptors in the basket may be related to synchronization of basket cells, either self-inhibition or facilitation within the basket formation, or presynaptic suppression of the inhibitory action of basket cell on Purkinje cell. The presence of GABA autoreceptors in the cerebellum is proposed on the basis of the findings presented here. It is also suggested that GABA receptors other than the muscimol type demonstrated here may exist and may be localized by means of other GABA agonists. These studies together summarize some of the recent approaches that we have used to investigate neurotransmitter and other chemical localizations in the cerebellum.

Recent studies on the mammalian cerebellum indicate that a number of other neuroactive substances exist and coexist with GABA in neurons, in particular the Purkinje cells. Motilin-like immunoreactivity is found in Purkinje cells [19a] alone and in coexistence with GABA. Motilin has been demonstrated to have depressant effects on cerebellar nuclear neurons [19b]. The amino acid taurine]19c, d] as well as peptides, demonstrated by β-endorphin-, enkephalin-, gastrin-cholecystokinin- and somatostatin-like immunoreactivity is present in Purkinje cells as well [19e]. These observations open new vistas for understanding chemical encoding in the cerebellum and the roles played by other neuroactive substances in their cooperation with GABA to produce neural communication.

Acknowledgments. This work was supported in part by U.S. Public Health Service Grants NS14740 and NS03659; Louise Harkness Ingalls Fellowship on Parkinson's Disease from the Massachusetts General Hospital; an Alfred P. Sloan Fellowship in Neuroscience. Presented during the author's tenure as White House Fellow and Staff Assistant to the Secretary of Defense at the Pentagon, Washington, D.C.

The author thanks Mr. Howard Cook and Ms. Joyce Barton for photographic and technical assistance.

Abbreviations. GABA, γ-aminobutyric acid; *GABA-Tase,* GABA transaminase; *PAP,* peroxidase-antiperoxidase; *cGMP,* guanosine 3′,5′-cyclic monophosphate; *cAMP,* adenosine 3′,5′-cyclic monophosphate; *SP,* substance P.

References

1. Barber R, Saito K (1976) Light microscopic visualization of GAD and GABA-T in immunocytochemical preparations of rodent CNS. In: Roberts E, Chase TN, Tower DB (eds) GABA in nervous system function. Raven Press, New York, p 113
2. Beart PM, Johnston GAR (1973) GABA uptake in rat brain slices: inhibition by GABA analogues and by various drugs. J Neurochem 20:319–324
3. Beaumont K, Chilton W, Yamamura HI, Enna SJ (1978) Muscimol binding in rat brain: association with synaptic GABA receptors. Brain Res 148:153–162

4. Bloom FE, Hoffer BJ, Battenberg EF, Siggins GR, Steiner AL, Parker CW, Wedner HJ (1972) Adenosine 3′,5′-monophosphate is localized in cerebellar neurons: immunofluorescence evidence. Science 177:436–438
5. Brehm L, Hjeds H, Krogsgaard-Larsen P (1972) The structure of muscimol, a GABA analogue of restricted conformation. Acta Chem Scand 26:1298–1299
6. Brodal A (1967) Anatomical studies of cerebellar fibre connections with special reference to problems of functional localization. Prog Brain Res 25:135–173
7. Chan-Palay V (1973a) Cytology and organization in the nucleus lateralis of the cerebellum: the projections of neurons and their processes into afferent axon bundles. Z Anat Entwicklungsgesch 141:151–159
8. Chan-Palay V (1973b) Afferent axons and their relations with neurons in the nucleus lateralis of the cerebellum: a light microscope study. Z Anat Entwicklungsgesch 142:1–21
9. Chan-Palay V (1977) Cerebellar dentate nucleus, organization, cytology, and transmitters. Springer, Berlin Heidelberg New York
10. Chan-Palay V (1978a) Autoradiographic localization of γ-aminobutyric acid receptors in the rat central nervous system using ^{3}H-muscimol. Proc Natl Acad Sci USA 75:1024–1028
11. Chan-Palay V (1978b) Quantitative visualization of γ-aminobutyric acid receptors in the hippocampus and area dentate demonstrated by ^{3}H-muscimol autoradiography. Proc Natl Acad Sci USA 75:6281–6284
12. Chan-Palay V (1979a) Immunocytochemical detection of substance P neurons, their processes and connections by in vivo microinjections of monoclonal antibodies: light and electron microscopy. Anat Embryol (Berl) 156:225–240
13. Chan-Palay V (1979b) Combined immunocytochemistry and autoradiography after in vivo injections of monoclonal antibody to substance P and ^{3}H-serotonin: coexistence of two putative transmitters in single raphe cells and fiber plexuses. Anat Embryol (Berl) 156:241–254
14. Chan-Palay V (1980) Recent advances in the morphological localization of γ-aminobutyric acid receptors in the cerebellum by means of ^{3}H-muscimol. Prog Brain Res 51:304
15. Chan-Palay V, Palay SL (1977) Ultrastructural identification of substance P cells and their processes in rat sensory ganglia and their terminals in the spinal cord by immunocytochemistry. Proc Natl Acad Sci USA 74:4050–4054
16. Chan-Palay V, Palay SL (1978) Ultrastructural localization of γ-aminobutyric acid receptors in the mammalian central nervous system by means of ^{3}H-muscimol binding. Proc Natl Acad Sci USA 75:2977–2980
17. Chan-Palay V, Palay SL (1979) Light and electron microscope immunocytochemical localization of cyclic GMP, evidence for involvement of neuroglia. Proc Natl Acad Sci USA 76:1485–1489
18. Chan-Palay V, Wu J-Y, Palay SL (1979) Immunocytochemical localization of GABA-transaminase at cellular and ultrastructural levels. Proc Natl Acad Sci USA 76:2067–2071
19. Chan-Palay V, Yonezawa T, Yoshida S, Palay SL (1978) Gamma-aminobutyric acid receptors visualized in spinal cord cultures by ^{3}H-muscimol autoradiography. Proc Natl Acad Sci USA 75:6281–6284
19a. Chan-Palay V, Nilaver GT, Palay SL, Beinfeld MG, Zimmerman EA, Wu J-Y, O'Donohue TL (1981) Chemical heterogeneity in cerebellar Purkinje cells: Existence and coexistence of glutamic acid decarboxylase-like and motilin-like immunoreactivities. Proc Natl Acad Sci USA 78:7787–7791
19b. Chan-Palay V, Ito M, Tongroach P, Sukarai M, Palay SL (1982) Inhibitory effects of motilin, somatostatin, leucine- and methionine-enkephalin, and taurine on neurons of the lateral vestibular nucleus: Their interaction with gamma-aminobutyric acid. Proc Natl Acad Sci USA 79:3355–3359
19c. Chan-Palay V, Lin L-T, Palay SL, Yamamoto M, Wu J-Y (1982) Taurine in the mammalian cerebellum: Demonstration by autoradiography with ^{3}H-taurine and immunocytochemistry with antibodies against the taurine synthesizing enzyme, cysteine-sulfinic acid decarboxylase. Proc Natl Acad Sci USA 79:2695–2699
19d. Chan-Palay V, Palay SL, Wu J-Y (1982) Sagittal cerebellar microbands of taurine neurons. Immunocytochemical demonstration by using antibodies against the taurine synthesizing enzyme cysteine-sulfinic acid decarboxylase. Proc Natl Acad Sci USA

19e. Chan-Palay V, Palay SL (1982) Neuropeptides in the cerebellum: Cortical and nuclear neurons with β-endorphin-, enkephalin-, gastrin-cholecystokinin and somatostatin-like immunoreactivity. Proc Natl Acad Sci USA
20. Coons AG (1958) Fluorescent antibody methods. In: Danielli JF (ed) General cytochemical methods. Academic Press, New York, p 399–422
21. Cummings R, Eccleston D, Steiner A (1977) Immunohistochemical localization of cyclic GMP in rat cerebellum. J Cyclic Nucleotide Res 3:275–282
22. Curtis DR, Duggan AW, Felix D, Johnston GAR (1971) Bicuculline, an antagonist of GABA and synaptic inhibition in the spinal cord of cat. Brain Res 32:69–96
23. Dalstrom A (1968) Effect of colchicine on transport of amine storage granules in sympathetic nerves of rat. J Pharmacol 5:111–112
24. Eccles JC, Llinás R, Sasaki K (1966) The inhibitory interneurons within the cerebellar cortex. Exp Brain Res 1:1–16
25. Eccles JC, Ito M, Szentágothai J (1967) The cerebellum as a neuronal machine. Springer, Berlin Heidelberg New York
26. Enna SJ, Collins JF, Snyder SH (1977) Stereospecificity and structure-activity requirements of GABA receptor binding in rat brain. Brain Res 124:185–190
27. Enna SJ, Beaumont K, Yamamura HI (1978) Comparison of ^{3}H-muscimol and ^{3}H-GABA receptor binding in rat brain. In: Fonnum F (ed) Amino acids as chemical transmitters. NATO Advanced Study Inst. Symp. Plenum Press, New York, p 487
28. Eugster CH (1969) Chemie der Wirkstoffe aus dem Fliegenpilz (*Amanita muscaria*). Fortschr Chem Org Naturst 27:261–321
29. Ferrendelli JA, Kinscherf DA, Chang MM (1975) Comparison of the effects of biogenic amines on cyclic GMP and cyclic AMP levels in mouse cerebellum in vitro. Brain Res 84:63–73
30. Ferrendelli JA, Steiner AL, McDougal DB, Kipnis DM (1970) The effect of oxytremorine and atropine on cGMP and cAMP levels in mouse cerebral cortex and cerebellum. Biochem Biophys Res Commun 41:1061–1067
31. Fertuck HC, Salpeter MM (1976) Quantitation of junctional and extrajunctional acetylcholine receptors by electron microscope autoradiography after ^{125}I-α-bungarotoxin binding at mouse neuromuscular junctions. J Cell Biol 69:144–158
32. Gobel S (1971) Axo-axonic septate junctions in the basket formations of the cat cerebellar cortex. J Cell Biol 69:144–158
33. Gould BB (1977) Topographic organization of the cerebellar nucleocortical projection in the cat. Anat Rec 187:592 (1977)
34. Gould BB, Graybiel AM (1976) Afferents to the cerebellar cortex in the cat: Evidence for an intrinsic pathway leading from the deep nuclei to the cortex. Brain Res 110:601–611
35. Hökfelt T, Ljungdahl A (1970) Cellular localization of labeled gamma-aminobutyric acid (^{3}H-GABA) in rat cerebellar cortex: an autoradiographic study. Brain Res 22:391–396
36. Hyde JC (1978) Electron cytochemistry of GABA-transaminase in rat cerebellar cortex, and evidence for multimolecular forms of the enzyme. In: Fonnum F (ed) Amino acids as chemical transmitters: NATO Advanced Study Inst. Symp. Plenum Press, New York, p 49
37. Johnston GAR, Krogsgaard-Larsen P, Stephanson AL, Twitchin B (1976) Inhibition of the uptake of GABA and related amino acids in rat brain slices by the optical isomers of nipecotic acid. J Neurochem 26:1029–1032
38. Krogsgaard-Larsen P (1978) GABA agonists and uptake inhibitors of restricted conformations: structure activity relations. In: Fonnum F (ed) Amino acids as chemical transmitters. NATO Advanced Study Inst. Symp. Plenum Press, New York, p 305
39. Krogsgaard-Larsen P, Johnston GAR, Curtis DR, Game CJA, McCulloch RM (1975) Structure and biological activity of a series of conformationally restricted analogues of GABA. J Neurochem 25:803–809
40. Ljungdahl A, Seiger A, Hökfelt T, Olson L (1973) (^{3}H)GABA uptake in growing cerebellar tissue: Autoradiography of intraocular transplants. Brain Res 61:379–384
41. Matsuda T, Wu J-Y, Roberts E (1973) Sodium dodecyl sulfate acrylamide gel electrophoresis of glutamic acid decarboxylase from mouse brain. J Neurochem 21:167–172

42. McLaughlin B, Wood JG, Saito K, Barber R, Vaughn JE, Roberts E, Wu J-Y (1974) The fine structural localization of glutamate decarboxylase in synaptic terminals of rodent cerebellum. Brain Res 76:377–391
43. McLaughlin BJ, Wood JG, Saito K, Roberts E, Wu J-Y (1975) The fine structural localization of glutamate decarboxylase in developing axonal processes and presynaptic terminals of rodent cerebellum. Brain Res 85:355–371
44. Mugnaini E (1972) The histology and cytology of the cerebellar cortex. In: Larsell O, Jansen J (eds) The comparative anatomy and histology of the cerebellum: the human cerebellum, cerebellar connections and cerebellar cortex. University of Minnesota Press, Minneapolis, p 201
45. Palay SL, Chan-Palay V (1974) Cerebellar cortex, cytology and organization. Springer, Berlin Heidelberg New York
46. Peters A, Palay SL, Webster H de F (1976) The fine structure of the nervous system. The neurons and supporting cells, 2nd edition. Saunders, Philadelphia
47. Ribak CE, Vaughn JE, Saito K (1976) Immunocytochemical localization of glutamic acid decarboxylase in neuronal somata following colchicine inhibition of axonal transport. Neurosci Abstr 11:796
48. Saito K (1976) Immunocytochemical studies of GAD and GABA-T. In: Roberts E, Chase TN, Tower DB (eds) GABA in nervous system function. Raven Press, New York, p 103
49. Saito K, Schousboe A, Wu J-Y, Roberts E (1974) Some immunochemical properties and specificity of GABA-α-ketoglutarate transaminase from mouse brain. Brain Res 65:287–296
50. Schousboe A, Wu J-Y, Roberts E (1973) Purification and characterization of the 4-aminobutyrate-2-ketoglutarate transaminase from mouse brain. Biochem 12:2868–2873
51. Shousboe A, Wu J-Y, Roberts E (1974) Subunit structure and kinetic properties of 4-aminobutyrate-2-ketoglutarate transaminase purified from mouse brain. J Neurochem 23:1189–1195
52. Sotelo C, Llinás R (1972) Specialized membrane junctions between neurons in the vertebrate cerebellar cortex. J Cell Biol 53:271–289
53. Sotelo C, Privat A, Drian MJ (1972) Localization of (^{3}H)GABA in tissue culture of rat cerebellum using electron microscopy radioautography. Brain Res 45:302–308
54. Steiner AC, Parker CW, Kipnis DM (1972) Radioimmunoassay for cyclic nucleotides. I. Preparation of antibodies and iodinated cyclic nucleotides. J Biochem 247:1106–1124
55. Sternberger LA (1979) Immunocytochemistry. 2nd edn. Wiley & Sons, New York
56. Tolbert DL, Bantli H, Bloedel JR (1976) Anatomical and physiological evidence for a cerebellar nucleocortical projection in the cat. Neuroscience 1:205–218
57. Van Gelder NM (1965) The histochemical demonstration of γ-aminobutyric acid metabolism by reduction of the tetrazolium salt. J Neurochem 12:231–237
58. Voogd J (1964) The cerebellum of the cat. Structure and fibre connexions. Van Gorcum, Assen
59. Wong F, Schousboe A, Saito K, Wu J-Y, Roberts F (1974) Glutamate decarboxylase and GABA-transaminase from six mouse strains. Brain Res 68:133–139
60. Wood JG, McLaughlin BJ, Vaughn JE (1976) Immunocytochemical localization of GAD in electron microscopic preparations of rodent CNS. In: Roberts E, Chasen N, Towers DB (eds) GABA in nervous system function. Raven Press, New York, pp 133–148
61. Wu J-Y (1976) Purification, characterization, and kinetic studies of GAD and GABA-T from mouse brain. In: Roberts E, Chase TN, Tower DB (eds) GABA in nervous system function. Raven Press, New York, p 7
62. Wu J-Y, Roberts E (1974) Properties of brain L-glutamate decarboxylase: Inhibition studies. J Neurochem 23:759–767
63. Wu J-Y, Matsuda T, Roberts E (1973) Purification and characterization of glutamate decarboxylase from mouse brain. J Biol Chem 248:3029–3034

Discussion

Krnjevic: Concerning the variability of GAD-immunostaining in Purkinje cells, McLaughlin and co-workers observed much stronger reaction using topical injections of colchicine.
Chan-Palay: Yes, we have observed this also. Not all Purkinje cells, however, were stained.
Mugnaini: With the new antiserum introduced by Oertel and co-workers, nearly all Purkinje cells are stained in the rat.
Krnjevic: Not everybody agrees that muscimol is selective for the receptor sites. There is some evidence that it may bind also to the uptake sites.
Chan-Palay: We have done a long series of studies not only with muscimol but also with isoguvacine and we use these in parallel with an uptake blocker such as nipecotic acid. There is conflicting evidence in the literature.
Korn: Would you rule out that some of your labeling may be presynaptic?
Chan-Palay: The EM studies indicate that the labeling is equally presynaptic and postsynaptic. Other agents, such as serotonin were exclusively presynaptic, but not the muscimol binding.
Balazs: I am very pleased about your localization of cGMP in astrocytes. This agrees with our biochemical data. However, I wish to express a warning: the antibodies do not show where cGMP is, but reveal sites where there is a concentration of binding protein.
Chan-Palay: In fact, these problems indicate that neurochemical studies should be paralleled by immunocytochemical studies.
Balazs: We are able to increase the cGMP level 400-fold in the cerebellum, and we do not find it when we look with the antiserum because with the electron microscope, it is the binding protein that shows with this method. Also, biochemistry indicates that GABA-transaminase is mainly a mitochondrial protein. In your pictures the mitochondria were negative. Could you explain why?
Chan-Palay: Yes, it has been shown that mitochondrial *fractions* stain positively with an immunocytochemical method. But we are working with tissue sections and we have to be careful. It may be that the enzyme is in mitochondria at the surface of the sections. We discard the surface of the slice, where the reaction might have been seen.
Balazs: In biochemical tests muscimol shows a high binding to glomerular particles. Is it possible that the reason why you see a high concentration of binding in the pinceau region, whereas biochemically we do not, is that the amount of the endogenous inhibitor may vary?
Chan-Palay: Yes, it is possible.
Marshall: Is it your interpretation that there are different GABA receptors on Purkinje neurons and cerebellar nuclear neurons?
Chan-Palay: Yes, they are different, and muscimol is not the best agent for detecting binding in the cerebellar nuclei. There must be other GABA analogues which may be more effective.
Marshall: In your slide of the cerebellar nuclei with GAD-antibody staining, there was no background which could indicate there were no Purkinje terminals in that region. Was this as unusual slide?

Chan-Palay: I showed that slide only to demonstrate the two small cells. The background staining is there.
Korn: Concerning the question whether muscimol binding sites at the pinceau and the electric field effect are somehow related, I wish to point out that there are no synapses in the pinceau. In the Mauthner cell system, we were unable to show that the field effect by itself can induce transmitter release. The pinceau remains a mysterious structure. Your findings are very interesting.
Chan-Palay: I am well aware of the controversies about GABA-binding sites. The field of GABA-receptors is blooming. We are now trying to plot binding sites for muscimol and other GABA analogues during different stages of development.
W. Oertel: First, I wish to thank Dr. Palay and Dr. Chan-Palay for the opportunity to present our work at this symposium. I will deal with a study on the immunocytochemical localization of GABAergic neurons in the rat cerebellar cortex using a new antiserum against rat brain glutamic acid decarboxylase (GAD) raised in the sheep. This antiserum detects one antigen in rat brain homogenate supernatant. We used the indirect peroxidase-antiperoxidase of Sternberger applied to floating Vibratome sections of aldehyde-fixed tissue. To test the antiserum, we selected the known GABAergic projection from the striatum to the substantia nigra. Seven days after injection of kainic acid in the striatum, which leads to degeneration of the striato-nigral pathway, the GAD-immunoreactivity in the substantia nigra was substantially decreased ipsilaterally, in accordance with biochemical measurements of GAD-activity. Our results in the cerebellar nuclei using this antiserum were presented yesterday by Dr. Mugnaini. In the cerebellar cortex we obtained staining of all the types of axon terminals proved to be inhibitory by electrophysiological techniques. In the slides presented, one can recognize immunoreactive stellate cell axons synapsing on dendrites of Purkinje cells and stellate cells, basket cell axons and Purkinje recurrent collaterals synapsing on Purkinje cell bodies and basket cell bodies, and Golgi cell axons synapsing on granule cell dendrites at the periphery of glomeruli. Basket axon terminals in the pinceau were also heavily labeled. Parallel fibers, climbing fibers and mossy fibers were negative. Immunostaining of the axon-terminals in the cerebellar cortex was usually obtained with dilutions of the antiserum 1:2000–4000. With antiserum dilution of 1:1500, the cell bodies and dendrites of Purkinje cells, Golgi cells and molecular layer interneurons were also labeled. Golgi cells showed the strongest immunoreactivity and were also labeled with higher dilutions of the antiserum. Granule cells and glial cells were negative. These results, thus, indicate that our antiserum specifically localized inhibitory neurons in the cerebellar cortex, both at light and electron microscopic levels.
Chan-Palay: Dr. Oertel, with these studies were you able to obtain long series of sections allowing extensive mapping of brain structures?
Oertel: Yes. Such a study is still in progress. We have already obtained many data on brain stem and forebrain indicating the existence of several systems of GAD-positive projection neurons in addition to local circuit neurons.

Structural and Functional Relationships Between Cerebellum and Catecholamine Systems: An Overview *

S. R. Snider and R. S. Snider

Introduction

A cerebellar role in the control of catecholamine (CA) systems is a concept which was developed only in the past decade. This report summarizes recent work from this laboratory, relates these findings to relevant publications from other laboratories, and attempts to interrelate the dopamine (DA) system and some cerebellar and caudate functions.

The description of the locus ceruleus (CL) pathway to the cerebellum by Swedish workers, including Hökfeld and Fuxe [20], pioneered extensive structural and physiologic studies on this noradrenergic projection. However, it was not until 1975 that Snider [43] described cerebellar efferent fibers to the LC. A year later [45] these studies were expanded to the DA system, showing cerebellar nuclear efferent projections to the ventral tegmental area (VTA)-substantia nigra (SN) in the ventral midbrain. Several more studies have appeared (Table 1). Chan-Palay [11] described both ipsi- and contralateral fibers from the nucleus dentatus (ND) to the LC while Mezey et al. [30] found efferents from the nucleus interpositus (NI) to the LC bilaterally. Sakai et al.]39] and Cedarbaum and Aghajanian [10] reported nucleus fastigii (NF) and dentate projections to the LC. In our studies on the rat and cat [45, 49], the NF projections were primarily ipsilateral to the LC and VTA, and the NI-ND pathway to the VTA-SN was primarily contralateral. Phillipson [36] described a pathway that was mainly contralateral to the VTA from the ND, while Simon et al. [40] found ipsilateral NI-ND efferents to the VTA in addition to bilateral projections from the VTA to the cerebellum. Mezey et al. [30] reported a pathway from the NI to contralateral A8, the DA cell group adjacent to the VTA-SN.

These anatomic studies furnished a basis for planning the biochemical and physiologic experiments on functional interactions of cerebellum and CA pathways with basal ganglia. The experimental protocols also took advantage of the large literature on fast ascending systems, probably cholinergic, which might exert some control, perhaps indirect, on slower or tonic actions of the monoamine systems. We were not unmindful of Kornhuber's [25] belief that the primary function of the cerebellum is control of saccadelike movements, while basal ganglia control tends to dominate ramplike slower movements. Ad-

* This research was financed in part by NINCDS Grant No. 15953 and the Parkinson's Disease Foundation. The skilled technical assistance of Mr. William Thomas, Ms. Vernice Jackson, Ms. Judy Glassgold, and Mr. Carl Miller is gratefully acknowledged

Experimental Brain Research, Suppl. 6

Table 1. Summary of reference anatomic papers on cerebellar pathways to catecholamine nuclei

Investigator	Technique	Animal	Pathway
Simon et al. 1979	HRP	Rat	NI/ND ipsi VTA bilat CBL
Phillipson 1979	HRP	Rat	ND contra > ipsi VTA
Mezey et al. 1979	Isotope	Cat	NI contra A8
Cedarbaum and Aghajanian 1978	HRP	Rat	NF bilat LC ipsi ND
Sakai et al. 1977	HRP	Cat	NF ipsi LC ipsi ND
Chan-Palay 1977	Isotope	Rat	ND ipsi > contra LC
Snider et al. 1976	HRP	Rat	NF ipsi VTA
	FH	Cat	NI/ND contra VTA/SN
Snider 1975	FH	Cat	NF ipsi LC

bilat, bilateral; *contra,* contralateral; *ipsi,* ipsilateral; *FH,* Fink Heimer technique; *HRP,* horseradish peroxidase technique; *LC,* locus ceruleus; *ND,* nucleus dentatus, *NF,* nucleus fastigii; *NI,* nucleus interpositus; *CBl,* cerebellum; *SN,* substantia nigra; *VTA,* ventral tegmental area

ditional areas of interest were anatomic parallels in reciprocal connections of the cerebellum with the LC as part of the NE system and of the caudate nucleus with the SN as part of the DA system. Since there appears to be extensive overlap between cerebellar and basal gangliar functions it should be possible to manipulate one or both of these sets of functions to compensate for deficiencies in the other and reestablish a balance which is necessary for the correction of movement disorders. Such speculations would have great merit if it could be shown that some aspects of Parkinson's or Huntington's disease resulted from imbalance of ramp and saccadiclike movements under striatal and cerebellar control.

Methods

In biochemical studies on chronic cerebellar lesions, male Sprague-Dawley rats of about 250 g were used. Rats were anesthetized with chloral hydrate and operations were performed in a stereotaxic apparatus. Lesions were made electrolytically [48, 49], and in one group (vermal cortex) by injection of kainic acid, 1 µg in 1 µl [50]. Controls were sham-operated except as indicated. Nuclear lesions involved the dorsal-rostral NF (medial lesions), or dorsal-rostral NI, and medial ascending fibers of the ND (lateral lesions). Cerebellar cortical lesions involved the anterior vermal or paravermal cortex. The extent of the lesions was recorded by gross dissection as well as microscopic examination of the lesion site. Lesions were up to 2 mm in their largest dimension, and cerebellar weights in lesioned groups were about 6% less than controls. Cerebral hemisphere weights differed by less than 1%.

Turnover of CA was measured by administering: (a) the tyrosine hydroxylase inhibitor, d,l-alpha-methyl-para-tyrosine methylester HCl (AMT) [1]; (b) the dopa decarboxylase inhibitor, NSD-1015, 100 mg/kg [7]; or (c) 2,6-labeled ^{3}H-tyrosine (New England Nuclear, Boston), 5μg/kg [53]. Turnover-rate calculations were based on, respectively, rate of disappearance of NE or DA, rate of accumulation of dopa, and rate of accumulation of ^{3}H-NE or ^{3}H-DA in each forebrain half or, in three experiments, in each caudate nucleus. Operated animals were carefully matched with appropriate controls prior to biochemical measurements.

Three weeks after operation, rats were killed by decapitation and the brain was dissected on ice into left and right forebrain, brainstem (including mesencephalon), and cerebellum. This dissection separates the monoamine cell bodies in the midbrain and pons from nerve terminal areas in neostriatum and diencephalon. Specimens were homogenized in iced 0.4 N perchloric acid and centrifuged. Amino acids and amines in the extract were separated by column chromatography using a strong cation exchange resin [38]. Gamma aminobutyric acid (GABA), NE, and DA were sequentially eluted and standard fluorimetric assays were used to determine each compound [2, 13, 27]; GABA was assayed by a modification of a enzymatic assay [13], and glutamic acid decarboxylase (GAD) activity was measured by a similar method by Cote [13].

In experiments requiring stimulation of tissues, focal hyperthermia (FBF) of small (1–6 mm^2) areas of cerebellum or caudate was used. Accuracy of warming and readout was above 90% in both rats and cats. For the experiments reported here, we successfully adapted thermistors of varying diameters, from 0.5 mm to 2.5 mm. In addition to their capability as temperature measuring devices, thermistors may be used for warming when significant current is passed. A filtered, regulated DC power supply was used which could be set at any range between 0–10 and 0–5 mA. The warming ranged from 2 to 15 mW with thermistors of 2 mW/°C dissipation constant. Temperature spread was measured directly in some experiments (Fig. 7) and could be readily calculated from heat dissipation rates, especially when two thermistors were used (Figs. 7, 8). During momentary current interruptions, resistance readings were taken as an additional control of tissue-temperature calculations. The thermistor, encased in Teflon tubing, was placed on the brain surface or manipulated with a stereotaxic device to interior brain sites, such as cerebellar nuclei. For chronic stimulation sterile precautions were used. The thermistor was held in place by dental acrylic and flexible coupling wires were attached. In all biochemical experiments, rats were alert and restrained only by the wires during 2–4 h of stimulation. In some of the cats used in chronic experiments (example in Fig. 10), coils were also used for warming as previously described [46, 47].

Sixteen cats were used in the acute electrophysiologic experiments. They were anesthetized for surgery with i.v. Surital and rapid surgical exposure of dorsal cerebellar and cerebral surfaces was done. A standard Kopf stereotaxic instrument was then used, and as the anesthesia lightened the animal was given Flaxedil and attached to a mechanical respirator. Local xylocaine (2%) infiltration of potentially painful sites was done at 1–2 h intervals. Bipolar surface electrodes were placed on the vermis, lobule V, and lateral crus I and II. Depth electrodes were placed in the NF, ND, and contralateral caudate head according to methods used by Maiti and Snider [28].

Results

In the biochemical experiments, the steady-state rate of turnover, i.e., of release and replacement, of NE and DA was used as an estimate of physiologic activity in CA pathways. This is based on the approximate proportionality under normal conditions between neuronal firing rate and rate of turnover of neurotransmitter in nerve terminals, which in the case of the major ascending CA pathways, are located in the ipsilateral forebrain. Activity of discrete areas of the cerebellum was altered acutely by thermal or electric stimulation, or in chronic experiments by electrolytic or kainic acid lesions.

Table 2. Gamma-aminobutyric acid (GABA) in left and right forebrain 3 weeks after left cerebellar lesion

	GABA (μmol/g) in forebrain	
	Left	Right
Unoperated control (5)	1.77 ± 0.04	1.75 ± 0.05
Sham-operated control (4)	1.65 ± 0.08	1.60 ± 0.05
Left cerebellar lesion (5)	1.62 ± 0.03*	1.59 ± 0.05*

Sham-operated rats had left posterior craniectomy without cerebellar lesion. Experimental group had electrolytic lesion of left paravermis similar to Fig. 4. Rats were sacrificed 3 weeks after surgery and each half of the forebrain was analyzed for GABA content. Shown is the mean ± S.E. of 4–5 values. * $P < 0.05$ *vs* control (2-tailed Student's *t*-test after analysis of variance)

Vermal lesions or stimulation resulted in ipsilateral effects. Contralateral values did not differ from controls except as noted. Reduced NE and DA turnover in the forebrain followed NF lesions or vermal cortical thermal stimulation, while enhanced turnover was found in rats with vermal cortical lesions or following fastigial stimulation (Figs. 2, 3). There was little effect of lateral cerebellar lesions on NE turnover (data not shown). However, lateral lesions did increase contralateral DA turnover if mainly cortex was involved, as did acute stimulation of ND (Fig. 4). Stimulation of vermal cortex decreased DA turnover (Fig. 3) but paravermal cortical stimulation had little effect (Fig. 4), possibly because the area stimulated by the 1-mm-diameter thermistor was small (Fig. 7) relative to the input to the NI and ND.

Since the physiologic experiments were based on interactions between the cerebellum and corpus striatum, additional data on forebrain GABA were obtained. There was a slight decrease in forebrain GABA concentration in rats with cerebellar lesions (Table 2). Additional data on GAD, a GABA-synthesiz-

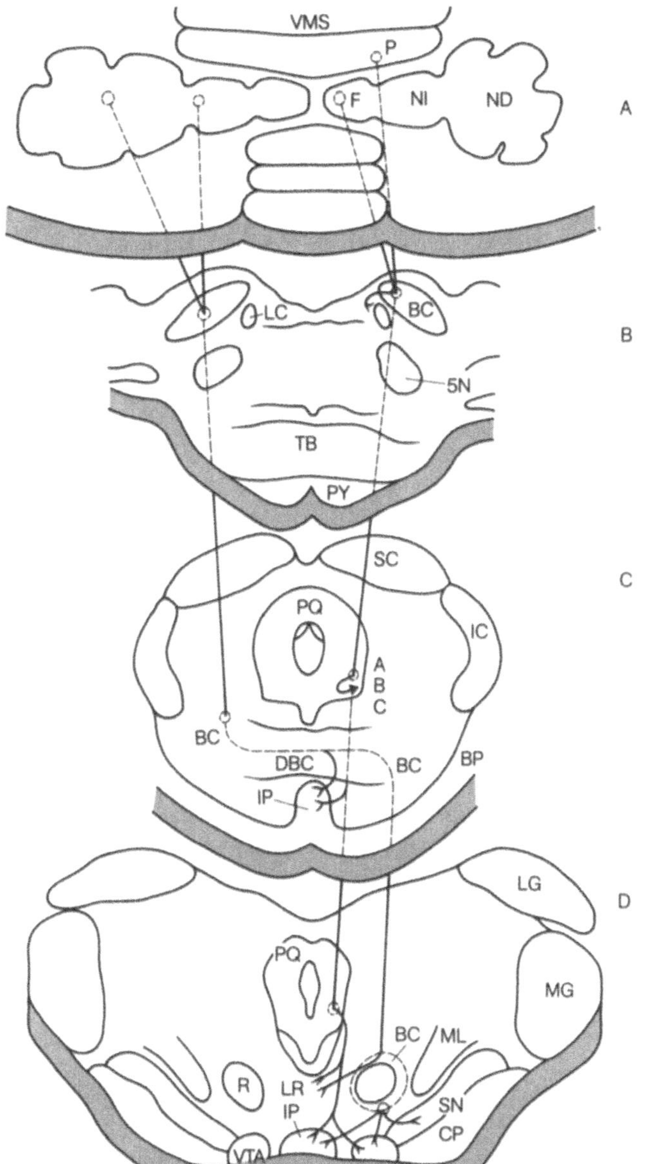

Fig. 1A–D. Cerebellar connections to locus ceruleus (*LC*) and substantia nigra (*SN*)-ventral tegmental area (VTA). **A–D** Cross sections of cat brainstem. *ABC*, accessory brachium conjunctivum; *BC*, brachium conjunctivum; *BP*, brachium pontis; *CP*, cerebral peduncle; *DBC*, decussation brachium conjunctivum; *F*, fastigii (nucleus); *IP*, interpeduncularis; *LR*, linearis rostralis; *LG*, lateral geniculate; *MG*, medial geniculate; *ML*, medial lemniscus; *ND*, nucleus dentatus; *NI*, nucleus interpositus; *P*, Purkinje cell; *PQ*, periaqueductal gray; *PY*, pyramid; *R*, red nucleus; *SC* and *IC*, superior and inferior colliculus; *VMS*, vermis; *5N*, fifth nerve (nucleus). Reprinted by permission of Academic Press, New York, Snider et al. [45]

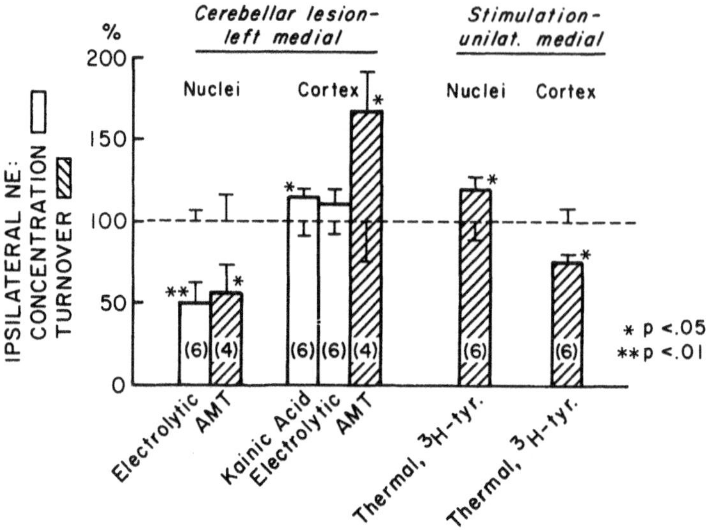

Fig. 2. Forebrain norepinephrine (*NE*) levels and turnover after unilateral medial cerebellar lesions or stimulation in rat. Electrolytic lesions of left nucleus fastigii (NF) or left vermal cortex, lobules IV and V, were made 3 weeks before sacrifice. Kainic acid, 1 μg in 1 μl, was injected into anterior vermal cortex 3 weeks before the lesions. Alpha-methyltyrosine (*AMT*), 250 mg/kg i.p. 1 and 2 h before sacrifice was used to measure disappearance rate and to estimate steady-state NE turnover in two groups with electrolytic lesions. Thermal stimulation of left or right NF or vermal cortex at 40 °C was used for 2–4 h. In these animals ^{3}H-*NE*, formed from ^{3}H-tyrosine, 5 μg/kg, i.p. 1 h before sacrifice, was measured in each half of the forebrain. In other groups, NE concentrations in each half of the forebrain were measured by a standard fluorimetric method and, in *AMT*-treated rats, disappearance rate was calculated by assuming a monoexponential decline of *NE*. Shown are means+S.E. of four to six experiments, expressed as percent control (ipsilateral/contralateral×100%). Control values: NE, 1.75 nm/g; NE turnover (AMT), 0.89 nm/g/h; ^{3}H-NE, 23.6 cpm. Kainic acid values from Snider and Snider [50]. Statistics by 2-tailed Student's t-test on right-left pairs. Differences vs *NE* values for unoperated control rats were significant in the two nuclear lesion groups and the AMT-cortex lesion group ($p<.05$, 2-tailed Student's t-test on grouped means). Lateral cerebellar lesions had only slight effects on forebrain *NE* [49]

Fig. 4. Dopamine (*DA*) levels and turnover in contralateral forebrain after unilateral lateral cerebellar lesions or stimulation. Electrolytic lesions of left nucleus interpositus (NI), medial nucleus dentatus (ND), and overlying cortex were made 3 weeks before killing; *AMT* was given to one group of operated rats as in Fig. 2. The dopa decarboxylase inhibitor, *NSD*-1015, 100 mg/kg i.p. 1 h before killing, was given to a second group, and dopa was determined in each forebrain half; ^{3}H-*DA* formed from ^{3}H-tyrosine was measured in caudate (*Cd*) in a third group of rats with nuclear lesions. Control values: dopa 3.02 nm/g/h; ^{3}H-*DA* (Cd) 26.2 cpm. Values for formation of ^{3}H-*DA* 30 min after unilateral electric stimulation of ND in cat are from Nieoullon et al. [33]. Data are expressed as percent of unoperated or prestimulation control values. Unilateral thermal stimulation of anterior paravermal cortex at 40 °C was used for 2–4 h as in Fig. 2

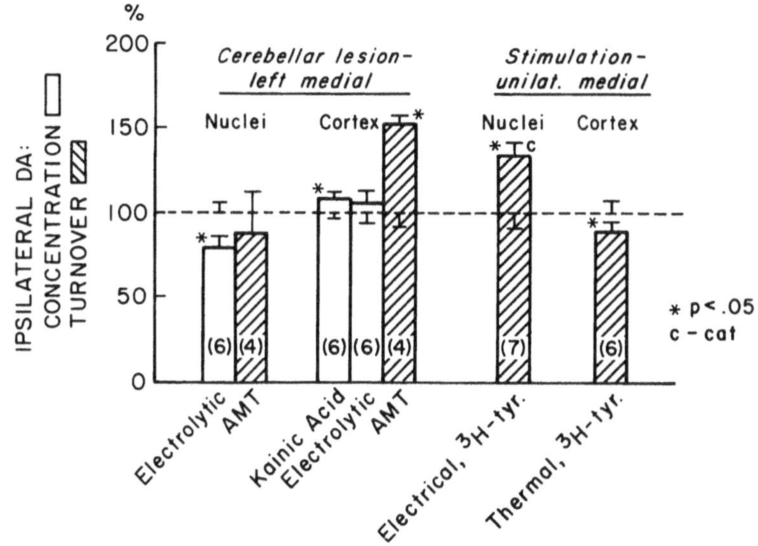

Fig. 3. Forebrain dopamine (*DA*) levels and turnover after unilateral medial cerebellar lesions or stimulation. Stimulation of NF was performed by trains of monophasic electric shocks, 0.2 Hz for 10 min, in cat; ^{3}H-*DA*, formed from ^{3}H-tyrosine, remvoed and delivered continuously via push-pull cannulae in the caudate nuclei, is expressed as percent of prestimulation value (data from Nieoullon et al. [33]). Procedures in other groups as in Fig. 2 except that *DA* and ^{3}H-*DA* were measured. Control vaules: *DA* 7.84 nm/g; *DA* turnover (*AMT*) 2.63 nm/g/h; ^{3}H-*DA* 34.9 cpm. Difference vs values for unoperated control rats was significant in *AMT*-cortex lesion group

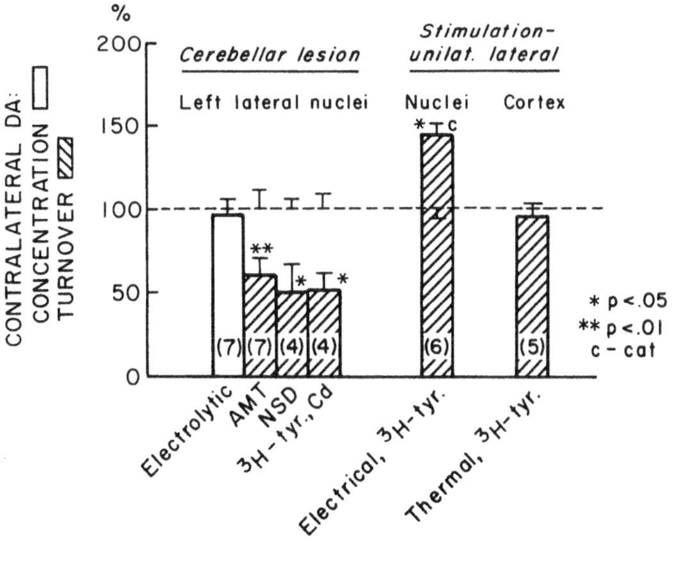

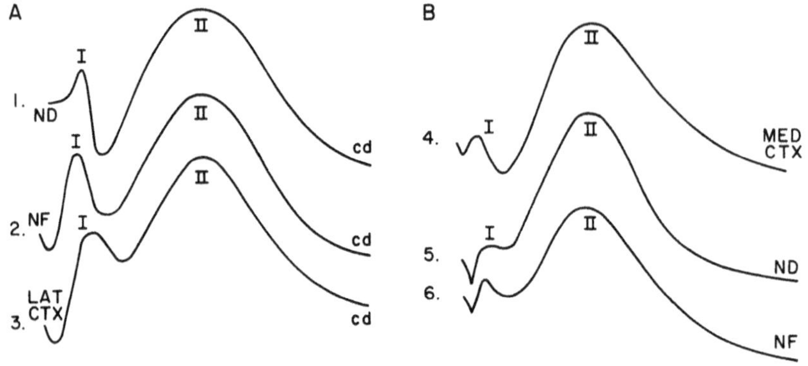

Fig. 5A, B. Cerebellar-caudate and caudate-cerebellar evoked responses. Evoked responses were recorded from cat lateral ventral caudate nucleus **A** T-3, and monkey medial cerebellar cortex $\mathbf{B}_4$, nucleus dentatus $\mathbf{B}_5$, and nucleus fastigii $\mathbf{B}_6$. Electric stimulation: in cat, $\mathbf{A}_1$ nucleus dentatus, $\mathbf{A}_2$ nucleus fastigii, and $\mathbf{A}_3$ lateral cerebellar cortex; in monkey **B** lateroventral caudate nucleus (contralateral to recording sites) for all three traces. Each curve is an average of five consecutive sweeps obtained from an acute animal. Each of the six curves shows a short latency peak (*I*) and a long latency peak (*II*). See also Table 3. *cd*, caudate nucleus; *ND*, nucleus dentatus; *NF*, nucleus fastigii; *MED CTX* and *LAT CTX*, medial and lateral cerebellar cortex

ing enzyme which reflects long term alterations in GABA metabolism [21], also suggest a real decrease. Forebrain GAD was 20% lower in operated than in control animals (11.5 ± 0.2 mmol $^{14}CO_2$ released/g wet wt./h; control $= 14.2 \pm 0.5$, $n = 6$, $p < .01$, no difference between sides). The tendency for forebrain GABA metabolism to decrease may be a consequence of some undetermined readjustment within the cerebellum [42] which is reflected in decreased striatal activity. Cellular location of GABA is uncertain but GABA levels in the corpus striatum are unusually high [13]. It is also possible that reduced GABA-mediated ac-

Table 3. Evoked response latencies between cerebellum and caudate

Stimulate		Record	Wave I peak latency	Wave II peak latency
A_1.	*ND*	Caudate	6–9	20–30
A_2.	*NF*	Caudate	5–10	18–27
A_3.	*Lat.Ctx.*	Caudate	5–12	18–30
B_4.	Caudate	*Med.Ctx.*	4–8	22–24
B_5.	Caudate	*ND*	5–6	18–22
B_6.	Caudate	*NF*	5–6	16–20

Range of latencies in milliseconds for cerebellum to caudate pathway (A_1, A_2, A_3; 4 cats) and caudate to cerebellum pathway (B_4, B_5, B_6; 2 monkeys. See text for details of procedure). Individual examples are illustrated in Fig. 5. Note differences in smaller first wave I and larger second wave II

ND, nucleus dentatus; *NF*, nucleus fastigii; *Lat.Ctx.*, *Med.Ctx.*, lateral or medial cerebellar cortex

tivity preceded the reduction in DA turnover (Figs. 3, 4), but it seems unlikely that the cerebellum contributes directly to the GABAergic innervation above the midbrain.

The biochemical studies provide additional support for the existence of ipsilateral and contralateral pathways to ascending CA systems from medial and lateral cerebellar nuclei, respectively (Fig. 1). They suggest that these pathways have an excitatory effect and that they may be inhibited by topographically related cerebellar cortex.

These studies also facilitated the adaptation of physiologic experiments to initial anatomic findings. Physiologic investigations focused on DA systems because of their known relation to motor function. The following stimulation experiments were performed: (a) Evoked caudate responses induced by electric stimulation of cerebellum, (b) evoked cerebellar responses induced by electric stimulation of caudate nucleus, and (c) chronic FBF stimulation of caudate head or cerebellum with EEG recording in various brain sites.

Evoked response data from ten cats and two immature *Macaca mulatta* monkeys are summarized in Fig. 5 and Table 3. The curves A1, A2, A3 in Fig. 5 (recording site: caudate nucleus, stimulation site: cerebellum) show more similarities than differences. In each trace there is a small, short-latency wave (I) and a larger, longer latency wave (II). Comparison of first peaks indicates A3 is larger than A1 or A2, which is interpreted as activation of a greater population of fibers and cells in the caudate nucleus. All the data are consistent in showing two populations of responses (early and late) in the caudate head, which result from cerebellar stimulation. The curves, B4, B5, B6, of Fig. 5 differ in that the stimulating and recording electrodes are reversed, and the data represent caudate projections to the vermis, NF, and ND. The small first wave has been interpreted in a similar experiment [15] to indicate mossy-fiber responses and the large second wave activity in fibers leading to climbing-fiber terminals.

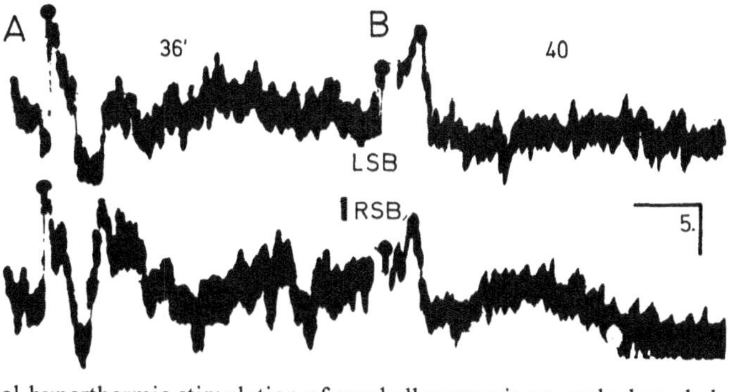

Fig. 6 A, B. Effects of focal hyperthermic stimulation of cerebellar vermis on evoked cerebellar activity. Surface temperature 36 °C **A**, and 40 °C. **B.** Electrodes were placed in left (*LSB*) and right (*RSB*) superior brachium for recording evoked responses. Single electric pulses (5 V, 0.1 ms) were applied to the cerebellar cortex in the focally warmed area. The effects of electric stimulation are shown in A (*upper* and *lower* tracings) and the combined effects of electric and FBF stimulation are shown in B (*upper* and *lower* tracings). Focal hyperthermia enhances cerebellar activity [46, 47]. It is not known how such changes alter the responses shown in **B.** *Calibration: horizontal,* 5.0 ms; vertical, 5×50 mV

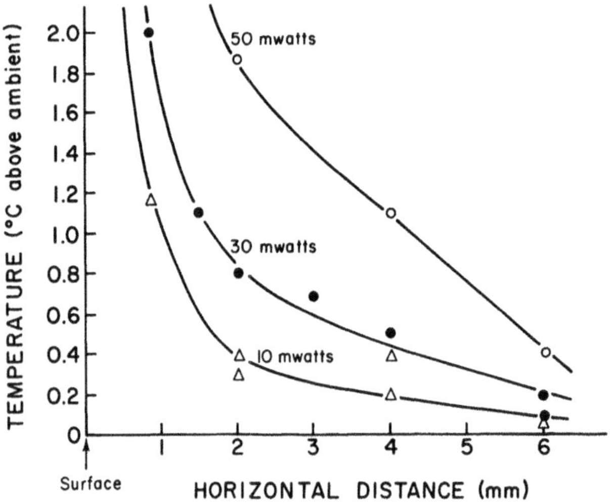

Fig. 7. Temperature spread in rat brain during focal warming. Temperatures were recorded with a thermistor probe at indicated distances from a heat-generating, 5 KΩ, 1-mm diameter, thermistor ("surface") at three levels of warming (10, 30, 50 mW). Recording and stimulating thermistors were placed on the cerebral cortical surface through burr holes 2 mm from the midline. Results from two anesthetized rats are combined in the figure. Temperature decrement is approximately proportional to the reciprocal of the distance. Temperature-distance curves for the cerebellar surface of anesthetized rat and cat were similar. Somewhat higher rates of heat dissipation and less lateral spread of temperature were usual in alert, free-moving animals but significant warming of the contralateral cerebellum was infrequent

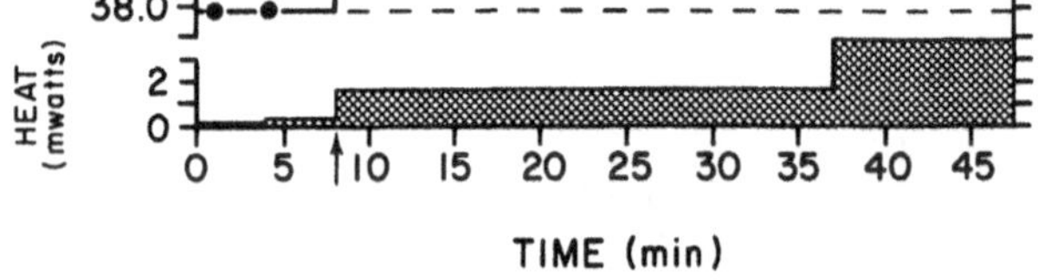

Fig. 8. Temperatures of caudate nuclei during left caudate warming in cat. Bilateral, 3-KΩ, 2-mm diameter thermistors were placed over caudate nuclei bilaterally. The right thermistor was used to record temperature, and heat to the left thermistor was increased three times in the period shown. At 1.4 mW (*arrow*) there was a rapid increase in left caudate temperature. A gradual decrease in temperature occurred during the next 20–30 min, although the temperature on the right was unchanged and thermal energy supplied to the thermistor was kept constant. The increased rate of heat dissipation may be caused by an increase in local blood flow. EEG recordings from the same animal are shown in Fig. 9

Additional information on the effects of chronic stimulation of the striatum was obtained by focal warming (FBF) stimulation of the caudate. The methodology for FBF of the caudate was similar to that for the surface of the cerebellum remove although thermistors were more often used for stimulation (Figs. 6, 7, 8; ref. [46]). Figure 9 demonstrates some acute effects of this procedure on an unanesthetized cat. When focal warming (+ 0.2 °C) was applied to the left/caudate head, spontaneous electric activity began to increase in amplitude and the fast frequencies were replaced by synchronous slower frequencies (second pair of tracings). Additional elevation of temperature (1.3 °C) induced further amplitude increases in the 6–9/s sharp waves and increased synchronization (third pair of tracings). When the electric activity of the warmed caudate in this pair of tracings is compared with that of the unwarmed side, and both compared with the uppermost pair (prior to warming), the significant increase in amplitude can be readily appreciated. With cessation of warming (lowermost pair of

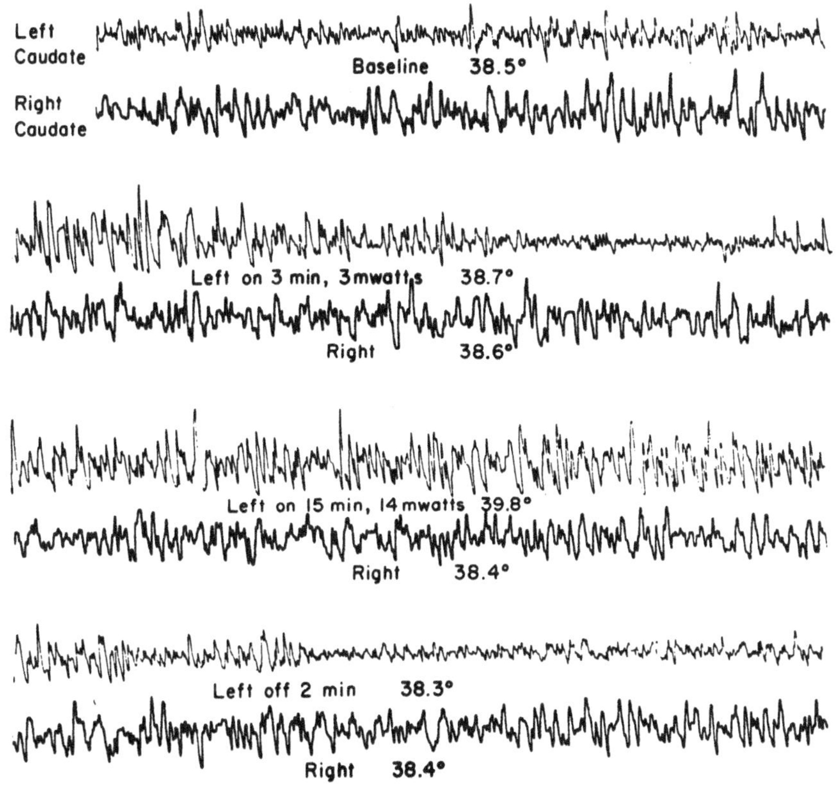

Fig. 9. EEG bipolar recordings from left and right caudate during left caudate warming. Records were obtained from cat in Fig. 8 during relaxed wakefulness. *Uppermost pair* show left-right caudate EEGs before induction of focal hyperthermia (FBF). The *second pair* of EEGs show early changes in left caudate activity induced by focal warming of 0.2 °C (from 38.5 to 38.7 °C) for 3 min. In the *third pair* of tracings, a prominent sustained increase of amplitude and frequency is seen after 15 min of FBF to 39.8 °C. The *last pair* of tracings show caudate activity after FBF was withdrawn. The EEGs are similar but not identical to the baseline tracings

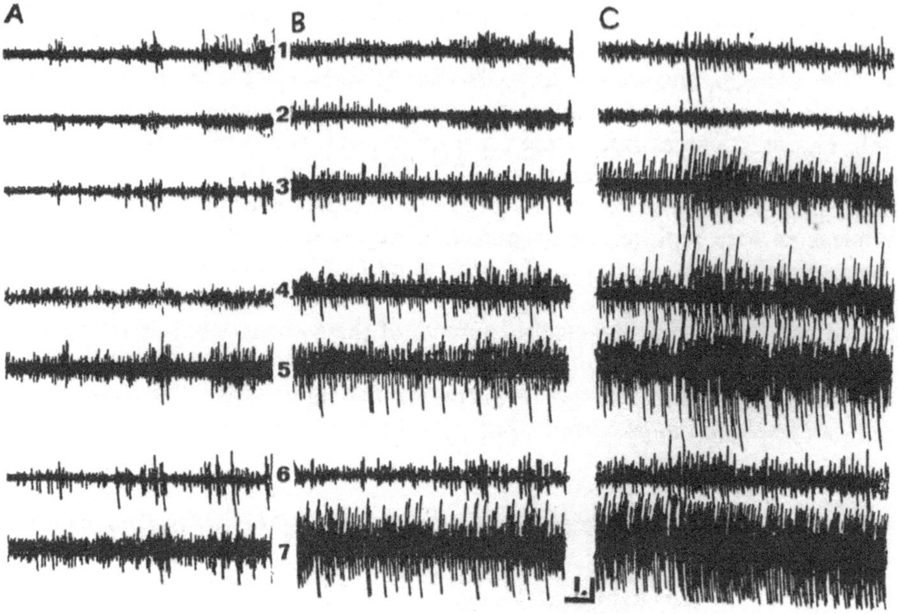

Fig. 10A–C. EEG tracings from multiple brain sites before and during chronic caudate warming. Records were taken in an unanesthetized free-moving cat implanted with seven electrodes and thermodes 7 weeks previously. **A** Control without focal warming (FBF); **B** after 9.5 h FBF to 40.5 °C (about + 2 °C) of left caudate nucleus; **C** after 4 days FBF of left caudate nucleus. The tracings were taken from: *1*, left amygdala; *2*, left hippocampus; *3*, left sensorimotor cortex; *4*, right anterior vermis; *5*, right nucleus fastigii; *6*, left nucleus ventralis lateralis; and *7*, left caudate head (*lowermost* tracing). Increased amplitude and frequency is especially prominent in the stimulated left caudate (channel *7*) as well as in nucleus fastigii (channel *5*), vermis (channel *4*), and sensorimotor cortex (channel *3*). There are only slight changes in limbic area (amygdala)

tracings) left/caudate activity when recorded as EEG tracings returned to prestimulation levels. These and related experiments demonstrated the effectiveness of the method for acute stimulation of the caudate and provided a basis for extending the work to chronic animals.

The 7-channel EEG tracings (Fig. 10) are representative of data obtained from four cats in which the effects of chronic unilateral caudate warming were studied over periods up to 22 days. During 9 h of warming there was unquestionable increase in caudate activity (channel 7) and increases of small amplitude in the NF and vermis as well as sensorimotor cortex. The series of EEG tracings in Fig. 10C were taken after 4.5 days of continuous caudate warming and show additional enhancement of caudate activity along with further increases in the NF, vermis, and sensorimotor cortex. Smaller elevations are seen in ventralis lateralis thalami while the limbic areas (amygdala, hippocampus) show only slight change. These data demonstrate the effectiveness of chronic FBF stimulation on the caudate nucleus, and they show that the cerebellum may be more prominently involved than the cerebrum or thalamus.

Discussion

The morphological and chemical studies have emphasized some parallels between the caudate and cerebellum. For example, unlike the cerebral cortex which has direct efferents to the brain stem, cerebellar cortical efferents synapse upon nuclear cells with cholinergic output to the ventralis lateralis (VL) plus intralaminar thalamus. Caudate-nucleus efferents synapse in the nucleus (globus) pallidus with strong cholinergic output to the ventralis anterior (VA) and intralaminar thalamus. Both the cerebellar cortex and caudate nucleus have high levels of acetylcholine and GABA and both have important reciprocal connections with catecholamine systems. The serotonin connections are especially interesting since the same nucleus (B7, B8) sends efferent fibers to both the cerebellum and caudate nucleus. (Additional details on these connections are given by Chan-Palay [11].)

Major pathways are summarized in Fig. 11 and two circuit categories are emphasized: (a) reciprocal connections of the monoamine systems with the cerebellum and basal ganglia, and (b) loop circuits not utilizing the monoamines as primary neurotransmitters. The following discussion reviews the evidence for these circuits and relates data on CA systems presented above to existing information on cerebellar-basal ganglia interactions.

Descending Pathways

Anatomic studies on possible descending pathways from basal ganglia to the cerebellum are numerous. Pathways from the caudate nucleus and globus pallidus to olivary nuclei have been more extensively studied [52]. Fox and Williams [15, 16], Gresty and Paul [19], and Oka and Jinnai [34] have described cerebellar responses following caudate stimulation. The responses are similar to those shown in this chapter (Fig. 5A). Difficulties in interpretation of the data have arisen because of collaterals to the caudate from cerebral efferents in the internal capsule. We favor the interpretation of Oka and Jinnai [34], who believe that the short-latency, so-called mossy-fiber response results from collaterals of corticopontine fibers and that the longer latency response is the result of collateral activation of olivary nuclei. Chronic cortical lesions to induce degeneration of cortical efferents reduced or eliminated the responses. However, a discrepancy still remains since Fox and Williams [16] noted that the longer latency responses pass through the SN while the shorter latency ones pass through the midbrain just dorsal to the red nucleus. If Oka and Jinnai [34] are correct then the descending cortical efferents should be located in the internal capsule and cerebral peduncle. The dilemma could be resolved by a careful study with one of the anatomic labeling techniques.

The origin of a second descending pathway not related to the monoamine pathways may be either the corpus striatum or globus pallidus, with efferents via the tegmental nucleus of the pontine region [24], which has reciprocal connections to the cerebellar cortex. Such connections require additional study [56] since there is little evidence for pallido-rubral and nigrorubal fibers (although

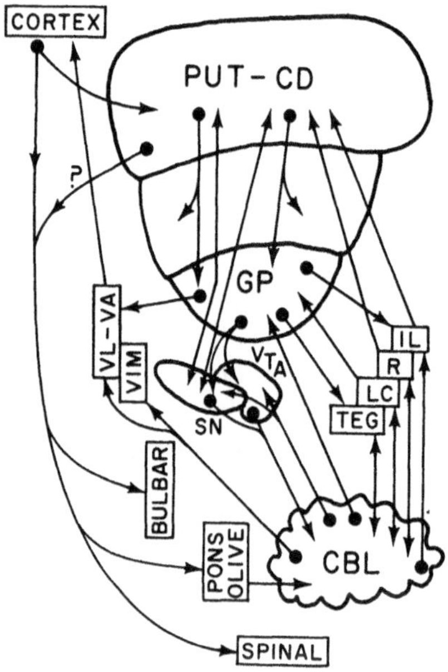

Fig. 11. Connections of cerebellum, monoamine systems, and basal ganglia. The wide-ranging overlapping connections of basal ganglia and cerebellum are grouped into (a) the monoamine loops, and (b) loops which exclude the monoamines as primary transmitters. The diagram emphasizes connections of structures interposed between cerebral cortex and lower reticular formation and several thalamo-cortical relays are not included. *BULBAR*, midbrain and medulla; *CBL*, cerebellum; *CD*, caudate; *CORTEX*, cerebral cortex; *GP*, globus pallidum; *IL*, intralaminar thalamus; *LC*, locus ceruleus; *PONS* and *OLIVE*, pontine and olivary nuclei; *PUT*, putamen; *R*, raphe nuclei; *SN*, substantia nigra; *TEG*, midbrain tegmentum; *VA*, ventralis anterior; *VIM*, ventralis intermedius thalamus; *VL*, ventralis lateralis thalamus; *VTA*, ventral tegmental area

the rubrocerebellar loop is widely recognized). No known function has been assigned to the pallido-tegmenti-pedunculo-pontinus (compacta) loop nor have cerebellar connections to it been established.

Ascending Pathways

An ascending nonmonoamine pathway from the ND to the globus pallidus has been described by Carpenter and Stevens [8] and Carrea and Mettler [9]. A more frequently described pathway is that of cerebellar nuclei to intralaminar thalamic nuclei [22], hence to the corpus striatum [32]. Mehler and Nauta [29] believe that the centruum medianum (CM) sends fibers to putamen while the centralis lateralis and parafascicularis project to the caudate. It must be significant that the cerebellum projects via the brachium conjunctivum to at least two of the three intralaminar nuclei; globus pallidus efferents to the CM are widely recognized [29].

The tracts from the cerebellar nuclei to the VL and ventralis intermedius (VIM) have been frequently described and need no additional documentation. Recognition is given to prominent pallidal projections to the ventral thalamic group, primarily to the VA but overlapping with cerebellar efferents in the VL [23].

In our studies, at least two groups of ascending fibers are indicated if the latencies of evoked responses in the caudate are used as an indicator (Fig. 5). The widest spread and fusion of waves are seen when the cerebellar cortex (Fig. 5, A3) rather than the nuclei is stimulated. Considering the fast conduction rates of cerebellar efferents to the thalamus (see Fig. 11) wave I could follow one of several paths: (a) CBL → IL → CD/, (b) CBL → GP → IL → CD/, (c) CBL → GP → SN → CD.

Possibilities for wave II include the monoamine pathways, since their conduction velocities may be as slow as 1.0 m/s. In each of the following, latencies longer than 18 ms can be predicted: (a) CBL → LC → CD, (b) CBL → R → CD, (c) CBL → SN/VTA → CD. Interpretation becomes complex when thalamic nuclei (VA, VIM, VL) and their connections to motor and premotor cortex are considered. For example, what is the latency of (a) CBL → VL or VIM → cerebral cortex → CD, or (b) CBL → GP → VA → cerebral cortex → CD? If the answer proves to be – it overlaps the monoamine systems – then neurochemists and neurophysiologists have many busy laboratory periods ahead.

The functional significance attached to these pathways is slowly emerging. There is general agreement that the cerebral motor and premotor areas receive highly integrated data from them that can be rapidly processed [12, 23]. In higher mammals, these systems when combined with parallel circuits from the cerebellum and pallidum converging on intralaminar thalamic nuclei emphasize the complexity and extent of interactions between the cerebellum and striatum.

Focal Hyperthermic Stimulation

In two groups of experiments reported here, focal warming stimulation (FBF) was used on the caudate nucleus in acute (Fig. 9) and chronic (Fig. 10) free-moving animals. The advantages of the FBF methods are: (a) electric pulses are not necessary to enhance activity within the caudate nucleus, (b) the troublesome features of metallic electrodes reacting with brain tissues and membranes during chronic stimulations are avoided. Focal warming of the caudate nucleus with as little as 1.3 °C above ambient temperature elevated EEG amplitudes as much as 100% in the frequency range of 6–10/s (Fig. 9). Abnormal discharges were not seen. Earlier studies [46, 47] on FBF-induced changes showed enhanced multiunit activity in the cerebellum. Figure 6 demonstrates effects on evoked reponses. These studies were then extended to the DA system (Figs. 3, 4). Cholinergic agents such as oxotremorine or physostigmine enhance, whereas anticholinergic drugs diminish, the release of striatal DA [4], indicating that a cholinergic influence may activate the nigro-striatal DA pathway. Bartholini and Stadler [4] also point out that there may be an extrastriatal site of action of acetylcholine, and we suggest the cerebellar efferent system of fibers to the SN may contribute to the cholinergic input; most but perhaps not all of the fibers in the brachium conjunctivum are cholinergic.

Despite its complexity some progress has been made in relating the functions of the DA system to disorders of movement and posture [3, 4, 6, 21, 26, 37, 44]. By contrast, it is more difficult to assign defined functions to the serotoninergic and the noradrenergic systems. Smith and Sweet [41] emphasize the complexity as follows: "central 5-HT and NE systems seem designed to integrate, regulate or perhaps 'tune' the whole range of cerebral functions by switching . . .".

Electroencephalogram changes in several forebrain and brain stem sites resulted from chronic FBF stimulation of the caudate nucleus. Progressive increase in amplitude of caudate activity was the most prominent and consistent finding, but of greater interest was the enhancement of cerebellar activity (Fig. 10, channels 4 and 5) with only slight increase in the VL. Figure 11 summarizes pathways, the activity of which may be altered by caudate stimulation. Ventralis lateralis may be involved secondarily through the cerebellum while the intralaminar nuclei may be activated more directly, both by the cerebellum and the globus pallidus. All of these nuclei could participate in cerebral activation. Some supporting data are available from Ishida's studies [22]. He was able to stimulate the NF and obtain increased unit activity in the intralaminar thalamus. Feger et al. [14] also reported excitation of nigral single units following either peripheral nerve or cerebellar surface stimulation and inhibition of the same units by motor cortex or caudate stimulation.

Some Interactions with DA Systems

The above physiologic data also have biochemical support since opposing actions of the cerebellum and cerebrum on DA metabolism have been found by Glowinski et al. [17] and Nieoullon et al. [33]. During acute electric stimulation of the cerebellum there was enhancement of ^{3}H-DA efflux from caudate, while inhibition resulted from stimulation of the cerebrum. The specific pattern of ^{3}H-DA efflux with stimulation of the ND was increase in the contralateral caudate and decrease in the ipsilateral caudate, and with NF stimulation was increase in the ipsilateral caudate and no contralateral effects. Additional studies on single-unit activity in the SN and caudate during ND or NF stimulation are clearly indicated.

In rats, chronic cerebellar cortical lesions resulted in increased NE and DA turnover while nuclear lesions produced the opposite (Figs. 2, 3, 4). Like the stimulation experiments, these results indicate an alteration of activity in catecholaminergic pathways. In the case of the NE system, interruption of the reciprocal connections between the NF and LC [43] could explain the decreased level and turnover of NE following NF lesions, while vermal cortical lesions could increase the firing rate of LC neurons by disinhibition of the NF. The latter could contribute to the increased spinal fluid levels of NE in patients undergoing electric stimulation of the anterior cerebellum for epilepsy [55]. Retrograde effects, mediated via LC afferents to the cerebellum, on NE pathways to the forebrain may be present but are less likely to be important in chronic experiments of 3 or more weeks (see ref. [49]). A direct effect of lesions on NE or DA cell bodies is unlikely since such neurons have not been identified in the cerebellum of the rat, and no morphological changes in the LC, SN, or VTA were found after chronic lesions in previous studies [45, 48, 49]. Therefore, at least part of the effect on NE and possibly DA may be mediated by functional alterations in the direct cerebellar pathways to the pons and ventral midbrain (Fig. 1). In the case of the DA system, indirect effects of lesions or stimulation on DA pathways to the forebrain, mediated by parallel non-CA ascending pathways such as the multisynaptic cerebellar projections to the caudate nucleus (Fig. 11) also are likely.

In earlier studies, systemic injection of the DA agonist, apomorphine, in rats with lateral or medial cerebellar nuclear lesions resulted in ipsiversive or contraversive rotation [49], indicating, respectively, contralateral or ipsilateral supersensitivity of striatal DA receptors. The unidirectional turning elicited by apomorphine was prevented by levodopa pretreatment (unpublished data). In addition, rats with cerebellar nuclear lesions showed increased sensitivity to the hypokinetic effect of the DA antagonist, haloperidol [49]. Conversely, intrastriatal apomorphine was reported to elicit an increase in the cerebellar cyclic GMP, an indication of stimulation of cerebellar cortical neurons [5]. These biochemical and pharmacologic results, along with the anatomic and electrophysiologic findings (Figs. 1, 5, 10), strongly argue for specific functionally important relationships of the cerebellum with DA pathways and striatum. The parkinsonism syndrome (bradykinesia, tremor, rigidity, postural disorder) cannot be fully reproduced in experimental animals or in man by lesions of the nigrostriatal pathways alone. Based on observations in monkeys with interruption of ascending cerebellar or DA pathways, several groups have suggested that functional abnormality of cerebellar efferents also is required [3, 31, 35, 37]. The role of the cerebellum in tremor has been established by the studies of Narabayashi [31] and others on VIM thalamus. Levodopa can alleviate the resting component of cerebellar tremor in the monkey [18], suggesting that a resting tremor associated with relative deficiency of brain DA may result from cerebellar lesions. Conversely, both lesions and electric stimulation of the cerebellum have been reported to increase DA turnover in humans [51]. Surgical manipulation of the cerebellum would be unlikely to increase brain DA turnover in Parkinson's disease because of degeneration of DA neurons. However, it is of interest that vermal atrophy has been found in a small number of patients with schizophrenia [54] since some symptoms of this disease may be due to an increase in brain DA.

Summary

A) Anatomic evidence indicates reciprocal connections between (a) cerebellum and locus ceruleus, (b) cerebellum and substantia nigra-ventral tegmental area, and (c) cerebellum and raphe nuclei. Cerebellar and pallidal pathways converging on ventral and intralaminar thalamic nuclei are described and some functional relations with catecholamine systems given.

B) Biochemical evidence is presented for the functional significance of these connections: (a) unilateral, cerebellar, medial nuclear lesions reduced dopamine (DA) and norepinephrine (NE) turnover in ipsilateral forebrain, (b) unilateral cerebellar lateral nuclear lesions reduced DA turnover in contralateral forebrain, (c) unilateral vermal cortical lesions increased NE and DA turnover in the ipsilateral forebrain, and (d) focal hyperthermic or electric stimulation of cerebellar nuclei increased forebrain NE and DA turnover in acute experiments.

C) The physiologic effects of focal hyperthermic stimulation of the cerebellum and caudate nucleus are given along with alterations of electrical activity in the cerebello-striato-cerebellar loop.

References

1. Anden N-E, Corrodi H, Fuxe K (1969) Turnover studies using synthesis inhibition. In: Hooper G (ed) Metabolism of amines in brain. pp 38–47
2. Atack CV (1973) The determination of dopamine by a modification of the dihydroxyindole fluorimetric assay. Br J Pharmacol 48:699–714
3. Barbeau A (1976) Progress in understanding and treating Parkinson's disease. Can J Neurol Sci 3:81–84
4. Bartholini G, Stadler H (1976) Neurotransmitter interaction in the basal ganglia: relation to extrapyramidal disorders. In: Birkmayer W, Hornykiewicz O (eds) Advances in parkinsonism. Hoffmann-LaRoche, Basel
5. Biggio G, Guidotti A (1977) Regulation of cyclic GMP in cerebellum by a striatal dopaminergic mechanism. Nature 265:240–242
6. Brownstein MJ (1979) Biochemical anatomy of the extrapyramidal system. In: Fuxek, Calne D (eds) Dopamine, ergots and motor function. Pergamon Press, New York, pp 33–43
7. Carlsson A, Davis J, Kehr W, Lindqvist M, Atack C (1972) Simultaneous measurement of tyrosine and tryptophan hydroxylase activities in brain *in vivo* using an inhibitor of the aromatic amino acid decarboxylase. Naunyn Schmiedebergs Arch Pharmacol 275:153–168
8. Carpenter M, Stevens G (1957) Structural and functional relationships between deep cerebellar nuclei and the brachium conjunctivum in the rhesus monkey. J Comp Neurol 107:109–164
9. Carrea RM, Mettler FA (1955) Function of the primate brachium conjunctivum and related structures. J Comp Neurol 102:151–319
10. Cedarbaum JM, Aghajanian GK (1978) Afferent projections to rat locus ceruleus as determined by a retrograde tracing technique. J Comp Neurol 178:1–16
11. Chan-Palay V (1977) Cerebellar dentate nucleus, organization, cytology and transmitters. Springer, Berlin Heidelberg New York
12. Delong MR, Georgopoulos AP (1979) Physiology of the basal ganglia – a brief overview. Adv Neurol 23:137–153
13. Fahn S, Coté L (1968) Regional distribution of gamma-aminobutyric acid (GABA) in the brain of Rhesus monkey. J Neurochem 15:209–213
14. Feger J, Jacquemin J, Ohye C (1978) Peripheral input to substantia nigra. Exp Neurol 59:351–360
15. Fox M, Williams T (1968) Responses evoked in the cerebellar cortex by stimulation of the caudate nucleus in the cat. J Physiol (Lond) 198:435–450
16. Fox M, Williams T (1970) The caudate nucleus-cerebellar pathways: An electrophysiological study of their route through the midbrain. Brain Res 20:140–144
17. Glowinski J, Nieoullon A, Cheramy A (1978) Regulation of the activity of the nigrostriatal dopaminergic pathways by cortical, cerebellar and sensory neuronal afferences. Adv Biochem Psychopharmacol 19:75–87
18. Goldberger M, Growden J (1971) Tremor at rest following cerebellar lesions in monkeys: effect of L-dopa administration. Brain Res 27:183–187
19. Gresty MA, Paul DH (1975) Responses of fastigial nucleus neurons to stimulation of the caudate nucleus in the cat. J Physiol (Lond) 245:655–665
20. Hökfelt T, Fuxe K (1969) Cerebellar monoamine nerve terminals, a new type of afferent fiber to the cortex cerebelli. Exp Br Res 9:63–72
21. Hornykiewicz O, Lloyd K, Davidson L (1976) The GABA system and function of the basal ganglia and Parkinson's disease. In: Roberts E, Chase T, Tower D (eds) GABA in nervous system function. Raven, New York, pp 479–486

22. Ishida Y (1977) Intralaminar thalamic responses to somatic and fastigial stimulation: cortical inhibition and its blockade by strychnine in cats. Neuropharmacology 16:163–170
23. Kemp JM, Powell TPS (1971) The connections of the striatum and globus pallidus: Synthesis and speculation. Philos Trans R Soc London [Biol] 262:441–457
24. Kitai ST, Kiyohara T, Kennedy DT, Preston RJ (1974) Intracellular analysis of antidromically and synaptically activated nucleus reticularis tegmenti pontis neurons. Experientia 30:1420–1421
25. Kornhuber HH (1974) Cerebral cortex, cerebellum and basal ganglia: An introduction to their motor functions. In: Schmidt FO, Worden FG (eds) The neurosciences, third study program. MIT Press, Cambridge, pp 267–279
26. Krnjevic K (1975) Electrophysiology of dopamine receptors. Adv Neurol 9:13–24
27. Laverty R, Taylor KM (1968) The fluorometric assay of catecholamines and related compounds: improvements and extensions to the hydroxyindole technique. Analyt Biochem 22:269–279
28. Maiti A, Snider RS (1977) Modifications of caudate spindles and seizures by cerebellar stimulation. Int J Neurol 12:120–135
29. Mehler WR, Nauta WJ (1974) Connections of the basal ganglia and of the cerebellum. Confin Neurol 36:205–222
30. Mezey E, Kios J, Palkovits M, Szentagothai J (1979) Efferents of the interpositus nucleus in the cat. In: Fanardjian VV, Hayrapetian AA (eds) Neuronal mechanisms of integrative action in the cerebellum. Armenian Academy of Science, Yerwan, Armenia
31. Narabayashi H (1974) Possible role of cerebellar circuits in parkinsonian symptoms. Confin Neurol 36:292–301
32. Nauta WJ, Domesick VB (1979) The anatomy of the extrapyramidal system. In: Fuxe K, Calne D (eds) Dopamine, ergots and motor functions. Pergamon Press, New York, pp 3–22
33. Nieoullon A, Cheramy A, Glowinski J (1978) Release of dopamine in both caudate nuclei and both substantia nigrae in response to unilateral stimulation of cerebellar nuclei in the cat. Brain Res 148:143–152
34. Oka H, Jinnai K (1978) Common projection of the motor cortex to the caudate nucleus and the cerebellum. Exp Br Res 31:31–42
35. Pechadre J, Larochelle L, Poirier L (1976) Parkinsonian akinesia, rigidity and tremor in the monkey. J Neurol Sci 28:147–157
36. Phillipson OT (1979) Afferent projections to the ventral tegmental area of Tsai and interfascicular nuclei. HRP study in rat. J Comp Neurol 187:117–144
37. Poirier LJ, Filion M, Larochelle L, Pechadre JC (1976) Physiopathology of tremor and rigidity. In: Birkmayer W, Hornykiewicz O (eds) Advances in parkinsonism. Editiones Roche, Basel pp 217–235
38. Prasad ALN, Fahn S (1973) A simplified method for the simultaneous determination of the biogenic monoamines, their precursors and metabolites. Trans Am Soc Neurochem 4:105
39. Sakai K, Touret M, Salvert D, Leger L, Jouvet M (1977) Afferent projections to cat locus ceruleus as visualized by HRP technique. Brain Res 119:21–41
40. Simon H, LeMoal M, Calas A (1979) Efferents and afferents of the ventral tegmental-A10 region studied after local injection of ^{3}H-leucine and horseradish peroxidase. Brain Res 178:17–40
41. Smith BH, Sweet WH (1978) Monoaminergic regulation of central nervous system function. II. Serotonergic systems. Neurosurgery 39:257–272
42. Smith R, Mosko S, Lynch G (1974) Role of various brain areas in recovery from partial cerebellar lesions in the adult rat. Behav Biol 12:165–176
43. Snider R (1975) A cerebellar-ceruleus pathway. Brain Res 88:59–63
44. Snider R, Maiti A (1976) Cerebellar contributions to the Papez circuit. J Neural Sci Res 2:133–146
45. Snider R, Maiti A, Snider S (1976) Cerebellar pathways to ventral midbrain and nigra. Exp Neurol 53:714–728
46. Snider R, Thomas W, Snider S (1978) Focal brain hyperthermia. I. The cerebellar cortex. Experientia 34:479–481

47. Snider R, Thomas W (1978) Focal brain hyperthermia: Evoked responses in sensorimotor cortex. Exp Neurol 61:516–526
48. Snider S, Snider R (1977) Phenytoin and cerebellar lesions. Similar effects on cerebral catecholamine metabolism. Arch Neurol 34:162–167
49. Snider S, Snider R (1977) Alterations in forebrain catecholamine metabolism produced by cerebellar lesions in the rat. J Neural Transm 40:115–128
50. Snider SR, Snider RS (1979) Kainic acid: enduring alterations in cerebellar morphology and in cerebral catecholamine and GABA concentrations after cerebellar injection in the rat. Neurosci Lett 12:339–342
51. Tabaddor K, Wolfson LI, Sharpless NS, Cooper IS (1978) Ventricular fluid homovanillic acid and 5-hydroxyindoleacetic acid concentrations in patients with movement disorders. Neurology 28:1249–1253
52. Walberg F (1956) Descending connections to the inferior olive. J Comp Neurol 104:77–173
53. Waldeck B, Snider S, Brown R, Carlsson A (1975) Studies on the synthesis and subcellular distribution of dopamine in the rat adrenal medulla. Naunyn Schmiedebergs Arch Pharmacol 287:1–10
54. Weinberger DR, Kleinman J, Luchins D, Bigelow L, Wyatt R (1980) Cerebellar pathology in schizophrenia. A controlled postmortem study. Am J Psychiatry 137:359–361
55. Wood JH, Ziegler MG, Lake CR, Sode J, Brooks BR, Van Buren JM (1977) Elevations in cerebrospinal fluid norepinephrine during unilateral, alternating and bilateral cerebellar stimulation in man. Neurosurgery 1:260–265
56. Woodburne RT, Crosby EC, McCotter RE (1946) The mammalian midbrain and isthmus regions. Part II. The fiber connections. J Comp Neurol 85:67–92

Discussion

Eccles: If you want to get back from the striatum to the cerebellum, there is a pathway through the thalamus and the cerebral cortex. One has, therefore, to consider those circuits also. I think that they are active all the time and may be involved in reprogramming of movements.

Snider: If is difficult to analyze movements, particularly movement disorders. There is evidence for a complete loop from the catecholamine system back to the cerebellum. Although we had some problems with this study, we think also that there is a closed catecholamine loop. So there is a double system of projections from the cerebellum to the forebrain, which seems to complicate our understanding of cerebellar function.

Beitz: There is an additional pathway to be taken into consideration; namely, one linking ventral tegmental area, substantia nigra, periaqueductal gray, inferior olive and from there to the cerebellum.

Snider: Yes. Walberg many years ago suggested a link between striatum and inferior olive, although at that time he thought of this as a direct pathway. We now know this is not the case.

Chan-Palay: Has warming of the cortex the same effect as cooling?

Snider: No. Focal hyperthermia is a form of stimulation of the nervous system. Historically it is the oldest form of stimulation. Raising the temperature between 1° and 3 °C, always remaining below 42 °C, is very effective in increasing metabolism and neuronal activity.

The Future of Studies on the Cerebellum

J. C. Eccles

Introduction

I am grateful for the invitation to give this lecture. It was doubtless motivated by the idea that I am now so distanced from my period of intense involvement in cerebellar studies that I can have some perspective in my relationship to the cerebellum. From 1962 to 1975 I was fully engaged. It was my scientific life. And this stressful period can be viewed critically and dispassionately in retrospect from the vantage point of 5 or more years later. I can hope that this perspective gives me some insights into the present state of cerebellar science, which has been so fascinatingly displayed in this present conference, and that I can make suggestions relating to its future.

Let us consider first the exquisite design of the cerebellar cortex as a laminated rectangular lattice, a structure built with a precision only exceeded in biology by the insect eye and its connectivities. A theory of the cerebellar cortex has to incorporate this design as a key feature, and moreover has to account for the convergence onto each Purkinje cell of two quite distinctive inputs, that from the mossy-fiber input with the immense divergences (8000) and convergences (100,000) and that from climbing fibers where the divergence number is about 10 and the convergence number is 1. This extraordinary double innervation has been maintained through all the exigences of evolution from primitive cerebella to the great efflorescence in mammals and birds. It is particularly remarkable that, when the cerebellar hemispheres were developed in step with the cerebral hemispheres, the inferior olive hypertrophied also. The cerebral efferents had to travel down to the medulla oblongata to excite the newly developed inferior olivary neurons for the essential climbing-fiber input to the cerebellar hemispheres.

It has long been recognized that the mammalian cerebellum has three principal components, and that they are distinguished by their connectivities. With the evolutionary development of the primates there has been a progressive increase in the cerebellar hemispheres. They account for 88% of the human cerebellum with the pars intermedia and the vermis sharing the remaining 12%. These three components will be considered in turn. I would regard it as of the greatest importance to investigate the primate cerebellum because such studies relate particularly to the human cerebellum and provide a basis for understanding clinical disorders of the cerebellum. Furthermore such studies open the way to discriminative investigations on the extremely complex interactions occurring in the cerebral control of movement. One can expect that the greater the evol-

Experimental Brain Research, Suppl. 6

utionary differentiation of function, the greater will be the opportunities for discriminative investigations into fundamental problems raised by the cerebello-cerebral interactions.

The Role of the Cerebellar Hemispheres and the Nucleus Dentatus in Voluntary Movement

At the outset I would like to make reference to a very comprehensive survey of problems in cerebrocerebellar actions that has just been published [35]. There have been important advances since the comprehensive review by Evarts and Thach [17] more than a decade ago. Let us begin by attempting to outline the happenings when we carry out a voluntary movement, as for example quick flexion of a finger. Electric recording from the scalp displays an incrementing negativity over the precentral and parietal cortices on both sides that begins about 0.8 s before the electromyogram of the finger flexor, the so-called readiness potential [9]. After about 0.4 s the precentral readiness potential becomes asymmetric, being larger on the crossed side, and at about 0.05 s before the onset of the electromyogram there appears a negative potential localized over the area of the motor pyramidal cells that bring about the movement, the so-called motor potential.

Quick movements are called ballistic because, like a projectile out of a cannon, there is no control once they have been initiated by the discharge of the motor pyramidal cells. The importance of ballistic movements will be appreciated when it is recognized that they are the quick movements employed in playing a percussion instrument such as a piano and in typing. The total duration of such movements is no more than 0.2 s. As demonstrated by Desmedt and Godaux [10] the fastest feedback controls from the contracting muscle are too late to modify the course of the ballistic contraction programed by the discharge down the pyramidal tract. Thus for accurate execution of ballistic movements there must be a complete preprograming of the motor pyramidal discharge. The principal circuits engaged in this programing are outlined in Fig. 1. From the mental initiation in the association cortex there are circuits both to the basal ganglia and to the cerebellum. Our special concern will be with the cerebrocerebellar circuits that are outlined in Fig. 2 for the connectivities of the cerebellar hemisphere. It should be stated that the long duration of the readiness potential is attributable to it being a freely willed action with no triggering stimulus. Much shorter times are involved in reactions to a signal, or to ballistic movements that occur in some learned sequence as in typing or piano playing.

It has been shown in primates that wide areas of the association cortex project to the cerebellar hemisphere and the dentate nucleus of the opposite side. The strongest inputs to the dentate nucleus come from Brodmann area 6 [the premotor and the supplementary motor area (SMA)], with also inputs from the frontal, cingulate, and temporal cortices [3]. In a very comprehensive study of cerebellar cortical responses Sasaki et al. [47] carefully differentiated the mossy-fiber from the climbing-fiber responses. These responses were evoked by stimulation of the frontal association cortex (areas 8 and 9), the premotor area, 6, and

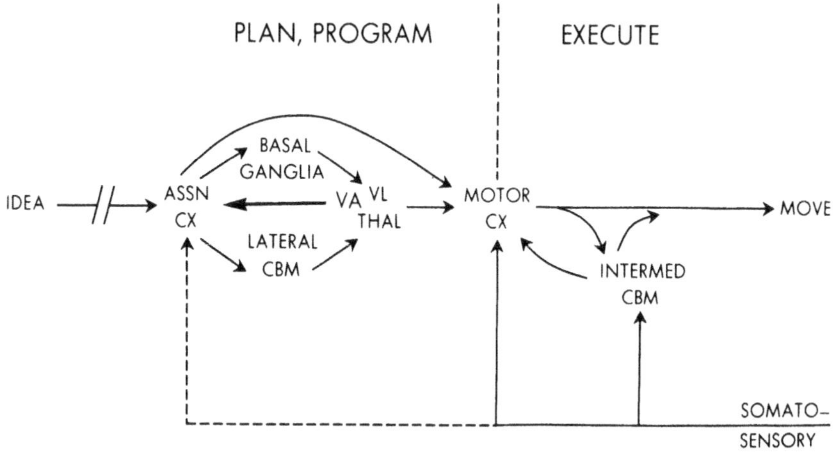

Fig. 1. Diagram showing pathways concerned in the planning, execution and control of voluntary movement. *ASSN CX*, association cortex; *lateral CBM*, cerebellar hemisphere; *intermed CBM*, pars intermedia of cerebellum. Full description in text. Allen and Tsukahara [4]. *CF*, climbing fiber; *GrC*, granule cell; *IO*, inferior olive; *IP*, interpositus nucleus; *LPrC*, large pyramidal cell; *LRN*, lateral reticular nucleus; *MF*, mossy fiber; *PC*, Purkinje cell; *PF*, parallel fiber; *PN*, pontine nucleus; *PT*, pyramidal tract; *RN*, red nucleus; *RST*, rubrospinal tract; *SPrC*, small pyramidal cell; *VA(thal)*, ventro-anterior thalamic nucleus; *VL(thal)*, ventro-lateral thalamic nucleus

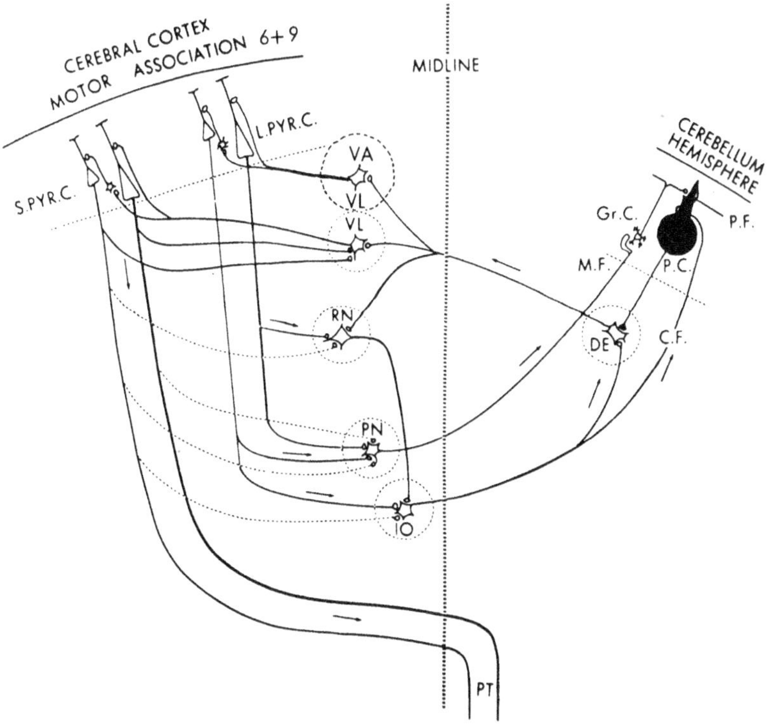

Fig. 2. Cerebrocerebellar pathways linking association and motor cortices with the cerebellar hemisphere. *DE*, nucleus dentatus. In the red nucleus only a small cell is shown. Abbreviations see Fig. 1

the parietal association area, 5. Area 9 and 6 were particularly potent in evoking climbing- and mossy-fiber responses. However, it was also found that the forelimb zone of the motor cortex, 4, effectively projected to the cerebellar hemisphere [47], so the dotted lines suggesting these projections in Fig. 2 could be converted into continuous lines.

The converse projection fron the dentate nucleus to the contralateral cerebral cortex has been found to go not only to the motor cortex, 4, but also strongly to the premotor area 6 (including the SMA) and also to the frontal association area 9 [46, 48]. There is direct evidence that these projections are mediated by the ventralis lateralis (VL) and ventralis anterior (VA) thalamic nuclei as indicated in Fig. 2.

It is of particular interest that there are these neural pathways with the potentiality for acting as reverberating circuits between wide areas of the cerebral association cortex (ASS CX) and the cerebellar hemispheres (CBH). In the original concept of the open-loop operation of the cerebrocerebellar communication [4] the pathway would be:

ASS CX → CBH CX → Dent.N. → VL →MCX → PYR.T. → MOVE.

The cerebellar fashioning of the preprogramed instruction to the motor cortex was restricted to a single operation. Now we have to envisage the operation of reverberatory loops between the ASS CX and the CBH, with the possibility of involving the motor cortex at all stages:

ASS CX → CBH CX → Dent.N. → (VL) → MCX → PYR.T. → MOVE
↑———————————————— ↘ (VA)

It is now possible to recognize that the readiness potential is not simply due to a buildup of activity in the association cortices with a simple open-loop projection to the CBH and the basal ganglia before the signal goes to the motor cortex for initiating the preprogramed movement (cf. Fig. 1). During the readiness potential we may suppose that there is an on-going reverberatory circuit operation to the CBH, i.e., closed loops, so that they are given continuous ongoing opportunities to participate in the preprograming. It will be appreciated that during the readiness potential of 800 ms duration [9] there will be ample time for many replays of these reverberatory loops, perhaps in some patterned sequence. In accord with this idea is the finding that with complex integrated movements, as in articulation of a word, the readiness potential is up to 1.5 sec in duration [24]. It may thus be conjectured that in learned skills programs of movements are stored in connectivities both in the cerebellum and in the association areas of the cerebral cortex. Recent studies on the responses of dentate neurons during trained movements reveal a complexity in accord with these concepts [50].

There are here immense and challenging opportunities for investigation. In particular the experiments of Sasaki et al. [46, 47, 48] should be developed by recording the responses of single neurons in the cerebral and cerebellar cortices. Already this has been done for the dentate nucleus [3], where the neurons displayed a complicated sequence of inhibitory and excitatory responses, as would be expected from interaction of impulses in the inhibitory Purkinje axons and in the excitatory axon collaterals from both the pontocerebellar fibers (not shown in Fig. 2) and the olivocerebellar fibers. The study of single neurons in the ASS CX would be valuable in relation to the superficial and deep negativities reported by Sasaki et al. [46, 48], which may relate to the excitation of pyramidal cells in laminae 3 and 5, the former possibly being projectors to the association cortex and motor cortex, the latter to the cerebellum. Evidently we are only at the beginning of our attempt to give a comprehensive account of the cerebrocerebellar interactions in voluntary movement.

This analytic work will be a great value in attempting to understand and to develop further the investigations of Thach [49, 50] on the responses of cerebellar nuclear cells and motor cortical pyramidal cells during voluntary movements of a trained monkey. There is good evidence in general that dentate neurons discharge before the motor pyramidal cells, which would be in accord with the circuits of Figs. 1 and 2. However, it would be advantageous to have the responses to trained ballistic movements so that the timing of onsets could be more discriminative. An important new study has been that of Mano [33] on the responses of Purkinje cells during trained movements. With a variety of movements Purkinje cells begin to discharge well before the onset of the movement, which is in accord with Fig. 2. It is suggested that the circuits of Fig. 2 be tested in every aspect of trained movements by the analytic procedures of Allen et al. [2, 3] and Sasaki et al. [46, 47, 48]. A most important study would be to apply the techniques of Thach [49, 50], Mano [33], and Robertson and Grimm [41] to areas of the frontal lobe that are known to receive reciprocal connections from the cerebellum as indicated in Figs. 1 and 2. In view of the radio-Xenon findings reported below [43, 44] the SMA should be the prime target, but also the remainder of the premotor cortex, 6, and the association cortex, 9, should be explored. According to the hypothesis that these areas preprogram movements, it would be expected that impulse discharges would precede the cerebellar (cortical and nuclear) responses. The motor cortical discharges would be expected to be still later. However, the SMA and 6 can discharge directly to area 4, but evidently not effectively, else the readiness potential would be much shorter.

The Role of the Pars Intermedia and the Interpositus Nucleus in the Control of Movement

In the primate brain the main second component of the cerebellum, the pars intermedia, is small relative to the greatly evolved CBH, which form about 88% of the human cerebellum. Nevertheless an important role can be assigned to the pars intermedia and its associated interpositus nucleus. Allen et al. [2] made a systematic study of the projection to the interpositus nucleus from the cerebral cortex of monkeys. In contrast with the dentate nucleus [3] there was a projection to almost all of the interpositus neurons (85%) from the sensorimotor cortex, which was more than twice the percentage for dentate neurons. Reciprocally, the projection from area 6 (premotor plus supplementary motor) was much less, and the other association areas were ineffective. These findings are in general accord with the hypothesis [4, 12] that the pars intermedia of the cerebellum is principally concerned in updating the discharge pattern from the motor cortex down the pyramidal tract, acting in this way like the control on a target-finding missile (cf. Figs. 1 and 3).

Both the mossy- and climbing-fiber inputs to the pars intermedia are generated by axon collaterals from the pyramidal tract fibers (Fig. 3), and the return circuit via the interpositus nucleus goes directly to the motor cortex in a closed-loop manner. In further contrast to the CBH the pars intermedia has another mode of operation (Fig. 3), receiving input from peripheral nerves and via the rubrospinal pathway acting directly on the spinal motor centers without the loop through the cerebral cortex. Apart from this reciprocal peripheral connection of the pars intermedia there is no sharp distinction in the cerebro-cerebellar circuitries for these two components of the cerebellum. The manner

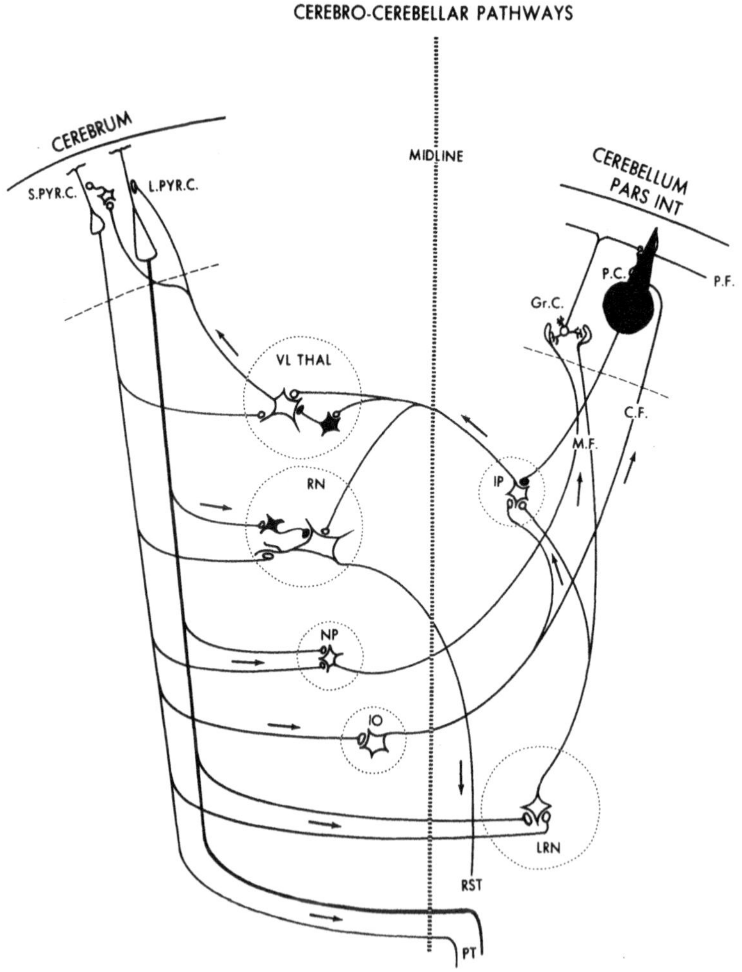

Fig. 3. Pathways linking the sensorimotor areas of the cerebrum with the pars intermedia of the cerebellum. Full description in the text. Abbreviations see Fig. 1

in which their activities mesh together in the control of movement raises many problems for experimental investigation.

Experiments of the type conducted by Allen [2], Sasaki [46], and their colleagues should be attempted with implanted electrodes in order to eliminate the depressant effects of anesthesia. The experimental investigations of Thach [49, 50] and Mano [33] could be carried out with monkeys trained in ballistic movements. When studying the timing of neuronal discharges relative to a ballistic movement, there should be investigation of the association cortex of the frontal lobe, the premotor, and SMA divisions of area 6 and also of area 9. Already there has been a preliminary study [6] showing that SMA neurons usually fired 150–200 ms before the muscle contraction, but unfortunately there was no recording of neurons of the primary motor cortex or of the cerebellar cortex and nuclei.

On the basis of the conjectural cerebrocerebellar interactions in preprograming and updating movements (Fig. 1), it would be expected that neurons of the frontal association cortex, 9, 6, SMA, would discharge before the neurons of the CBH and the dentate nucleus and the neurons of the pars intermedia and the interpositus nucleus would be still later, even following the motor cortex discharge. It is not possible to evoke the readiness potential with monkeys because there is the necessity for a freely willed movement with no triggering stimulus. However, the method used for contingent negative variation could be applied in a study of the relative timing of neurons of the frontal association cortex in comparison with discharges of neurons in the CBH, the dentate nucleus, and the motor cortex. Furthermore, it may be possible to record from the human premotor cortex during the carrying out of freely willed actions generating readiness potentials.

Investigations on Cerebral Blood Flow in Relation to Voluntary Movement

Studies of human cerebral blood flow by the radio-Xenon technique have now advanced to a high level of precision and reliability with simultaneous recording at 254 sites over one hemisphere. Using this technique Roland et al. [43] have provided most important evidence on the role of the SMA in preprograming movements. When subjects were mentally carrying out a program of fast complex movements of the fingers without executing them [controlled by the zero level of the electromyograms (EMGs)], there was an increased blood flow of about 20% in the SMAs of both sides. When the finger movements were actually carried out, the blood flow to the SMA and the contralateral motor area for the fingers was increased to about 30% above normal and to about 20% in the contralateral somatosensory area of the hand and 10% in the premotor area. On the other hand the blood flow to the SMA was but little increased during forceful routine flexions of the fingers, though it was then high to area 4 and the sensorimotor and sensory areas for the hand. Much the same effects were observed during sustained isometric contraction of finger against thumb. It was concluded that in new and intricately patterned movements the SMA is developing the programs for the motor activity, i.e., SMA → motor cortex just as in Fig. 1.

Unfortunately timing was not possible with this technique. It was further shown by the blood-flow technique [44] that the premotor area, 6, is used in establishing a new motor program or in modulating an already existing program.

The Vermis and Fastigial Nucleus and the Cerebellar Relationship to Posture and Simple Automatic Movements

The third component of the cerebellum, the vermis, presents many interesting problems for the future. Though it is not prominent in the primate cerebellum, it is larger than the pars intermedia. Although mainly related to the spinal cord functions of muscle tone, posture, and the simpler automatic movements, it has a strong rostral projection via the various components of the VL thalamic nucleus as described by Carpenter and Batton (this volume, p. 250). These connections revealed by modern labeling techniques should be investigated electrophysiologically in order to discover the full range of rostral projection from the fastigial nucleus. Only a minor, rostral projection occurs via the medial reticular nucleus [16]. Sasaki (reference [45], Figs. 8, 9) depicts the VA VL connections but also connections to the nonspecific thalamus center median (CM) and intralaminar nuclei (ILN). From there it can be presumed to be distributed to the cerebral cortex, to the limbic system, and the basal ganglia. This rostral projection of the cerebellar vermis to the limbic system and possibly to the raphe nuclei presumably provides the pathway whereby continuous vermal stimulation through implanted electrodes greatly benefits many psychotic patients (personal communication R.G. Heath and J.R. Smythies). There is control of maniacal violence and schizophrenics can be restored to a normal life. There should be a study of the effects of a similar vermal stimulation in monkeys both in normals and in animals with induced psychoses.

By a systematic study of various peripheral inputs into the cerebellum and associated nuclei [11] it was possible to trace the sensory inputs to the cerebellum (pars intermedia and vermis) and thence to the interpositus and fastigial nuclei with their further projections to the red nucleus and the medial reticular nucleus and so down to the spinal motor centers. The interaction of the mossy- and climbing-fiber inputs was investigated for a wide range of skin and muscle inputs. Afferents from joint receptors require more study. Also to be integrated into this cerebellar control of posture and simple automatic movements are the inputs from the vestibular and neck receptors with their pathways down the vestibulospinal and reticulospinal tracts. These have been extensively investigated by Wilson [51] and Peterson [40].

It should be possible to develop comprehensive hypotheses of the vestibulospinocerebellar controls of posture under a wide variety of imposed movements and stresses. One can predict that computer modeling could be developed to give a very effective simulation of the operations of the cerebellospinal controls of tone and posture, and so would lead to further insights into the mode of operation of the cerebellar circuitry. The last review of the spinocerebellar system would seem to be some years ago [11]. Since that time there has been a great increase in knowledge. An up-to-date review is urgently needed.

It is a general principle that reliability of computation in neuronal systems is secured by having many neuronal lines more or less in parallel with, at each stage, divergence and convergence so that there is automatic averaging. This principle should serve as a guide in attempting to fashion models of cerebellospinal function. A most challenging situation is that the spino-olivary projections by climbing fibers to the vermis and pars intermedia are arranged in sagittal strips about 1–2 mm across [38], each strip representing a special functional connectivity. This would suggest a series of computing areas in parallel. Yet the parallel fibers that stem from the mossy-fiber input are each about 6 mm in length [37]. Even if the mossy-fiber and the climbing-fiber inputs are in register, which often occurs [11, 38], the parallel fibers excited by the mossy-fiber input will exert an excitatory action on Purkinje cells of climbing-fiber strips adjacent to the strip corresponding to that of the mossy-fiber input and even on strips one further removed. There is at present no explanation of the functional significance of this distributed arrangement. It is one of the enigmas in attempting to give meaning to the dual input to all Purkinje cells by mossy and climbing fibers. It would seem that the mossy-fiber input is the principal driving force in Purkinje-cell performance because the rate of climbing-fiber inputs is so very low, usually 1–2/s, while the background firing rate of Purkinje cells is usually 50–100/s in unanesthetized animals. These considerations give basic support to the hypothesis that the role of the climbing fiber is to induce plastic and trophic changes in Purkinje cells, as will be described in the next section.

The key role of the cerebellum in controlling the discharge of gamma motoneurons [23] and so of the muscle-spindle loop control of alpha motoneurons will be an important component in the eventual solution of cerebellar action at the spinal level. Another factor may be the cerebellar influence on Renshaw cells, which seem to be specially concerned with the responses of the more distal muscles of the limbs with their finely graded responses.

Cerebellum and Motor Learning, Plastic Properties, and Trophic Influences

It is my thesis that the cerebellum is concerned in the enormously complex organization and control of movement, and that throughout life we are engaged in an incessant teaching program for the cerebellum, particularly in the earlier years. As a consequence it plays a key role in all the remarkable tasks involved in skilled movements. Somehow its immense neuronal structure and the special features of its design would be accounted for by its evolution for this plastic performance.

Marr [34] made a notable advance when he proposed that the climbing-fiber input to Purkinje cells provided the instruction for selecting from the enormous number of parallel-fiber synapses on a Purkinje cell (more than 100,000), with the consequence that a small fraction of these synapses was potentiated. He postulated that there would be hypertrophy of those parallel-fiber synapses activated at about the same time as the climbing-fiber activation of that cell. Thus conjunction would lead to selection, and with adequate repetition of the conjunction there could be developed a considerable and lasting hypertrophy of the parallel-fiber synapses, so that their excitatory action could substitute for the climbing-fiber activity on that Purkinje cell. Marr's hypothesis has two important features. It gives a key significance to the numerous parallel-fiber synapses on a Purkinje cell, since they provide the population from which selection is made in some learning process. It accounts for the dual innervation of all Purkinje cells – by mossy- and climbing-fiber inputs – and for the finding that these two inputs tend to come from the same source, i.e., a peripheral source in a restricted region of skin of muscle or a specific central region, i.e., of the primary motor cortex to Purkinje cells of the pars intermedia.

I reviewed the evidence for this conjunction-selection hypothesis of learning some years ago [13]. Experiments on the vestibulo-ocular reflex by Ito and associates [27, 29, 30, 31], by Robinson [42] on rabbits and cats, and by Gonshor and Melvill Jones [21, 42] on humans and cats gave empirical support, but there were several disturbing features when it came to detailed interpretation. The critical time for conjunction of climbing-fiber with parallel-fiber interaction remained undefined. In particular, the temporal relationships between the observed climbing-fiber and mossy-fiber inputs did not suggest some fairly sharp conjunction time such as would be expected on the original hypothesis [34]. Since the time of my review [13], there has been empirical evidence for the alternate hypothesis of mossy-fiber–climbing-fiber interaction proposed on the basis of perceptron theory by Albus [1]. According to this hypothesis conjunction results not in potentiation, but in depression of the parallel-fiber synapses, i.e., selection is by depression not potentiation.

Gilbert and Thach [20] trained monkeys to compensate for movements produced by standard forces randomly applied by a torque motor to flex or extend the wrist. In the learning procedure the force applied in one direction was increased or decreased, necessitating a learned adjustment. It was of great interest that many Purkinje cells in the intermediate lobe had a climbing-fiber input at 50–150 ms after onset of each trial with the changed load. The response to the changed load was learned in 12–100 trials, and at the same time the climbing-fiber input reverted to its initial low random frequency. During this learning procedure there was usually some slowing of the simple-spike responses of the Purkinje cells from their high base rate of about 100/s. This slowing was interpreted as a learning response in accord with the Albus hypothesis [1]. However, the observations on such Purkinje cells continued for little more than 100 trials [20], which would be about 250 s. It would seem that the published results can be regarded as giving no more that suggestive support to the Albus hypothesis. Much more extensive investigation is needed in this most difficult field. The one clear result is that in the learning of a novel task there is a increase in the climbing-fiber input to Purkinje cells [20]. This finding is in accord with the evidence of Ito and Mijishita [29] that the learned changes in the vestibulo-ocular reflex to compensate for head rotation were greatly reduced after ablation of the inferior olive. However, with the vestibulo-ocular reflex there is evidence of complex phase relationships [19] and that the increased climbing-fiber activity in the learning process is associated with a depression of the simple-spike activity [28], which is in accord with the Albus hypothesis [1].

It can be concluded that in this most important field of cerebellar learning we as yet know very little, perhaps no more than that the inferior olive with its climbing-fiber input to Purkinje cells plays a key role. The elegant investigations of Ito and associates [27, 29, 30, 31] and of Gonshor, Melvill Jones, and Robinson [21, 22, 42] have the great advantage that learning processes can be studied for many hours or days in a stabilized preparation. Yet they cannot give information on the time relationships that must form an essential component of the postulated climbing-fiber influence on the parallel-fiber synapses. Since the climbing fiber activates the whole of the Purkinje-cell dendrites, the basis of selection must be in a specific time relationship, as is implicit in both the Marr [34] and Albus hypotheses [1].

I would like to suggest that an experiment be designed that would give precise control of the climbing-fiber and parallel-fiber inputs to Purkinje cells. This was attempted when Marr visited Buffalo in 1970. With stimulation of the inferior olive, sites of strong climbing inputs could be found in the anterior lobe of the cerebellum. Surface stimulating electrodes excited a parallel-fiber volley projecting to such a site and a penetrating microelectrode recorded the depth profile of Purkinje-cell activation by that volley. Then there was conditioning by many seconds of repetitive stimulation of both the inferior olive and the parallel fibers at some chosen interval of conjunction on the Purkinje cells. There were some encouraging results with a sustained increase in the parallel-fiber activation of the Purkinje cells, but in other cases there was no effect or even depression. The weak point of the experiment was that with our techniques we could not rely on maintenance of the exposed cerebellar cortex in a steady state for more than 1 h. If learning is due to a synaptic growth process [14, 18], then many hours of reliable recording will be necessary. Furthermore, there will have to be empirical determination of the optimum interval for conjunction which Marr [34] left undefined, and also of the frequency of the conjunction stimulation. This should not be above 10/s, which is the maximum discharge rate of climbing fibers.

An alternative method would be to investigate the spine synapses on Purkinje cells for the hypertrophy demonstrated by Fifková and van Harreveld [18] for the synapses on the granule cells of the hippocampus. It should be possible to have a climbing-fiber input to almost all Purkinje cells in a zone and to project into that zone a parallel-fiber volley of maximum strength. After the conditioning – conjunction stimulation the animal could be sacrificed at 2, 4, 6, 8 h and the spine synapses examined by electronmicroscopy. Controls would be provided by an adjacent lobule. This is a laborious study, involving planimetric measurements of thousands of spines, but it is capable of providing direct information on a most important problem.

Besides these postulated plastic changes induced by climbing fibers on Purkinje cells, there are also trophic influences that provide a most exciting challenge. It is now well established that in the young animal climbing-fiber innervation of Purkinje cells is necessary for the full growth of the dendritic tree [5, 32].

Recently Ito and associates [28] have opened up a more complex trophic operation. Destruction of the inferior olive results within a few hours in a severe diminution of the inhibitory action of Purkinje cells on their target nuclei with evidence for a depletion of the inhibitory transmitter substance, gamma aminobutyric acid (GABA). This effect is selective, being restricted to those Purkinje cells innervated by the destroyed zone of the inferior olive. It does not occur when olivocerebellar impulses are blocked by tetrodotoxin (TTX). Thus it would seem that the inferior olive exerts a trophic influence on Purkinje cells enabling them to produce adequate inhibitory transmitter substance. This new type of trophic influence merits a rigorous critical investigation.

Cerebellar Investigations Specially Related to Observations on Clinical Cerebellar Lesions

For over a decade Brooks and his associates [7] have systematically investigated the effects of reversible inactivation of the cerebellar nuclei, dentatus or interpositus, on the trained motor performance of monkeys. This work bears a close relationship to clinical lesions of human subjects, but has the advantage that the inactivation is produced by cold and is reversible. Brooks [7] relates these findings to the comprehensive account of cerebellar dysfunction published by Gordon Holmes [26] some 40 years ago. I also [12] in a similar manner have attempted to show how far the experimental investigations can be correlated with the insights of Holmes [26]. I concluded:
"In appraisal of the attempt to account for the symptoms of cerebellar lesions in the light of our modern knowledge, I am cognizant of the great deficiencies in this knowledge. There has been a successful analysis of the neuronal interactions in the cerebellar cortex, but this does not help to any appreciable extent in the attempt to develop an understanding of the mode of operation of the cerebellum in the control of movement. At the best it can form the basis for building models. ... The immensity of the neuronal machinery and the amazing finesse and reliability of its performance completely escapes our comprehension. I am sure that Holmes would have felt that we have not advanced very far beyond the explanations he was able to develop before the analytical successes of recent times. The understanding of cerebellar function can be attempted only when there have been synthetic studies to match the analytical. But this is an age where analysis attracts the attention and the rewards! The much more demanding and visionary task of synthesis is being attempted in far too few laboratories."

Postscript. I have omitted reference to an immense range of important work on the cerebellum: neurochemistry, neurotransmitters, neuroembryology. In particular there has been almost no reference to microscopic anatomy of the cerebellum that has been so superbly illustrated and described by Palay and Chan-Palay [39] and by Chan-Palay [8]. Microstructure will continue to be essential in our efforts to understand the cerebellum as a neuronal machine [15]. On the basis of the microstructure the electrophysiologic studies were made very easily and quickly. In some 4 years the main features were known [15]. But the manner of operation of the cerebellum in motor control is a much more demanding discipline, as has been displayed in the various sections of this review.

References

1. Albus JS (1971) A theory of cerebellar function. Math Biosci 10:25–61
2. Allen GI, Gilbert PFC, Marini R, Schultz W, Yin TOT (1977) Integration of cerebral and peripheral inputs by interpositus neurons in monkey. Exp Brain Res 27:81–99
3. Allen GI, Gilbert PFC, Yin TCT (1978) Convergence of cerebral inputs onto dentate neurons in monkey. Exp Brain Res 32:151–170
4. Allen GI, Tsukahara N (1974) Cerebrocerebellar communication systems. Physiol Rev 54:957–1006
5. Bradley P, Berry M (1976) The effects of reduced climbing and parallel fibre input on Purkinje cell dendritic growth. Brain Res 109:133–151
6. Brinkman C, Porter R (1979) Supplementary motor area in the monkey: activity of neurons during performance of a learned motor task. J Neurophysiol 42:681–709
7. Brooks VB (1979) Control of intended limb movements by the lateral and intermediate cerebellum. In: Asanuma H, Wilson VJ (eds) Integration in the nervous system. Igaku-Shoin, Tokyo New York, p 321
8. Chan-Palay V (1977) Cerebellar dentate nucleus. Springer, Berlin Heidelberg New York
9. Deecke L, Grözinger B, Kornhuber HH (1976) Voluntary finger movements in man. Cerebral potentials and theory. Biol Cybernet 23:99–119
10. Desmedt JE, Godaux E (1978) Ballistic skilled movements: Load compensation and patterning of the motor commands. In: Desmedt JE (ed) Cerebral motor control in man: long loop mechanisms. Karger, Basel, p 21
11. Eccles JC (1973) The cerebellum as a computer: patterns in space and time. J Physiol (Lond) 229:1–32
12. Eccles JC (1977) Cerebellar function in the control of movement (with special reference to the pioneer work of Sir Gordon Holmes). In: Rose FC (ed) Physiological aspects of clinical neurology. Blackwell Scientific Publications, Oxford London, p 157
13. Eccles JC (1977) An instruction-selection theory of learning in the cerebellar cortex. Brain Res 127:327–352
14. Eccles JC (1979) Synaptic plasticity. Naturwissenschaften 66:147–153
15. Eccles JC, Ito M, Szentágothai J (1967) The Cerebellum as a neuronal machine. Springer, Berlin Heidelberg New York
16. Eccles JC, Nicoll RA, Táboříková H, Willey TJ (1975) Medial reticular neurons projecting rostrally. J Neurophysiol 38:531–538
17. Evarts EV, Thach WT (1969) Motor mechanisms of the CNS, cerebro-cerebellar inter-relations. Ann Rev Physiol 31:451–498
18. Fifková E, van Harreveld A (1977) Long-lasting morphological changes in dendritic spines of dentate granular cells following stimulation of the entorhinal area. J Neurocytol 6:211–230
19. Ghelarducci B, Ito M, Yagi N (1975) Impulse discharges from flocculus Purkinje cells of alert rabbits during visual stimulation combined with horizontal head rotation. Brain Res 87:66–72
20. Gilbert PFC, Thach WT (1977) Purkinje cell activity during motor learning. Brain Res 128:309–328
21. Gonshor A, Melvill Jones G (1976) Short-term adaptive changes in the human vestibulo-ocular reflex arc. J Physiol (Lond) 256:361–379
22. Gonshor A, Melvill Jones G (1976) Extreme vestibulo-ocular adaptation induced to prolonged optical reversal of vision. J Physiol (Lond) 256:381–414
23. Granit R (1970) The basis of motor control. Academic Press, London New York
24. Grözinger B, Kornhuber HH, Kriebel J (1975) Methodological problems in the investigation of cerebral potentials preceding speech: determining the onset and suppressing artefacts caused by speech. Neuropsychologia 13:263–270
25. Harvey RJ, Porter R, Rawson JA (1977) The natural discharges of Purkinje cells in paravermal regions of lobules V and VI of the monkey's cerebellum. J Physiol (Lond) 271:515–536
26. Holmes G (1939) The cerebellum of man. Brain 62:1–30
27. Ito M (1976) Cerebellar learning control of the vestibuloocular mechanisms. In: Desiraju T (ed) Mechanisms in transmission of signals for conscious behaviour. 26th International Physiological Congress, New Delhi, Amsterdam, Elsevier

28. Ito M (1980) Roles of the inferior olive in the cerebellar control of vestibular functions. In: Courville J, de Montigny C, Lamarre Y (eds) The inferior olivary nucleus – anatomy and physiology. Raven, New York, pp 367–377
29. Ito M, Mijishita Y (1975) The effects of chronic destruction of the inferior olive upon visual modification of the horizontal vestibulo-ocular reflex of rabbits. Proc Jap Acad 51:716–720
30. Ito M, Shiida T, Yagi N, Yamamoto M (1974) The cerebellar modification of rabbits horizontal vestibulo-ocular reflex induced by sustained head rotation combined with visual stimulation. Proc Jap Acad 50:85–89
31. Ito M, Shiida T, Yagi N, Yamamoto M (1974) Visual influence on rabbit horizontal vestibulo-ocular reflex presumably effected via the cerebellar floculus. Brain Res 65:170–174
32. Kawaguchi S, Yamamoto T, Mizuno N, Iwahori N (1975) The role of climbing fibers in the development of Purkinje cell dendrites. Neurosci Lett 1:301–304
33. Mano N (1979) Analyses of cerebellar Purkinje cells activity in relation to the direction, position and velocity of wrist tracking movement. In: Massion J, Sasaki K (eds) Cerebro-cerebellar interactions. Elsevier/North Holland Amsterdam, p 163
34. Marr D (1969) A theory of cerebellar cortex. J Physiol (Lond) 202:437–470
35. Massion J, Sasaki K (1979) Cerebro-cerebellar interactions. Elsevier/North Holland, Amsterdam
36. Massion J, Sasaki K (1979) Cerebro-cerebellar interaction: solved and unsolved problems. In: Massion J, Sasaki K (eds) Cerebro-cerebellar interactions. Elsevier/North Holland, Amsterdam, p 261
37. Mugnaini E (1976) Organization of cerebellar cortex. Exp Brain Res Suppl 1:8–19
38. Oscarrson O (1976) Spatial distribution of climbing and mossy fiber inputs into the cerebellar cortex. Exp Brain Res [Suppl] 1:36–42
39. Palay SL, Chan-Palay V (1974) Cerebellar cortex: cytology and organization. Springer, Berlin Heidelberg New York
40. Peterson BW (1979) Reticulo-motor pathways: their connections and possible roles in motor behaviour. In: Asanuma H, Wilson VJ (eds) Integration in the nervous system. Igaku-Shoin, Tokyo New York, p 185
41. Robertson LT, Grimm RJ (1975) Responses of primate dentate neurons to different trajectories of the limb. Exp Brain Res 23:447–462
42. Robinson DA (1976) Adaptive gain control of vestibulo-ocular reflex by the cerebellum. J Neurophysiol 39:954–969
43. Roland PE, Larsen B, Lassen NA, Skinhøj E (1950) Supplementary motor area and other cortical areas in organization of voluntary movements in man. J Neurophysiol 43:118–136
44. Roland PE, Skinhøj E, Lassen NA, Larsen B (1980) Different cortical areas in man in organization of voluntary movement in extrapersonal space. J Neurophysiol 43:137–150
45. Sasaki K (1979) Cerebro-cerebellar interconnections in cats and monkeys. In: Massion J, Sasaki K (eds) Cerebro-cerebellar interactions. Elsevier/North Holland, Amsterdam, p 105
46. Sasaki K, Kawaguchi S, Oka H, Sakai M, Mizuno N (1976) Electrophysiological studies on the cerebello-cerebral projections in monkeys. Exp Brain Res 24:495–507
47. Sasaki K, Oka H, Kawaguchi S, Jinnai K, Yasuda T (1977) Mossy fiber and climbing fiber responses produced in the cerebellar cortex by stimulation of the cerebral cortex in monkeys. Exp Brain Res 29:419–428
48. Sasaki K, Jinnai K, Gemba H, Hashimoto S, Mizuno N (1979) Projection of the cerebellar dentate nucleus onto the frontal association cortex in monkeys. Exp Brain Res 37:193–198
49. Thach WT (1975) The timing of activity in cerebellar dentate nucleus and cerebral motor cortex during prompt volition movement. Brain Res 88:233–241
50. Thach WT (1978) Correlation of neural discharge with pattern and force of muscular activity, joint position, and direction of intended next movement in motor cortex and cerebellum. J Neurophysiol 41:654–676
51. Wilson VJ (1979) Electrophysiological and dynamic studies of vestibulospinal reflexes. In: Asanuma H, Wilson VJ (eds) Integration in the nervous system. Igaku-Shoin, Tokyo New York p 167

Subject Index

Techniques in Neuroanatomical Research

Editors: C. Heym, W.-G. Forssmann
1981. 165 figures. XIII, 395 pages
ISBN 3-540-10686-3

Contents: General Research Methods in Neuroanatomy. - Light Microscopical Research Methods in Neuroanatomy. - Electron Microscopical Research Methods in Neuroanatomy. - Investigation of Living Nervous Tissue. - Subject Index.

Techniques in Neuroanatomical Research is a detailed presentation of selected methods the neurobiologist needs for conducting morphological studies. The formulae and practical introductions provided for each technique allow even non-morphologists to acquire them easily. Each chapter concludes with an extensive bibliography to enable the reader to broaden his knowledge while at the same time introducing him to the works of leading scientists in the field.

A. G. Brown

Organization in the Spinal Cord

The Anatomy and Physiology of Identified Neurones

1981. 148 figures. XII, 238 pages
ISBN 3-540-10549-2

Contents: Spinal Cord Organization: An Introduction. - Axons Innervating Hair Follicle Receptors. - Axons Innervating Rapidly Adapting Mechanoreceptors in Glabrous Skin. - Axons Innervating Slowly Adapting Type I Mechanoreceptors. - Axons Innervating Slowly Adapting Type II Mechanoreceptors. - Spinocervical Tract Neurones. - Relationships between Hair Follicle Afferent Fibres and Spinocervical Tract Neorones. - Neurones with Axons Ascending the Dorsal Columns. - Other Dorsal Horn Neurones. - The Organization of the Dorsal Horn. - Afferent Fibres from Golgi Tendon Organs. - Afferent Fibres from Secondary Endings in Muscle Spindles. - Relationship between Group IA Afferent Fibres and Motoneurones. - Appendix 1: Methods. - Appendix 2: Nomenclature. - References. - Subject Index.

Organization in the Spinal Cord is not just a text on spinal cord anatomy and physiology, it is also a description of results obtained using the intracellular injection of HRP, together with other complementary experiments, on selected axons and neurones, specifically on the larger cutaneous axons and dorsal horn neurones and on the larger muscle afferent fibres and motoneurones. This book presents a sufficient amount of new material for review and assessment to suggest that the time has come in a complete rethinking of structural-functional relationships in the mammalian central nervous system.

Springer-Verlag
Berlin
Heidelberg
New York

GPSR Compliance

The European Union's (EU) General Product Safety Regulation (GPSR) is a set of rules that requires consumer products to be safe and our obligations to ensure this.

If you have any concerns about our products, you can contact us on ProductSafety@springernature.com

In case Publisher is established outside the EU, the EU authorized representative is:

Springer Nature Customer Service Center GmbH
Europaplatz 3
69115 Heidelberg, Germany

Batch number: 10761697

Printed by Printforce, the Netherlands